"This detailed text was created to advance an ongoing necessary evolution of current rehabilitation practice. Utilizing realistic case examples and opportunity for personal reflection, it serves as a complex, 'deep-dive' resource manual for developing holistic humanistic healthcare practices for 'post normal' times. It pragmatically outlines the nuts and bolts of a model of true health care that offers practitioners examples of practice models based on an alternative to those currently utilized, which were created from an outmoded linear science that reflects a 'fix-it' mentality of disease and disability management. This manual offers an evidence-based foundation of how to provide patient care emphasizing authentic health care that is comprehensive and relational, where the patient is sovereign, and all systems coordinate and cooperate to offer comprehensive holistic care."

—*Carol M. Davis, DPT, EdD, MS, FAPTA, Myofascial Release Physical Therapist, Integrated Physical Therapy and Wellness, Professor Emerita, Department of Physical Therapy, University of Miami Miller School of Medicine*

"This book is the most important and relevant collection of expert perspectives on integrative rehabilitation. I highly recommend this book for all healthcare professionals and even to patients. The breadth of collective knowledge and depth of experience brings together the most comprehensive wisdom on integrative rehab practice in print. This book is an empowering read and the experiential pauses throughout the book make the learning 'hands on.' Through stories and cases, the authors beautifully weave the importance of the whole person into the care of the physical body while recognizing the power and complexity of the mind and spirit in the healing process."

—*Mari Ricker, MD, Associate Professor, Family and Community Medicine, Director of Integrative Medicine in Residency, Andrew Weil Center for Integrative Medicine*

"The use of storytelling in this text brings each chapter alive, engaging the reader in a practical and accessible way no matter the profession or environment you are working in. With a focus on cultivating psychological flexibility in relationship to science, within ourselves and with our clients it serves a purpose at various levels of the mind-body-environment connection. The authors humbly create a case for embracing uncertainty which is embedded within IRP. Therefore, whether you are wanting to cultivate fresh eyes and clearer sight into your experience as a rehab practitioner or have just entered the field, then this is a valuable new resource for that creation to begin."

—*Louise Sanguine, OTR/L, Occupational Therapist, Adolescent Addiction and Mental Health Outpatient Therapist, AB, Canada, Occupational Therapy Consultant, Simply Counseling Services and Imagine Psychological Services, AB, Canada*

"This is a totally unique book that should be read by a range of professionals. Health professionals, students going through training in any healthcare field, public health professionals, politicians, and of course people that experience anything less than acceptable levels of health should read it. The first part of this book suggests a new base/concept/context for health. As it is stated in the book, not 'piling a new set of tools onto existing practice patterns…[but a] new orientation at the base.' I could not agree more. It is time that we stop 'band aiding' a healthcare system that is not working towards healthy citizens and communities… Part 1 should be read and re-read to ground the reader in the editors' vision of a new health care that will bring forth healthier citizens and communities."

—*Staffan Elgelid, PT, PhD, GCFP, RYT 500, C-IAYT, NBC-HWC, Professor in Physical Therapy, Nazareth College*

"*Integrative Rehabilitation Practice* is the first book of its kind to apply the powerful mind-body concepts of Integrative Medicine to the field of rehabilitation. It is a Call to Action for all rehab professionals! This comprehensive text allows clinicians to 'walk the walk' of an integrated approach within our respective professions. The 'Body-as-Machine' paradigm has served us well in solidifying skills in the 'bio' component of rehab medicine. 'YES/AND' is a tool that is expounded on throughout the text to embrace our 'bio' history AND develop a whole person approach so as not to undervalue ourselves and our patients by offering a reductionistic view on health… There are no easy solutions or cookie-cutter approaches… With curiosity and humility, IRP serves as a guide and a resource to create the best possible future for yourself and all those you serve. As you embrace IRP, step into the future of rehab!"

—*Carolyn Vandyken, PT, Registered Physiotherapist, Physio Works Muskoka, Pelvic Health Physiotherapist, Educator, Advocate, Researcher, Co-Founder, Reframe Rehab*

"This book is the expression of an important evolution in creating the necessary bridge between mind and body and emphasizes the importance of interdisciplinary and transdisciplinary care. With this book, the authors set out a new course for future-oriented rehabilitation care. The focus is not purely on the functional aspect of care but also on optimizing the well-being and empowering of the individual… Inviting people to the integrative rehabilitation practice is not always about finding a direct solution; it is rather about helping people to start a dialogue… Everyone in clinical practice will find something to suit his or her taste, regardless of his or her theoretical or therapeutic background. Moreover, this book provides food for thought and that is what a good book should do. Reflection is the basis of successful and quality care in the rehabilitation sector."

—*Em. Prof Michel Probst, PT, PhD, Department Rehabilitation Sciences KU Leuven, Belgium, President of the International Organization for Physical Therapy in Mental Health*

"This book is a missing contextual link that can be used for medical and other healthcare students about integrative medicine and care. The book is well-organized and the exercises deepen the flow. I believe every person who has the opportunity to serve others in health care would benefit tremendously from reading *Integrative Rehabilitation Practice*. This book reminds us of the many beautiful ways we are able to interact with each other and how very powerful each interaction can be."

—*Anne E. (Annie) Weisman, PhD, MPH, LMT, Director of Wellness & Integrative Medicine, University of Nevada, Las Vegas, School of Medicine*

"Person-centered care has long been a buzz word in health care. Transitioning from the biomedical model into an integrated and complexity model is challenging, and can feel so wide it's impossible to see round. This book is a great introduction to some complex theories and will give you a wide, flexible framework to develop your practice within. Opening up the 'thinking space' to nurture collaboration and tailor individualized, meaningful care. In short, it will help you do your job."

—*Laura Rathbone, BA, BSc, MSc, MCSP, MACP, HCPC, Advanced Physiotherapist, Consultant and Educator, specialized in complexly presenting pain conditions*

"*Integrative Rehabilitation Practice* is a landmark book for the rehab professions, particularly physical therapy. This book provides us, educators in academic and clinical settings, with critical depth to concepts where we often just scratch the surface. While we talk about taking a wholistic approach to patient care and integrating all body systems, the socio-cultural-behavioral systems consistently receive little curricular attention and limited research funding, yet fully understanding the lived experience of the patient is central to all clinical care. The chapters provide sound evidence of important concepts and models that have direct clinical application. Concepts like social determinants of health and application of the ICF model are detailed in ways that make them come 'to life' for all learners, students and faculty. This book will have a transformative influence."

—*Gail M. Jensen, PT, PhD, FAPTA, FNAP, Professor of Physical Therapy, Vice Provost for Learning and Assessment, Creighton University*

"In this book, Matt Erb and Arlene Schmid seek to define and describe the complexities and philosophy of *Integrative Rehabilitation Practice* with success. In addition to great detail among the chapters regarding specific therapies with case examples, there is a refreshing experiential component that will surprise and enlighten readers."

—*Bridget Chin, MD, MA, Assistant Professor, Michigan State University College of Human Medicine, Clinical Instructor, Harvard Medical School/Spaulding Rehabilitation Network, Adjunct Lecturer, University of Michigan/Metro Health Hospital*

"*Integrative Rehabilitation Practice* is more than a textbook. It is a living, breathing, and crucial guide to truly integrate the mind and body in a medical realm that has long only attended to the physical. As an Integrative Physician myself, I was astounded at the attention to not only how to cultivate an integrative practice within the provider's practice, but to the integration of that work within the provider themselves. Studying this book is an alive experience as the reader is encouraged throughout to weave the teachings into their own selves and not just be a passive learner. The guidance found in this work expands the integration of the mind and body to a new level and will no doubt forge a deeper path for Integrative Medicine within all of health care."

—*Tanmeet Sethi, MD, Fellowship Director and Faculty, Swedish Cherry Hill Family Medicine Residency, Assistant Professor, University of Washington Medical School, Seattle, WA of related interest*

Yoga and Science in Pain Care
Treating the Person in Pain
Edited by Neil Pearson, Shelly Prosko and Marlysa Sullivan
Foreword by Timothy McCall
ISBN 978 1 84819 397 0
eISBN 978 0 85701 354 5

Touch is Really Strange
Steve Haines
Illustrated by Sophie Standing
ISBN 978 1 78775 710 3
eISBN 978 1 78775 711 0

Yoga Therapy as a Creative Response to Pain
Matthew J. Taylor
Foreword by John Kepner
ISBN 978 1 84819 356 7
eISBN 978 0 85701 315 6

INTEGRATIVE REHABILITATION PRACTICE

The Foundations of Whole-Person Care for Health Professionals

Edited by **Matt Erb** and **Arlene A. Schmid**

Foreword by Victoria Maizes

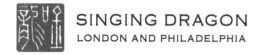

SINGING DRAGON
LONDON AND PHILADELPHIA

First published in Great Britain in 2021 by Singing Dragon, an imprint of
Jessica Kingsley Publishers

An Hachette Company

1

Table 1.2 is reproduced from Gosnell *et al.* (2017) with
kind permission from Guildford Press.
Figure 12.1 is adapted from Haskenkamp *et al.* (2012) with
kind permission from Wendy Haskenkamp.

Front cover image source: Britt Freda.

A CIP catalogue record for this title is available from the British Library and the
Library of Congress

ISBN 978 1 78775 150 7
eISBN 978 1 78775 151 4

Printed and bound in the United States by West Publishing Corp.

Jessica Kingsley Publishers' policy is to use papers that are natural, renewable
and recyclable products and made from wood grown in sustainable forests. The
logging and manufacturing processes are expected to conform to the environmental
regulations of the country of origin.

Jessica Kingsley Publishers
Carmelite House
50 Victoria Embankment
London EC4Y 0DZ

www.singingdragon.com

Contents

Disclaimer

For *health care professionals*: You are encouraged to seek professional supervision or mentoring to support clarity and safety in the delivery of whole-person care. Each professional must determine their capacity and the applicability of the material to their scope of practice.

For *health care consumers*: The information contained in this book is not intended to replace the services of trained medical professionals or to be a substitute for medical advice. The integrative rehabilitation approach described in this book may not be suitable for everyone to utilize. You are advised to consult with trained medical professionals on any matters relating to your health, and in particular on any matters that may require diagnosis or medical attention.

Foreword

Matt Erb, Arlene Schmid, and their colleagues have written an important book that will be of great value to practitioners and patients alike. As society grapples with how to address chronic pain, they encourage a larger frame within which to view its treatment. This paradigm, named integrative rehabilitation practice, considers a human being as much more than a highly sophisticated machine in need of fixing; instead a person is seen as a dynamic, evolving, storytelling organism with biopsychospiritual needs.

Through patient cases, a broader history, and an expanded set of therapeutic tools, the authors encourage a discovery process. Each person is understood to have a unique story that helps define who they are and begins to shape a potential therapeutic journey. I am honored to have been invited to write a foreword.

As a long-standing advocate of integrative medicine, I share Matt and Arlene's perspective in arguing for a richer definition of the human experience. However, I have also faced its importance from hard personal experience. In 2013, I became one of the 40% of Americans who lives with persistent pain when I developed thoracic back pain. To date, I have been treated with acupuncture, chiropractic, physical therapy, osteopathic manipulation, massage therapy, and postural therapy. I have done trauma-releasing exercises, yoga, breathing exercises, and guided imagery. I have taken anti-inflammatory medicine, herbal remedies, and a rare opioid.

Why did my pain begin and what has led to it continuing for the past seven years? What is the best way to manage it? What acts to trigger worsening pain and what helps to ease the pain? How much do I limit my life due to anticipatory pain? These questions define how I have approached the pain. In some cases, I have found valuable clues or answers; in others, mystery remains.

Those of you in the field will have heard versions of this story before. Multiple tries of multiple therapies and still the pain returns. If there is anything unique about my story, it is that I have had the resources and the desire to pursue integrative rehabilitative therapy. I bring with me the attitude that each time I am a patient, I learn something of value, not only for myself, but also for the patients I serve.

What part of the pain is in my mind and what part is in my body? Once you read Matt and Arlene's book you are likely to push back at such a question and point to the inability to dichotomize. The pain is simultaneously in brain and body. Similarly, on hearing a seven-year history of pain, with multiple therapies tried, you are likely to believe the solutions will be complex.

Included in this text are a variety of thoughtful questions and reflections. These will be useful to add to your armamentarium. They are likely to elicit poignant stories from your patients; this in turn may change how you approach patient care. The stories contained in the chapters that follow are almost certain to touch your heart and are intended to take you into the experience of integrative rehabilitative practice.

Having shared a bit of my story, I would like to add several additional questions.

On the personal level: Say a miracle occurred, you have advanced ten years into the future, and your pain has markedly diminished or completely disappeared. What would have happened? What changed in your life? What story would you tell? This "miracle" question comes from the motivational interviewing approach. It may be useful to jettison yourself far enough into a future where you are free of pain and work backwards.

On the societal level: If you were the health care czar, what practices would you cover? Most of the care I received was not covered by my medical insurance. Chiropractic and physical therapy were two exceptions. The rest of my care was paid for out of my pocket and cost thousands of dollars each year. Many do not have the opportunities that I had and yet my back-care program was almost certainly significantly less expensive than any recommended back surgery, which would likely have been covered by my insurance.

Finally, to enhance your relationship with those who treat you: What questions would help you to feel seen and understood? Is there anything else that you consider important? (I ask this last question of all my patients at the end of my history taking.) Even if you are not asked, please bring these concerns forward. They will help your treating provider better focus on your needs.

I am confident that this textbook, depicting a rich integrative paradigm, a wide range of therapeutic options, and a healing philosophy, will resonate with patients and practitioners alike. I hope that practitioners broaden their practice to embody integrative rehabilitative practice and that their patients experience them as partners.

To all readers, I wish you well on your healing journey.

Victoria Maizes, MD
Andrew Weil Endowed Chair in Integrative Medicine
Executive Director, Andrew Weil Center for Integrative Medicine
Professor of Clinical Medicine, Family Medicine and Public Health
—University of Arizona

Acknowledgements

First, as priority, the editors, authors, and reviewers thank *all of those individuals in the role of patient whom we have worked with and learned from.* These individuals have been our most cherished teachers. While we may not have always realized it at the time, patients have taught us much of what we present here, and the authors have been deliberate in reflecting patients' voices across the pages of this book. Thank you! Many of us have been in the role of patient too, deepening this understanding of mutual learning in health care.

Next, the editors wish to thank each of the contributing authors in order of appearance: Matthew J. Taylor, PT, PhD, C-IAYT, Daniel Winkle, MD, Andra DeVoght, PT, MPH, Todd E. Davenport, PT, DPT, MPH, OCS, Bronwyn Lennox Thompson, MSc(Hons), PhD(Cant), DipOccTh(CIT), Noshene Ranjbar, MD, Shelly Prosko, PT, C-IAYT, Geoff Sittler, OTR/L, BCN, Kellie Finn, MS, C-IAYT, ERYT-500, Betsy Shandalov, OTR/L, C-IAYT, Peggy Ninow, OTR/L, SEP, CHTP, Leslie Davenport, MA, MS, LMFT, Rachelle Palnick Tsachor, MA, CMA, RSMT, Irena Paiuk, MscPT, BPT, CMA, Molly J. Lahn, PT, DPT, PhD, Margaret Gavian, PhD, Marlysa Sullivan, PT, C-IAYT, Dena Rain Adler, BEd, MA, ATR, Sherril Howard, MS, CCC-SLP, Alicia L. Barksdale, MS, MT-BC, NMT, Brigid Titgemeier, MS, RDN, LD, IFNCP, Cheryl Van Demark, PT, C-IAYT, and James S. Gordon, MD. Each individual spent countless hours compiling their experience, wisdom, and a solid base from the existing research. Collectively they present an integral view of various topics that provide insight into the larger landscape of our lives, health, and healing processes. We are deeply grateful for them sharing their time and resources with us in this landmark venture. Together, the editors and authors collectively thank family, friends, and colleagues who contributed in many ways to this book's origins and development across time. We also wish to thank Victoria Maizes, MD, for the Foreword.

Beyond the review and editing process of the co-editors, the content of this book has been peer-reviewed. We extend gratitude to the following individuals for reviewing chapters and providing valuable feedback as follows: Karen Alexander, PhD (Chapters 1, 3, 6, 9, 25, 26); Matthew J. Taylor, PT, PhD, C-IAYT (Chapter 11); Mary Lou Galantino, PT, MS, PhD, MSCE, FAPTA (Preface, Chapters 1, 15); Stephen Bezruchka, MD, MPH (Chapter 4); Beth Nauman-Montana, MLIS (Chapter 4); Shelly Prosko, PT, C-IAYT (Chapters 4, 11); Daniel Winkle, MD (Chapter 2); Anjali Goel, MD

(Chapters 3, 7); Marlysa Sullivan, PT, C-IAYT (Chapter 5); Bronwyn Lennox Thompson, MSc(Hons), PhD(Cant), DipOccTh(CIT) (Chapters 6, 16, 17); Joe Tatta, PT, DPT, CNS (Chapters 8, 25); Dena Rain Adler, BEd, MA, ATR (Chapter 9); Emily Rich, MOT, OTR/L (Chapter 10); Rebecca Kloberdanz, MPH, OTR/L (Chapter 12); Betsy Shandalov, OTR/L, C-IAYT (Chapters 14, 18); Robin Bourjaily, MA/W, E-RYT 500 (Chapter 15); Kathie Swift, MS, RDN, LDN, FAND, EBQ (Chapter 22); Geoff Sittler, OTR/L, BCN (Chapter 24); Sharna Prasad, PT, DPT (Chapter 25, Appendix B); Tom Hyland Robertson, DC (Chapter 23); Mark Kargela, PT, DPT, OCS, FAAOMPT (Chapter 23); Laurie Hyland Robertson, MS, C-IAYT (Chapters 1, 19); Susan M. Mingils, MM, MT-BC (Chapter 21); John Weeks (Appendix A); Leah Fabiano Smith, PhD, CCC-SLP (Chapter 20); Andra DeVoght, PT, MPH (Chapter 26), Marianne H. Mortera, PhD, OTR/L (Chapters 1–27).

Matt Erb: As lead developer and co-editor of this project, I wish to thank James S. Gordon and the entire Staff and Faculty of The Center for Mind-Body Medicine (CMBM) for pioneering a collectivist approach to sharing evidence-based mind-body medicine with the world. Additionally, I wish to acknowledge my CMBM colleague and dear friend Jerrol Kimmel whose encouragement to develop a book became a key energy that moved it forward.

Arlene Schmid: As co-editor, I wish to thank the many clients, mentors, and researchers whom I have worked with to study integrative rehabilitation practice, specifically yoga, for multiple populations. I am thankful that Matt Erb approached me to be a co-editor for the endeavor; this book is an excellent and much-needed contribution to the literature.

Editors' Note

A JOURNEY

The editors and authors of this book are inviting you on an exploration and adventure! The journey ahead can be seen as both discovering new landscapes and seeing one's existing landscape with clear and fresh eyes. Like any big journey, knowing where we are at the start, how we got there, where we are going, and what we have to accompany us along the way are crucial to any successful undertaking.

Section One of this book aims to present contextual understandings and increased capacity for health-care professionals to navigate whole-person care. Chapters 1–7 are foundational to a working definition of integrative rehabilitation practice (IRP) and include multiple important topics related to health care and models of rehabilitation.

In Section Two, we explore and discover ways that support enacting IRP. This exploration includes skills and experiments employed from the fresh, expanded, and contextual paradigm brought to you in Section One. The skills presented are capable of supporting the potential for greater autonomy, well-being, and/or healing processes for ourselves and those we serve equally.

No two experiences of this journey will ever wholly be the same. Make it your own. Be careful to not fall into a "rose-colored glasses" state. Stay alert to acknowledging a mix of positives and challenges. Section Two encourages the use of clinical approaches that lead from a primary focus on presence, relationship, and support for larger processes.

As you proceed, a stance of "beginner's mind" will be helpful. As such, consider leaving behind preconceived notions of what all of this might look like. Similarly, it is important to consider the idea that each of us is in charge of our effort, but not necessarily the outcomes. Our relationship to the "outcome" matters. Here it becomes important to be aware of our tendency to deploy clinical "tools" or techniques in a "just fix it already" way that reinforces a common, often-hidden tendency—the "normal" but problematic tendency for avoidance or aversion. Without calling this to awareness, we miss the importance of valuable clinical reasoning constructs that must underlie the use of any such tools or techniques. Clinical reasoning underpins both the *nature of* these "tools" that we have chosen to present, as well as why and how the tools are utilized within an experiential learning model. In other words, look for an understanding that underscores being mindful not to just throw them into an existing toolkit without changing the base stance from which you work. "Skills for supporting and navigating" reflects this shift in intention. More on this throughout the book...

In Section Three, we explore several key examples of going deeper into models that can hold the whole of IRP...and that can expand the reach of IRP toward public health efforts. Section Three gives opportunity to dive deeper into: yoga therapy as an emerging standalone profession; group-based and community-oriented care approaches—something largely missing in our increasingly individualistic societies; and advocacy for increased utilization of IRP. Advocacy is directed towards addressing public health efforts for integrated health-care systems and integrative care models in support of individual and societal mental (and thus physical!) health.

HEART ADVICE FOR CHALLENGING TIMES

We are living in an age of exponentially expanding information and an accelerating rate of change. Contemporary thought is appraising and reappraising the philosophical foundations of health care. Emerging approaches increasingly inquire into the phenomenological (the study of consciousness), epistemological (how we come to know), and ontological (the metaphysical nature of being) underpinnings of health care. Such inquiries are seen as not just valid, but critical for growth and transformation of not just the individual, but also the larger living systems that we form, experience, and participate in.

Navigating the complexity of life and information in the context of your personal and professional process, and the myriad relationships within that, can be challenging. Our exploration is designed to assist you in adopting a foundation rooted in awareness and informed by knowledge and skills that are embedded within a whole-person and heart-centered approach. Such an approach aims to support the navigation of our contemporary version of life complexity, and ultimately the formation of wisdom.

As we will explore in Chapter 3, the rates of burnout of health-care professionals are increasing. The concept of "caring for the caregiver" reflects another broad goal that is embedded within each approach illuminated. By exploring our own personal processes through an experiential lens that assists in connecting previously disparate dots, we lay a solid foundation for:

- reducing burnout by bolstering our innate resilience
- the enhancement of your own unique way of serving others, as being required to fit a mold adds stress, trickling down into the quality of care
- an expansion into concepts of interdependence between living systems
- the exploration of "relationship"—with self, others, and one's environment.

THE AUDIENCE

While a number of the authors of and contributors to this book are steeped in the professions of occupational and physical therapy, we have contributions from many other professions. This includes: physicians specializing in both physical medicine and mental health, and who practice from a mind-body integrated lens; a speech-language pathologist; an art therapist; several psychologists and mental health professionals; a music therapist; public health professionals; and several yoga therapists. Unfortunately, we were unable to represent all relevant professions as authors, but many other professions will equally find this book of use. Other relevant professions include: nurses, social workers, recreational therapists, vocational rehabilitation therapists, chiropractors, massage therapists, primary care doctors, psychiatrists, other physicians, and various behavioral and mental health professionals. Complementary and integrative health (CIH) practitioners will also find value. In essence, any professional (and even some patients and/or laypersons) interested in integrative medicine (IM), mind-body medicine, the biopsychosocial (BPS) model, and/or improving health care in general are welcome here! Critics and doubters from any field or background are welcome too!

The material presented draws from a mix of evidence-based, science-informed, experiential, intuitive, historical, and contemporary material. Material is illuminated by philosophy, psychospiritual concepts, and the wisdom traditions which continue to evolve as contemporary practitioners intuitively rediscover and repurpose healing principles.

In this book we present a practical and foundational approach to whole-person support in rehabilitation. Our effort is not meant to be an exhaustive literature review; however, many key studies and findings from research are presented to underscore IM and IRP as devoted to scientific inquiry.

Research and information in general are expanding at an astronomical rate. Often by the time a book is published, the references are considered outdated. For this reason, we have done our best with the current state of information to present an approach that is geared towards advancing the prevailing treatment paradigm. This will change too, as we are ever-evolving in our personal and professional lives. If hindsight was available as foresight, we may have written a completely different book! Alas, this is not possible, and so we present from our current level of awareness, experience, and understanding in the hope that it proves useful to you, the reader.

We approach our work with humility and willingness to learn, grow, and transform together. We ask you, the reader, for your forgiveness for that which we do not yet see or understand. Teach us! We invite your knowledge and wisdom to mix with ours to co-create better ways of being and working with people on their very real and very human journeys; towards a definition of well-being that ameliorates our shared experience of suffering. We hope others will take this effort and improve upon it.

DON'T JUST TAKE OUR WORD FOR IT

We believe experiential learning is the best way to bring any information alive. Experiential learning supports embodiment, action, and motivation to bring it alive in the delivery of health care. As such, throughout this book we have built in *experiential pauses*. These pauses allow you, the reader, to reflect, experiment, and discover your own truths and applications of the material that we offer in the words of this book. The words are not the way, rather they point the way. Words are chosen for a reason and reflect an intent. Listen for the intent. Consider taking the time to complete each experience. Repeat. Reflect. Repeat again.

Each person's experience of this journey is going to look different and is equally important to anything that we as authors and editors might offer. Consider that your own creation out of the material has great potential. This comes with a full invitation to critically review, accept, and/or reject...and in the process, to evolve into your own version of it.

CLOSING (OPENING) WORDS

There are no experts here, only various levels of experience and understanding mixing together; in continual process. In this, we are co-creating and learning to continuously reinterpret and reappraise...everything. And, all process is enhanced by flexibility. *Welcome* to what we intend to be a flexible process of mutual learning! We are glad to meet you on this path...

Preface from a Physical Therapist

Matt Erb, PT

Physical therapy (PT), or physiotherapy as it is known outside of the US, found me in what I prefer to see as an act of fate. After graduating with an undergraduate degree in biology, I enrolled in veterinary school, only to arrive at an early crisis of psyche, questioning what I was destined to do with my life. Looking back, I now see that this "crisis" (decisive point) was touching into already present biobehavioral patterns developed from earlier life stress. A friend who was already attending physiotherapy school said that she thought I might like the profession. On what felt like a whim (and that was rooted in a sense of urgency to medicate the discomfort and confusion I was experiencing) I took a leave of absence from veterinary school and was accepted into PT school. Within a week of starting the PT program I knew it was part of the path I would pursue, but not for the reasons I thought at the time. Looking back, I believe the interest in working with animals, followed by the interest in working with the complexity of the human body, were both ultimately rooted in desire for connection and my own version of the hero's journey of healing and transformation. Every little detail and facet of the path along the way has been well suited to mirror and messenger larger processes. I believe this will continue to be the case.

I discovered quickly upon graduating that there were gaps in how I experienced people and their "physical" problems, and what I had been taught in school. I recall a series of lectures on the psychosocial facets of patient care that gave lip service to the need to address psychological and social factors but that offered negligible practical strategies to do so. The course was experienced as "that's nice"—information with an emphasis on passing a test and not a person to care for. My other courses reflected "doing to" much more than understanding the patient's experience.

The extent of my early education in mind-body medicine came from basic training in biofeedback and reading a book on holistic therapies in rehabilitation. These early components pointed towards something emerging, but not yet formed. There were many unconnected dots that fell short in helping me adequately navigate the reality and complexity of human experience—especially the role of all things "mind" within the processes of the body. As we will see, the integration of mind and body into a more uniform construct is increasingly demanded in health care as science catches up with ancient wisdom teachings.

I have devoted my career to understanding human experience and behavior in relationship to that which manifests in the body and there remains as many unanswered questions as those answered. In the context of wisdom teachings on health and healing, it serves us to say that truths are being rediscovered and re-presented through the contemporary scientific lens. The ones that have been revealed to me have illuminated an improved way of working with illness and disease within myself and others. This has included insight into the ways in which I relate to my environment and, more broadly, a perspective on the nature of human suffering and ways to improve my relationship to that suffering.

While I by no means have all of the answers, I have gradually discovered and co-created a more integral way of working within my field that engages and serves the complexity of each person. This has not been solely of my own doing—and has arisen from the interaction of numerous impersonal sources of information, knowledge, and wisdom.

My personal journey, which has included a series of slender threads and synchronicities, has led me into this project as a heartfelt effort in the service of an intention: to consciously contribute to the amelioration of human suffering. With that backdrop, and as the developer, a contributor, and a co-editor of this project, I have aimed at presenting a flexible guide in support of the ongoing co-creation of a more holistic and mind-body integrated approach.

Preface from an Occupational Therapist

Arlene Schmid, PhD, OTR, FAOTA

I was lucky, as I found occupational therapy (OT) while I was still in high school. My cousin was in OT school at the time, and I wrote a paper about kids with disabilities and quickly figured out that OT was the way to go. I, of course, learned in school that OT is considered to be holistic and that we treat the whole person: mind, body, and spirit. But I really struggled with what holistic meant or how I could treat the whole person while working in a hand clinic or in a skilled nursing facility with little time dedicated to each client.

Right after I graduated from OT school in Buffalo, New York, I got on a plane and moved to Hawaii, where I lived and worked for five years. My life was changed! I learned what it was like to be surrounded by people from all around the Pacific Basin and how to truly consider culture during my OT treatment. Most importantly though, I found yoga (oh, and also my sweet husband and amazing friends, but this story is about yoga). There was not much yoga or anything like it in Buffalo at the time, but yoga and other aspects of integrative care (Tai Chi, acupuncture, different types of massage) were everywhere in Hawaii. I tried a yoga class, and then another, and then quickly I was hooked—which is often the case with yoga. I did some basic yoga trainings and started to use yoga in my clinical practice, with clients in different settings from different cultures. I worked in skilled nursing facilities, long-term rehabilitation, an inpatient adolescent psychiatric unit, and an outpatient hand clinic. Somehow, almost magically, yoga kept helping different people in different ways. I had to know more.

I made the emotional decision to leave Hawaii and pursue my PhD, with the simple plan of researching yoga for people with disabilities, wanting to prove that yoga could be integrated into OT and rehabilitation. I wanted to show that yoga was a way to be truly holistic and treat the whole person, regardless of the disability, disease, or setting. And I am lucky enough that I now get to do this every day. I have now been researching yoga for 15 years and I love what I do. Every study tells us new things, but importantly every single study tells us that yoga is both feasible and beneficial for all of our clinical populations. An important finding has been that yoga is great, but yoga alone is not enough. We have now developed and tested programming where we merge yoga with group OT or group education for multiple populations. These merged interventions, or where we are integrating yoga into OT (think IRP), lead us to our strongest results.

I feel so lucky that I found yoga—or that yoga found me. I have since been trained as a yoga teacher so that I can better understand the complex philosophical underpinnings of yoga that impact our interventions and our delivery. I have had the opportunity to take a deep dive into yoga, and I have learned so much. And now I have the opportunity to co-edit this important book—and I have learned so much! Matt, the co-editor, has the knowledge and ability to connect the dots and found the perfect author for each chapter. I have read the chapters multiple times and continue to learn from each—and this is changing my day-to-day life and influencing how and what I teach OT students. I hope that you, the reader, have the opportunity to learn as much as I have, and to allow this new knowledge to be integrated into your life and your rehabilitation practice.

FOUNDATIONS OF INTEGRATIVE REHABILITATION PRACTICE

The content of Section One aims to build a foundation for integrative rehabilitation practice (IRP)—one that reflects a paradigmatic transformation in how we understand, relate to, and approach health care and rehabilitation. The presented content demands gradually building capacity for complex and contextual thinking and clinical reasoning, and then applying it across the entirety (intra-individual, inter-individual, collective, organizational, and systemic) of health care and rehabilitation processes.

Disclaimer: Across this book, we present descriptions of individuals and their experiences. These presentations and details are a compilation of the authors' and editors' shared clinical experiences. Any details relevant to specific persons such as gender, name, and age are purely coincidence. In a few cases, permission for the use of specific material has been obtained.

Recommendation: The editors and authors encourage you to obtain a personal process journal to document your journey through this book. There are many experiential learning opportunities that ask you to document your responses. Further, every chapter ends with a request to lay out an active response to the material. As part of your journal, we invite you to document anything that comes up for you as you read—including judgments, criticisms, and concerns. We aim towards a process of mutual learning and growth in support of enhanced, person-centered health care.

The Landscape

Matt Erb, PT and Arlene Schmid, PhD, OTR, FAOTA

SEEKING QUALITY OF CARE

The current biomedical model and system of health care emphasizes an approach that focuses on the physical basis of disease. This model has been successful at treating acute injury, many surgical interventions, and the management of some illnesses. The science that informs the biomedical model continues to evolve and present life-saving discoveries. Simultaneously, the biomedical model does not adequately address the roots of chronic disease, many of which have origins in lifestyle factors and the impact of post-industrial changes, such as: food changes, increased sedentary lifestyles, and toxic stress. Ralph Snyderman, Chancellor Emeritus at Duke University, said: "What we have now is a 'sick care' system that is reactive to problems."[1] In the US, in 2012 about half of all adults had one or more chronic health conditions.[2] A focus on ameliorating symptoms in a health-care system with limited and/or poor utilization of resources leads to missed opportunities for comprehensive and relationally focused models of well-being. Patients feel the gap and are seeking to fill it on their own, often through "complementary and alternative medicine" (CAM) approaches. At the same time, in the US, more than half (53.1%) of office-based physicians across specialty areas recommended at least one complementary health approach to their patients during the previous 12 months.[3]

Due to challenges around the language and construct of CAM, the NIH's (National Institutes of Health, US) center on the topic changed its name to the National Center for Complementary and Integrative Health (NCCIH). In the US, the term "complementary and integrative health" (CIH) is preferred and used most often. Health-care practices that are perceived as falling outside the biomedical model include ongoing research by NCCIH and are estimated to be an industry worth $30 billion per year in the US alone.[4]

The various labels (CIH, CAM, biomedical, and integrative) are not without criticism, politics, opinions, and emotion. This is welcome, as it compels us to examine our beliefs and foster clarity as we optimize self-care. Ultimately, our efforts must focus on the preferences and needs of the individuals that we are serving over our own current belief systems. A number of approaches that historically fall under the CIH label (yoga, meditation, mind-body medicine, nutrition) have emerging evidence and blend well into mainstream health care. Their presence is partly due to increased patient demand and partly due to the establishment of integrative medicine (IM) as a board-certified physician specialty in the US where this evidence-based approach to health care continues to expand. Bridges are being built and previous distinctions and lines are blurring.

Any approach must be examined from the lens of complexity and held to a critical inquiry into the "if, how, and why" such approaches may yield a positive outcome. This is where a distinction between "integrative" as a *model of humility* versus integrative as an overly reified belief system enters. In the latter case, a professional can form an identity with the label of their approach which becomes indistinguishable from other belief systems that may be operating from faulty assumptions. Thus, it misses the understanding of complexity and emergence. As such, CIH approaches may be included within a spectrum of an integrative approach if supported by evidence and well matched to a patient's preferences and needs. We therefore seek to focus this book on a foundational picture of working with the whole person as the root of "integrative," as opposed to the notion that it is necessarily about something "alternative" or "complementary." If defining principles are applied, care can be offered from the integrative construct, regardless of setting/system or techniques/modalities. Preferably, if the concepts used to define integrative care become innate to the delivery of health care, such labels will fall aside.

The purpose of our exploration has the intention of improving quality of care. Our purpose is not to suggest specialness (dichotomize good/bad), nor to lead people into over-identification with labels. As the Advisory Commission on Consumer Protection and Quality put it: "Exhaustive research documents the fact that today, in America, there is no guarantee that any individual will receive high-quality care for any particular health problem. The health care industry is plagued with overutilization of services, underutilization of services and errors in health care practice."[5] There are many factors that impact quality of care, especially from the patient's perspective.[6] Health-care professionals must listen closely to the patient experience to gain insight. Research indicates that better patient care experiences and inherent goals driven by intention are associated with improved adherence to chosen treatment options, better clinical outcomes, and less health-care utilization.[7]

TEARING DOWN COMPLEXITY AND PUTTING IT BACK TOGETHER

The topic of patient experience is complex. Many challenging factors interact to determine patient perception of quality care.[8] The IM movement is built upon researching, understanding, and supporting that which serves fundamental needs and substrates of human experience and healing processes. IM includes an exploration of what, for each individual, supports safety, nurturance, and empowerment; what best supports individuals' unique blends of experiences, conditions, relationships, beliefs, cultures, and more. Talk about complexity!

Perhaps for ease, the preceding facets are often split off or ignored altogether, though they directly influence the manifestation and course of any health or disease state. This splitting is inherent in our tendency to separate mind from body. Such separation is challenged in integral thinking. As such, *non-dual thinking* is needed. Non-dual thinking is the adoption of a "both/and" perspective when facing questions, concerns, concepts, and challenges. This is compared to the tendency to engage either/or thinking. Is health a situation of either body or mind? It is always both. A shift here serves to ignite creativity and wisdom in yourself and your work, and we will continue to encourage non-dual thinking around most any question that arises.

Rehabilitation has been reduced to various degrees, such as a focus on physical, occupational, or other labeled constructs. As we will see, this previously necessary reduction has, in many cases, inadvertently compromised care, reducing the whole person to the labels of "a knee," a vocational goal, or an otherwise stigmatizing status. Even "therapy" can imply deficit, dysfunction, or wrongness that leads to objectifying or diminishing another.[9] These dynamics represent a challenge to cultivating the full potential that rehabilitation can offer. IM, rooted in the concept of an integral whole, helps complete a fuller picture of what rehabilitation means, while maintaining necessary boundaries and professional integrity.

As noted in a creative book on, well, creativity, the rehabilitation professions are under great pressure to innovate and evolve in order to cater to a growing market of sophisticated and informed consumers who are increasingly responsible for paying for their services.[10] On the heels of Dr. Matthew J. Taylor's work, the focus of our efforts in this book is to present a novel construct of clinically oriented *integrative rehabilitation practice* (IRP) as one avenue that can help navigate the multiple challenges of complexity. Such complexity brings us into three important defining questions.

- What exactly is integrative medicine (IM)?
- How does the IM movement inform our efforts in this book to define IRP?
- How does IRP relate to the growing lip service being given to *biopsychosocial* (BPS) care?

Let's take a look…

INTEGRATIVE MEDICINE

The University of Arizona Center for Integrative Medicine (UACIM) describes IM as "healing-oriented medicine that takes account of the whole person, including all aspects of lifestyle. IM emphasizes the therapeutic relationship between practitioner and patient, is informed by evidence, and makes use of all appropriate therapies."[11] UACIM describes the following defining principles of IM.

- "Patient and practitioner are partners in the healing process.
- All factors that influence health, wellness, and disease are taken into consideration, including mind, spirit, and community, as well as the body.
- Appropriate use of both conventional and alternative methods facilitates the body's innate healing response.

- Effective interventions that are natural and less invasive should be used whenever possible.
- Integrative medicine neither rejects conventional medicine nor accepts alternative therapies uncritically.
- Good medicine is based in good science. It is inquiry-driven and open to new paradigms.
- Alongside the concept of treatment, the broader concepts of health promotion and the prevention of illness are paramount.
- Practitioners of integrative medicine should exemplify its principles and commit themselves to self-exploration and self-development."[12]

Other academic centers, such as Duke University, offer similar definitions.[13] Ultimately, the integrative construct is not new. Many ancient and indigenous healing systems that evolved across disparate geographic locations and time are rooted in integrative constructs, regardless of whether they have been defined using contemporary formats.

The word *integrative* is defined as "serving or intending to unify separate things."[14] In general, *integration* refers to concepts of unity or consolidation, i.e., the integration of parts into a whole. Both *integrative* and *integrated* are adjectives of integration— representing being composed of a whole. Going further, *integral* implies a constitution of the whole with other parts or factors as not being omittable or removable. As such, IM promotes an integral approach that navigates health care in a way that frames and supports each person's experience as representing a complex whole. We are whole. Already.

IM is grounded in the World Health Organization's (WHO) definition of *health*: "a state of complete physical, mental and social well-being and not merely the absence of disease or infirmity."[15] The WHO Traditional Medicine Strategy includes stated support for the integrated, safe, and effective use and research of both traditional and integrative models.[16] The preceding definition is equally consistent with the salutogenic model—an approach that focuses greater attention on factors that support health and well-being than on deficits and perceived problems.[17] *Salutogenesis* engages in exploration of positively framed relationships between health, stress, and coping patterns. Salutogenesis implies an approach that cultivates an underlying sense of order, predictability, and meaning as a backdrop within one's experience regardless of the degree of perceived chaos, disorder, or distress in one's present experience. In other words, well-being can exist despite the presence of a disease state and whether a problem is fixable or not.

In one sense, we have had to create our contemporary idea of well-being. "Remember" can be broken apart into "re-member"—to put things that have been taken apart back together again into a new whole. IRP sees remembering as an ongoing process of co-creation—something that is demanded to fit the rapidly changing conditions of our world.

The preceding notions of health are fundamental within the IM approach. An IM approach posits going even further by encouraging attention to a "fix-it" paradigm, first described as "doing to" versus "being with" by Dr. Matthew J. Taylor.[18] When a fixer/

fixee dynamic is brought to awareness, hierarchical power imbalances (helper/helped) are uncovered.[19] The fixer/fixee dynamic implies that the fixee is "broken" and can be repaired by the fixer. This misses the participation of the patient in facilitating their wholeness, and the importance of relationship and co-creation in the healing process. Additionally, both professional and patient questions of "Why?" and "How?" can be reframed when this dynamic is brought to light. This reframe opens us to the possibility of moving beyond "Why?" and towards "What can I learn from this and how can I be in the best possible *relationship with* this experience?"

THE BIOPSYCHOSOCIAL MODEL

How is IM related to the growing call for a BPS approach? BPS is a general model of care, positing that biological, psychological (i.e., thoughts, emotions, and behaviors), and social factors all play a significant role in human functioning in the context of disease or illness. The BPS view of health was first defined in 1977.[20] Delineations of the BPS model as relates to various topics such as pain came later.[21]

Often missed in looking at the origins of the BPS model is the understanding that it was presented as rooted in relationship: "...clinical study begins at the person level and takes place within a two-person system, the doctor-patient relationship."[22] As we will see moving forward, it also takes place in the larger context of the systems and environments that individuals are embedded within.

The BPS model is increasingly expanded to include the influence of individual spiritual beliefs and practices. The first incidence of this in the literature appears to be by Sulmasy in 2002,[23] where the notion of a *biopsychosocialspiritual* (BPSS) approach was presented in the Western health-care context.

Unfortunately, without additional concepts and definitions, both the BPS and BPSS models may fall short of *integral*, as they are often viewed and/or delivered in a compartmentalized, fragmented fashion.[24] For example, the listed components of BPS/BPSS models tends to be thought of as separate things. "Because of their etiological complexity, it is implausible to expect any one explanation (e.g., neurotransmitter dysregulation, irrational thinking, childhood trauma) to fully account for mental disorders."[25] Insert "any health condition" in place of mental disorders. "No portion of the BPS model has a monopoly on the truth."[26] Ultimately, while our endless search to "know why" will continue, we must stop searching for any absolute "why." This includes any reduced tendency to seek purely physical, psychological, genetic, etc. explanations for a manifestation. These challenges are embedded across society, and shifting collective beliefs and understanding is needed.[27] Consider how rearranging the order of BPS to read *socio-psycho-biological* places the model in a framework of relationship first, and could potentially change the meaning and how people might perceive it.

The IM construct includes and then builds upon all these concepts to include additional considerations. Calling out the aforementioned fix-it dynamic is a defining aspect of our view of integrative care. Additional topics that assist in defining IRP include *living systems theory*, *non-duality*, *emergence*, and *enactivism*. We will delineate these further as we move through this book. For now, let's start with living systems theory.

LIVING SYSTEMS THEORY

Living systems theory is a general theory about how all living systems "work," maintain themselves, and change. In short, living systems are open, self-organizing systems that have characteristics of life and interact in an inseparable way with their environment. This takes place by means of continuous flow of information and energy exchange. Living systems can be simple (a single cell) or complex (an organization).

Living systems depend upon the interacting processes of systems and subsystems to survive. Integrative care seeks to explore and support, in non-harming ways, the myriad processes informing living systems. These processes can be conceptualized as levels and entry points within a whole. Take stress for example. Stress can arise from many sources, such as mental, emotional, physical, nutritional, social, and environmental. Mitigation of stress through any one of these facets has influence within the larger whole, even if not immediately detectable. As such, throughout this book we use the construct of an integral sense of the whole of each person's unique experience of body-mind-environment (BME). Integrative care posits complexity and interconnectivity across levels both within and between individuals and their environments. With the development of this understanding comes the implication of the need to seek out improved ways of exploring, engaging, and supporting various levels within each person's life, in salutogenic (positively framed) support of well-being as earlier defined.

Figure 1.1 reflects upon how the various levels of consideration are often relegated to specific scientific disciplines, and is intended to convey dynamic interactions within and between these levels. The depiction of levels is itself limiting, so remember to take these as relative and contextual. Table 1.1 below contemplates this model of levels in relation to reductionism versus holism.

Table 1.1: Comparing Reductionistic and Integral Tendencies

Reduction	Integral
Evaluating, studying, and/or explaining from or focused on addressing mostly from one level	Contemplating, considering the whole
Focused on parts/components	Working from and supporting from above and/or below levels
Tends to be more apt to look down levels to explain causality	High context orientation including the larger picture of where an individual has come from and what the individual is a part of (environments)
Individualistic	Adds collectivist considerations

Adapted from Greg Henriques[28] and Kennon Sheldon[29]

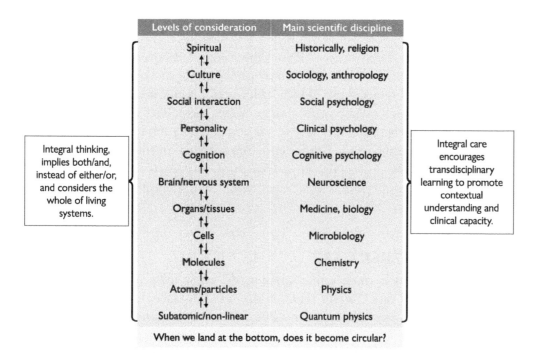

FIGURE 1.1: INTEGRATING LEVELS AND DISCIPLINES
Adapted from Greg Henriques[30] and Kennon Sheldon[31]

REDUCTION

It is important to not see reductionism as "bad." It serves our scientific disciplines well. Think "both/and" here too. We can work from a more microscopic (the focus of most health-care professionals' core academic training) and a more macroscopic approach (the focus of this book) at the same time. When looking at the limitations of one paradigm, as the saying goes, we do not need to throw the baby out with the bathwater. The integrative approach encourages health-care professionals to evolve and transform their practices to fuller constructs by building upon the foundation of their professional training. This supports a greater sum of parts. Even holism as a concept can be reduced, leading to assumptions and causing one to miss the benefits of working "down" a level.

Finally, we must consider the idea that a form of "reduction" in relationship to complexity *is* useful: simplicity. Reduction from the complexity of a whole is often necessary in research and teaching, though may inadvertently contribute to deficits in care delivery and/or invalidation of the patient's experience. Is it possible to support the whole without overwhelming ourselves and others with too many complex considerations? The ability to translate complexity into simplicity, a learned skill in teaching and clinical practice, offers us a way.

Experiential pause: Take a moment and, if it's comfortable, close your eyes. Become aware of your body and your breath. Now, think of a time when you were feeling stressed, down, or upset…allow this memory to form just a bit…when was it? How old were you? Now, do you recall if your mind sought an answer to the question "Why?" Was that answer simplified? Did your mind try to pin it on a simple chemical imbalance in the brain and ask: "I wonder if I need a medication?" Or if the stress was around a physical symptom, did your mind seek a simplified cause and solution? This tendency is common. It is easy to fall into quick-fix mode. Now take a little longer to contemplate the same experience through a lens of complexity. What else was happening in your life at this time? Were prior experiences or patterns carrying influence? Was there physical, mental, emotional, social, or nutritional stress at work? Other factors? Consider jotting down any ideas or insights in your process journal.

PERSON-CENTERED CARE

We are moving away from an authoritarian model where the provider takes the lead, to *patient*-centered care. *Patient*-centered care can be conceptualized even further in the context of *person*-centered care (PCC). Thomas Kitwood, an early advocate, described PCC as: "a standing or status bestowed upon a human being by another/ others, in the context of relationship and social being. This care implies recognition, respect, and trust."[32] PCC is defined as "a holistic (bio-psychosocial-spiritual) approach to delivering care that is respectful and individualized, allowing negotiation of care, and offering choice through a therapeutic relationship where persons are empowered to be involved in health decisions at whatever level is desired by that individual who is receiving the care."[33]

Within the preceding definition, Morgan and Yoder emphasize the attributes of holistic, individualized, respectful, and empowering.[34] Patients are seen as equal individuals with capacity to participate actively in their health and health-care experience. PCC is personalized, enabling, and built upon principles of choice, dignity, humility, and respect. Trusting, following, and supporting each person's narrative is vital.[35] PCC is innate within the IM model. For health-care providers, these ideas suggest an approach focused on: "selecting and delivering interventions or treatments that are respectful of and responsive to the characteristics, needs, preferences, and values of the person or individual."[36] As such, IM includes fundamentals of *health coaching, motivational interviewing*, and the *transtheoretical model of change*.

In IM, dynamics of power, influence, and fixing must be brought to awareness. Mentioned earlier, the presence of fixer/fixee roles implies that it is the responsibility of the professional to fix the patient's experience. This dynamic inhabits an authoritarian space, creating a power imbalance. Power can be seen as influence which may be intended or unintended and that may show up in various forms such as force, manipulation, persuasion, or authority. For the latter, authority can be seen in various constructs such as "coercive," "legitimate," "competent," and, of great importance in health coaching models, "personal authority" or "agency."

Two interdependent individuals exploring their experiences in relationship reflects a better stance aimed at restoring a power balance and contributing to the potential for the emergence of greater personal authority. This in turn has potential to contribute to healing processes and/or the emergence of well-being. Here, *emergence* refers to how collective properties arise from the properties of interacting parts from both higher and lower levels on the living system construct. In other words: "the whole is greater than the sum of the parts." We often lose sight of the whole that we each are. This book is deliberate in laying out concepts and strategies to support "parts," with an eye toward the sum of parts from which the whole emerges. Figure 1.2 demonstrates an evolution from the current model to guiding concepts embedded in the working construct of IRP.

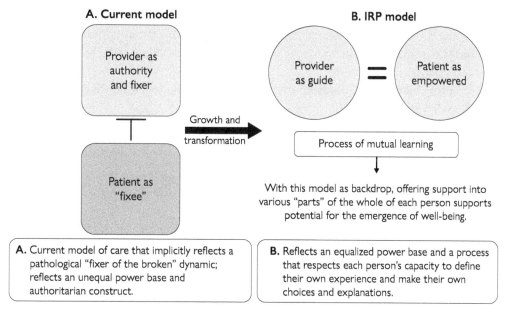

FIGURE 1.2: IRP—A MODEL OF MUTUAL LEARNING

PROCESS ORIENTATION

The transtheoretical model of change explains the nature of complex *processes* within health and human behavior.[37] In doing so, this model highlights the need to deliver care from a position of humility, especially as it relates to "outcomes." Introducing any treatment or intervention, which must first be self-selected with informed consent, may interact with other conditions to influence an endless array of possible outcomes. Further, understanding the nature of change becomes especially relevant when the care model requests or requires active participation outside of the encounter, such as is demanded with lifestyle medicine.

A process-oriented view of health demands that care be approached with awareness that there are extensive factors, many of which may be unknowable, that influence the trajectory of living systems. Without the humility that comes with this understanding, professionals of any kind may reify faulty belief systems around causality. This can lead to the inadvertent harm that comes if the unconscious dynamic of patient blame arises. An example is when a "failure to improve" is passed off as a failure on the part of the patient—or lack of "compliance." It is entirely possible that a "non-compliant" presentation will have improvement or resolution of a health condition. Equally, the most compliant patient, who does everything suggested to get better, may end up in an experience of disease progression. Is it possible to realize wholeness in either case?

THE PRACTICE OF INTEGRATIVE REHABILITATION

The word rehabilitation comes from the Latin prefix *re-*, meaning "again," and *habitare*, meaning "make fit"—to make fit, again. Wordplay: perhaps: "The restoration of a better condition"? How about: "To return to one's original fitness and innate status of well-being"? Do these expansions point to spiritual or existential notions? Something beyond the immediate restoration of an apparent state of disrepair? We will cultivate that discussion as we go along!

In putting all the concepts from the preceding sections together, we call for the use of IRP to denote a therapeutic approach that:

- focuses on supporting self-referential processes and self-care principles for practitioner and patient equally, within a safe container of relational attunement that includes an understanding of principles of *co-regulation* (one person's ability to regulate physiological state positively impacts the other's state and ability), mutual learning, and interdependence
- favors a phenomenological heuristic that supports the embodied lived experience of the patient and supports each person's capacity to come to know, understand, and define their own experience, treatment preferences, needs, and wisdom
- operates with humility that recognizes that there are many courses and "outcomes" that may emerge from a complex mix of both knowable and unknowable determinants within and between each individual's integrated BME experience
- aims to improve our collective ability to advance the implementation of systems in support of understanding, collaboration, and deepened ways of working with our shared human experience
- is less concerned with clinical techniques as being "solutions" or "fixes" and more concerned with seeing them as skills and experiments supportive of larger processes
- is capable of promoting salutogenic well-being
- includes and supports self-selected spiritual considerations
- uses the most appropriate interventions from an array of both biomedical and CIH disciplines to help people progress towards experiences of health and well-being
- emphasizes evidence-informed practice and considers how this interacts with the art of health care as well as individual patient beliefs, experiences, and preferences.

Experiential pause: Ask yourself: "What did I just hear these authors say?" Explain to yourself, and if possible, to another person. Then repeat. Often.

CONTINUUM CARE

As you will see, IRP treatment approaches include an emphasis on mind-body skills integration as they inherently fit the preceding principles. However, emphasis within the care approach falls on a continuum of relative need within the physical, psychosocial, and/or environmental subcategories. This continuum is influenced by the nature of each condition, individual needs, historical factors, prevailing conditions, and more. If you have a nail in your foot, you are probably going to have it surgically removed, get a tetanus shot, and support wound healing. If you are severely depressed due to the stress of a recent divorce and child custody battle, you are likely going to focus greater support on psychosocial factors. However, providing space for the mind and for psychosocial support in predominantly "physical" presentations, and not forgetting the profound relevance and role of the body in predominantly "psychological" presentations, reflects an approach and understanding that guides IRP.

VALUES FOR IRP

To demonstrate a set of values that reinforces these ideas, a think tank focused on family therapy professionals laid out a set of values focused on collaborative practices.[38] We believe these values (Table 1.2) lie in support of the development of the IRP construct.

Table 1.2: Declaration of Values

We value this:	More than this:
Pluralism—differences of view 1. Acknowledging multiple "truths" 2. Responsiveness to particularities in context 3. Exploring multiple social realities 4. Exploring multiple cultures, contexts, interactions, and influences	Singularity—of view 1. Holding to a singular firm belief 2. Applying generalities (including diagnosis) 3. Searching for a single reality 4. Privileging specific cultures and contexts over others
Flux—differences of state 1. Facilitating the emergence of new identities 2. Regarding every interaction as mutual influence 3. Recognizing people as persons embedded in relationships 4. Experimenting with transformational restorative justice practices	Static—fixed states 1. Stabilizing fixed or rigid identity/identities 2. Assuming neutrality and objectivity with potential for unidirectional influence 3. Treating people as separate individuals 4. Implementing traditional retributive justice practices
Opening space—expanding choice 1. Living with curiosity 2. Opening space for enlivened possibilities 3. Inviting others to entertain change 4. Proactively including others (while respecting their possible choice to remain apart)	Closing space—removing choice 1. Living with certainty 2. Closing space for problems to persist 3. Imposing change interventions on others 4. Passively and/or actively excluding others from participating

We value this:	More than this:
Responsibility—generativity	Deficit focus—constraint
1. Noticing resources, competencies, and possibilities	1. Identifying and diagnosing deficits, dysfunctions, and limitations for correction
2. Anticipating potential effects of resource use and developing sustainable ecologies	2. Utilizing profitable resources without consideration of the consequences
3. Assuming collective responsibility and accountability	3. Projecting responsibility and specifying to whom it belongs; judging others
4. Enacting an ethics of caring and privileging restorative justice	4. Applying moral judgements and retributive justice

Reproduced with permission from Gosnell et al. (2017)[39]

PERSON-CENTERED LABELS AND TERMS

Across the remainder of this book, the nuances of labels and terms is important to acknowledge. In particular: "patient," "client," or "person"? At a minimum, a shift away from "treating a diagnosis" to "working together with another person" is important. Historically one might hear: "We have a heart attack in bay 1" or "You have a back pain waiting in room 2." Such language reduces a person's experience to a label that may come with preconceived notions or assumptions that add harm to the nature of the interaction. Never forget that you are serving a whole person, not "treating a diagnosis."

In looking at these words, *patient* comes from *patior*, meaning "to suffer"—one who suffers. *Client* comes from the Latin word *clinare*, which means "to lean," which may be taken as "to lean on another." However, the contemporary use of the word client reflects someone who receives a professional service. As noted above, the health-care system, in recognizing that the patient's experience of care was frequently reported as negative, formulated the notion of *patient-centered care*. The aim was to recognize that the individual's needs and preferences, within a model of shared decision making, included attention to a spectrum of levels. These levels include emotional, mental, cultural, social, socioeconomic, and more. Sound familiar? This is within the basic definition of integrative. Often, however, the system is still run with a power differential that fails to provide a forum for deep listening to the patient's needs, beliefs, and preferences for care, let alone the whole of their experience. Enter: the *person-centered care* as earlier defined. This language comes closest to the intent of integral care as it aims to support a non-authoritative approach to processes of self-discovery and emergence.

Throughout this book, you will see variations on the use of these words and concepts based on individual use from the contributing authors. We invite you to not get bogged down nor attached to these or other semantics. Instead, recognize that the backdrop of each contributor's use of these terms falls back to the core intent of respecting, guiding, supporting, and serving each person as a sacred individual.

CHALLENGES AND GROWING EDGES FOR IRP

Journeys are best undertaken with balanced and realistic perspective. Challenges, better framed as *growing edges*, exist in moving towards whole-person care. These growing edges have been delineated in a way that is specific to the IM movement[40] and come in categories: individual, systemic, intra-professional, and inter-professional dynamics. These edges equally apply to IRP as a derivative of the IM movement.

Across the book, insight into these growing edges will be developed. For now, consider the individual level. For many, there exists a tendency to avoid stressful or uncomfortable truths and experiences—even when they might benefit us or others.[41] We will add to this understanding in the concluding chapter of this book as a launching point for taking this work out into the world.

> **Experiential pause:** Take a little time and jot down anything that comes to mind that might be uncomfortable to you in approaching integrative, whole-person care. As you go through the book, continue to add to this list anything that you read that generates discomfort. Then ask if the discomfort is calling you into a truth, action, or response of some kind.

In the ideal situation, the health-care consumer and professional are partners in addressing the complexity of factors contributing to one's health experience, above and beyond the suppression of specific somatic symptoms. Specific to rehabilitation therapy professions, similar challenges and proposed solutions for advancing psychosocial integration have been delineated.[42] These challenges and opportunities include categories of professional education, clinical practice/care pathways, and policy issues (Table 1.3). While the extent to which such dynamics apply may vary based on profession and individual capacity, they provide a solid talking point for examining considerations for moving towards whole-person care.

IRP is transdisciplinary. *Trans* implies over or beyond and in the context of IRP reflects the emergence of a discipline that *transcends* the boundaries of traditional disciplinary perspectives.[43] IRP as transdisciplinary requires a foundation of knowledge from a number of disciplines (the relevance of inter-professional education) *and* the ability to work together with others (patients, colleagues) to relate the considerations that arise from various disciplines (perspectives) into a coherent whole—all towards the purpose of well-being.

As we approach the reality of challenges within IRP, we must be prepared to ask if including numerous levels of inquiry across disciplines results in a disheveled, ungrounded, or "wishy-washy" approach. Seemingly helpful approaches must be examined with numerous possibilities in mind, such as regression to mean, natural course, placebo effect, faulty perception, and errors in logic.[44] These topics, and more, must be considered as part of context.

Table 1.3: Addressing Challenges to Whole-Person Care

Area	Example strategies
Academic	Professional organizations* working in collaboration with academic programs to advance the inclusion of evidence-based integrative constructs; processes for updating licensure exam content to parallel rapidly changing evidence and clinical trends
Clinical	Established post-professional training and/or certification/credentialing options; clearly define scope of practice and referral patterns
Policy	Educate payors on both the need for, and evidence basis of, integrative care approaches and tools; establish coding, billing, and documentation standards
Organizational	Address barriers within organizations to support whole-person care initiatives
Sociocultural	Widespread education on topics such as mind-body integration, the role of social-emotional, and/or cognitive-behavioral facets of pain
Individual	Identify barriers within individual practitioners such as discomfort with engaging psychological dynamics, time constraints, cost barriers, etc.

* Examples include the Academic Consortium for Integrative Medicine and Health and the American Congress of Rehabilitation Medicine.

Adapted from Keefe, Main, & George[45]

DO NO HARM

Similarly, we must ask if the IRP concept inadvertently justifies a confused situation of "anything goes" that leads people into possible harm. In yogic teachings, the concept of "ahimsa" reflects the intent of non-harmfulness. Or, as Hippocrates wrote, *primum non nocere*, which is the Latin translation from the original Greek for "first do no harm." We must remain conscious, realistic, open, and humble to operate from these valued intentions when working with the whole of each person. As such, we will continue to discuss the topics of evidence, scope of practice, person-centered care, and boundaries as we go along.

Next, we must ask if we need to now be an expert in everything? No. It is reasonable and appropriate that health-care professionals take into consideration the psychophysiological and sociological factors associated with health. There are safe and effective ways of providing support within each profession's scope of practice. This does not mean each provider becomes a psychologist, social worker, or physical "expert." Each profession and each inter-related scientific discipline are assuredly needed. Instead, we are talking about acknowledging, validating, and supporting foundations of the whole person. If a patient is already working with multiple disciplines, such an approach is capable of reinforcing similar messages received from different disciplinary perspectives.

In considering the question of boundaries in whole-person practice and how this interacts with the goal of supporting fundamental human needs, it is relevant to note that, in many cases, access to or utilization of all available providers and disciplines is limited. In some cases, utilizing such care is actively avoided by the patient due to stigma or other reasons. As such, basic competency for whole-person support across domains supports quality care. The purpose here is not to water down therapy, effectively losing quality, but rather to improve quality by provision of therapeutic experiences that engage each person's lived experience. We seek to acknowledge and support the larger landscape of our lives, as is appropriate, and in a self-selected, safe, and informed approach. We will continue to address the topic of boundaries and safety across the book.

Finally, IRP must be mindful to avoid simply piling a new set of tools onto existing practice patterns.[46] Rather, IRP reflects an entirely new orientation at the base. Any tools, techniques, or skills that follow are shared from that base. The content of this book is deliberate in assisting in addressing this "new" orientation.

WRAPPING UP AND OPENING FORWARD

Ultimately, we are not doing anything "new" in the sense that wisdom is already established in this world. Perhaps, we are co-creating a repurposed form of wisdom for health care in modern times. We are several thousand years into scientific inquiry and we might say we still don't understand a single thing! Science, in one sense, doesn't serve us well without the right stance: life is complex, and…sacred. What would it be like to return to our roots? What are those roots? Can we re-member parts, put them back together?

IRP aims to deepen. We might call it "depth rehab"—going deeper in ourselves, in our clinical reasoning, and through invitations to others to look deeper into their health experience. Depth comes with responsibility. As we move forward, we must continually ask: "How do we define the various terms of IRP? How do we define their boundaries and their interrelationships?" IRP, aware of and encompassing many considerations, is about having a broad appreciation for the various levels of analysis in human behavior. IRP seeks to inquire into multiple determinants to health (see Chapter 4). When appropriate, and within each professional's knowledge and training, IRP seeks to support awareness and transformation around multiple levels.

We will continue to address these questions as we move ahead. For now, consider that IRP is first and foremost about approaching care from a fundamentally human perspective, guided by ethics, values, an emphasis on relationships, and the lived experience of each person. Mutually exploring what is right for each person at each point in time is vital. Magic might be defined as just the right amount of energy, at just the right time, for just the right purpose; IRP, in this light, can be seen as being about magic.

If we approach our work from the stance of "me fixing you," instead of a bidirectional and mutually beneficial relationship, we miss the larger truths of our shared humanness. Expanding on the idea of relationship will become increasingly important. IRP is rooted in improving the many types and forms of "relationship" in our lives. As such, relationship does not just apply to the interaction between two people. We must also consider relationship with ourselves, our body, our symptoms, our diagnosis, our environment, our situations, our experiences, and more. Examining these forms of relationship supports the sense of interdependence in our lives.

Finally, IRP supports the examination and cultivation of these relationships with principles of understanding, respect, appreciation, and acceptance. When we approach care from this sacred lens of relationship: "we are mentored into the understanding that when we are serving another, we are serving ourselves; when we are serving ourselves, equally we are serving all others."[47] Come along as we "open forward"…

Experiential pause: Having read this chapter, identify and write down at least one actionable item of interest to you. In doing so, consider ways in which applying the material first to yourself, and then to patients, might serve those who come to you for care.

RESOURCES

–   For a deeper look into the nature of transdisciplinarity, see: http://integral leadershipreview.com/7072-transdisciplinary-reflections.

CHAPTER 2

Creative Wisdom

Matthew J. Taylor, PT, PhD, C-IAYT

Further disclaimer: The adoption of an integrative rehabilitation practice (IRP) is a double-edged sword. The one edge will prime you to experience and identify suffering in yourself and others more acutely and accurately. Mercifully, the other edge will foster a deeper resilience and capacity to care. You have been cautioned.

OVERVIEW

This is the chapter where I am supposed to orient you to how IRP is situated in both the field of creativity and the wisdom traditions. A tall order by any stretch, and besides, I have written/edited entire books on both topics.[1] If you are like me, there's nothing worse than an info-dense early chapter in a book or the first hour of a seminar. I won't do that to you.

Instead, as someone who may be just a little further down the road of trying to practice integratively, allow me to take care of myself first, and then, hopefully, you as well, by trying to write a rehabilitative chapter that is "fit to live in." That, by the way, is the whole book: care for you first and then others. Ours and the subjective, first-person experiences of those we serve in IRP are to be made primary. Literally putting the order of priority upside down, on its head so to speak, from traditional practice's third-person "objectivity" (sic) and detachment, is paramount.

So, let's see what that looks like and how it feels, shall we? I will share my present experience as our context, and then, from there, demonstrate how your exploration of IRP will firmly plant you in the leading edge of creativity, as well as the wisdom traditions.

MY EXPERIENCE

I am typing this at the kitchen table of my best friend from physical therapy (PT) school. We'll call him the General, my nickname for him because when we were both serving our obligation from the US Army/Baylor University, that's how he would get past our battle-hardened bureaucratic receptionist: "This is General K, may I speak to Cpt. Taylor, please?" Unfortunately, he's sitting on his couch behind me, watching a third hour of home fix-up television, tapping his right foot and rubbing his left thigh. This is his day, every day.

You see, he turned 62 last week and has now been medically disabled for five years with dementia from cumulative traumatic encephalopathy (CTE) due to his college football days. Do you get the same lump in your throat and nauseating turn in your belly that I do as I type these words? He's down to barely being able to follow single step commands, never initiates conversation, is fully incontinent, and is socially isolated. I am grateful he knows to flash his impish smile when I make a bad joke with a certain tone, but that's all I and his family have of the General we love. I'm here giving respite care for ten days so his wife, his full-time caregiver, can participate in an across-a-state bike ride with their youngest daughter, a fourth-year medical student. The General has two other daughters, and three grandchildren who only know him in this condition. Now I am angry. How are you?

Bear with me a bit more; I promise to tie this all together, but for now, feel the feelings my account invites you to experience. Their four cats weave around the table. Did I mention I hate cats and am allergic to them? I make this respite visit twice a year across country because I love my friend and his wife. It's what I know he'd do if our roles were reversed. It demands of me responses that no book knowledge, PhD, logical argument, or moral standing can provide. It is part of how I learn who I am. And it hurts. Bad. Now tears.

OK, Taylor…tie this together. The General's wife is caught in a double bind. He has a disability policy that pays their bills. If she places him in long-term care with his veteran's benefits, she loses that income, and that includes their ability to make house payments. She can't afford in-home care either. He's fallen twice in the past month and she had to call for lift assist from the first responders (he's 6' 2", 220 lbs.). I can see his movement degradation, to include a moderate-assist sit-to-stand transfer, a narrowing base of support, slower cadence, decreased stride length, and I am pretty sure that's now classic pill-rolling with both hands as we walk their block several times a day. How do we respond to this one single case report as IRP providers? How did these friends get here? What is driving the circumstances and what will the future hold? Is there a way to ease the suffering for his family, their shrinking circle of friends, fellow parishioners, and neighbors as care fatigue arrives? If ever there was a need for both creativity *and* wisdom, I think we are there in this circumstance. Allow me to now use this suffering and hopefully transform some part of it as context that enriches your experience as you read this and the following chapters on IRP.

OUR LARGER CIRCUMSTANCES

The General's story will serve as our skeleton to flesh out where we stand today regarding creativity and wisdom in our rehabilitation professions. Consider this list of how we'd have traditionally looked at their situation (evaluate the individual, assess, limit treatment goals to within the patient's skin, then execute treatment plan and intervene, re-assess, repeat) versus what exists right now (all of the above plus economics, politics, resources, etiology, advocacy for patient and family, prevention in larger community, etc.). So how does an integrative practitioner approach something like the General's situation creatively and with wisdom? In other words, how do we fulfill our definition of rehabilitation, to make a life "fit to live in"? What is required of us and what resources can we access to create a better possible future? I am going to suggest that in addition to wisdom and creativity, priming ourselves to increase our compassion is essential for advancing our IRP. Fortunately, all three share common foundational principles, so it isn't as daunting as it may appear. Let's begin.

ADOPTING A LENS METAPHOR

Swapping lenses, converging and diverging, and zooming in and out are useful metaphors for IRP. Probably the only lens metaphor we won't use is the "rose-colored" glasses… this is hard, hot, dusty, sweating work and those lenses will all need regular cleaning! We begin by zooming out to observe a wider context of our life today. We are embedded in a wider environment that affects what is possible for all of us. We are living in a world with climate change, environmental crises, the rise of autocrats, a teetering sick-care system that falls further behind in quality and cost, shifting world allegiances, etc. Oh, and there's the General's situation: a society that worships (every Saturday in autumn) a violent affair where mostly men of color trade their futures for providing entertainment in a multi-billion-dollar industry within a system that doesn't equitably reimburse them, is without guaranteed health care, and dwindling to no social support after they "graduate." That same industry denies responsibility and the legions of fans are either ignorant about the risks or just don't care. What is going on?

Well, if you have been out of school over ten years, you were trained in a literally different "world" and almost all of us were taught from that same world: now termed "normal times" (NT).[2] Quite quickly, the present rapidly changing world now has us deeply embedded into what is referred to as post-normal times (PNT). PNT is marked by complexity, chaos, contradictions, uncertainty, progress, modernization, efficiency, virtues, and (ethical) imagination. NT for the General would have been the culture of "be a team player," "winner takes all," community rallies to support one of theirs in need, affordable health care, social safety nets, etc. NT is basically the opposite (at least for privileged groups) of PNT: predictable, orderly, certainty, coherent, traditions, "moral standards," and historical precedents to reference when needing to solve new problems (i.e.: What worked last time this happened?).

Can you see how NT isn't the General's circumstance today dealing with his traumatic brain injury (TBI)? All of these wider issues come to bear on the General's specific plight. If we're truly going to "make fit to live in" and prevent future occurrences, what is addressed in rehabilitation can't stay within the literal boundaries of their home. There are much broader issues to "rehab." Our advocacy and activism is therefore part of the complex responses needed to fuel the imagination required in this PNT example. There aren't historical models of caring for a family in these circumstances, nor randomized controlled trials (RCTs) to guide us, nor attentive governmental or insurance bureaucrats to make changes. We need to bring forward or create a unique response in this PNT. The example I often use for rehabilitation professionals that is even closer to home and personal is to invite you to put on your "pain treatment" lens. For me, in 1981 pain treatment was pretty straightforward and "normal": find the offending tissue, correct it through activity, medication, through surgery, or with modalities. If it didn't work, the patient was probably just a bit "off" and either needed psychiatric care or to be caught symptom magnifying. Pretty brutal in hindsight.

Today we are describing pain as an emergent phenomenon that is complex, often with contradictory descriptions and with a myriad of systems influencing the experience to include many intra-systems and the environments within which the individual is embedded and enacts. And each month pain gets a good deal more complex. Consequently, in this PNT we can find ourselves asking about pain:

- What's this BPSS (biopsychosocialspiritual) stuff?
- I can do the "B" in BPSS but how am I to attend and treat the PSS?
- I vaguely remember something about the immune system, but it had nothing to do with pain?
- And glial cells?
- Neuroplastics?
- Endocannabinoids?

…Ay caramba! Does anyone else hear within you a voice calling out: "I want my RCTs, plastic spine with the red herniated disc, and certainty back please…and so does my patient!"?

ZOOMING IN TO YOU

We need to apply that same PNT lens to any other aspect of rehabilitation as well. How do we successfully navigate now from NT to PNT? (Realizing most new graduates are still being taught the NT material because of faculty and national testing inertia.) I guess we'd better call in "creativity and wisdom" to cope with PNT. Don't get me wrong. I don't mean "cope" in a negative way such as "not coping." Instead, as Cairns, Montuori, and Beech (2001) describe, in "real" life there are paradoxical and conflicting meanings and interpretations that are commonplace, and most must be held simultaneously and in paradoxical dissonance without conflict or a need for synthesis.[3] That is also the use of "coping" in this chapter. Cairns *et al.* further argue against the notion of the "will to unity," where someday this PNT will all get tied together in a neat new NT bundle of unity and cohesion again.[4] Rather, we need to understand that this won't be the case, and instead seek to follow the "rainbow" of IRP of thinking/acting—being ephemeral and transitional in nature, of many colors/permutations, with no fixed location in space and time, having no end, and certainly no "right" way to be an integrative rehabilitation practitioner. Does that take some pressure off you ever knowing for "certain" how to practice? Seems like now would be a good time to explore both creativity and wisdom as containers to hold this mess.

WISDOM AND CREATIVITY

Which would you start with? Creativity and then wisdom? Or wisdom followed by creativity? I'm thinking that creativity without wisdom can be a problem...think Auschwitz gas nozzles that look like showerheads...yikes! Wisdom it is then...

Wisdom

Wisdom is a huge topic, so this cursory introduction is only designed to support our IRP adventure as foundational, but I hope it also piques your interest in exploring wisdom further someday. To deal with that enormity, let's call in Socrates, or at least his method of teaching with pointed questions.

- Who said these subjects of creativity and wisdom aren't so tough?
- So, what is wisdom?
- Do you consider yourself wise?
- Do you consider your profession part of a wisdom tradition? Why or why not?
- Can wisdom be acquired? If so, how?
- Can patients be wise? Grow in their wisdom? Is that related to our rehab goals? How?
- Does one have to be smart to be wise?

This guy has a lot of questions.

Well OK, here are some answers.

- A: No one who ever seriously began to study creativity or wisdom.
- A: The definition follows below.
- A: Only you can say whether you consider yourself wise...and whether you are or not is another question!
- A: If your profession isn't part of the wisdom traditions, what does that imply? Oops, another question.
- A: Yes and no is the answer to "Can one 'acquire' wisdom?"
- A: How we and those we serve can be primed to become wiser is described below.
- A: No, intellect or smarts are neither sufficient nor necessary in and of themselves.

When I began to research wisdom for my book, I didn't realize wisdom had a formal field of study several decades old. That is, there are people who are actually working to define/refine what wisdom is, its history of development, and how it relates to other subjects. And guess what? Wisdom appears to be...come on, say it: complex, emergent, part of both an individual experience and a larger species arc of development, dependent on circumstances, and on and on. A PNT thing again.

To save word count, here's some of that cursory coverage I promised. I found Walsh's

(2015) attempt at constructing a working definition to be an outstanding and full-text free-access gem.[5] After he reviewed the many facets of wisdom, his definition of wisdom in general is:

> Wisdom is deep accurate insight and understanding of oneself and the central existential issues of life, plus skillful benevolent responsiveness.

For those who like math better than the humanities:

> W = ((Deep + Accurate) Insight / ((Oneself + Existential Issues) × Understanding) + (Skillful + Benevolent) Responsiveness)

For me, that definition was that one jigsaw puzzle piece that leads to a breakthrough in completing a large chunk of the puzzle. What would it take for rehabilitation professionals like ourselves to be part of the wisdom tradition? How are we not part of it individually and as a collective right now?

By "central existential issues of life" Walsh is referencing the big questions.

- What's the meaning of life?
- Why is there suffering?
- Is there something larger than myself that I am part of?
- What is death?
- How should I be and act based on those answers?

You know, those ponderings that are so foundational, but generally glossed over and "assumed" in every aspect of life, to include religion and graduate education. So, let's pause and ponder, shall we?

> **Experiential pause:** Slowly reread, out loud several times, whichever version of the definition of wisdom above most appeals to you. Notice which words grab at your attention more than some of the others. Sit with each of those words by themselves for about ten soft breaths, moving to the next and noting what arises with your attention to each. Stories, emotions, feeling, sensations, etc. Once you are finished with your list of words, sit quietly for two to three minutes and see if you can sense the "whole" of the definition…not remembering the words literally, but softening into experiencing just the entire definition with blurred consideration. Then finish this experiential pause by again slowly reading the entire definition out loud and noting how that experience is compared with your first experience of reading it as just more text in this chapter. What, if anything, changed and why?

Creating a frame for studying wisdom

Now that we are settling in with the uncertainty of the PNT of wisdom, unfortunately for those wanting certainty, I have even more questions. Luckily, a preview of the proposal for this entire book suggests there may be at least partial answers and practices to support our inquiry into these and other questions. For our part, allow me to suggest these answers to the Socratic questions posed earlier that can serve as a framework or scaffolding of concepts onto which you can apply the new ideas and processes that lie ahead.

- **What else is there to wisdom?** Libraries of possibility. Walsh (2015)[6] condensed some of the wisdom traditions into four large sub-types of wisdom that I mention here to entice you to explore each in your experience.
  a. **Practical**: is skillful benevolent responsiveness to the central existential issues of life. This suggests both skill acquisition and mastery in performance to address real-world challenges.
  b. **Conceptual**: is deep, accurate, rich, and integrated understanding of oneself and the central existential issues of life. The concepts that undergird practical wisdom.
  c. **Intuitive**: is deep, accurate intuitive insight into oneself and the central existential issues of life. Intuition can be used in several ways, but Walsh employed it to indicate rapid, automatic, implicit information processing where one just knows without being able to precisely map the concepts or causal factors for why they understand so deeply and accurately.
  d. **Transconceptual**: is deep transconceptual insight into oneself and the nature of reality. Transconceptual insight arises as a direct apprehension of the fundamental nature of reality and identity, which may then lead to further conceptual insights.

These four large sub-types of course influence one another, occur in varying degrees for individuals, and all build to support the general wisdom definition. Chances are you have either personally experienced each type or observed a wise clinician or client exhibiting the sub-types. Again, as an emergent phenomenon, there isn't a prescription or formula per se to arrive at each sub-type. The whole of the wisdom tradition practices rather primes the participants to foster such emergence. Don't bother buying "Six Easy Steps to Wisdom"…that would be unwise.

- **How do we/our professions become part of the wisdom tradition?** We begin through our personal practices as outlined below, and then take our transformed selves back into our larger communities and create new possibilities. Easy to say, a bit more challenging to do, but that's what each of we authors is hoping to share.
- **How are we not part of it individually and as a collective right now?** This is quite easy. In my yoga experience, I have come to value that discernment process of reality referred to as "Neti, Neti"…not this, not that. Which is the same way I describe how I became a physical therapist: the process of subtraction (not medicine, not engineering, etc.). The exercise then becomes one of asking: "Does my profession [fill in the aspect of the wisdom definition] or not?" For instance, I would ask: "Does the usual PT practice in clinics today reflect deep and accurate understanding of the therapist, to include limitations in BPSS understanding and self-care?" On average I would say: "Not in my experience." How about: "Assess

and intervene on the psychosocial components affecting the client's condition with skillful, benevolent responsiveness"? Again, the same answer from me.

> **Experiential pause:** Break down the above definition of wisdom and apply it to the facets of your profession, tabulating the affirmatives and the netis. Write down your response. Once you are finished, just gaze at your results, extend your exhales for about three minutes, and note your experiences to include thoughts, emotions, somatic responses. This is a first step toward wisdom for you and your profession.

And, there's nothing wrong with many "not this, not thats"…they illuminate where we need to grow and develop skill. When we do, both individually, and collectively, then we will by definition have moved deeper into a wisdom practice and identified where creativity will be required at both levels. Fortunately, many of the remaining chapters, not coincidentally, will take us in those directions as integrative rehabilitation practitioners.

- **What about acquiring wisdom? And, can we and those we serve be primed to become wiser?** Walsh (2015)[7] notes that wisdom emerges both on an individual level and through a collective evolutionary arc over time. In the article, he describes how the many wisdom traditions create environments and hold space for the emergence of wisdom through both teachings and practices. There isn't a "Six Easy Steps to Wisdom" protocol because it is a complex, emergent human experience. So, beware anyone, to include me, selling you such a solution. They are all called disciplines for a reason, and require continual, dedicated attention and practice. In summary: "Shortcuts to Wisdom" is for fools. The good news is, like creativity ahead, we can prime for emergence through embodied practices that will have many entry points for our professions. Then we let that "systems emergence" thing unfold. Before you head off into the book for those discoveries, we need to weave in related creativity concepts and weed out a few misperceptions around creativity.

Application of wisdom to the General's circumstances

In NT, this would be where I would tell you (instruct: place into you) how these wisdom principles would apply for you as a rehabilitation professional. As just noted, however, that isn't the "IRP Way." Instead, I want to try to educate (educare: draw out from within) your best answer. So, try the following exercise around wisdom and the General's circumstances before we tackle creativity.

> **Experiential pause:** In awareness that it is now PNT, can you identify reasons why my instructing you with "the" answers wouldn't be a wise thing for me to do? [Hint: Use the definition.] Are my skills, resources, relationships, profession, etc. the same as yours? Why does that matter, if it does? Will your "depth and accuracy" be different

than mine? How so? Is there "a" solution to his challenges? Might you have skills and resources to allow for some different and possibly "better" process to emerge from this complex situation? Are our virtues and ethical imaginations the same? What differences might arise and which virtues or imaginations would be more skillful and benevolent in responding to them? Grab your journal, make a T-column, left column titled "Me" and right column titled "Matt" (the columns creating a contrast between my and your resources/experiences), and spend some time drawing out answers based on your reflections around these questions. No grades or right answers. The only way to fail is by skipping this activity. Does that illuminate the need to trust your answers rather than mine?

Can you imagine that our care would differ dramatically in some respects? But would either one be the "best"? Could we even predict a best? (And there sure isn't an RCT to inform us.) I know you aren't his best friend. You don't have 40 years of experiences together with him and his family. Our professions may differ, and our educational experiences surely do. You probably (and for good reason) wouldn't dedicate considerable personal funds to assist the family as I have. And on, and on. The important point to this exercise is that it offers a framework or process of inquiry whereby you can use wisdom features to guide *your* evaluation and reflection on any tough question ahead (i.e., life's existential questions). This process then becomes one way to "cope" successfully in the PNT sea of uncertainty. More ways will follow.

Those last two sentences might not be all that comforting. Anybody else missing NT certainty about now? Sardar (2010) offers some consolation, stating that to cope with this complexity and diversity of options, we need to adopt humility (I and my profession's best benevolent responses are all fallible), modesty (there is no right answer, this process will be an ongoing, iterative process without a set endpoint), and accountability (I am accountable to myself, those I serve, and ultimately the entire planet in selecting my responses).[8] To cope in this way requires not just imagination, but also an ethical imagination that isn't dependent on rote responses, legalistic prescriptions, or protocols. This imagination does function while respecting laws, codes of ethics, and practice acts. *And*, ultimately, of highest priority is our advocating for the one we are serving and their family. Sardar's ethical imagination won't necessarily provide coherent guidance, because PNT's nature brings us back to contradictions. Oh, now I'm hearing some sad country lyric about "How I miss my certainty, won't ya please come home?" Hang on, I hear that train whistle coming down the line…

Creativity

How does our preparing to get primed to be wise relate to creativity? I think we understand that, as in this example of the General's situation, something new is going to need to be created. In this section using the above wisdom scaffolding as a framework, we will add creativity concepts as additional support upon which the rest of the book can rest.

Before we do that, let's consider two very related concepts that serve as practice/praxis for both creativity and wisdom application: transdisciplinarity and transformative learning. Never mind that I spent five years of my life and a ton of money on these topics as my doctoral pedagogy, I'm including them because they are really useful for developing an IRP and in clinical practice!

Transdisciplinarity is a form of inquiry and *transformative learning* is an outcome of the inquiry, each having many of their own textbooks. Alfonso Montuori (2010) offers an excellent introduction to both.[9] He was my dissertation chair and advisor, and I have been forever grateful for his introducing me to them, as it is the spine of this entire chapter, as well as our collective inquiry into IRP.

Transdisciplinarity is not multidisciplinary, where a problem is approached from a number of different disciplines. It isn't interdisciplinary either, where one discipline uses other disciplines' approaches. Nor does it replace any of the methods of inquiry, but it brings them additional insights not otherwise available. Can you see how this might be useful in PNT? Montuori outlines four key facets of transdisciplinarity.

- The focus is inquiry driven as it seeks to understand the underlying assumptions of disciplines without rejecting their knowledge (including but not limited to scientific method research), while developing *pertinent* knowledge for acting in the world. Consider how often you have paged through a journal of knowledge but failed to find anything that solved a problem or changed your practice pattern.
- Transdisciplinarity is understood to be a process of constructing knowledge by appreciating meta-paradigms versus mining knowledge from a single paradigm. See any utility in this inquiry for BPSS inquiry?
- Through the above then, can we hold unique contexts and discover new connections? Think about the General's circumstances.
- Most importantly, the process honors the integration of the inquirer (you) as being legitimate authority (that leg of evidence-based medicine called clinical mastery) and essential in…come on, what's this section subtitle? Creativity!

This transdisciplinary process then transforms (changes the root/form) knowledge base, grounded in pertinent, real-world solutions that weren't available in any one discipline and wouldn't have been discovered in inter or multidisciplinary approaches. Aka, transformative learning: the outcome being shifting perspectives to reveal new, practical ways of behaving and being in the world. Not just adding to a knowledge storehouse, but transforming the frame *and* practice/praxis of the learner. This of course only comes about if the inquirer understands themselves before they can understand the world. There's that wisdom definition again. There are also huge political implications when we enact both of these for ourselves as inquirers, but also when we create these inquiry skills for our clients. The shift in power is reversed, looking inward for authority, knowing that in PNT and in developing wisdom, that is the first step. That does not discount all of the valuable knowledge from outside the inquirer, for the process then requires integration and enactment into one's unique circumstances. This should be a familiar refrain from the previous chapter and will certainly be echoed throughout the rest of the book.

Note of caution: All of this relativism, meta-paradigm surfing, and minimalizing binary disjunctions can pretty easily lead into a postmodern fragmented nihilism if we aren't careful (What's the point? Nothing is true; Why try? etc.). If complexity and emergence is going to make certainty and predictability so, well, uncertain, do we just throw up our hands in despair? Not at all. In fact, beware that tendency and understand that in our coping we are looking to decide on and skillfully execute benevolent meaningful action as best we can in coherence with our values. We just now appreciate the uncertainty that was always there, hold the uncertainty, and relax into what was always happening anyway. The cycle then is iterations of practice, feedback, adjustment, and more practice. This time, however, we aren't blaming or grasping for certainty or solutions, but easing into the process with less stress and suffering while supporting our clients with an ease that is comforting versus frantic or frustrated.

Quick start guide to creativity

Now as we dive deeper into creativity directly, another important consideration is the metaphor for creativity that can be found in music—specifically in jazz that my dissertation chair, Alfonso Montuori, PhD, often employs.[10] As a jazz musician knows, when you are improvising it is important to be comfortable when trying out different approaches without being perfect, so try applying this to the material ahead in this book. Your variance from convention isn't an "imperfection." The variance is not because you cannot read the "reality" of the "text" music—analogous to the "original" composer's score/some "right way to practice rehabilitation." And it also is not because you wish to subvert and reject the tenets and traditions of your profession in favor of anarchy. Rather, reality grounded in wisdom suggests we all need to proceed with humility, adopting what may appear to be an anarchistic approach in which there is diminished concern for the law and order of the score (protocols/appeals to RCTs), but without resorting to chaos or nihilism. And this is another skill that you have always practiced to some degree. Now, we can proceed by fully embracing the improvisation while inviting the client to relax into the same, softening into successfully coping rather than executing "the" strategy or some rigid defined course of action.

Therefore, the focus of this book is on presenting a construct of IRP as one avenue that can help us cope with so many challenges (self-pay/payment models/documentation nightmares, restricted visits, etc.). *Integrative* is defined very broadly as "serving or intending to unify separate things" beyond the skin of the client and points the way towards the meaning of *holistic*. Holistic refers to the complexity of the whole person, to include the relationships of that person to a long host of contextual levels and environments. This unity of so many separate things should then simultaneously hold contradictions without resolution or unifications, but with the integrity of a tight jazz trio improvising through the night.

Experiential pause: How about a little support in this sea of uncertainty? OK, try these on and use them regularly to blend into the band. Adopt the habit of answering questions with either a "both/and" or "yes, and..." to break away from the habit of consulting some exact score/answer. This works well to broaden perspective when facing questions, concerns, concepts, and challenges versus our tendency and training to engage in binary, certainty thinking and answers. For example: "Will this make my pain worse?" "Yes, it may, *and* you now have these tools to give yourself relief." Or: "Is it bad that I keep having my attention wander during exercise?" "It isn't optimal, but it is normal *and* every time you notice that it has wandered and you return to paying attention you are building your ability to have more choices and control in moving." Now try asking yourself the top three questions you get at work and practice with these tools.

Good, how is that? What's fun is that this then serves the capacity to ignite creativity and wisdom in yourself and your work, and simultaneously address the goals and needs of the person you are serving. That's where we're headed shortly.

That perfection thing

Before we finally arrive at creativity, we need to address a common question that reflects an underlying urge for being perfect. That question is: "Doesn't this mean I have to be an expert in all of these disciplines and scopes of practice?" Remember the definition of transformative learning: fostering a new world view, practical utility, and the resultant change in behavior to adapt (create) in this new PNT. Yes, transdisciplinarity draws from many fields as far-ranging as evolutionary biology, individual and social psychology, public health, wisdom teachings, and spiritual practices. While some may choose to advance their career through integrated roots, the short answer is: No you don't have to be an expert in them all. We carry great potential for transdisciplinary competency in areas that are within the grasp of any rehab professional. Rather, focus on becoming a relationship expert...dot connector...doctor of context. Keep in mind humility, modesty, and accountability, but you can safely drop the perfection thing.

Finally, creativity

In the year I was born, Barron (1958) reported that creativity requires unusual respect for forces and phenomena that appear chaotic, confused, and irrational.[11] What a perfect practice in PNT. He also later listed five broad traits of creative individuals, which, as you will sense, reflect our needs both individually and collectively in navigating PNT.[12]

- An independence of judgment rather than conformity.
- A tolerance for ambiguity rather than a need for certainty.
- A preference for complex thinking rather than polarized, simplistic oppositional thinking.
- Androgynous behaviors with clarity on gender attributes and roles rather than an authoritarian or patriarchal preference.
- A preference for complexity of outlook and a tolerance for asymmetry rather than symmetric, constrained possibilities.

I hope the wait to see why the editors felt we needed to address these two topics early on was worth it. While creativity is a hot topic these days, most descriptions being touted (to include brain imagery studies) are very mechanical approaches of proper "ingredients," to try to explain creativity or at least how new ideas come along. Yes, these descriptions all have useful components, but from a PNT perspective, they still yearn for that predictable, prescriptive certainty that falls well short of fully holding the mystery and messiness of creativity. And once more, word count constrains us to the briefest of introductions and focus on utility versus an entire textbook.[13] Just beware any clickbait titles such as "The Five Steps to Creativity." Therefore, we'd better just dispel some common myths and tie the current version of creativity understanding to clinical application. Then I'll introduce broad domains that can prime us for further emergence of wisdom and creativity, before sending you off into the rest of the book.

Myths and misunderstanding about creativity

Let's begin by dispelling the big one:

- **You need to learn to be creative…**we already are, and we are always creating. The concern is, are we aware of what we're creating and whether it is skillful and benevolent? To think or behave as if we or those we serve are not creative is an impediment to creating a better future. Challenge and edit that narrative.
- **There isn't enough time or resources to be creative**: Again, you are always creating, so the concern should be what you are creating with your time and resources. Deadlines and limited resources can actually facilitate creativity.
- **Creativity means anything goes**: No, true creativity includes novelty and practicality/utility in the real world. Violating laws or practice acts doesn't include that requirement. Evidence-based medicine practiced in the way it was intended is a vessel for creativity.
- **Only certain people are creative**: See the first point. We and those we serve are all creative. Have you listened to their stories as to why they didn't adhere to their home program?
- **Creativity is a skill you learn or acquire**: Creativity is a complex, emergent phenomenon in all of life, not just human beings, and in all humility, we don't know much yet about creativity. Yes, we can prime ourselves for the emergence, but beware the linear, mechanistic prescription for acquisition of creativity.
- **Creativity is the life of the lone genius and arises in isolation**: The lone genius (almost always male by the way) is a myth, and current best constructivist understanding of creativity holds that its emergence is very context sensitive. To claim otherwise is disempowering and an affront to providers and consumers of our services.
- **Creativity is visible in patterns of brain activity**: We're back to humility and the need to surrender certainty. We don't understand creativity or the brain, yet we claim images are creativity. Really?
- **Creativity is easy or simple**: If Einstein said it was 10% inspiration and 90% perspiration, believe him. Creativity is not the easy road, but it is a rich, full way to travel through life. It also has two parts: the idea, and then the implementation. Without

both a novel idea and implementation, it isn't creativity, and the implementation is the 90% perspiration that often requires wholly new skills and behaviors.

- **I need to be creative with this patient**: Can you sense the reductionism and disempowerment for both of you in this statement? IRP attests that it is never not the case that you and the client are creating.
- **Creativity is threatening**: Disruptive, inconvenient, and often addressing power imbalances? Yes. If it is grounded as skillful benevolence, it is also a form of social justice and the role of an advocate. Expect resistance and potential conflict with others and policies. Do it anyway.
- **Creativity is taught in our core academic professional programs**: Really? Send me some examples. Next…
- **Creativity requires expertise**: See the earlier perfection subsection. Some research suggests that expertise can be an impediment and therein lies the value of the inter-professional collaboration.
- **Creativity is activities like brainstorming and lateral thinking**: Those are practices that can prime, but are not creativity per se.
- **Creativity is the innovation of something new or better**: No, it is value sensitive and there's an entire field of study around malevolent creativity. No values or the wrong values, no wisdom practice.

Contained above, can you see then what might be potential barriers to creativity for you personally and your profession more broadly? How then do we support clinicians in priming for creative capacity? Fortunately, it is the practices of the individual that then affect systems change. So when we as individuals practice as IRP, we are in fact priming both ourselves and the larger systems for change. Phew, it is nice to get a two for one. Let's look at the domain practices next.

Priming for creativity

Creativity in rehabilitation is our (yours and the client's) participation more fully in practices that facilitate the emergence of a renewed flourishing of our being at "home" in our circumstances. Me[14]

Halifax's (2012) six domain practices to prime for compassion were the foundation for the textbook on creativity for rehabilitation professionals.[15] These same practices prime for creative emergence in your life and practice.[16] She placed two on each of three axes. The practices are a heuristic process of ongoing iterations and reassessments, without an endpoint. Each domain informs the others, requires the others, and learns from the others. This is consistent with emergence in complex systems, and results in no prestatable order or outcome. Sure sounds like PNT, so it is a great fit. After this introduction, there will be an example for context and your employment of the practices. The domains are as follows and the order is for convenience of memory only as they are each of equal importance.[17]

- **Attentional/Affective axis (A/A axis)**: These practices enhance mental balance, to include concentration, emotional regulation, and allocating mental processing resources. Our ability to direct and sustain attention on both our own and the client's mental state makes it possible to accurately recognize the presence of suffering with a sustained, selective focus that could otherwise be lost with misdirected (inaccurate) attention or loss of affective balance.

- **Intentional/Insight axis (I/I axis):** These practices of focused attention utilize the intention to be compassionate that then generates insights about the suffering, the suffering's origins, and how to transform suffering in a creative emergence. These cognitive dimensions of experience interact in conjunction with the other axes. Reciprocally, intention and insight also prime attention and affective balance (i.e., I intend to sustain attention on my intention to attune to my and their affect in order to gain insight…).

- **The Embodiment/Engaged axis (E/E axis):** What we sense, how we move, and why we move are essential to our effectiveness and our creative capacity. Science has revealed how attention, practice, and behavior alter both function and structure of our very anatomy and physiology via neuroplasticity, epigenetic function, and the exhibition of altruistic behaviors, including compassion. This experiential E/E axis celebrates these new facts and demands our engagement (responsiveness) with all domains to prime the greatest number of emergent possibilities. In short, we need our body and we need to act in responsiveness, hopefully with skill and benevolence.

Let's apply this to the General's situation for continuity. Attention training is essential for me: to sustain attention to his and his family's needs over a long period of time; to note when I lose attention to them being physically distant; to note when I project my needs over theirs, etc. My training to sense both my own affect and theirs develops my ability to note when our interactions aren't satisfying needs, are generating unintended (note intention) outcomes, or are distracting from the present moment and missing key information (insight) that is arising right now. I experience all of this through my lived body experience (embodiment) as I engage with them, which then demands new attention, reassessing intentions, yielding new insights, etc. Can you feel the cycles and interweaving?

But let's not just stop at my skin or theirs; what else needs to be addressed and learned from this rehabilitation (make fit to live in) to evoke healing and prevention of future suffering? What engagement is required to address social and systemic structures that created this situation and continue to generate this harm today and tomorrow? Is it my responsibility to not support those systems or actively work against them as IRP? When colleges are building $1,000,000,000 football facilities, do I have an obligation to not participate at that or the professional level? How about educating in my local community from peewee football on up? Do I offer training services at the games to feed my rehab practice? Do I wear a helmet when I ride my bike? Allow my children to participate in football? I think you are getting the drift, right? There aren't any right answers devoid of context for me or you. Or the General and his family. But our depth of accurate insight demands many layers of skillful, benevolent responses. And that's how creativity and wisdom dance in us as we navigate PNT.

CONCLUSION

This brings us to the conclusion of this chapter, which I suspect has been, in the words of my first yoga therapy instructor Joseph Le Page, "Something new and completely different" than its predecessors and the remainder of the book. I believe you now have a sturdy frame to construct the one, unique way you will embody and enact IRP.

If you get bogged down or frustrated along the way, please circle back to refresh your context; knowing that confusion, uncertainty, and contradiction are genuine signposts that you are heading in the right direction. In fact, in transformative learning, the first step is to create a safe learning space. The second step is to introduce a disorienting dilemma, which is when your world view stumbles upon a situation that it is unable to hold or explain. That naturally leads to "I don't know" and "both/and" as our mantra. Carry on.

You might ask: "What exactly is our role as integrative rehabilitation practitioners in PNT?" The answer of course is: "We don't know…we are not there yet, but this book will serve as a guide and resource." We need your diversity and for you to step into your power as an important thread in the weave of creating a best possible future for the General, and all of those you serve…now.

> **Experiential pause:** Having read this chapter, identify and write down at least one actionable item of interest to you. In doing so, consider ways in which applying the material first to yourself, and then to patients, might serve those who come to you for care.

CHAPTER 3

Defining the Need

Matt Erb, PT and Daniel Winkle, MD

OVERVIEW

There is a need for integrative care in rehabilitation. There are many reasons for this need, including but not limited to: stress; the prevalence of pain in our lives; the growing challenge of comorbidity; high rates of burnout in healthcare workers; and the mind-body disconnect that keeps us from moving towards greater wholeness.

In general, we see an entrenched split between mind and body in our culture. While some may be conscious of this fact, most are not. In healthcare, the biomedical delivery system operates through highly specialized and compartmentalized professions, which inadvertently sidesteps the challenge of treating body and mind as integrated; splitting mind and body leads to deficits in care. The concept of *embodied mind* challenges us to re-examine divisions and compartmentalizations, and instead find helpful ways of exploring the myriad of spiritual, religious, and philosophical views on consciousness, mind, and spirit, all in relationship to the body.

A starting point lies in asking, what exactly is mind? Dr. Dan Siegel, a physician, psychiatrist, and researcher at UCLA, suggests mind has several defining features: subjectivity, consciousness, information processing, and self-organization. He defines mind as being both embodied and relational, a self-organizing and emergent process that regulates the flow of energy and information within an individual and between individuals.[1] Let's break this down.

- The mind is embedded in the body and one's experience of it. It is only in and through the body that we experience ourselves and the world. Conscious awareness and one's subjective experience of that comes through the lived experience of the body. More on this in a bit.
- The mind is *relational*, meaning the very mechanism of mind is built upon relating. We might say that the mind's job is to interpret and respond—to create a meaningful story out of the information it receives and experiences.
- What about self-organizing? This suggests mind has an innate, spontaneous drive for order, and does not rely on control by any particular external agent.

- Emergent? This brings us back to living systems theory (see Chapter 1), as the term emergent suggests an ongoing process of coming into being—seen as the very nature of living systems. Additionally, emergence occurs when a living system has properties that its parts do not have on their own. These properties emerge from the way that parts interact to form the larger picture of the whole of the organism/being.

In Dr. Siegel's defining principles, we have "within and between," suggesting that mind exists not just within an individual, but in the space between that individual and others. In Chapters 8 and 9 we will define this *relational space* and present strategies for building and supporting interpersonal relationship. The relational part of Dr. Siegel's definition includes other levels such as relationship to one's physical environment,[2] to one's body or body part(s), to one's diagnosis, to any component of experience, or to oneself as a whole. This fuller view of relating is consistent with integrative rehabilitation practice's (IRP) advocacy for an integral look at body-mind-environment (BME).

THE EMBODIED MIND

There is continuous and inseparable interplay of all that we label mind and all that we label physical. The fact that there are fields of *physical* therapy (or *physical* medicine in general) and *psycho*therapy is an excellent example of how the historical separation of mind and body has led to disciplinary entrenchment of the treatment of mind and body apart from one another.[3]

As described in a book exploring creativity in rehabilitation,[4] the very definitions of our professional disciplines reinforce a false dichotomy; i.e., we separate the physical health professions from mental health ones. This does not mean that either physical or mental health approaches are not important or are misguided. Each approach brings innate value. It *does* mean that more attention must go to the rehabilitation of the mind-body relationship directly.[5] This is best achieved through an exploration of the whole, instead of taking a reductive view of the parts. Doing the latter often represents the "fixer of the broken" disease model in contrast to a model of fostering well-being that might be realized regardless of state, experience, or outcome.

To explore the subject of mind-body relations further, we are required to touch on the philosophical dilemma embedded in this topic. The academic field of *neurophilosophy* presents a vast array of beliefs around the origins of mind and the nature of consciousness itself. These beliefs range from pure *materialism* (the stance that consciousness/mind is explainable solely by material constructs in the workings of the brain and body) to pure *dualism* (the stance that consciousness/mind is a phenomenon that is wholly distinct from the body). Somewhere in between, and potentially useful in clinical care, lies the idea that all things mind (thoughts, beliefs, personality, feelings, etc.) are found to have physiological correlates, regardless of whether the mind is seen as having a non-linear (metaphysical) quality or not.

An example of how we inadvertently split the psychological, social, and environmental from biology in the biopsychosocial (BPS) model is underscored in recent attempts to frame and study the problem. In a paper examining neural correlates of chronic pain, Vachon-Presseau *et al.* state: "In its current form, the BPS model is built on fragmented evidence taken from different disciplines, and—remarkably—lacks integration between psychosocial components and underlying biology."[6] The authors state: "a systematic approach of linking such concepts with brain biology has, to our knowledge, not been undertaken. Here, we unravel and inter-relate components of BPS by combining psychological, personality, and SES (socioeconomic) factors with measures of resting state functional connectivity to begin to define a unified perspective of chronic pain."[7] Finally, comments like: "The neurobiological underpinnings of chronic pain psychology/personality also remain relatively unknown…"[8] are made throughout the paper. These comments reflect that such notions of mind are embodied. This approach, while not named in the paper, precludes the need to debate the actual nature of mind. In the end, the neurophilosophical construct of *mysterianism*—the notion that "we simply don't know"—is also useful as it underscores a stance of humility. In integrative care, musings into the origin of individual consciousness, psyche, or spirit are left to each person to define and interpret for themselves.

With this debate aside, there is ample evidence from the inter-related fields of psychoneuroimmunology and mind-body medicine (MBM) that affirm physiological correlates for components of mind such as thoughts, beliefs, emotions, and memories. The psychophysiological research into mechanisms underlying placebo and nocebo responses also underscore this point.[9] From this foundation, we argue that regardless of the origin of consciousness, psychology is embedded in biology. We also argue that the mind is distributed into the whole of the bodily experience, hence our work is informed by the concept of "the embodied mind." This necessarily implies our call for a greater capacity in rehabilitation medicine to explore and support processes of mind in direct relation to that which is manifest in the body.

Experiential pause: Without adjusting or moving the body in any way, shift your attention to the felt sense of your body. Notice every facet of its current position. Notice the multitude of sensations that can be brought into conscious awareness—joints, muscles, skin, internal sensations from tissues and organs…the whole-body sensation. What do you notice? Where does your attention land? And, how does the current state of the body reflect your attention, mood, focus, or energy level as facets of the embodied mind? Now, ask the body if it would like a change? What would support the various levels of attention, mood, focus, energy level, and more? Does it need a movement break? Does it need a postural shift? How is the breathing pattern? Listen carefully. Respond slowly, staying aware. You may wish to jot down any insights from this experiential in your journal.

BREAKING DOWN BARRIERS WITH MBM

While technically an accurate term for mind-body, *psychosomatic* comes with conceptual, pragmatic, and moral dilemmas.[10] Kirmayer and Gómez-Carrillo state:

> Psychosomatic explanation invokes a social grey zone in which ambiguities and conflicts about agency, causality and moral responsibility abound. This conflict reflects the deep-seated dualism in Western ontology and concepts of personhood that plays out in psychosomatic research, theory and practice. Illnesses that are seen as psychologically mediated tend also to be viewed as less real or legitimate.[11]

These authors go on to discuss the ways in which an integral, ecosocial, and multilevel approach can address these dilemmas. You, the reader, are encouraged to take a side trip (see Resources at the end of the chapter) to deepen your understanding of the profound relevance of these topics. Having suggested this, we note that the IRP approach presented in this book has aimed to name these challenges and support grappling with them.

When approached from a non-dual lens, MBM is vital to this effort. MBM is a steadily expanding academic and clinical field rich in subtopics and research.[12] A growing body of work supports the presence of a unified psychophysiological framework of functionally and anatomically interconnected brain-body networks that present a picture of affect, behavior, and cognition integrated with somatic states.[13] MBM supports the understanding that physiological patterns underlie mechanisms of stress and resilience and play critical roles in both mental and physical illness, in comorbidity, and in recovery.[14] Hence, MBM offers a valuable foundation within IRP. While our biomedical model is needed and effective for many scenarios, the model tends to fall short at addressing roots of chronic disease. IRP assists by embracing a practical approach to the reality of complexity. This includes consciously addressing the larger context of illness in relationship to topics such as life history, unique psychobiological factors, and present conditions (physical and social environment).

Recently, following an introductory presentation on MBM delivered to physical therapy students, anonymous feedback included: "Some of the content is relevant for treating patients whose symptoms are purely in their head, but in terms of most patients with actual musculoskeletal impairments, these treatments have little utility." The topic of the mind-body split and tendency to perceive it from the either/or lens had already been specifically addressed in the content of the presentation, yet was still present to a startling degree in this feedback. In addition to demonstrating the extent to which mind-body duality is enculturated in our society, this example underscores a need to identify and bridge gaps in translation.

In rehabilitation medicine, there is a growing call to recognize the potentially negative impact of over-reduction and mind-body splitting in clinical care. Several authors have emphasized the following points:

- Not all psychosocial factors are indicative of a mental health disorder requiring assessment and treatment by a dedicated mental health professional.
- Psychosocial factors are not distinct from biological factors.

- The categorization of interventions into "physical" versus "psychological" creates limitations for what clinicians deem to be within their scope of practice.[15]

Taking these statements as foundational, we can say that, beyond the presence of mental health comorbidity, individuals experiencing what is predominantly categorized as a physical versus mental health issue still benefit from an integral lens on BME interactions. The development of transdisciplinary models that assist professionals in understanding and contributing to positive transformation within the many multidirectional BME relationships is needed. This may seem like a lofty goal; however, the general integrative medicine (IM) movement has laid the foundation for this capacity. The IRP approach is built upon the concept of a higher-order system of care that emphasizes realistic self-care, wellness, and healing of the whole person as primary goals. Such care must occur within the container of a compassionate, relationally attuned patient-provider relationship.[16]

Finally, in our culture of quick fixes, we see a general impatience for results. We want relief, and we want it now. MBM and the other tools and concepts presented for consideration as part of IRP represent *slow but powerful medicine*. This means we must give a message of patience, commitment, and realistic expectations from the start. We must also call out the possibility of an unconscious interpretation that instruction in mind-body and self-care skills means: "If you just relax and think positive, then you will be healed."

SELF-CARE IN CONTEXT

MBM includes a focus on the relevance of self-care. Self-care includes a large range of activities such as exercise, meditation, rest, nutrition, prayer, and social activity to name just a few. Embedded in self-care is the construct of self-efficacy, which has been shown to play a pivotal role in health including in relation to persistent pain.[17]

Self-care is often approached as an individualistic construct. In IRP, self-care expands to include a view of self-care as affecting relationships and rooted in interdependence. Further, self-care that acknowledges the balance of giving and receiving in relationship can have positive health effects.[18] These ideas reflect *self-care in context*.

MBM places self-directed care at the center of healing. Similarly, rehabilitation generally intends to influence a person's self-efficacy. However, care delivery often misses the intersection of psychological, social, and spiritual factors with one's bodily/physical/physiological experience. Mind-body and self-care approaches emphasize guiding patients toward an authentic, self-selected, and values-based version of their own self-care. Further, the larger influences that interact with self-care capacity are considered. Engaging self-care in context helps create individualized healthcare. When this care is delivered with enactive compassion (recall Chapter 2),[19] positive effects such as pain reduction can be realized.[20] Finally, when self-care in context is applied to professional and patient equally, it reflects mutual processes of self-discovery. This can be a turning point in the practitioner-patient relationship from a relatively dependent relationship into one that is empowering for both parties.

PUBLIC HEALTH, COMORBIDITY, MULTIMORBIDITY, AND SYNDEMICS

The IM and IRP movements address public health concerns such as the complexity of chronic illness and comorbidity. There is an epidemic of co-occurring somatic and mental health challenges. These dynamics challenge us to examine relationships and underlying shared biological constructs.

The IM/IRP approaches support the Chronic Care Model,[21] the Substance Abuse and Mental Health Services Administration's Primary and Behavioral Health Care Integration (SAMHSA PBHCI) program,[22] and the Primary Mental Health Care Model.[23] We contend that a failure to adequately and safely address the topics that arise in MBM, such as comorbidity and the other challenges laid out in this chapter, contributes to public health epidemics. IRP stands in support of public health as it: focuses on addressing contributing factors; favors prevention and lifestyle medicine approaches; and addresses the contributions of societal and organizational structure in the process. Stay tuned for a deeper dive into social determinants of health in Chapter 4.

The prevalence of comorbidity is significant. For example, researchers report that persons diagnosed with major depressive disorder (MDD) have significantly higher rates of chronic disabling (66% versus 43%) or nondisabling (41% versus 10%) pain.[24] Respondents with comorbid MDD and disabling pain also have significantly poorer health-related quality of life (HRQL), greater somatic symptom severity, and higher prevalence of panic disorder than other respondents. Given that, individually, musculoskeletal conditions and depression have the largest estimated effects on disability at both the individual and population levels,[25] the importance of the association is amplified. A gap exists between these findings and the allocation of healthcare resources, where these two conditions receive lower funding allocation relative to the disability impact of other conditions.[26]

Other researchers report similar associations between pain and depression, as well as comorbidities of chronic pain with post-traumatic stress disorder (PTSD), anxiety disorders, and insomnia.[27] Specific to PTSD, the Shared Vulnerability and Mutual Maintenance models have delineated the degree of symptom overlap between PTSD and chronic pain.[28] This includes the frequent presence of anxiety, hyperarousal, avoidance behavior, emotional lability, and elevated somatic focus; both PTSD and chronic pain are characterized by hypervigilance, attentional bias for stimuli, and an exaggerated startle response during states of negative affect.[29]

We must be careful in considering these associations: correlation does not imply causality. However, their coexistence necessitates further examination of relationships and shared physiological correlates. Seen in Figure 3.1, these relationships include interdependent changes in neurochemistry, autonomic activity, the hypothalamic-pituitary-adrenal (HPA) neuroendocrine axis, faciliatory and inhibitory nociceptive physiology, and inflammatory and immune processes.[30]

Taking just one of these interacting components, chronic autonomic dysregulation as indexed by measures such as heart rate variability (HRV) is increasingly proposed to play an important role in these relationships.[31] A recent meta-analysis determined that HRV is a viable marker of top-down inhibitory processes,[32] and the relationships between HRV, psychiatric illness, and other comorbidities (e.g., diabetes, obesity, arthritis, neurocognitive diseases, dental disease, cancer) are being elucidated.[33] Ongoing research is needed to discover interactions between HRV and risk factors such as age, smoking, diet, activity level, and confounding factors like medication use.

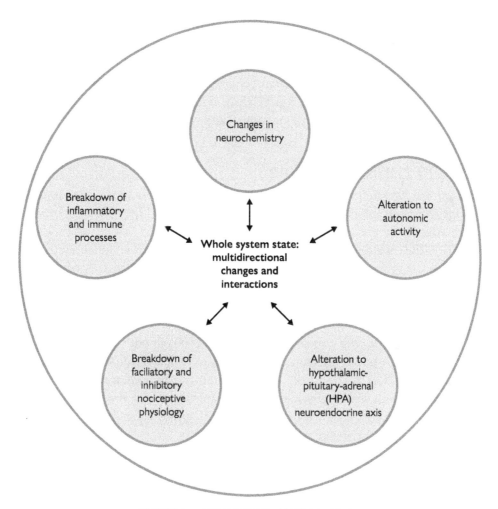

FIGURE 3.1: WHOLE SYSTEM INTERACTIONS
© Embody Your Mind

In examining comorbidities, additional relationships emerge. The reader is encouraged to review relationships between mental illness, psychosocial functioning, chronic disease,[34] shortened lifespan,[35] poorer care,[36] and both somatic neglect and iatrogenic effects from medication use.[37]

Beyond physical/mental health comorbidity, *multimorbidity* (the presence of multiple, chronic health conditions simultaneously) is a growing challenge in healthcare, calling for the type of skilled generalist capacity that comes with integrative care training.[38] Going further, a *syndemic* is a synergistic epidemic, and is more than a convenient synonym for co- or multimorbidity. The hallmark of a syndemic is the presence of two or more disease states that adversely interact, negatively affecting health trajectory and increasing vulnerability, and that are made more deleterious by the experience of adversities and inequities.[39] Towards the latter, and as we will build upon in the next chapter (which looks at sociocultural determinants of health), IRP approaches disease and illness as biosocial in nature. The syndemics model of health is consistent with IRP's use of a BME complex where interacting, co-present, or sequential conditions are studied in relationship with interacting individual, social, and environmental factors that either promote or diminish the negative effects of disease interactions. This emergent approach reconfigures conventional understandings of diseases as distinct entities in nature, separate from other diseases and independent of the social contexts and environments in which they are found. Instead, all these factors are seen to interact synergistically in various and consequential ways, having a substantial impact on the health of individuals and whole populations.[40]

PAIN AND THE NEED FOR IRP

While we will explore pain across the book and in particular in Chapter 16 on pain science/therapeutic education, an introduction is warranted here because, more than any other topic, the prevalence of persistent pain may be seen as a poster child for the call for IRP. The epidemic of persistent pain has become interwoven into both the opioid medication dilemma and the topic of comorbidity. The estimated 16% of Americans who have mental health disorders receives over half of all opioids prescribed in the US.[41]

In 2011, the Institute of Medicine (IOM) published a historic report, *Relieving Pain in America*. The report suggests that at least four of every ten American adults live with chronic pain, with annual costs exceeding $500 billion.[42] The report presented the frequency of co-occurring pain conditions, now called Chronic Overlapping Pain Conditions (COPCs).[43] The COPC phenomenon can be explored using a similar mind-body model of shared physiological mechanisms as seen above when exploring comorbidity. In general, healthcare systems are failing to adequately meet the needs of persons experiencing persistent pain conditions.

Pain is commonly defined as: "An unpleasant sensory and emotional experience associated with actual or potential tissue damage, or described in terms of such damage."[44] More recently, several authors proposed pain as: "a mutually recognizable somatic experience that reflects a person's apprehension of threat to their bodily or existential integrity."[45] We can see in these definitions the need to apply integrative constructs. The inclusion of physical, emotional, and existential components implies exploring pain experience from multiple lenses instead of solely the reduced structural lens. There is a current tendency to reduce pain to both a perception and a location (the brain). While simplification can be helpful in teaching about pain when it normalizes and validates, it also carries the risk of stigmatizing the patient experiencing pain (see Chapter 6 for more on stigma). If we use the "both/and" lens we can consider that pain is *both* a sensation in the body *and* processed by the brain. Going further, in integral thinking, pain is an experience within *the whole organism integrated system* and the *individual experiencing that system*.

One lens that is rarely considered is the understanding that pain presents a social threat to one's well-being. As a vital part of one's experience, pain can challenge basic human needs including:

- the need for autonomy and an experience of empowerment
- the need to belong socially
- the need for fairness and justice.[46]

Figure 3.2[47] demonstrates these considerations by placing the individual into social/relational and even larger sociocultural contexts, underscoring BME interactions and relationships as relevant within a person's pain experience. As an example of the outer ring, socioeconomic status (income) has been associated with chronic pain, the individual's psychology, and underlying neurophysiology.[48] It is critical that rehabilitation professionals understand how such dynamics are intimately intertwined in multidirectional relationships within the whole of the individual's experience and do not over-assign causality. This includes temporality—considering what this looked like before onset of pain and following it, but without assuming causality. This context is applicable to any health challenge.

In regards to functional impairment and disability caused by pain, various domains linked to the International Classification of Functioning, Disability and Health have been identified: nociceptive drivers, nervous system dysfunction drivers, comorbidities drivers, cognitive-emotional drivers, and contextual drivers.[49] It is important that a clinician acquire skills to: consider the interacting facets within and between each domain and still see the whole; identify where relative support might be offered; and in doing so, provide an integrative treatment approach within the scope of practice/expertise that respects inter-professional considerations and does not add inadvertent harm.

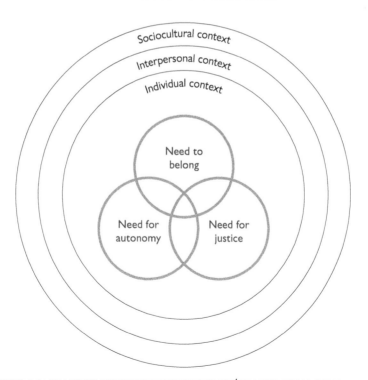

FIGURE 3.2: EXAMPLE INFLUENCES WITHIN PAIN/HEALTH EXPERIENCES
Adapted from Karos[50]

To build on the notion of these relative domains in relationship to mind-body processes, we know that psychological factors play a role in pain processes.[51] Pain is associated with shared meanings including threat/danger, cognitive meanings focused on long-term implications, and existential meanings such as hopelessness.[52] These factors do not imply causation, but rather reflect that, out of parts, the whole of experience emerges. Cognitive constructs, such as thoughts, beliefs, and perceptions, are each just one "part." Emotion, prior experience (conditioning), physical and social environment, and more are other ingredients. Figure 3.3 provides an example, using a soup recipe analogy, of how various relevant components may come together as part of one's health experience (including but not limited to pain) at any given point in time. Perhaps most vital in relationship to IRP is the last item in the figure: unknowable factors.

"Unknowable factors" leads us to a *dispositional theory of causation.* This practical theory describes the use of dispositions to see causes not as events necessitating an effect in isolation, but rather as phenomena that are highly complex and context sensitive and that tend toward an effect.[53] Hence, health experiences, including pain, emerge in unpredictable ways.[54] The ability to co-create a "map" of the larger landscape of a person's life and experience can afford shared understanding and decision making based on the complexity of possible factors. This must be done gently and mindfully, without reducing the person's experience to any particular component. Furthermore, when component parts are supported in the container of a therapeutic relationship, it changes the recipe and creates possibility for a shift in the trajectory of the experience. The nature of the dynamics can shift a trajectory either towards worsening/crisis or towards greater well-being.

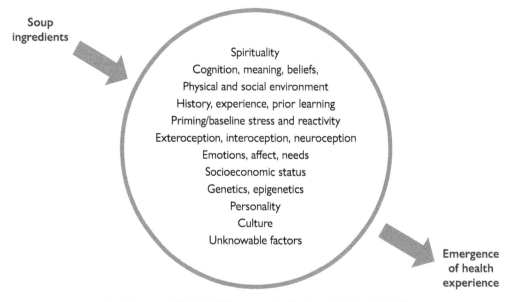

FIGURE 3.3: SOUP RECIPE ANALOGY OF HEALTH EMERGENCE
© Embody Your Mind

Figure 3.4 demonstrates a conceptualization of a sample individual with persistent pain. Note as you review the figure how this representation focuses on perceived limitations. It is critical that a "strengths and resources map" (Figure 3.5) also be created. Focusing solely on limiting factors adds distress. Finally, Figure 3.6 shows how the resultant combined factors may influence the trajectory of the person's health away from greater crisis towards greater well-being. *Note that this integrative approach can apply to all health conditions, not just pain.*

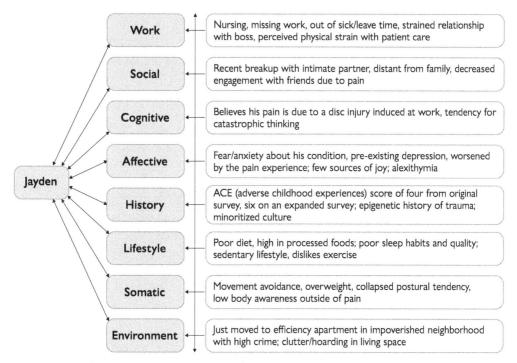

FIGURE 3.4: CHALLENGES MAP: BIDIRECTIONAL ARROWS BETWEEN
JAYDEN AND THE COMPONENTS REFLECT AWARENESS OF, RELATIONSHIP
TO, AND ASSIGNMENT OF RELEVANCE TO THESE DYNAMICS
Adapted from Low[55]

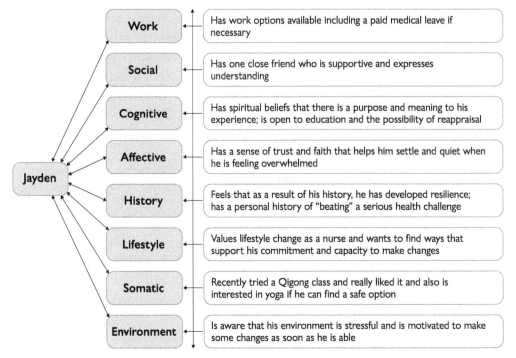

FIGURE 3.5: RESOURCES MAP: A STRENGTH-BASED ASSESSMENT
TO FRAME POSSIBILITY AND DIRECTION

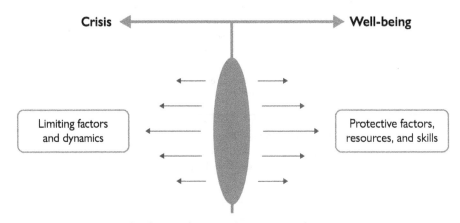

FIGURE 3.6: SHIFTING BME TRAJECTORY TOWARDS WELL-BEING
Adapted from Low[56]

PAIN AND IRP

Contextually, "pain" can be framed through a larger lens of not just physical pain, but also emotional pain/distress, mental pain/anguish, and wisdom teachings that explore spiritual pain in terms of human suffering. While beyond the scope of this chapter, valuable new frameworks rooted in integral thinking in relation to pain are emerging, and the reader is invited to take a side trip to learn more[57] (see Resources for a full text link).

For now, consider the following points as examples of broadening into a larger, contextual approach to pain.

- Pain is not just personal, it is universal.
- Pain is mysterious and unpredictable.
- Pain can be approached as "vital and sacred"—a protector, a teacher, and a motivator, as well as a seed for compassion.

Pain can motivate us to seek social resources, in part because revealing pain to others can elicit social support.[58] This must be weighed against the potential threat to social status and environment. Pain also presents opportunity for choice in terms of how to deal with one's experience of pain. This includes the possibility to shift away from our tendency to focus on "Why is this happening?" towards "How am I going to be in the best possible relationship to this experience of pain?" Pain presents a forum for exploring and challenging innate tendencies for avoidance, aversion, or resistance. These tendencies can add psychobiological tension within the system and the person's experience of it. The possibility of applying principles rooted in acceptance, commitment, and a less reactive/judgmental state of mind presents itself for consideration. Introducing such constructs must be done gently and with full awareness of risk to marginalize, minimize, or imply self-blame.

Pain can be examined through the wisdom teaching that suffering is connected to a tendency to form unconscious attachment to feeling good and a tendency to experience discomfort from a place of aversion/resistance. The old saying "What you resist is more apt to persist" is rooted in this construct. On the other side of the coin, if you form attachment to the "up" state, as soon as it is gone, you grasp, and suffer more.

Pain self-management affords a solid example of need for specific mind-body skills and tools, such as breath control, body awareness and body relationship, movement and exercise, applied mindfulness principles, lifestyle changes, and cognitive-behavioral tools. These tools are offered in support of improved well-being and not solely from the stance of making pain go away. The latter approach leads the individual to use such skills in a way that inadvertently reinforces the aversion/avoidance tendency. Research shows improvements in well-being when an approach consistent with IRP is utilized for persons living with persistent pain.[59]

The current state of pain research suggests there is not always (usually not) going to be a purely physical fix, thus a need for IRP. Even when physical change (movement, exercise, posture, surgery) is needed, it remains vital to acknowledge the larger landscape of each person's life. When considering mind and body, it is *always* both/and—perhaps on a relative spectrum, but always with a lens on both.

The state of pain research reminds us to inquire: Where is relative support or transformation needed the most? What combination of entry points for support will optimize potential for a positive shift in the trajectory towards healing? Examples on the list include physical, environmental, nutritional, chemical, mental, emotional, social, spiritual, and energetic.

Experiential pause: The preceding concepts are not intended to be reserved solely for pain as the primary challenge in a patient's life. Reread the preceding with other health challenges and symptoms in mind—physical, mental/psychological, emotional, existential... Include, if applicable, any health challenge that you are facing or have faced in the past; look for any insights as well as any aversion or resistance and use that to help you begin to formulate your own understanding of and approach to working with a larger view of and approach to health promotion.

STRESS AND THE NEED FOR IRP

Stress is another key example of why we need IRP. Stress is ubiquitous in our lives, and while we are designed to navigate stress in various forms, we have an epidemic of high, unrelieved, and/or prolonged stress states that are known to contribute to a wide range of chronic health challenges. Stress is often underestimated and overlooked, but sometimes overestimated too.

Developmentally, stress is both normal and necessary. Experiences such as a skinned knee or being separated from parents support building stress tolerance and resilience. This is especially true when the stressful experience occurs within a nurturing environment with empathetic caregivers who provide support and validation. However, when biological systems develop under high or sustained stress, the future function of physiological systems can be affected, increasing future risk of developing health problems.[60] The phenomenon of adverse childhood experiences (ACEs, explored in more detail in Chapter 4) reflects the potential consequences of early-life stress exposure. Similarly, there is growing evidence that processes of early-life attachment (caregiver relationship) play a pivotal role in how one experiences one's body, environment, relationships, and health across the lifespan.[61]

Stress, independent of age or history, is implicated in health challenges.[62] Stress may burden the systems that achieve stability in the body, or homeostasis, through physiological and/or behavioral change. If there is an ACE history, stacking effects may be occurring. The concept of priming is useful here. "Priming" is rooted in the idea that an organism's baseline (historical) sensitivity and reactivity within the continual interplay of present BME interactions is of relevance to consider and explore in an integrative approach. One interesting example of this comes from a study that used a driving simulator to mimic a sudden car accident. Similar to watching movies where we react to what we are viewing (mechanisms of mental imagery), in the study ~20% of participants developed pain, and for some of those (~10%) it persisted one month after the simulation. The study's results suggested that the development of pain in this condition was potentially linked to baseline emotional stress/reactivity and psychological profile.[63] Similarly, researchers examined the rates of neck pain in demolition derby drivers. The study demonstrated, despite repeated physical whiplash, very little prevalence of neck pain.[64] We must ask why these scenarios are observed, and explore the BME factors in these cases.

Allostasis is the term used to describe the process by which the body responds to stressors in order to regain homeostasis. High or prolonged stress negatively affects allostasis. The increased allostatic load that comes with unrelieved stress carries the risk of mechanisms of neurophysiological dysregulation; for example, where an overall increased excitability and/or decreased inhibitory activity is seen.[65] Stress can also: have negative impacts on inflammatory, endocrine, and immune processes; influence gene expression; and diminish the system's overall capacity for physiological regulation.[66] More on these topics in Chapter 7.

Finally, when we combine the challenge of stress on health with MBM, we see that skills training provides the possibility of improving the flexibility and range for biobehavioral regulation. Inducing relaxation is part of this; however, the message of relaxation must itself be held in context—it does not fix everything, it does not demand 24/7 calm, and it does not forgive us from having to be present to the challenges of our lives. Towards the latter, we must be alert to the possibility of oversimplifying relaxation and/or inadvertently deploying it in a way that increases experiential avoidance, something we will explore across the book.

BURNOUT

As we move to close this chapter, a final topic deserves attention in underscoring the need for IRP: burnout. There have been unprecedented changes in healthcare. Often, demand is high, and resources are poorly distributed. Burnout is increasing across healthcare professions. The factors influencing burnout are numerous, complicated, and linked to the larger topic of social determinants in health.

Burnout affects not just you, the professional, but the patient experience. It is a matter of intersubjective experience that carries implications across community and societal levels. In examining burnout, it is vital to keep in mind that placing sole responsibility on the individual professional to solve burnout, while failing to examine the role that systems, organizations, and politics play, will fall short of an effective solution. This is also true of other dynamics in healthcare. In Chapter 4 we will cover social determinants of health in more detail.

In approaching burnout, the typical response is to suggest "improved self-care." While each individual plays an important role within their experience, we are a social species. Ask yourself: How might a lens of *community care* be useful? The concept of community care directs attention towards the healing of interacting living systems. An individual department in a hospital and the larger corporation managing the hospital are both examples of interacting living systems. This is part of the healthcare professional's environment, and BME exists in interdependence. Therefore, any notion of "caring for the caregiver" must consider context and multidirectionality. In the reality of our present healthcare environment, we must discover and co-create a "both/and" approach to this challenge: supporting individual capacity for protective factors that buffer against burnout, while simultaneously contributing to systemic transformation.

In evaluating burnout, it is important to address the potential for stigma around the concept of *provider wellness*. Some people might suggest that healthcare providers are privileged, and so ask why they need to focus on themselves. Consider the following points.

- Patients treated by healthcare professionals with burnout have decreased quality of care, increased medical errors, decreased satisfaction, and overall worse outcomes.
- Patients with chronic disease are less likely to follow instructions of healthcare professionals who are burned out.
- Students in healthcare education who have better well-being have higher rates of empathy and better ability to connect with patients.
- For healthcare professionals, burnout contributes to relationship difficulties, alcohol and other substance use, depression, and suicide.[67]

These points suggest that well-being of the professional directly supports the quality of relationships and the health of patients. This in turn supports community health and other constructs of interdependence. The ancient Sufi poet Rumi is often quoted as saying: "Never give from the depths of our well, but from the overflow." Self-care supports acting in service by giving the best of you, and not from the depleted place of what's left of you.

> **Experiential pause:** Take a moment, close your eyes, and bring your current workplace to mind. Imagine yourself moving through the environment like a typical day at work. Notice your body as you do this. What do you notice? How do you feel? Is the energy of the environment and your experience of it fast or slow, high or low, dense or light? What emotions are evoked in association with your workplace? Write down what comes to you.

As with Jayden's challenges/opportunities assessment, there are numerous factors within the professional environment (and our experience of it) that may shift one towards either crisis or well-being. Drivers include: workload, access to resources, control and flexibility, meaning in work, social support at work and/or home, organizational culture/values, and work-life integration.[68] If we look deeply into these drivers, we see how they tap into fundamental human needs that an individual cannot redress through self-care alone.

So, why do we need IRP for burnout? First, we suggest that we contribute to systemic change by being change agents—both in our own self-care, but also in our advocacy for systems change. Applying tools such as mind-body medicine skills to ourselves supports innate mechanisms of resilience, enhances well-being, contributes to our ability to guide others into the same processes, and lays a base for advocacy work.

Second, we are reminded of an important point from Chapter 1. A shift towards IRP does not always mean a drastic change in what you do, but rather in the why and how you do it. After acquiring a sense of how the patient understands their health challenge (covered in Chapters 7 and 8), functional education and skills training (Section Two) become important tools. Seeing one's experience in context assists in relieving pressure from the pervasive and unsettling question of "Why?" Building capacity for contextual understanding alongside self-care skills supports de-emphasizing the tendency to overly focus on any one piece of content, as is often done.

Third, the burden that comes from feeling that you must fix or solve another person's experience is reduced. We are often taught that we must identify the "cause" of the problem. Undoing this dynamic does not forgive us of our need to diagnose or identify medical red flags. Think both/and—we rigorously attend to biomedical evaluation guidelines and simultaneously honor and embrace the "not knowing" that comes with complexity and the uncertainty that it often implies.

WRAPPING UP

We have presented a foundation of concepts that inform and define the need for IRP as a valuable approach geared towards enhancing quality in healthcare. Applying the principles embedded in IRP supports a wide range of topics, including the underpinnings of persistent pain, stress, comorbidity, and burnout. There are more topics that underscore the need for IRP, which you will see woven throughout pages of this book. Look for them and define the need for whole-person care yourself—out of your own experience. Equally, challenge or improve upon these ideas as you see even better ways forward. Our hope is that the approaches and practices we advocate for in this book will become so embedded across individual, academic, and professional systems such that the word "integrative" will no longer be necessary. Integrative care will simply be the norm and will no longer need to be identified as such.

> **Experiential pause:** Having read this chapter, identify and write down at least one actionable item of interest to you. In doing so, consider ways in which applying the material first to yourself, and then to patients, might serve those who come to you for care.

RESOURCES

- For more on the conceptual, pragmatic, and moral dilemmas surrounding mind-body explanation, read the paper by Kirmayer and Gómez-Carrillo at: www.ncbi.nlm.nih.gov/pmc/articles/PMC6699606.

- For a closer look at the idea of an enactive, phenomenological approach to pain, read the Stilwell and Harman paper here: https://link.springer.com/article/10.1007/s11097-019-09624-7.

CHAPTER 4

Upstream Influences

Andra DeVoght, PT, MPH and
Todd E. Davenport, PT, DPT, MPH, OCS

BACKGROUND
Connecting the dots

Integrative rehabilitation practice (IRP) aims to improve clinicians' ability to connect the dots between body-mind-environment (BME). Patients present as individuals with rich and often complicated life histories, conditions, experiences, and stories—all of which hold valuable context around contributing or complicating factors that both shape health and affect rehabilitation/health-care outcomes.

In this chapter, we zoom out and investigate the effect that social determinants of health (SDOH) have on health over the course of one's lifetime and across generations. SDOH include interdependent social, economic, political, cultural, and environmental factors. For simplicity in this chapter, these factors are collectively referred to as SDOH or "social conditions" and are seen as a vital part of the "E" in the BME framework. We will investigate the relationships between SDOH, behavior, and biology to illuminate new approaches to health care.

The World Health Organization's Commission on Social Determinants of Health defines SDOH as: "the conditions in which people are born, grow, live, work, and age, and the wider set of forces and systems shaping the conditions of daily life."[1] While medical care is one of the determinants of health, it is worth noting that clinical care is, by far, not the most influential one. In fact, it is estimated that clinical care accounts for only about 10% of variation in premature death.[2] Beyond the societal risk factors listed above, additional SDOH include employment, housing, discrimination, food security, neighborhood safety, and transportation. Social conditions, in turn, are shaped by the distribution of money, power, and resources at global, national, and local levels.[3] These dynamics underscore the focus of IRP on context, as well as humility.

Social epidemiology

The field of social epidemiology examines how social factors affect individual and population health to understand the mechanisms and patterns of disease. The examination involves a study of advantages and disadvantages in individuals and populations that confer protection or risk, respectively. This requires examination of *societal* risk factors (aka SDOH), as opposed to the tendency to focus predominantly on *individual* risk factors. Examples of individual risk factors are smoking, sedentary lifestyle, diet, and stress. Examples of societal risk factors include poverty, racism, lack of educational opportunities, and domestic violence. Exposure to these risk factors often contributes to poor health outcomes.[4] Individual risk factors are largely shaped by societal risk factors.[5] The choices people make are restricted to the set of options that is available to them.

Health is the result of many causal streams

A useful way of viewing SDOH is through the metaphor of a stream. The water of the stream contains both risk factors and protective factors. The quality of the headwaters impacts downstream health. We must understand what is going on upstream to effectively care for what is manifesting downstream.

A related public health parable reinforces the understanding that unseen factors exist as root causes of health effects in individuals and populations.[6] In this parable the protagonist spots a person drowning in the river. The protagonist saves that person and then notices several more people also drowning. After saving these people, the protagonist heads upstream to find out why the people fell into the river.[7]

There are several versions of the parable demonstrating the challenges associated with action. One version holds that the protagonist found a broken guardrail and no sign to indicate the danger of falling in the river. They alerted the town council which repaired the guardrail and installed a warning sign, preventing more people from falling in. Other versions hold that the protagonist became such an expert at performing rescues, stayed so busy rescuing, or became so exhausted from performing rescues that they never identified why people fell into the river. This story demonstrates a fundamental tension that exists between managing current cases of disease (downstream rescues) and preventing new cases of disease (upstream action).

This SDOH parable presents important terms for describing "location" within a causal stream of health. *Proximal* anatomical structures are situated nearest to the origin, and *distal* anatomical structures are located farthest from the origin.[8] Similarly, the concepts of proximal (near) and distal (far) can be used to describe a location along the causal pathway toward a health outcome.

Proximal (downstream) causes are located closer to the health outcome in a longitudinal stream. They commonly focus on pathophysiology and are a common target of clinical reasoning. For example, death or disability secondary to myocardial infarction (MI) may have an obstruction of the left descending coronary artery as the proximal cause.

Distal (upstream) causes are located farther away from the health outcome in a longitudinal causal stream. Continuing to use MI as an example, distal causes may occur at the individual level, such as hypertension. However, environmental and social contributors to MI may have been laid down much earlier, forming a potent distal health outcome. For example, a combination of issues may interact to increase the risk of future coronary heart disease: psychosocial distress from an intolerant location,[9] sedentary lifestyle secondary to the lack of opportunities for active transportation,[10] and an unhealthy diet from limited availability of plant-based foods.[11] Thus, a variety of endemic (cultural, political, economic, legal, and regulatory) factors may influence the disease course. Further, historical factors such as levels of exposure to childhood adversity, which interact with SDOH, are known to contribute to cardiac health.[12]

Collectively, these statements suggest three interacting ideas. First, our health outcomes, both positive and negative, are biological manifestations of the social constructs into which we are born, live, work, and play. Second, the timing and duration of these exposures has relevance to preventing the disease state that may result from them. Third, when an individual is experiencing illness or injury we are trained to look for and address the most immediate or proximal cause. Consideration of mitigating influences on the potential negative impacts from the various SDOH must inform both downstream and upstream approaches to health promotion and constructs of well-being.

Building the case for an outside-in approach to health

What factors exert the greatest influence on health? Is it the genes we inherited? Is it the quality of medical care received? Is it the choices we make and the behaviors we demonstrate each day? Or is it the social conditions into which we were born, live, work, and play? An analysis of several studies helps us to answer these questions according to patterns of premature deaths in the US.[13] This analysis was conducted to determine the relative influence of individual versus societal factors to the incidence of premature death. The authors attributed 5–15% of the variance in risk to medical care, compared to 16–65% for individual behavior patterns and 15–46% for social circumstances.[14]

The data tells us that very little of our risk for premature death is determined by our access to medical care. Yet, medical treatments continue to be highly researched and incentivized. The prevailing approach to health is "inside out," involving a focus on processes that occur within a person, such as pathophysiology, to promote beneficial changes to health. Instead, most of our health is based on our individual behaviors and social circumstances, with the latter heavily structuring the former. Considering IRP, we must think about health from "outside in" through a careful consideration of social risk factors on health and deliver a model of care that addresses these larger contexts in the best possible ways.

SDOH influence health differently throughout the life course

Figure 4.1 reflects a socioecological model that reflects the complexity of BME in relationship to SDOH. These layers are best seen as a whole—interdependent and interacting in health-promoting or diminishing ways across each individual's life course.[15]

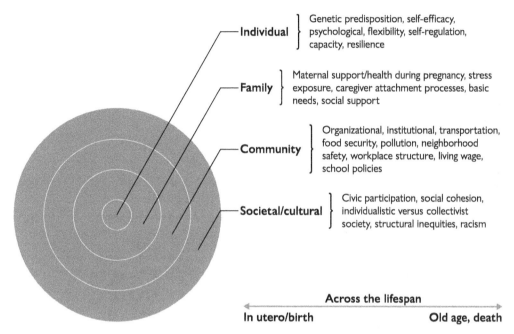

FIGURE 4.1: SOCIOECOLOGICAL MODEL OF RISK FACTORS
Adapted from Bronfenbrenner[16]

Each person's unique SDOH shape their health trajectory in different ways across the life course. There are various critical windows of biological development when an organism is developing rapidly into greater complexity. During these windows, exposures to risk and/or protective factors can be more or less potent from the perspective of either causing or preventing a disease.[17] Such exposures may occur years or decades prior to the onset of symptoms; thus are considered upstream or distal causes on a *temporal* scale. *Biological programming* is the enduring effect that exposure to risk or protective factors during a critical period has on the structure and function of organs, tissues, and body systems at later points in time.[18]

A life-course approach to understanding disease is one that looks back across an individual's or a population's life experiences; even across generations for clues to current patterns of health and disease.[19] It inherently challenges the model of adult lifestyle factors as the predominant risk factors and invites a broader perspective on the development of chronic diseases.

Experiential pause: Take a moment to pause and reflect on the section you just read. Try to notice the sensations in your body as you consider the following reflection questions: What can you do with this information? Is it beyond the scope of your practice to address it? Does it affect your patients? Do you discuss it with them? Why? Why not? If possible write down your insights and have a discussion with colleagues about your answers.

THE MANY LAYERS AND SETTINGS OF SDOH
Family
Adverse childhood experiences

In the 1990s Felitti and colleagues[20] studied the impact of adverse childhood experiences (ACEs) on later health patterns. The results of this landmark study identified strong associations between ten categories of adversity and subsequent physical, mental, and behavioral health challenges. The categories included *abuse* (psychological, physical, and/or sexual), *neglect* (physical and/or emotional), and *household dysfunction* (substance abuse by a household member, mental illness in a household member, violent treatment in the home, criminal behavior by a household member, and parental divorce). Participants' health status was then analyzed in relation to level of exposure before age 18. For each item marked, a "point" was given to determine the individual's "ACE score." Health outcomes were measured by the number of deaths, hospitalizations, outpatient visits to a health-care provider, emergency department visits, and pharmacy utilization.

ACEs are common and tend to cluster, and exposure tends to beget further adversity. Over half of participants reported at least one ACE and one-quarter of participants reported at least two ACEs. Exposure demonstrates a graded effect on health.[21] For example, participants reporting four or more ACEs had a 4- to 12-fold increased risk for alcoholism, drug abuse, depression, and/or attempting suicide. An ACE score of four or more also carries a 2- to 4-fold increase in smoking, poor self-rated health, 50 or more sexual partners, sexually transmitted infection, as well as a 40–60% greater level of physical inactivity and obesity than participants reporting no ACEs.[22]

ACE exposure is positively associated with the frequency of adult diseases including ischemic heart disease, cancer, chronic lung disease, skeletal fractures, and liver disease.[23] The original ACEs study brought the health effects of childhood adversity into the public discourse and has spurred extensive subsequent research. Since the original study, the categories of adverse experiences and the number of risks/outcomes have expanded.[24] Participants in the original study were mostly white, college-educated, and employed with health insurance, which demonstrated that ACEs may impact people from all socioeconomic positions. However, ACEs occur more often within populations experiencing greater socioeconomic disadvantage[25] or minoritized populations.[26]

The ACEs study provides us with valuable information regarding the health effects of family and household dysfunction but it does not measure the effects of adverse community, cultural, and societal conditions which result in poor health outcomes despite the absence of family and household dysfunction (ACEs) and vice versa. It has been estimated that 15–20% of the association between the number of ACEs and adult health risks were attributable to socioeconomic conditions in adulthood.[27] In fact, the health effects of three ACEs (exposure to household violence, parental divorce, and residing with a person who was incarcerated) were entirely explained by an individual's socioeconomic position (SEP) in adulthood. Conversely, the health effects of other ACEs are not significantly affected by SEP. Child physical, emotional, and sexual abuse also were significantly associated with several adult health risks but socioeconomic conditions explained only a small portion of these associations.[28] Adversities in the form of ACEs or adverse community, cultural, and societal conditions are significant contributing factors to health disparities. Efforts to reduce these disparities and promote health equity must consider these upstream drivers of poor health.

We must consider not just the health effects of exposure to ACEs and trauma but also the reasons why these damaging experiences are so prevalent in our society in the first place. The adverse health effects of such exposures are not to be seen as an individual or a community weakness or moral failing. The disparity in exposure to ACEs and trauma is commensurate with the disparity in the adverse health outcomes for those individuals and communities, yet many individuals experience shame and blame for their poor health, even in health-care settings. (See Chapter 6 for a closer look at how shame and stigma interact.) Biobehavioral responses to stress are best seen as rooted in adaptive psychophysiological strategies that promote survival.[29] The need for an individual or a group to utilize these survival strategies may exert an unnecessary toll on their health, but it is in no way a moral failing that their survival instincts were activated during times of adversity. Such understandings assist in destigmatization while bolstering individual and collective resilience.

Positive childhood experiences and resilience

The study of resilience and *strength-based* approaches must be inseparable to any exploration of ACEs. This includes the recognition that supportive societal conditions have potential to mitigate the potentially negative biological influences that can arise from ACE exposure or other SDOH. Examples include support for maternal mental health, neighborhood and school safety, and child resilience characteristics.[30]

Recent research reveals a set of specific positive childhood experiences (PCEs) that have potential to counteract the deleterious effects of ACEs.[31] These PCEs include having:

- felt able to talk to their family about feelings
- felt their family stood by them during difficult times
- felt safe and protected by an adult in their home
- enjoyed participating in community traditions
- felt a sense of belonging in high school (not including those who did not attend school or were homeschooled)
- felt supported by friends
- had at least two nonparent adults who took genuine interest in them.

The interaction between adverse and positive experiences at the levels of family, community, and society shape individuals' coping strategies. The relevance of coping strategies will also be explored further in Chapter 6. In sum, IRP, in relation to these topics, intends to gently and safely shed light on the health effects of adversity and maladaptive coping mechanisms while simultaneously working to build protective factors through therapeutic interventions.

Attachment styles influence the stress response

Attachment styles may be linked to SDOH via ACEs. The quality of attachment an infant develops with its primary caregiver in early life is influenced by a family's social circumstances and in turn influences the long-term health outcomes of the infant.[32] Attachment theory suggests that there is an innate, biological system of behaviors that provides protection from danger by keeping individuals in close proximity of their caregiver or other attachment figure.[33] The experiences of attachment in early infant-caregiver relationships establish a reference for future interpersonal behavior which can be described by attachment style: secure, insecure-avoidant, insecure-preoccupied, or insecure-fearful.[34] Each attachment style presents an inclination toward different mechanisms of self-regulation through anxiety or avoidance behaviors.

Researchers found a wide range of associations between ACE exposure, attachment style, and later health influence, such as accelerated cellular aging, the perpetration of sexual violence, and the development of disordered personality.[35] Further, Lin and colleagues[36] found that the association of ACEs with later somatic symptoms was stronger when levels of attachment anxiety were high and lower when secure attachment was present. Three types of biological responses also have been linked to insecure adult attachment styles that may mediate observed health outcomes: altered hypothalamic-pituitary-adrenal responses, cardiovascular responses, and immune responses.[37] Insecure adult attachment is also linked to risky health behaviors such as alcohol use, riskier sexual behaviors, poorer eating habits, less physical activity,[38] and less use of health-care services among individuals with three or more chronic illnesses.[39]

Maternal and intergenerational stress influences health

The SDOH can begin to influence health long before childhood or infancy. Maternal stress can be transmitted in utero, potentially leaving a lasting imprint on the stress response of the child.[40] Examples of adverse societal conditions that contribute to maternal stress include poor nutrition, domestic violence, discrimination, and poverty.[41]

The Fetal Origins Hypothesis was first developed over 35 years ago with the discovery of the correlation between low birthweight and mortality from ischemic heart disease.[42] This led to the later discovery that undernourishment during gestation leads to lasting changes in fetal metabolism that contributed to adult disease.[43] These findings spurred the formation of the International Society for Developmental Origins of Health and Disease (DOHaD). The DOHaD theory supports the importance of the mother's womb as the first environment for the fetus. It is important to keep in mind that the mother is not wholly responsible for the environment of the womb—the current and past social conditions in which the mother has lived affect the environment of the womb and therefore the neurophysiological development and health of the fetus.[44]

Looking even further upstream, stress has been demonstrated to be passed on intergenerationally. Such transmission is not just in the passing down of social conditions and/or behavioral learning, but also by epigenetic mechanisms.[45] Epigenetics means "on or around" the genes and it is the process by which genetic expression is changed by both health behaviors and *the environment*.[46] The environment provides the signals for genes to express themselves in large or small ways, or not at all. The science of epigenetics will be covered further in Chapter 7. For now, consider how these topics underscore complexity in health. While we can't change the past that may be influencing our patient's present health, context informs present-day strategies for health promotion—an aim of IRP. We must "look back, but not stare."

Work

Work environments impact health

Inequality in the workplace, manifested as a hierarchical power structure, has been shown to cause negative health effects. The landmark Whitehall studies conducted in the 1950s and again in the 1990s on British civil servants illustrated these negative health effects of hierarchical working conditions. The main findings of the Whitehall studies[47] include:

- stress is caused by a combination of high demand and low control
- social support at work improves health
- an imbalance of effort and reward harms health
- job insecurity harms health
- wider social networks are important for health
- control in life outside of work is important for health.

Community and society

Social gradients and health

Just as hierarchal work conditions affect the health of workers, hierarchal societal structures affect the health of populations. Health follows a social gradient.[48] One long-studied social gradient, introduced earlier, is SEP as measured through wealth/income, education, and occupation. SEP is a measure that represents an individual's or a population's level of financial, social, cultural, and human capital resources. SEP is an indicator of one's access to resources—money, social networks, material goods, educational opportunities, leisure, and power, all of which shape exposure to risk factors and protective factors.

The social deprivation that may come with low SEP can be considered a form of structural classism. The graded relationship between SEP and health points to a dose-response nature. Some argue that there might be reverse causation and that poor health is a driver of low SEP. While poor health is certainly a contributing factor in SEP, studies have shown that the primary direction of influence is from low SEP to poor health.[49]

Babies born with low birthweight are more likely to be from low SEP families,[50] suggesting the negative effects of low SEP start in early life and can persist into old age.

A high level of socioeconomic inequality in a population has a negative effect on the health of everyone, not just those of low SEP. Of note, people of low SEP are likely to experience worse health than people of high SEP. People of high SEP living in a society with high inequality will fare worse on health indicators than their counterparts living in a society with low inequality. Similarly, persons with low SEP living in a society with low inequality demonstrate better health outcomes than their counterparts in a society with high inequality.[51] High levels of inequality in a society contribute to the conditions that fuel threat perception and aggression. It is in these conditions that "isms" and "phobias" thrive: racism, sexism, minoritization, xenophobia, and discrimination based on gender, sexual orientation, neurodiversity, disability, and more. Such dynamics increase tension, aggression, and shaming/blaming and reduce the protective effect of supportive social networks.

PHYSIOLOGY—TRAUMA, TOXIC STRESS, AND ALLOSTATIC LOAD

SDOH can be sources of resilience or sources of toxic stress. In Chapter 3 we introduced the relevance of stress and allostatic load (AL) to IRP, including the core of mind-body medicine. Stress occurs on a spectrum from positive to tolerable to toxic; with variable influence on childhood development and/or adult health.[52] *Toxic stress* is stress that is either extreme or persistent enough that it exhausts the body's coping mechanisms. Accumulated toxic stress could lead to increased AL over time. The previous sections illustrated some of the potential sources of toxic stress that can lead to increased AL if they remain unchecked by protective factors that promote physical, psychological, and emotional safety.

Trauma may be a source of extreme physical, psychological, and emotional stress. The study of trauma has many subtopics, such as: shock trauma, vicarious/secondary trauma, historical/intergenerational trauma, developmental trauma, and complex trauma, to name a few. An individual history of trauma may or may not lead to a diagnosis of post-traumatic stress disorder by current psychiatric criteria, but nonetheless warrants an understanding of trauma-informed care (presented in Appendix B).

The degree to which a stressor causes an increase in AL is influenced by mechanisms of threat appraisal. SDOH carry high potential to increase or decrease the level of threat that an individual experiences. An individual's response to danger is dependent on their perception of the degree of danger and the availability of resources that will mitigate it. This determination is not predominantly a conscious, cognitive appraisal. *Threat appraisal* is shaped throughout the life course by social circumstances and it influences both the degree of physiologic response/AL and the behavioral strategies utilized to manage the experience of threat (or potential future threats). Maladaptive threat appraisal is considered a risk factor for toxic stress and its related health effects.[53] Pathways of influence for the preceding relationships are presented in Figure 4.2.

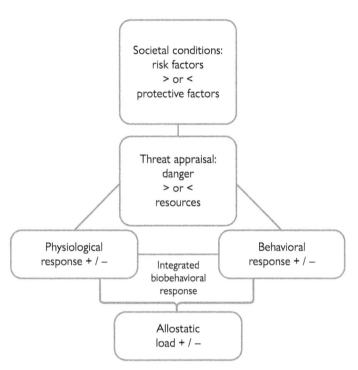

FIGURE 4.2: SOCIETAL CONDITIONS AND THREAT APPRAISAL INFLUENCE ALLOSTATIC LOAD

While further scientific underpinnings to toxic stress and AL will be covered in Chapter 7, several points are timely to elaborate here. Contributions to increased AL arise from social adversity. For example, beyond ACE exposure, immigration- and race-related burden of disease has been demonstrated.[54] Unmitigated AL affects all body systems and is associated with early all-cause mortality.[55] In sum, high, prolonged, and/or unmitigated stress from ACEs and other SDOH can impair the function within the integrated psychophysiological framework[56] that is necessary for self-regulation in the face of the demands of BME interactions. It is vital that any efforts to enhance personal responsibility for the management of stress be placed into a broader context of health equity and SDOH. In other words, *community-oriented* care represents the upstream look at our current tendencies to emphasize *self*-care.

Experiential pause: Can you think of a patient who experiences a great deal of real or perceived danger on a regular basis? Perhaps it is associated with their body, their pain, their medical providers, the police, their boss, or other relationships? Try to understand where that perception of danger comes from. Consider the impact on their body, their mind, and the condition they are seeing you for. Can you address the effects of toxic stress and allostatic load in a meaningful way through the care you provide? Use your journal to document what comes to mind.

INTEGRATING SDOH INTO CLINICAL PRACTICE
Taking action

What does all of this mean for health-care providers? How can the delivery of medical care make good use of this science? We suggest that IRP practitioners be equipped with the best tools to care for the person experiencing illness or injury while also participating in "upstream" efforts. There is a growing movement to adopt this perspective in health-care delivery and in the training of health-care providers. *Structural competency* is a concept described by Hansen and Metzl that:

> radically rejects the exclusive focus on individual responsibility for one's own health outcomes and replaces it with public responsibility for creating the conditions needed for health and well-being. And it radically transforms the relationship between medical professionals and the communities they serve from one of arrogant authority over patients to recognizing the competencies and expertise patients and their communities offer. It requires, as well, alliances with other disciplines and movements for social, economic, and environmental justice to have the capacity to achieve structural change.[57]

This section suggests a framework for IRP to operationalize this lofty and important vision.

Biomedical care largely focuses on symptom remediation and sometimes on behavioral/lifestyle counseling instead of addressing the complex challenges that lie upstream, despite evidence that these approaches have largely not proven effective.[58] The benefits of downstream interventions are limited because health behaviors are embedded into the social, economic, and cultural context. Health behaviors are more likely to improve when the social and environmental conditions are such that healthy choices are the *easy choices*, not the harder or more expensive ones.

It is important to keep in mind that the environments we live and work in carry *affordances*—possibilities afforded by the nature, conditions, and materiality of the environment.[59] Moving from one environment to another can change affordances and thus stress and health.[60] However, changing environment is not always possible. We have already emphasized that the choices people make are subject to the choices available to them. The concept of affordances thus also comes with an important understanding: the affordances that our environments offer is partially contingent upon having the skills to utilize available resources as well as to relate to/navigate current conditions to the best of our ability. The latter does not forego working for change towards improved environments in advocacy for others and for ourselves.

Integrative rehabilitation professionals can be a powerful voice for change in these environmental and social conditions, and also carry great potential to support individuals in navigating their environments with greater skill. In doing so, we must understand that the risk/gain assessments we and our patients make around health behavior are often unconscious. Motivation may be more apt to arise from a combination of perceived low risk and high gain, as well as low effort, time use, cost, and practicality.

The remaining sections introduce approaches to rehabilitation practice that connect dots between upstream (outside in, distal) and downstream (inside out, proximal) perspectives. These examples provide a framework for looking at critical windows of development, the various sources of risk or protection during those windows, and the enduring effects on future health. This perspective gives us meaningful ways to communicate with patients about the multiple layers of health in order to paint a fuller picture of their health and resilience. This picture can then be drawn upon to help a patient understand their health in the context of their life story and also leverage strengths and resources for patients to draw on and reinforce.

Education and validation matters

We assert that medical providers, including rehabilitation providers, are in an ideal position to create public awareness about the SDOH in a way that can facilitate both collective social and individual behavioral change. The IRP approach advocates going beyond solely symptom remediation to include the development of patients' understanding of their health status in the context of their life course and past/present SDOH. This outside-in perspective can lead to understanding, insight, action, and advocacy on the part of the patient and the provider. IRP is deliberately designed to support this reality through innovative practice models that involve upstream actions, as well as enhance the nature and types of downstream interventions.

Patient care, practice management, community involvement

Consideration of the SDOH is likely to instigate out-of-the-box thinking among some providers. In this section we summarize Andermann's framework for taking action on the social determinants of health in clinical practice. Andermann presents health-care providers with methods that can be implemented at the levels of *patient care*, *practice management*, and *community involvement*.[61]

Patient care

Social and economic disadvantage exists in all communities. Sometimes it may be hidden as in the case of domestic violence or child abuse. It may be current or historical. A patient may presently be in a safe environment with their needs met, but may have had severe exposure to adversity in their childhood that is affecting their adult health. A provider's adherence to a strict biomedical approach and failure to consider a patient's exposure to social challenge may result in unnecessary or ineffective intervention. Any efforts towards health behavior change must account for SDOH and the way these factors interact with individual factors.[62]

Similar to an understanding that an ACE screening process by itself may be therapeutic due to a validating effect, helping a patient understand their health experience within the context of their life course carries potential therapeutic impact. For example, neglecting to inquire about sexual violence when evaluating pelvic pain or family/household dysfunction when evaluating childhood abdominal pain or asthma are oversights that could prevent a patient from discovering the optimal path toward healing. Providers can learn to weave SDOH history questions into the patient interview and ongoing care in order to add greater depth and breadth to their understanding of the patient's health condition.

- **Identify hidden or obvious social challenges**: Ask patients about social challenges in a sensitive and caring way. The topic can be introduced by way of simple education about the links between exposure to stressors and various poor health outcomes. A basic explanation of allostatic load can open a doorway to ask patients if they are experiencing any undue stressors in their life. It is also an opportunity to describe resilience and protective factors and offer to connect the patient with resources that can help them build these. We will have more on weaving education and collaborative interviewing together in upcoming chapters. There are also a growing number of screening tools to aid providers in gathering this information; however, providers are encouraged to familiarize themselves with the content and engage in *direct* inquiry with the patient over the course of evaluation and ongoing care (Table 4.1).

Table 4.1: SDOH Screening Tools

Example social risk factor screening tools
Health Related Social Needs (HRSN): A screening questionnaire that can inform patients' treatment plans and referrals to community services. Additional information about the screening questionnaire may be found at: https://nam.edu/wp-content/uploads/2017/05/Standardized-Screening-for-Health-Related-Social-Needs-in-Clinical-Settings.pdf.
Protocol for Responding to and Assessing Patient Assets, Risk and Experiences (PRAPARE): A modularized toolkit that describes major steps to implement a new data-collection initiative on socioeconomic needs and circumstances. Providers may locate additional information at: www.nachc.org/research-and-data/prapare.
Your Current Life Situation (YCLS): A questionnaire assessing needs in six domains (economic stability, education, social and community context, health and clinical care, neighborhood and physical environment, and food). More information can be found at: https://sdh-tools-review.kpwashingtonresearch.org/screening-tools/your-current-life-situation.
Adverse Childhood Experiences (ACEs) Questionnaire: Providers can either familiarize themselves with the questions in order to aid in the interview process regarding childhood risk factors that guide clinical decision making or obtain non-diagnostic screening tools such as Center for Youth Wellness ACE-Questionnaire (CYW ACE-Q Child, Teen Self-Report). For adults, while the original/full questionnaire was designed for research, versions of it are routinely used in clinical settings as a springboard for discussion. Health-care practices are encouraged to adopt tools based on the needs of their patient population and clinical workflow. More information can be found at the Center for Healthcare Strategies website: www.chcs.org/media/TA-Tool-Screening-for-ACEs-and-Trauma_020619.pdf.
HealthBegins Upstream Risk Screening Tool and Guide: This social needs screening survey contains questions on education, employment, social support, immigration, financial strain, housing insecurity and quality, food insecurity, transportation, violence exposure, stress, and civic engagement. More information about this instrument is available at: https://sirenetwork.ucsf.edu/tools-resources/mmi/healthbegins-upstream-risk-screening-tool.

Southern Kennebec Healthy Start Resilience Questionnaire (SKHSRQ): This is an example of a commonly found tool that was designed to balance perspective and promote discussion in relation to the original ACE survey questions. The text of the survey can be found at: www.ashlandmhrb.org/upload/documents/ace/finding_your_resiliency_score.pdf.

The SKHSRQ was developed by a group of early childhood service providers, pediatricians, psychologists, and health advocates, who modeled the questionnaire after the original ACE survey questions. This survey was developed for parenting education, not for research purposes, and has not been tested for reliability and validity. Resilience surveys continue to be developed. A review of other resilience surveys can be found at: www.ncbi.nlm.nih.gov/pmc/articles/PMC3042897.

- **Recognize and address the influence of privilege and oppression**: Social norms, culture, gender, sexual orientation, race, class, and other topics intersect and interact with SDOH.[63] Figure 4.3 (adapted from Pauly Morgan[64]) presents topics vital to understand and address in efforts to support whole-person care that is individualized, sensitive, and responsive to stress from these domains. IRP aims to support this level of understanding. A necessary starting point is provider education about the obvious and hidden ways these dynamics may impact patient experiences. The topics found in Figure 4.3 apply to the succeeding sections on practice management and community involvement as well.

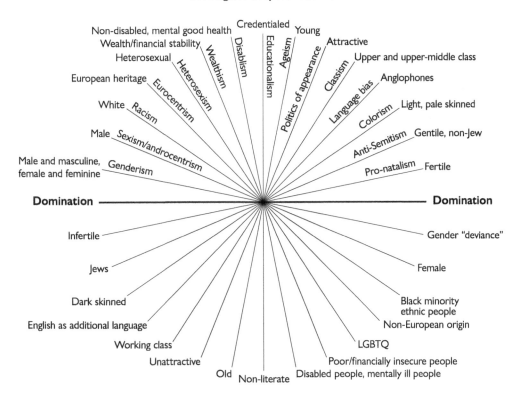

FIGURE 4.3: TYPES OF PRIVILEGE AND OPPRESSION
Adapted from Pauly Morgan[65]

- **Social prescribing**: Providers can make appropriate referrals to benefits and services that support patients' social challenges. Advocating for patients' social needs may include medical-legal partnerships, advocacy in schools or workplaces, or advocacy in health-care interactions if other essential providers are not recognizing the relevance of social challenges. Providers can include social needs in the development of treatment plans and goals. ICD-10 coding has Z codes for social conditions that providers can include in billing/reporting to document the complexity of need and support social interventions that are linked to better health outcomes.
- Additionally, and found throughout this book, we advocate for **clinical interventions that address the whole person and promote protective factors**. These include:
  - interventions that do not overly reduce or compartmentalize patients' "parts" and experiences
  - strength-based interventions that recognize innate wholeness and build resilience rather than instill fear or the sense of being "broken" (recall salutogenesis from Chapter 1)
  - mind-body interventions that promote adaptive self- and co-regulation, sensory-motor-cognitive development, sleep, healthy relationships, nutrition, and physical activity
  - interventions that reduce stigma and improve social cohesion/reduce isolation such as group medical visits and group-based offerings
  - interventions that include the patient's family, friends, or community in order to build social networks and reduce isolation.

Practice management

Changes at the level of practice management influence patient care and get care to the populations that need it most.

- **Inequity-responsive care** requires practice management to recognize health disparities and take steps to provide services that are accessible to those experiencing social and economic disadvantage. Examples include a commitment to billing insurance plans including Medicare and Medicaid and offering sliding fee scale/pro bono options.
- **Trauma-informed care** ensures an understanding of the experience and effect of trauma and violence on individuals and communities.[66] See Appendix B.
- **Contextually tailored care** reflects the needs of the community by being in an accessible location; offering extended hours, language interpretation, or childcare; or offering services in settings beyond the clinic such as schools or community organizations.
- **Care that demonstrates cultural humility** is relevant, meaningful, and self-selected for each individual based on their culture, beliefs, and values.[67] The principles presented by Ranjbar *et al.*[68] as applied to psychiatric care are easily extrapolated to rehabilitation practice.

- We also suggest that integrative rehabilitation providers attempt to structure their practices in consideration of the following.
  - **Critical windows of development, during which the effects of allostatic load are likely to have the most potent negative, long-term effects**: This could include services for pregnant women, children, adolescents, and families that address the stress that may contribute to or complicate their condition.
  - **Promote healthy relationships**: This could include modeling compassionate communication or working with dyads, families, or groups to build social cohesion and diminish the fallacy that we need to heal by ourselves.
  - **Interdisciplinary collaboration**: Collaborating across disciplines validates the complex nature of human suffering for the provider and the patient. Collaboration enables providers to understand their patients in greater depth and reduces the amount of compartmentalization that can happen when patients' experiences are reduced to fit the scope of practice of the provider they are seeing.

Community involvement

Medical providers can have a powerful voice in communities and thereby contribute to social change that promotes health and reduces health disparities. Andermann[69] suggests the following actions.

- **Partner with community groups, public health, and local leaders**: Health-care providers can participate in community-wide initiatives that provide services where they are most needed (e.g., violence prevention programs in schools), create health-promoting infrastructure (e.g., bike paths, parks, green spaces), or advocate for public policy that reduces health risks (e.g., banning soda vending machines in schools).
- **Use clinical experience and research evidence to advocate for social change**: Health-care providers can engage in advocacy and social change by influencing public opinion and participating in local and national efforts to create conditions that reduce health inequities (e.g., progressive taxation, basic income, affordable childcare, family planning).
- **Get involved in community needs assessment and health planning**: Community-oriented primary care is a model of integration of public health and primary care that is a form of "community diagnosis" and "community treatment." It is an innovative approach to meeting the most pressing needs of a community whereby primary care providers and partners collaborate to meet the needs of disadvantaged patient groups. "Community-oriented rehab practice" is considered a valuable component of IRP.
- **Use community engagement and empowerment to transform social norms and beliefs**: Community engagement can facilitate the development of community-wide conversations and actions that lead to the amelioration of societal norms and structures that have negative health effects on communities. Providers can

encourage patients toward social action and civic participation as a means to improve population health. It is important that providers start with their own self-reflection about their biases and assumptions.

In addition to Andermann's suggestions for addressing SDOH in the context of patient care, practice management, and community action,[70] Hansen and Metzl[71] suggest three more levels of action: individual, policy, and research. The individual-level intervention involves awareness and mitigation of one's own implicit biases.[72] Policy-level actions involve collaborative efforts to advocate for changes in local or national policies that affect health, for example universal health care. Research-level interventions include innovation in study designs that investigate the effects of structural factors on health and health care.

> **Experiential pause:** Imagine what these suggestions would look like in your work environment. Who are the individuals and organizations in your community that you would collaborate with? What would be the first step to take to implement any of these recommendations? Write down your answers.

Barriers to implementing a SDOH approach to clinical practice

Andermann et al.[73] identify five barriers to adopting a SDOH approach in clinical practice.

- Predominance of the medical model bias and imperative to treat (linked to the fixer/fixee dynamic).
- Possible reluctance among patients to disclose social determinants due to history of stereotyping and discrimination in clinical care.
- Lack of time for clinicians to engage in SDOH screening and lack of reimbursement for care that addresses SDOH.
- Lack of knowledge among clinicians about resources in the community that may be necessary to properly address SDOH.
- Uncertainty among clinicians about concrete actions to address SDOH and the absence of communities of practice to support each other in these efforts.

Additionally, the authors of this chapter recognize the following barriers.

- The scope of practice limitations that might prevent providers from engaging in work that overlaps with the scope of practice of other disciplines (i.e., mental health, public health). IRP is deliberate in addressing this topic (see Chapters 1, 6, and 26 in particular).
- Deficits in academic education, partially linked to the need to "teach the test."
- Lack of postgraduate training opportunities and experiential learning in SDOH and IRP.
- Lack of revenue to engage in this work.

- The question of medical necessity—will interventions to address SDOH be considered medically necessary, billable services by IRP?

Experiential pause: Which of these barriers can you mitigate? Who will you collaborate with to do so? Take a few moments to imagine what it would be like for you and your patients if these barriers were removed. What does that feel like?

SDOH HAVE NO IMMINENT "CONCLUSION"

Illness is complicated, especially chronic illness. Within this complexity lies tremendous opportunity if we are willing to consider upstream factors that can be both drivers and complicating factors affecting the health conditions we seek to ameliorate. When we consider and act on SDOH, we inherently begin to address health inequities. Rehabilitation professionals can be agents of social change while simultaneously engaging our patients in a therapeutic process that invites them to do the same. We underestimate ourselves and our patients if we only offer a reductionist perspective on health.

Informed by a perspective of the impact of SDOH on health, and in partnership with their ally integrated rehabilitation practitioners, patients may be more able to put their health into context and advocate for their well-being in a way that reveals more paths toward healing. This can be validating for patients and may lift some of the burden from the individualistic culture's tendency to blame and shame people for their experience of disadvantaged circumstances and/or their health conditions. Patients may be more able to make committed lifestyle changes that address the root causes of their illness, and/or they may become stronger advocates for themselves and others.

We can look upstream, think outside of the box, and continue to co-create innovative practice models that connect the dots between social circumstances, behavior, and biology. Let us move forward together to tap into the huge potential that exists for both individual and collective healing to take place by developing willingness and capability to have these conversations.

Experiential pause: Having read this chapter, identify and write down at least one actionable item of interest to you. In doing so, consider ways in which applying the material first to yourself, and then to patients, might serve those who come to you for care.

CHAPTER 5

Whole-Person Clinical Reasoning

Bronwyn Lennox Thompson, MSc(Hons),
PhD(Cant), DipOccTh(CIT)

SEEING PEOPLE AS WHOLE

Every person has a story to tell about discovering their illness. A story about how they went looking for someone to help, found someone, and worked out what to do. Their story is told in a setting: of a community, a landscape, a history, and a future. Their story is populated with other people, activities they're doing, things they've stopped doing, a sense of time, and a pace. Their story involves thoughts, emotions, and what they do next. When that person comes to see us, they bring their story as well—but what do we see when we look at them? Do we see an arm? A belly? Do we see a daughter? A partner? A parent? A weekend warrior? A worrier? A woman?

Our job as health professionals is, first, to do no harm; then, to support recovery so the person in front of us can be who they want to be and do what they want and need to do. This can best be done if we answer important questions: "Why is this person presenting to me in this way, at this time, and what is maintaining their predicament?" and "What can be done to reduce this person's distress and disability?"

The process of asking these questions—and what we do with the answers—is clinical reasoning. *Clinical reasoning* may be defined in several ways. Rogers[1] describes it as the: "thinking processes used...when planning, conducting and reflecting on...practice." Daly's[2] definition describes the process as: "the acts of determining a diagnosis and prognosis and making a therapeutic decision for a particular patient"; and goes on to describe a: "self-correcting cycle of learning in which understanding mediates between experience and judgement in gaining new knowledge." Clinical reasoning involves gathering and organising information to generate hypotheses about what might be going on. Sometimes we quickly recognise what we see, and the process can seem intuitive (known as Type 1 reasoning), while other times the process is slow, analytic, and logical (known as Type 2 reasoning). Possibly, both forms of thinking operate together.[3] In both types of reasoning, background knowledge known by the clinician is combined with the patient's information and organised for diagnosis and treatment planning.

Medical clinical reasoning processes are well known, but diagnosing is not as singular a process as we might think. Sturmberg and colleagues report that "most primary care consultations result in non-specific diagnoses,"[4] meaning that the focus for consultation is in the space beyond diagnosis and prognosis to what McKenzie, Pierce and Gunn describe as: "an integrative and patient-centred approach…[of] guiding patients through complexity to promote health."[5] Most rehabilitation is in this "integrative and patient-centred" space beyond diagnosis and prognosis, where we guide people towards health and where we often deal with uncertainty and ambiguity.

Concepts and approaches for clinical reasoning are presented in this chapter to help clinicians navigate what another person may want and need from health care. This chapter begins by discussing person-centred health care, the distinction between a disease and being ill, and why the process of seeking help is important for clinicians to understand. A distinction between making a diagnosis and developing a case formulation is made, along with suggestions for ways clinicians can develop their treatment plan in collaboration with the person seeking help.

[W]HOLISTIC HEALTH CARE = PERSON-CENTRED HEALTH CARE

Health and illness emerge from the interactions of many levels (e.g., physical, emotional, cognitive, social, etc.) within the whole of each person. In this book we previously defined integrative health care, and we can see the similarities between holistic health care, person-centred health care, and integrative health care. Two people may have the same disease, for example influenza or COVID-19, but *experience* the disease in different ways depending on many factors such as their age, other health problems, their personal vulnerability to viruses, or their living situation.

While we may be comfortable with the idea of holistic or integrative health care, it is evident that when it comes to clinical reasoning, we find it far more difficult to synthesize psychosocial and spiritual considerations than we do biological or physical factors. The assessment processes we use may focus primarily on identifying a diagnosis, or the biological disease we assume caused the problem. But we fail to integrate unique factors that led this person to see this clinician for this problem at this time. Angelina's experience may help at this point:

> Angelina is 23 and has been having episodes of neck pain over the past two years. She thinks it's related to falling off a horse, and although she didn't seek treatment at the time, she has limited her riding since then. She's working in a responsible job managing a retail store and has been achieving good sales figures. Recently her neck pain has been bothering her more than usual, and she's been having trouble getting comfortable at night. In the morning, it's been hard to turn her head to reverse her car. She's noticed that putting her arms up to do her hair is quite uncomfortable, and she's expected to be well groomed in her managerial role. At night when she gets home after work, she's not comfortable sitting in her lounge chair, and she's even stopped going to the gym because she feels it aggravates her neck pain. Her partner is unsympathetic and has told her just to keep going to the gym because "You can't go wrong getting strong," but Angelina feels he's

being simplistic and minimizing her distress. She's particularly worried about an upcoming conference where she will need to drive for two hours to get to the venue, sit for the whole day, and then drive for two hours to get home again.

Why has Angelina presented in this way at this time, and what might be maintaining her predicament? What can be done to reduce her distress and disability?

A diagnosis might identify that Angelina has some minor osteoarthritic changes in her spine—perhaps a bit earlier than we'd expect for a woman of 23 but still a common finding. However, a diagnosis cannot tell us why she has decided that *today* is when she seeks help for her neck pain. A diagnosis does not tell us why she is not going to the gym, nor what is happening between Angelina and her partner. We are left unsure of how Angelina is making sense of her experience and what she needs from her interaction with us. When we think about how to help her, how can we be person-centred?

> **Experiential pause:** Before reading any further, take a moment to note your thoughts about why Angelina is seeking help right now and what might be maintaining her current health predicament. What does she want from her encounter? What would you offer her, and how might this help to reduce her distress and disability? Write down your insights.

BEING ILL AND HAVING A DISEASE

Most of us assume that being ill involves some specific "disorder" of some part of the human body. We call this disease, pathology, or "dysfunction." We assume that the pathology produces the symptoms, and that all symptoms are attributable to a pathology. We may also assume that there is a linear relationship between disease → pathology → symptom/sign. We hold social expectations of those who develop pathology: they are victims of something that has happened to them, and therefore not responsible for having the disease; they are expected to seek help from appropriately trained people, adhere to the prescribed treatments, and return to normal health as quickly as possible. This is a simplistic view of the conventional biomedical model of disease.[6] However, there is much health-care activity that is not accounted for within this depiction of disease and treatment, such as the social and psychological factors known to shape the diagnostic process. For example, sociology of diagnosis scholars point out that what constitutes disease is shifting with the advent of diagnoses such as "pre-diabetes."[7] People given this diagnosis may be "at risk" of full-blown diabetes, but are currently healthy. Do they have a disease? What is their responsibility for following a treatment? What do we think of the person who doesn't follow their "pre-diabetes" diet and exercise programme? Do we consider the larger upstream determinants to health as covered in the preceding chapter?

The problems with a purely biomedical model of illness begin with the first assumption: that symptoms always indicate something wrong in the body. This is hard to fault at first, because our experiences of acute illness, for example a sprained ankle or the common cold, are reasonably well correlated with "disease." Yet when we examine the nocebo response, people receiving an inert substance for headaches drop out of randomized controlled trials because of adverse effects like nausea and drowsiness.[8] They are experiencing symptoms, yes—but is this disease? Probably not. Is it physiological? Yes.[9] Most of us will have had symptoms such as palpitations or unexplained nausea, but we generally appreciate these as temporary and unremarkable. Yet, we often believe the symptoms and signs we see in our patients, including our tests and examinations, are indications of disease. This may be true even though there is a wide range of "normal" in the population,[10] the response to the test may be a defence mechanism to an unusual situation,[11] and/or our testing may be inaccurate and unreliable.[12]

A further problem is that much pathology does not produce symptoms until late in the disease process. This is the rationale for screening programmes for breast cancer, cervical cancer, type 2 diabetes, and hypertension. With radiological imaging we recognise now that many people with disc prolapse experience no pain,[13] and the relationship between knee osteoarthritic changes and pain is inconsistent.[14] In other words, the relationship between disease and illness is complex.

What about the person who describes symptoms and illness, but for whom no structural or functional disorder can be identified? Our tendency to seek confirmation of *physical* hallmarks of disease relates to dichotomising health into "physical" and "psychological." This stance reflects the traditional mind-body disconnect.[15] However, current clinical testing procedures are not sufficiently well developed to identify "biomarkers" for conditions such as fibromyalgia or post-concussion syndrome.

The mind-body dilemma contributes to the challenges of agency and identification. As Wade[16] points out, when a person seeks health care they typically do not consider just the body part(s) as ill. Instead they consider *themselves* to be ill even when they believe the cause of their sickness lies within a bodily part or organ. "In other words, *illness* (sickness) is an attribute of a person, not of any specific part of the person."[17] [Italics added.]

Wade further remarks that while people may or may not have pathology present, the *disease* may not be the cause of the illness or may contribute only a *part* of the person's experience. The physiological changes that come with emotions and stresses, family responses, and other social demands are common factors embedded within any illness experience. A shift towards such contextual understandings of human behaviour is being seen across disciplines. For example, a valuable insight into distressing or troubling behaviour in ourselves or others comes from a "power threat meaning" meta-framework that is based on the core assumption that these are intelligible responses to adversities and their cultural and ideological meanings.[18] Finally, clinicians also need to consider adaptation factors that influence the impact of the person's symptoms on their experience of illness or disability, such as using spectacles to correct vision, or the existence of ramps to allow access to a building. In these instances, adaptations to the environment or aids to augment existing capabilities may enhance the person's ability to the point they may no longer identify as being disabled. In some cases, assistive devices may even provide a person with a competitive advantage, which some critics have argued with respect to amputees using "blades" in athletic track events.[19]

WHAT GOES IN, AND WHAT GETS EXCLUDED?

How can we approach the problem of finding out why this person is presenting in this way at this time, and what may be maintaining their predicament? How do we go about identifying what can be done about this person's distress and disability?

We need to have a process with both rigour and flexibility. Rigorous enough to ensure we can identify problems quickly and reliably, yet flexible enough to explore important parts of the person's presentation. Case formulation, a clinical reasoning approach used in clinical psychology and occupational therapy, can be used to expand on a diagnostic approach. Before describing case formulation in detail, we will consider a meta-framework that captures contextual elements in treatment seeking and receiving.

Benedetti,[20] a neuroscientist who studies placebo, describes four steps within the "doctor-patient" relationship (we can reinterpret this as meaning "clinician-patient" in our context). The steps are:

1. feeling sick
2. seeking relief
3. meeting the therapist
4. receiving treatment.

Benedetti's interest in all four of these steps lies in the "meaning response"[21] experienced by everyone, based on contextual sociocultural interpretations of what it means to be unwell and be treated. For our purposes, the four steps also provide clinicians with information about the person in context, how they made the decision to seek help now, and what they may be expecting from us. We will break down each step and consider important implications that may arise. Later, we discuss how to integrate this information into a clinical reasoning approach.

1. Feeling sick

As noted above, there is a difference between "feeling sick/being ill" and having a disease. It is possible to have a disease and be quite biologically compromised, yet not feel sick. It is usually only when a person feels sick, however, that they seek treatment, particularly when "feeling sick" is accompanied by interruptions to daily doing.[22] Feeling sick begins by interpreting interoceptive information (experiencing what the body feels like). This awareness arises from information conveyed by the sensory system (particularly the viscera) to the brainstem, limbic system (emotional correlates), and cortical structures via the nucleus tractus solitarius. Various structures and circuits seem to be crucial for representing what the body feels, and activity in these areas is associated with comparing expected body states with actual body states (predictive processing) and ultimately preparing body systems to respond to anticipated needs.[23] Importantly, social and psychoemotional contexts are thought to influence the weight and judgement given to these experiences, based on both learning history (especially from childhood; see Chapter 4) and current focus or goals. These processes are expectancies, beliefs, and/or attitudes that influence "priors" against which the actual sensory information is compared. Many parts of the brain process the differences between incoming sensory information and homeostasis, while simultaneously comparing those differences with expectations about what this means to that person at that time in that sociocultural context.[24]

Benedetti points out that feeling sick may involve many events: physical sensations, unusual changes in body presentation (such as skin colour change in jaundice, weakness in one side of the body in stroke, etc.), body temperature change, change in appetite, and sleep alterations. Clinicians, through measurements or examinations, can identify that something is not working within the normal range (such as blood glucose levels or joint cartilage changes). Together these experiences and measurements can engender negative emotions, and in doing so can increase symptoms while motivating action. Importantly, negative emotions and pain are tightly linked[25] so that whenever intensity is considered, so too must the person's negative emotions; they are inseparable.

Implications

For clinicians, this process means it is important to uncover the person's understanding of and feelings about what is going on. How did they first identify that something wasn't right? What did they first notice? What did they think was happening? What did they feel about it (emotionally)? Our most intimate relationships are found within the family, and families develop their own repertoire of beliefs and attitudes towards symptoms. Therefore, clinicians must consider the influence of family on the person's decision to seek treatment.[26] Awareness of sociocultural norms can inform us of common beliefs about what symptoms mean and how this is demonstrated by the person, for example stoicism in people living in rural farming communities.[27]

We must be open to cultural awareness; first of our own cultural practices and beliefs, and then of other cultures. The need becomes clear as we recognise that practices and beliefs are learned from infancy, are often implicit, and exert strong influences on how we each recognise and interpret "feeling sick."[28] We may be unaware of our own cultural assumptions until we encounter someone from a different cultural background. We may think of this person as "other" and their practices "unusual," but we must remember that, to that person, our cultural practices are "other" and what we assume is normal may be "unusual" to them. Culture is not limited to ethnicity, but can be extended to all groups such as families, communities, sporting groups, motorcycle groups, or business organisations.

2. Seeking relief

When we are ill, we are motivated to reduce discomfort—or at least, suppress it. Benedetti[29] states that this involves brain reward mechanisms and he argues that the drive to seek relief is comparable to the drive to reduce hunger or thirst. There is an innate motivation to escape unpleasant experiences of feeling sick, although *how* we go about this will vary.

As children, we seek relief from feeling ill from our parents or caregivers. They, in turn, follow cultural norms to find a healer, someone who holds specialised knowledge about ways to enhance health. It is easy to see that healers in early times could be those with access to spiritual powers and special herbs, and who could perform potent rituals to alleviate the sense of "wrongness" experienced by a person when they are ill.[30] From childhood illness experiences, we learn who to see, and when, because this behavioural repertoire is both highly emotional and modelled by those we most closely follow.[31] Treatment seeking is a strongly rewarded behaviour: when we are distressed and uncomfortable, the effect of someone taking control and offering comfort can quickly reduce the sense of helplessness. This is operant conditioning at its most powerful.

Seeking and receiving relief is influenced by whether a person seeks treatment, when they do, and from whom, and is tempered by many contextual factors:[32] financial, stigma,[33] gender, and previous health-care experiences.[34] While it is common to assume that people seek *treatment* for the *disease*, people experience *illness*, not disease, and they may be looking for other things from this encounter. For example, the person may want comfort, a listening ear, someone to take control of the situation, an answer to "What is wrong with me?", and/or guidance about the future.

Implications

Clinicians must recognise that people seek treatment for many different reasons. It is tempting to assume that the person sitting in front of us is looking for a diagnosis, and a treatment "fix" that returns them to a prior sense of normal, but this view is simplistic—and easy for both the patient and professional to presume. Part of the work of a clinician is to find out what the person expects or wants from the clinical encounter. From there, clinicians must establish to what extent this expectation can be met—and respond accordingly. This involves taking the time to listen not only to the patient's words, but also to what they are *not* saying. It requires asking questions sensitively to hear the meta-messages that words alone may not convey. It almost goes without saying that it is crucial to give the person enough time to feel that the clinician is interested, caring, and competent. Where the health problem is not immediately life-threatening, taking the time to allow the person to tell their story has support from narrative medicine as a humanising tactic against the tide of health care that focuses on the disease alone.[35] Chapters 7 and 8 will take us much deeper into how to work with this vital concept.

3. Meeting the therapist

The moment a person meets a clinician is what Benedetti describes as: "a special and unique social interaction in which the therapist represents the means to suppress discomfort."[36] He goes on to describe the mechanisms at work: trust, hope, compassion, and empathy. We seek others, perhaps to replicate the early bonding we experienced as infants. Attachment theory (covered in Chapter 4) extends Benedetti's discussions to describe the tasks that therapists must undertake to help the person make sense of their situations, in light of their attachment experiences in childhood.

While attachment theory helps explain the impact of early life experiences on feelings of security and belonging, the theory does not explain why humans throughout the world have sought help from what we can call "shamans." Shamans were responsible not only for spiritual health, but also for physical and emotional health. Shamans drew on knowledge of herbs, spiritual beliefs, and ritual to offer advice to people who were "feeling sick." People in the community associated shamanic practices with social bonding and a sense of belonging. When a shaman exhorted an illness to be gone—and it went—it seems reasonable to assume that the shaman also became known as a healer, particularly when illness was thought to have solely spiritual origins.[37] Modern clinicians have inherited similar status.

The seeds of what we call the "meaning response" or placebo response develop from the special regard we hold for healers. We have adopted the term meaning response because it clarifies what it is patients are responding to.[38] When a person meets a clinician, a sense of trust may (or may not) develop almost immediately.[39] Patients and clinicians evaluate one another, with patients seeking a sense of empathy, warmth, and competence in the clinician, while clinicians reciprocate in their evaluation of the patients' trustworthiness.[40] Gender, age, stature, and ethnicity all influence the "meet the therapist moment." In relation to pharmaceutical intervention, placebos are inert substances, so any clinical response when they are administered must be to "something else." Moerman and Jonas[41] point out that contextual aspects inherent within all clinical settings contribute to eliciting this response. They argue that it is the *meaning* inherent in the setting, the social role we have delegated to clinicians, the therapeutic ritual undertaken (what and how treatment is provided), and the neurobiological mechanisms involved in this specialised encounter that create this response. In fact, four requirements must be present for placebo to have any effect.

- The person must be aware that treatment is being given.
- The person must have some belief in the treatment.
- The person expects that the treatment will help, based on its reputation.
- This expectation enhances the body's own mechanisms for well-being.

In some ways, we can think of these factors as representing hope—anticipation that what is being done will improve health in the future.[42]

Implications

In the prior two steps, we've seen that we must cultivate awareness of the many hidden determinants occurring when a person seeks support. Similarly, and in context with clinical reasoning, there are hidden factors within the *clinician*. Clinical reasoning discussions typically consider explicit cognitions, but there is much that goes on beneath our conscious awareness. For example, Steinkopf[43] describes the tension between avoiding a person who is ill (to prevent contagion) and caring for them (to increase social bonding and inclusive fitness). Social processes in health and sickness serve to bias us towards, and away from, those who seek help. Clinicians are privileged to explore topics and undertake actions that other people may not. Alongside the prosocial adaptations (healing, listening, caring for) are factors that initially served to protect us from contagion but now may bias us towards avoidance. We can automatically perceive people who don't fit with "us," or the in-group, with a sense of disgust. Being different from the dominant culture,[44] such as being a different ethnicity or religion, and having a different appearance (weight,[45] height, disfigurement), mental health, and gender (being female in particular), can influence our judgements about pain and distress and what we should do about it.[46] Clinicians must recognise biases in themselves and take positive steps to limit the impact on clinical reasoning.[47]

4. Receiving treatment

Treatment is the period in which clinician and patient (hopefully) spend the most time. The quality of this time, marked by both the relational container that informs it and the types of treatments used, carries high potential for positive impact on outcomes. Throughout treatment, good clinicians work collaboratively with the patient to continually update their understanding of the areas of their life needing most attention and support. In this, whole-person clinical reasoning is ongoing and embedded into care and seen as a vital part of treatment itself.

We probably know the most about the time in which treatment is actively carried out. At least, we have researched the effectiveness of many treatments as compared with inactive treatments (placebo) and alternative active treatments. The meaning responses involved in receiving treatment cannot be readily disentangled from the actions of active treatments, especially in the case of rehabilitation. The result is that *all* treatments are enhanced if we actively manage expectations and maintain supportive interpersonal relationships. Darlow *et al.*[48] found that the ways in which we communicate with the person we seek to help, including the language we use, can have long-lasting effects. How we inform people about their options, and the good and not so good aspects of treatment, especially influence mood and pain.

Implications

An aspect of receiving treatment that merits discussion in a section on clinical reasoning is about what we do when our treatment isn't effective. How do we handle treatment failure? If we believe we've chosen the correct treatment for the person and their disease, *what* do we do when it doesn't help? *When* do we decide that a treatment is not working? Treatment rarely proceeds in a linear way, and clinical change processes are increasingly being examined.[49] Repeating an unsuccessful treatment while holding hope that it might work is undoubtedly doomed. The responsibility for choosing a treatment lies with the clinician, in collaboration with the person, yet it is not uncommon to find clinicians blaming the person for not recovering as expected.[50]

How do we manage our natural cognitive biases towards confirming our suspicions, identifying simple but wrong ideas, in what is a complex and ambiguous situation? Case formulation may offer us some ways out of this problem. Formulations provide several hypotheses and can incorporate multiple causal paths, as well as consider dispositions[51] as presented in Chapter 3. Factors influencing health may not be expressed, except when in combination with other factors in complex relationships that are not linear. Using a case formulation allows us to recognise the many factors present when a person "feels sick," and from a well-developed formulation we can generate many treatment options. For example, if our initial treatment was based on an assessment of muscle weakness and reduced motor control, but the person has not responded, we can begin a treatment based on an avoidance model. Perhaps the person has limited motor control because they are out of practice for that movement out of fear that doing it will increase pain. To test this hypothesis, we can begin using an exposure-based approach to movement: graded exposure for pain-related fear and avoidance is effective at reducing both disability and pain intensity.[52]

We must develop ways of considering our hypotheses as provisional so that we can respond flexibly if our treatments are not effective. Clinical reasoning strategies need to allow us to broaden the range of possible explanations beyond the simple and towards integrating many different possibilities, some from outside our own discipline. For this reason, transdisciplinary education and inter-professional teamwork are held as a gold standard in areas such as mild traumatic brain injury (concussion) rehabilitation, and persistent pain. The challenges then are about communicating across professional boundaries with the person seeking help as the key voice in the discussion. Recognising that the interpersonal elements of our clinical practice are crucial during treatment may mean we need to better develop our so-called "soft skills."

DIAGNOSIS AND CASE FORMULATION

Tying together the myriad factors involved in a person's health presentation involves clinical reasoning of two main types: diagnostic skills and case formulation. The rest of this section will discuss the differences and similarities between diagnosis and case formulation and identify strategies that may both make the clinical reasoning process collaborative and invoke a range of treatment options to offer.

Diagnosis is a system of grouping symptoms together, presuming that there is a unifying underlying explanation or cause. Case formulation, in comparison, is: "a narrative that integrates description and explanation of health problems."[53] Case formulations involve both diagnosis and explanation—the diagnosis identifies pathological processes involved (disease), while the formulation aims to explain its impact on the person (illness). In some professions, such as clinical psychology, case formulation is the dominant clinical reasoning approach.

WHAT IS DIAGNOSIS?

Maung[54] describes eight functions of conventional medical diagnosis, to which we will add a ninth.

- **Hypothesis**: A diagnosis is inferred from patient information, but usually there are several differential diagnoses, from which the clinician interacts to help direct treatment.

- **Explanation**: Diagnoses attempt to explain the information collected, in other words, summarise a causal link between the symptoms and the diagnostic label.
- **Prediction**: Diagnoses can be used to make predictions about the future outcomes for the person, including prognosis, complications,[55] and response to treatment.
- **Intervention**: Jutel identifies that the purpose of diagnosis is very often to indicate appropriate treatment(s).[56]
- **Denotation**: A diagnosis can be used in communication with other clinicians as a quick way to summarise "what is going on" in the person's body.
- **Classification**: Diagnoses represent a general form of the problem, and as Jutel says, diagnosis is "one of medicine's most powerful classification tools" used to inform public health policy, insurance, and clinical research.[57]
- **Normative**: A diagnosis functions to indicate that the person's state is abnormal, and that this is due to a disease, not a social or moral problem.
- **Semiotic**: Diagnoses can function as a "semiotic mediator" for the person, helping him or her understand and do something about their condition. A diagnosis can lead to a person reconsidering their goals, roles, and self-concept. The meaning of a diagnosis of, say, fibromyalgia has had such a profound effect on people that some doctors avoid giving the person this label for fear of it becoming a self-fulfilling prophecy.[58]
- **Social**: Finally, diagnosis functions to shape *social* responses to the person. Diagnoses allow clinicians to access private parts of the body that are not normally shared with others. By receiving a diagnosis, a person can access health care, mobilise social support systems, and alter their participation in daily life without violating cultural expectations: to be sick.

The explanatory strength of a diagnosis gives power to the above functions. If the diagnosis *explains* the patient data, it allows us to believe we have the correct diagnosis, appropriate treatment, and known prognosis. A diagnosis and treatment to address a single problem may, however, be inadequate to deal with the impact of *several* diagnoses and/or to address the contextual factors that explain why this person is presenting in this way at this time. Influential contextual factors are often in the psychosocial realm. For example, in our case vignette, Angelina may have minor osteoarthritic changes in her neck, but to understand why she has stopped going to the gym we must turn to psychological models of fear and avoidance,[59] and social responses from her partner.[60] To understand the best approach to treat the biological aspects of her neck pain requires taking the time to understand why she's making the decisions she is: What is her theory for her neck pain? Is she going to the gym for herself, or to please her partner?

Even when a person presents with a single health problem, Walton and Elliott[61] point out that drawing only on grouped comparisons, as in randomised controlled trials, risks over or under treating the individual. They suggest seven "domains" within which a musculoskeletal clinician can depict a person's susceptibility to risk: socioenvironmental, sensorimotor dysintegration, nociceptive/physiological, peripheral neuropathic, central nociplastic, emotional/affective, cognitive/belief. Together the clinician and patient synthesise the influence of factors that are most likely to be relevant. This strategy begins to approach a case formulation style of clinical reasoning, but does not extend to the explanatory and causal functions incorporated in a psychological case formulation style/approach.

CASE FORMULATION

Increasingly, case formulations are being adopted as a method of explaining disability.[62] In people experiencing persistent pain, a *biomedical* diagnosis is not particularly helpful because pain is a multidimensional phenomenon, with biopsychosocial factors interacting to form the *experience* of pain and the functional *effects* of having pain. Similarly, occupational therapists have typically considered that a biomedical diagnosis lacks the information needed to adequately describe disability or occupational performance deficit. Clinical reasoning processes need to go beyond diagnostic categories to consider both the whole-person construct and the notion of body-mind-environment (BME) in relation to living systems theory.

A case formulation or case conceptualisation can be an alternative or addition to diagnosis, and diagnoses can inform a case formulation. Case formulations provide an *ideographic* representation of the processes impacting the person's current health situation. By drawing on what is known about causal relationships between the factors that are present, the clinician and person create a series of possible explanations (hypotheses) to describe and explain how and why the person's situation has arisen and is being maintained.

A five-step process has been described when developing a case formulation.[63]

1. Detecting the underlying patterns.
2. Inferring causal mechanisms.
3. Developing a causal model.
4. Evaluating the causal model.
5. Writing the case formulation.

Detecting the underlying patterns

This part of the process involves working backwards from the presenting problems described by the person to proposed explanations or causes (abductive reasoning[64]). Abduction is a logical process of seeing a phenomenon (data) and working back to the most probable explanation/s.[65]

Clinical observations, test results, and information from the person represent data which we must sort into meaningful patterns. Often, many different explanations can be generated, and the clinician and person may have little idea as to which are the most plausible, parsimonious options with best explanatory breadth. For example, in our case vignette earlier, Angelina's painful neck and history of falling off a horse suggest a diagnosis of osteoarthritis in her neck based on her X-rays. Her pain has been getting worse recently and she is reducing her physical activity. We could hypothesise that she is also worried about what her pain means. We could add a further hypothesis that she is feeling stressed and this is in turn increasing her pain. As her pain increases, she may be worried that her neck pain indicates something seriously wrong, and that by reducing her activity level she is protecting herself from further harm. Any, or all, of these explanations could be contributing to why she is presenting in this way at this time, and while some of these hypotheses may not be readily recognised by the person, it is important to collaborate with Angelina to establish their relevance from her perspective.

Clinicians often work through various options in their minds during their assessment process as they ask questions, listen to the answers, and accept or reject possibilities as they proceed. Stanley and Campos[66] describe this as "an interplay between memory and imagination" and remark that clinical experience is the link between theoretical knowing (clinical thinking) and doing. They also identify that clinical reasoning is too complex for artificial intelligence programmes, because the process requires imagination—that abductive leap.

Expert clinicians begin the process of diagnosis and case formulation by integrating prior probabilities (facts and patterns we know from training) and clinical experience from "informed priors." Our effectiveness in this process is based on how well we've updated our informed priors over time and includes what we learn from journal articles, our colleagues, and our experience.

Inferring causal mechanisms

Stanley and Campos[67] describe two forms of abduction: "habitual," where the person knows a general rule and applies that existing rule to the facts as they are available to establish whether they provide a plausible explanation; and "creative," where there is no general rule, or the rule is unknown as yet, and the person must creatively generate a possible explanation. Because these explanations are provisional, all hypotheses need to both explain what is going on and be testable. If the hypothesis still holds after testing, we can conclude that it may be the explanation we are looking for.

The creative aspect of clinical work is how we conceptualise and organise the person's history, examination, and test results—how we ask about family history and work, interpret the physical examination and our observation skills, and finally, how we refine our testing in collaboration with the patient's feedback to arrive at a reasonable best guess from which to begin treatment.

In Angelina's case, we have evidence of osteoarthritic changes in her cervical spine, but on its own this isn't enough to explain why her pain has recently increased so much. The additional hypotheses about her stress levels, worry about the meaning of her pain, reason for avoiding movements, and so on are all testable as part of treatment. The informed and creative clinician will include these hypotheses as part of the case formulation.

Developing a causal model

Drawing the many possible contributing factors together involves creating an overall model of what may be influencing the person's decision to seek treatment at this time, and the impact of their experience on their illness. Models include various cognitive behavioural models,[68] a dispositions model,[69] discipline-specific models such as the Canadian Model of Occupational Performance,[70] and the "radar plot" approach,[71] along with many others. Many people have argued that an inter-professional approach is the preferred way to ensure all the various factors can be incorporated. This requires transdisciplinary capacity within each discipline, as well as a common vocabulary, and that all disciplines adopt a whole-person perspective.[72]

Evaluating the causal model

Evaluating the model begins with identifying the person's main concern, and in collaboration with the person and any other members of the health-care team. It can involve more clinical testing—is Angelina bracing as she turns her neck? Does she obtain a high score on pain-related fear and avoidance? It can also involve undertaking treatment—if she is feeling stressed, does problem-solving reduce her stress, and does this influence her pain? Carefully evaluating the impact of treatment on the areas of interest will shed light on those factors most likely to have contributed to her presentation, while eliminating any hypotheses found to be unsupported.

Writing the case formulation

Documenting the formulation is an ongoing process as hypotheses are tested, rejected, or accepted. At treatment completion, the model should consist of only those factors that have been shown to have an impact on the person's presentation. By writing the case formulation down, the person (and clinician) have a roadmap from which treatment for future illnesses can be started. It provides the person with information about their areas of strength and vulnerability.

ASSUMPTIONS AND CAUTIONS

As you move forward with this chapter and what follows, there are two important points to keep in mind when interacting with another person's experience and story:

Everything they have done to deal with their problem has worked at some point in their life, and if not their life, the lives of the people in their family and community. This means we must suspend any judgement made about the value of what the person has done. Our task may be to help the person think through the good and not-so-good consequences of any choices, in both the short term and the long term.

The person may not be able to describe aspects of why they have taken those actions. They may be unaware that they have made choices. Culture and "the way we do things" are deeply embedded, and we often fail to recognise that we hold certain assumptions until we encounter another person who has a different perspective.

These two points should remind clinicians to section off their personal and professional beliefs and values. Clinicians don't need to endorse everything the person currently believes, but it does mean that for a time we need to listen to *understand* rather than listen to *assess*. Once we have developed an understanding, and only then, we can work with the person to help them consider the implications of their choices and beliefs, offer alternatives, and support them to make decisions about what they will do next.

SUMMARY

Clinicians usually begin an assessment with an interview. This interview may be called the subjective part of the assessment: the time when the person can share their story and their concerns, and when their experience of being ill is explored. The term subjective may lead some clinicians to downplay its value. Using the information gathered in this part of the assessment only to guide test selection for diagnosis omits details of the person's illness experiences, their reason for seeking help at this time, and important outcomes the person is hoping for.

Using the framework drawn from Benedetti's depiction of treatment seeking, we can develop a nuanced understanding of why this person is presenting in this way at this time, and what may be maintaining their predicament. Doing so provides us with an understanding of the person's beliefs, concerns, priorities, and important contextual factors that will influence both satisfaction with our treatments and better, more relevant outcomes. Chapters 7 and 8 will paint additional pictures for translating these whole-person clinical reasoning principles into relationally focused and context-informed care.

> **Experiential pause:** Having read this chapter, identify and write down at least one actionable item of interest to you. In doing so, consider ways in which applying the material first to yourself, and then to patients, might serve those who come to you for care.

CHAPTER 6

Integrating Psychology in Practice

Noshene Ranjbar, MD and Matt Erb, PT

OVERVIEW

Albeit unintentionally, most rehabilitation disciplines have historically developed to fit into narrowed labels that contribute to the splitting away of psychological realities from the body. While these disciplines acknowledge the psychological facets of human experience and behavior, the majority of rehabilitation professionals are equipped to navigate these domains only to a small extent.

As explored in the preceding chapters, the pervasive splitting of psychosocial content from physical health conditions is rooted in a variety of factors that limit the possibility for a more integral understanding of body-mind-environment (BME). Together these dynamics give rise to gaps that need bridges. Perhaps most important is creating the bridge of safety (Figure 6.1) that is needed for exploring past and present psychosocial factors in relevance to the present health experience, without assigning causality and without stigma.

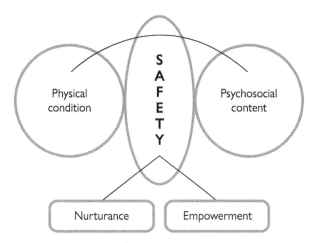

FIGURE 6.1: BRIDGE OF SAFETY

As an example, pain science and treatment, consistent with integrative rehabilitation practice (IRP), continues to advance towards transdisciplinary lenses and models.

The advent of "PIP"—psychologically integrated practice—also reflects these shifts in rehabilitation.[1] Such integrative-oriented care must not be relegated only to pain-focused clinical practice. A growing number of rehabilitation professionals who recognize the interconnectedness of mind and body are working from within the field to make it more transdisciplinary by expanding core education and clinical practice competencies. However, for the most part, entry-level professional programs are still tasked with "teaching to pass the exam," which has not caught up with the rigors that integrative care demands. The result is that inadequate space and time are devoted to building clinician capacity for psychologically integrated, whole-person practice.

In this chapter, we present a picture of human psychology and behavior from a normalizing view. Applying this integral lens to ourselves helps build capacity to naturally support others in exploring the many ways in which mind and body are intertwined. For this reason, this chapter includes many experiential activities and suggestions so you can practice applying these ideas to yourself in support of deepening your own self-development.

WHAT IS NORMAL?

There is a general societal tendency wherein many natural variations are excluded from the range of what is considered "normal." We overemphasize the narrow range of what tends to be acceptable as normal and in doing so fail to "normalize" (validate) uniqueness and the normalcy of the varied psychological realities of our lives.

Our needs, affect/feelings/emotions, communication, personality, coping, and cognitive processes range widely. Often these reflect, inflect, or develop in response to hidden determinants within health patterns. For example, a personality tendency might be labeled as disordered when in fact it is a natural adaptation developed as a stress-coping tendency. Another example: situation constraints predict behavior more strongly than does personality, IQ, or individual-level traits, challenging us to re-examine any notion we might have about "laziness," "adherence," or "compliance."[2] How do we cultivate contextual understanding of the potential relevance of such dynamics without making assumptions, looking down on, or falling into unhelpful analysis?

In this chapter, we provide a normalizing view of psychological patterns and behaviors, and underscore their interconnections within the whole. We present simple, practical, and effective ways of introducing support for each of them (ourselves first!) as vital to the development of an IRP approach.

LINKING NEEDS AND EMOTIONS

There are many variations on lists of core human needs. Most people jump to the category of physical well-being—we need food, air, shelter, rest, and so on. Yes. And what about relatedness, acceptance, appreciation, worthiness, and belonging? What about honesty, authenticity, and a sense of presence? Play? Peacefulness, beauty, meaning, or awe? What about choice, competence, independence, and freedom as reflective of autonomy? These examples of needs are consistent with self-determination theory's description of universal needs.[3] Seen earlier in Figure 6.1, and elsewhere in this book, we have presented safety, nurturance, and empowerment as important examples of universal needs. As healthcare professionals we must repeatedly ask how our delivery of care can assist others in meeting such needs.

Needs are intimately linked to *affect* (pre-personal/non-conscious intensity that includes a physiological arousal and valence[4]), feelings (personal/biographical categorization of affect), and emotions (outward/social display of the experience).[5] These details aside, the words are often interchanged and ultimately affect/feeling/emotion in turn informs or translates into behavior.

When needs are met, we are more likely to experience positive and prosocial emotions, such as gratitude, equanimity, excitement, generosity, or confidence. When needs are not being met, we become more likely to experience unpleasant emotions, such as frustration, fear, or despair. Met or unmet needs carry influence on the behavior we experience in ourselves and others. These dynamics may or may not be conscious to the individual. Such patterns play a key role in the healthcare relationship and experience. While some of what is enacted in any clinician-patient relationship is clearly informed by met/unmet needs outside of that relationship (for both), it is vital to attempt to provide a forum for meeting the needs that are relevant in a clinical encounter. Working from a foundation of understanding of just how intimately intertwined and powerful core human needs and feelings are, as practitioners we must optimize our approach and skills in how we communicate and relate to the individual seeking care.

EMBODIED COMMUNICATION

Deep down, we are all seeking validation, recognition, understanding, acceptance, and support. Many of these and our other needs are met in and through connection and relationship with others. Successful relationship and thus successful meeting of one's needs requires skillful communication to adequately and accurately convey one's experience. Communication involves both expressive (sharing, acting as in body language, conveying) and receptive (listening, receiving, understanding) domains, which are biologically linked to systemic physiological regulation.[6] Thus, there is profound therapeutic potential within our communication and interactions.[7]

Experiential pause: Think back to the last time you received healthcare. How did the communication dynamic between you and your care provider feel to you? Did you feel heard? Were you interrupted frequently? Were you given adequate time to share? Now, while still thinking of yourself as a patient, sense how the following styles of communication feel to you.

- When I heard you say __ ("that your back is trashed"), I wondered how that feels.
- What I think I heard you saying is __ (summarize what was shared), did I get that correctly?

- Is there more you'd like to share?
- You said: "This is stressful." Tell me more about that.
- When I heard about what you are experiencing, I felt concern that leads me to want to help you figure this out and find the right support for this problem. Before I offer anything from my experience, I'm wondering if you could tell me what you think might be wrong, if you have specific worries, as well as what you feel/believe might help.
- Is there anything else you need that can support you in your experience of this challenge?

Now document your thoughts about this experiential activity in your process journal.

As this book progresses, you will learn and experience principles of mindfulness (paying attention in a particular way to the present moment), body awareness (in self and other), and self-regulation (e.g., breathing). These ingredients are vital for the development of healthy relationship and effective, *embodied* communication, and are thereby foundational in IRP. Stay tuned. For now, we'll round out an overview of necessary topics for understanding and supporting the destigmatization of mental health needs and the normalization of human psychology and behavior.

A BIT MORE ON EMOTION

Have you ever wondered why the word feeling applies equally to the physical and emotional domains? Feeling is a somewhat generic word that can refer to emotion and sometimes not. Ask two people: "How are you feeling?" One responds: "I'm feeling sad and depressed; my dog died last week." Another: "I feel terrible. My back is painful, my head hurts, and my stomach is upset." Did the question distinguish which route to take?

Emotion derives from Latin, ex- → e- (out) + movere (move) = out-moving. A fun (and potentially insightful) way to look at emotion is e-motion, energy moving/in motion. Emotions are best approached as innately innocent and dynamic. Emotions are guides that alert us to our present condition and needs and that can assist us in navigating the complex energies that inform the continuously changing BME conditions.

Often, emotion is described as a state of mind; however, contemporary neuroscience (and relatively simple self-exploration!) reveals that emotion is inseparably linked to sensation, and thus to the body.[8] The development of extensive mind-body metaphors reflects this dynamic. Have you ever felt like you were shouldering a lot? Have you ever had a sinking feeling, or were not digesting a situation very well? This language is not coincidental. Pay attention to it, but do not assume causality. Let any relevance be self-revealed. An open-minded, contemplative stance (not analytical, pathologizing, nor diagnostic) serves as a springboard for somatoemotional awareness training. Finally, and as taught in Acceptance and Commitment Therapy (see Chapter 17), it is often our avoidance of a given unpleasant feeling/sensation (with accompanying thoughts and/or judgments) that creates the primary problem.[9]

Experiential pause: Find a comfortable position, where you can be undisturbed for a few minutes. Then, bring to mind, one at a time, each of the following emotions. Focus on discovering the felt sense of each one. How does that particular emotion "land" in the body? How and where do you feel it? Once you've completed this list, think of other emotions. After you are done, take a page in your journal, draw out a simple gingerbread person outline like the one shown, and then color in what you discovered. Use a unique color for each emotion that you've chosen.

- Anger
- Joy
- Fear
- Awe
- Sadness
- Competence
- Shame
- Disgust
- Surprise
- Other emotions…

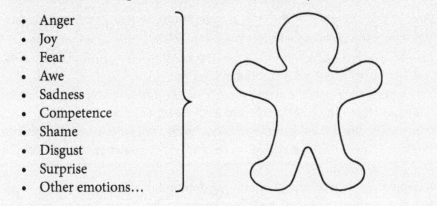

ANOESIS, AFFECT, AND ALEXITHYMIA

Anoesis is a term that describes the ability to experience emotion as pure sensation without the accompanying storylines. This is not an easy thing—to stay fully with an emotional experience and the bodily sensation that frames it without any reaction or response! Give it a try the next time you are feeling emotional. And, keep in mind that the goal is not to be completely unmoving to emotion 100% of the time. As just described, emotion often is seeking movement and expression. Emotions may also be alerting us to take action in support of meeting needs.

Introduced earlier, the word affect is sometimes used to describe the presence of arousal or activation and what might follow—feelings, the expression of emotion, and the way in which such a flow might inform behavioral response. For example, the presence or experience of a pure sensation may generate a positive or negative feeling that one assigns to it; the expression of an emotion or behavior may follow. These translations and responses often follow patterns that are highly individual and further linked to constructs of temperament, personality, disposition, intention, motivation, and movement.

You do not need to become an academic expert on these topics; however, cultivating a basic understanding of them is useful. What may be more important in clinical care is following Dr. Atul Gawande's advice[10]—cultivating the art of listening for and attuning towards the feelings underneath the words and the "presentation," including our own. This is accompanied by providing space for each person to become aware, acknowledge, and express their interior: *invitations to awareness and expression.* Just as difficulty with identifying and naming one's feelings (alexithymia) is associated with challenges such as anxiety, pain, and depression,[11] simple affect labeling, wherein individuals are supported in learning to name what they are sensing and feeling, carries potential therapeutic impact[12] (see Chapter 17 for more information).

Experiential pause: Part 1: Here are some clear, simple, yet powerful examples of invitations to awareness and expression that reflect a basic foundation for supporting emotion. Read each one and then imagine that you are with a recent patient offering these invitations.

- How is this experience of ___ (example: shoulder pain) making you feel? What does the experience bring up for you? What is its impact on you?
- How are you feeling right now? (If the response is solely a physical one, clarify: "OK, and what about at an emotional level?")
- When you talk about the stress you are under, what do you notice in your body? Are there any emotions linked to those sensations?
- I am wondering if there is some emotion happening for you around this?
- Wow, as I listen, this sounds like a very stressful experience. Would you like to share more about what this is like?
- It is important to receive support around the emotional impact of pain. Do you feel that you have adequate tools and resources for managing the emotional impact of your pain experience?

Part 2: Write down your answers to the following: How do these examples feel to you? What do you notice in your body as you imagine interacting with your patients in this way? Can you imagine how, beyond the words, your tone of voice and body language can dramatically change how the other person perceives and receives them? How would you tweak the language for greater ease and to match your own unique voice? Does any part of them bring up discomfort inside? If so, can you tell where that discomfort arises from?

EMOTION AND PAIN

Theory, philosophy, and scientific research are intertwined in the contemplation of most topics, including pain. This intertwining, which can also be described as "mixing levels," frequently brings up emotionalized opinions and can be a "rabbit-hole" topic. Some authors have indeed called pain an aporia (a mystery or topic without a clear path, passage, or way).[13] Regarding pain as an aporia is consistent with the suggestion, earlier in this book, to not overly reify anything—and to embrace mystery as a stance of flexibility in working with the lived experience of ourselves and those who come to us for support. Having said this, consider the following.

- Social rejection activates many of the same neurophysiological correlates involved in experiences of physical pain.[14]
  Pause and contemplate: What does one's social history and present social environment look like and how might this inform biological patterns? What affordances[15]

(resources) does one's social environment offer and how is this a part of the whole (BME)?

- Multiple researchers have demonstrated whiplash to be highly conditional, influenced by the stress response, and culturally sensitive.[16]

  Pause and contemplate: How does the shared possibility for victimization in our lives impact our health experience? How does perception of choice, autonomy, and control (and their neurophysiological correlates) interact here? How do cultural/collectivist beliefs across different populations influence individual health experience?

- Emotions are integral to the conceptualization, assessment, and treatment of persistent pain.[17]

  Pause and contemplate: Are we addressing this? If so, are we doing it in gentle, safe, and accessible ways that do not add harm, acknowledging this reality without shaming or blaming? Then, are we capable of going further into adequate support around this reality?

- Cultivating positive, prosocial emotions and behaviors can support physical health and pain management.[18] Here, context is demanded from us as healthcare professionals, as the suggestion of positivity may carry perils for some.[19] Stay tuned for more on this topic in Chapters 17 and 18.

  Pause and contemplate: How many of us consider hidden determinants when we interact with the behavioral patterns of those who come to us for help? Second, how do we support the cultivation of positive emotions and pro-sociality without it sounding like positive thinking alone will solve all one's problems, or "giving to others will help you manage your pain" (when the person you are supporting has substantial unmet needs)?

WHAT'S PERSONALITY GOT TO DO WITH IT?

Personality reflects how a person characteristically views themselves, how they view the world, and how they interact with the world to get their needs met.[20] Personality structure is largely in place by early childhood.[21] While it is often suggested that components of personality are immutable, it may be better to consider them as perhaps stubborn but potentially malleable with learning and experience.[22] Of the many models used to study human personality, the "big five" construct of personality (extroversion, agreeableness, openness, conscientiousness, and neuroticism) is one of the most utilized and examined in contemporary research. If you are not familiar, take a side trip now (see Resources at the end of the chapter).

There are associations between personality and emotional expression.[23] Further, these associations are linked to illness and disease biology, for example in irritable bowel syndrome,[24] lumbopelvic myokinematics,[25] and persistent pain.[26] Personality tendencies have been examined in association with a wide range of other topics, such as: resilience, prosocial behavior, learning style, physical activity level, sexuality, various pain conditions, sleep, obesity, overall quality of life, happiness across the lifespan, mental health treatment outcomes, and more.[27] Recent research examining a "light triad of personality" suggests that a loving and beneficent orientation toward others is able to predict life satisfaction and a range of growth-oriented and self-transcendent outcomes beyond existing measures of personality.[28] Because of these associations, it is vital that all rehabilitation professionals have some basic understanding of personality and its influence on health.

What about personality "disorders"? The term *personality disorder* intends to reflect cases where the trait(s) that make up a person's personality are inflexible and damaging, impair capacity for healthy relationships and/or work, and affect not just the individual but also those who interact with the individual.[29] Personality disorders typically come with a lot of stigma and assumptions, which is damaging, especially when the label influences professionals who lack a fuller understanding of the depth that informs the condition and how to support that depth. For further learning, see Resources at the end of this chapter. For now, it is vital to remember that *we all have personality characteristics on a continuum*. Normalization, understanding, and enactive compassion for ourselves and others are vital.

STIGMA AND SHAME

While attitudes vary across cultures, in general people consciously and unconsciously avoid the label of mental illness to avoid stigma, shame, and the harm that such a label may bring. This dynamic frequently leads individuals to decide not to open up or seek and fully participate in care.

Stigma

Two main categories of stigma-related harm have been defined:

- diminishment of self-esteem
- loss of social opportunity.[30]

Patterns of stigma follow a process: discriminable stimuli (signals) → cognitive mediators (in the form of stereotypes and relational dynamics) → behavior (discrimination). Take, for example, Massoud. Massoud appears disheveled in his dressing and hygiene habits (signal). He also experiences high anxiety that makes his patterns of social engagement seem unusual, i.e., not normal (signal). Massoud presents to a physician (Dr. W) who is unaware of the innate authoritarian power dynamics that his role as a doctor carries. Simultaneously, in reading Massoud's chart, Dr. W sees a comment from another clinician that states "question borderline personality disorder" due to a recent emotional outburst during a different clinical encounter. Having just read this in the chart, Dr. W approaches the session with an unconscious bias and nervousness rooted in the perception of possible relational tension (stereotypes). Massoud presents with complaints of abdominal pain, yet an implicit assumption is made by Dr. W that Massoud's symptoms are purely psychological. Dr. W fails to issue orders for several standard laboratory tests and suggests that Massoud follow up with his psychiatrist for medication management (discrimination). A month later, through an emergency room workup, it is discovered that Massoud has a gastric ulcer and he is also diagnosed with H. Pylori. Massoud is provided with treatment, suggestions for dietary changes, and home use of guided imagery for stress-response down-regulation. Massoud's gastrointestinal (GI) symptoms subsequently improve.

In examining Massoud's story, common errors are seen.

- While rarely explained clearly, the inference that symptoms are purely psychological ("all in the head") fails to acknowledge that when psychological factors are involved to any degree, this carries direct *biological* relevance/impact. Said another way, even when a condition is predominantly psychosomatic, it is still represented by neurophysiological correlates. The biomedical labels of MUS (medically unexplained symptoms) and functional neurological symptom disorder (FNSD) both reflect the complexity and challenge of safely and adequately supporting these dynamics with the possibility of stigma/shame in mind.[31]
- Second, we see a failure to recognize that Massoud's stress and psychoemotional patterns can be addressed and supported concurrently with the more biomedical facets (diagnostics, treatment options) of his care. That is, it is not *either* an ulcer/H. Pylori *or* purely psychological. Simultaneous attention to biomedical and psychosocial dynamics (which both equally carry biological influence) is not just possible but vital. Thus, the larger point is to engage with patients holistically and not just "integrate psychology" into care, which still implies a splitting that may carry stigma.

So how do we combat stigma? First, consciously work to become aware of the tendency to make assumptions and catch and combat the assumptions with an open mind. Second, as the second bullet above implies, continuously think and teach "both/and"— meaning that presenting complaints and symptoms always include a physiological level manifestation that is *coexisting and inseparable* from psychological/social/environmental factors. We must practice applying these efforts to both patients and ourselves. Validating and normalizing unique variations from person to person and culture to culture, instead of pathologizing psychology and behavior, will enrich our professional and personal experiences.

Shame

If someone is experiencing shame as an undercurrent to their experience, they will be more apt to:

- withdraw (isolate, hide)
- attack self (criticism, self-blame, self-harm behaviors, rigidity, judgment)
- attack others (blaming, projecting, reacting defensively)
- avoid (denial, self-medicating behaviors/strategies).[32]

Shame can be seen as an emotion that devours self-worth because it comes not from the sense that one has done something wrong, but that one *is* wrong or bad or broken at the core. As a result, experiences that might trigger the feeling of shame are often avoided. Shame may also be present in high-functioning (e.g., perfectionism) or low-achieving (procrastinating, indifferent, unmotivated, learned helplessness) tendencies. We must look below the surface to consider if/how shame may be interacting within ourselves and others' presentations, behaviors, and internal experiences. Ultimately, we must provide shame-countering messages and experiences. The whole of IRP is designed with this goal in mind.

> **Experiential pause:** Imagine you are sitting with a patient, and consider how you can enact each of the following concepts, pausing after reading each one.
>
> - Listening before teaching.
> - Frequently asking open-ended questions that allow the person to share more about their experience.
> - Normalizing the patient's experience or presentation instead of labeling/ pathologizing it.
> - Demonstrating patience rooted in understanding a person through the lens of longer-term life processes.
> - Holding awareness of one's own desire to help and how it can lead to an over-reduction of what the patient is experiencing in service to a "fix-it" approach that may add harm in unintended, hidden ways.
>
> Now, take a moment to document your answer to the following question: How do these ways of interacting support fundamental human needs and general psychological processes?

PERSONALITY AS A SPRINGBOARD TO DELINEATE SCOPE OF PRACTICE AND REINFORCE CONTEXT

It is vital when we explore the individual relevance of psychological subtopics in our work as rehabilitation professionals that we do so from a curious, caring, educational, and invitational stance. For most rehabilitation professions, diagnosing, analyzing, and/ or advising around specific psychological content is not called for. Additionally, unless you are a mental health provider who has specific training, IRP should not include taking people into regressive explorations and states. Instead, the aim is a focus on *present-moment* experiences and skills. The adage "Look back but don't stare" conveys the intent to stay with the present experience. If past events are impacting the present, we can of course acknowledge that fact, but we must stay focused in the present.

Further, and for example, if personality is affecting someone's health experience, create invitations for the person to self-define those traits rather than providing labels or names *for* them. These principles are true for the whole of each person's unique psychological variables. If more rigorous approaches are needed to assist a patient in unearthing and addressing the ways in which psychological dynamics may impede their ability to move towards well-being, referrals to dedicated mental health professionals are warranted.

Separate from defining scopes of practice, we invite *all* professionals to consider that some modes of interacting with another's experience—diagnosing/pathologizing, analyzing, advising, or regression—may add inadvertent harm. As discussed, when exploring shared needs and communication, we all seek to be seen, heard, and supported by our fellow human beings. We also seek mastery in relationship with our own experience. As such, the goal is to support processes of self-discovery and understanding of how our unique experiences (in this case, of personality) play a role within larger BME relationships. Help people see that they are whole.

While we are advocating for a broad view of what is considered "normal," there are behaviors that fall outside of "normal." Here, "outside normal" simply means "not working in this context" as all behavior has worked at some point in a person's life. Again, using personality as the example, if a troubling personality is present to the degree that it impairs the person's behaviors and functionality (including their ability to participate in therapy), your way of relating to the person is a first key site of therapeutic impact. Aim to look below the surface in a way that seeks understanding of the hidden determinants to that dynamic. Implicit acceptance and working with what the dynamic brings up in yourself goes a long way. Rehabilitation professionals are encouraged to think closely about whether/when referral to mental health resources is needed and how this might be received. Subsequently, the way in which any such suggestion is conveyed to the individual carries significant weight—it must be done in a respectful manner that reflects enactive compassion to minimize stigma and shame.

> **Experiential pause:** You are working with a person experiencing persistent pain. Take a piece of paper and write down examples of safe ways to present this person with the understanding that one's emotions and/or personality characteristics are represented by and interact with the biological underpinnings of pain. If you have studied pain neuroscience education (Chapter 16), you may already have some basic strategies. If you struggle with this, contemplate the relevance of context (Figure 6.2). We invite you to discuss this experiential pause and Figure 6.2 with your colleagues to deepen your ability to safely engage in self-appraisal—from a non-diagnostic, non-reduced, and non-judgmental lens. This applies to any facet of one's psychological landscape, not just personality.

In Figure 6.2, the upper component (soup recipe analogy) was seen in Chapter 3 to demonstrate complexity. Each of the many "ingredients" could be expanded upon as is shown for personality, creating an even deeper look into complexity. Various patterns within the whole may carry positive or negative valence. When identified and supported, transformational influence can shift the trajectory of health towards greater or lesser well-being.

It is vital to recognize that our use of personality as an example here aims to promote understanding and, ultimately, to *de-emphasize* (aka explore in relative context) it. Historically, efforts to explore associations between personality and pain have been reductionistic and stigmatizing. The reader is reminded that no one part is ever going to be causal in isolation and the whole must be held to maintain compassionate (and accurate) understanding. We are never "treating" a personality, an emotion, or any other part; instead, we are seeing these facets in context and supporting the whole.

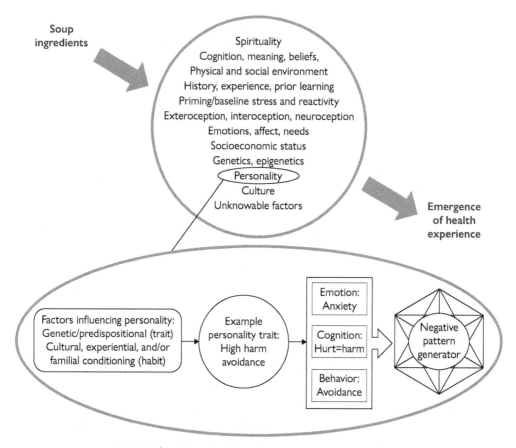

FIGURE 6.2: BREAKING DOWN INDIVIDUAL INGREDIENTS

Note: We have chosen to use the phrase "negative pattern generator" to represent concepts related to ACT's construct of "psychological inflexibility." Either term could carry a valence. In the context of this discussion, consider something along the lines of: "no longer effective biobehavioral patterns that benefit from the flexibility and adaptability gained in awareness and skills development." (See Chapter 17 for more on ACT as a model that supports the concepts presented here.)
Partially adapted from Conrad *et al.*[33]

THE DRIVE FOR PERSONAL AUTONOMY

Researchers have demonstrated the importance of empowerment and autonomy to human survival.[34] While further/specific research is needed, it is theorized that control and/or the perception of control directly contribute to neurophysiological processes of habituation/sensitization to one's external environment as well as to one's internal experience(s).[35] In mind-body medicine, researchers suggest that top-down inhibitory pathway influence is not constant, but continuously modulated, influenced by the level of vigilance or attention.[36] Brosschot refers to this as "cognitive-emotional sensitization,"[37] wherein forebrain products—the neurophysiological correlates of cognitions, emotions, attention, and motivation—have direct influence on sensation and systemic physiology.[38]

In essence, perceptions of both safety and control/autonomy/empowerment around one's experience heavily influence health processes and interact with personality to shape illness experience. A sense of control predicts survival.[39] It is therefore vital for the clinician to provide choice in treatment, thereby helping to foster the perception of control in the patient. Your task is to discover friendly, safe, and simple ways to assist each patient in strengthening the biological underpinnings of autonomy and the patient's conscious correlates to them.

Having said the preceding, no discussion of perceived control, empowerment, or autonomy is complete without recognition of the research and context presented in Chapter 4 on social determinants of health. External factors across levels of one's environment—such as work, family, organizational, and/or societal dynamics—carry direct impact.[40] Recall from Chapter 3 the discussion on stress. One component of stress comes from the perception of a lack of resources. We must individually and collectively ask: "Is my/our perception accurate? How can we meet needs and what action(s) can we take based on the answer to this question? Is the action an *internal* or *external* one? If external, to what extent can I change the conditions and circumstances that are contributing to disempowerment? If internal, how can I/we change my/our perceptions and beliefs if they are inaccurate?" Keep in mind that sociocultural differences in interpreting this construct (i.e., collectivist versus individualistic cultures) exist. The autonomy of a family unit may be prioritized over individual autonomy in a high-context, collectivist culture. For more on this, see Chapter 25 on the relevance of group-based health care.

> **Experiential pause:** Contemplate what ingredients support autonomy. Bring to mind your current clinical practice. What ways do you use to support the emergence of empowerment and how does this interact with the need for care and nurturing support? You might jot down your thoughts and/or explore this with a colleague. To assist your discussion, consider the following pointers and think:
>
> - experiential learning
> - provision of choice: not too little, not too much
> - balance between experiences of nurturance (which can include passive therapy components) with empowerment (active participation).

COPING AND STRESS

Coping can be conceptualized as the supportive actions, behaviors, or strategies that we consciously or unconsciously utilize to mediate perceived or actual stress, threat, discomfort, unpleasantness, or adverse experience.[41] Coping strategies can be seen as reflecting a person's sense of agency. The degree to which one sees oneself as an either active or passive agent in relation to the external environment, but also internally in relation to one's psyche and/or body, will be reflected in coping styles and strategies, thereby influencing health processes. This raises complicated moral questions around the topics of agency, responsibility, and the shame/blame dynamics explored earlier. While we are held accountable for events we cause through our intentional actions, we still deserve compassion when they lead to bad outcomes. And while we may be presumed to be excused for those things that just happen to us, we are still sometimes subjected to stigma and shame because of them. The presence of this tension "ensures that no matter how clearly we articulate holistic, integrative mechanistic theories of illness, patients and clinicians will continue to struggle with the social and moral meanings of affliction."[42]

In the context of coping, similar to the earlier contextual reminder that comes from Chapter 4 on social determinants of health, a person's real and perceived resources influence how stressful experiences are navigated. The relative presence or absence of affordances is then linked to cognitive patterns and emotional reactions.[43] As such, any consideration of coping strategies, options, and skills must understand that health equality ≠ health equity. While personal responsibility plays a key role in health, *the choices we make depend on the choices we have available to us.* In Chapter 3, we also discussed self-care in context. For some, certain facets of "self-care" may be a luxury. It is necessary to hold a broader understanding around the why and how coping patterns have come to be. This context informs the need for compassion, gentleness, and patience in the exploration of coping patterns. The possibility of transforming maladaptive coping into new resources may follow.

Experiential pause: How do you tend to cope?

Recall the core biology of stress, threat, and trauma responses. The constructs of fight/ flight/freeze/fright/faint have been translated into biobehavioral understandings and present us with a simple starting point for contemplating our own adaptive (and sometimes maladaptive) coping strategies. To these "f"s we will add some others to remind us to not "over-box" anything. In reality, our response to stress, demand, or suffering changes based on the changing conditions of BME. We might add "fold," "fawn," "fake," "friend," or "fatigue" to the list of responses; some examples are included in Figure 6.3. These examples are not absolute and will overlap in various combinations. Our coping patterns may have some foundational tendencies and can also shift over time. The point is to notice and compassionately work with our own tendencies first. It follows to then begin to offer safe contemplative invitations for others. In doing so, we present the opportunity for reappraisal and behavior change processes. Take a few minutes and examine the examples. If desired, add your own. Then, bring to mind recent stressful interactions or experiences in your life, sensing your way into awareness of your own coping tendencies. Inherent to many of these may be aversion to/avoidance of the unpleasantness of the experience.

Finally, consider how your strengths and positive qualities, including those that you intend, interact within the whole mix. Think (and feel) "both/and" here to assist in acknowledging your full humanity.

Fight	Flight	Freeze	Fold
Self-preservation, defensive	Retreat/withdraw	Feeling unreal, spacey	Helpless feelings
Aggressive feelings/behavior	Can't sit still, anxious	Dissociating	Turtle-shell strategy
Externalizing, controlling	Often internalizing	Poor body awareness	Nesting, isolation
High physical tension	Compulsive behaviors/"doing"	Gas/brakes at the same time	Hiding, aversion to living

Fawn	Friend	Fatigue	Fake
People pleasing	Reaching out	Lethargy	Acting "as if"
Fixing, helping, to a fault	Seeking support	Disinterest	Putting on a mask
Focus on others	Sharing, expressing	Procrastination	Pretending
Trouble setting boundaries	Nurturing tendencies	Oversleeping	Avoiding feelings

FIGURE 6.3: EXAMPLES OF COPING PATTERNS

STRANDS IN A WEB

Much of what we have presented here contributes to the foundations of understanding cognitive-behavioral processes. While we will dive into this topic in detail in Chapter 17, a few words are vital to weave a web to support this chapter. The cognitive level has numerous components unto itself: thoughts, beliefs, perceptions, and expectations. The thinking mind is assigned a lofty task—to make a sensible story out of all of it. No wonder our minds can run amok so easily. Cognition as a whole is woven into our behaviors; and linked into these patterns are feelings that are inextricably woven into needs. What an amazing web the mind is!

The mind is both an amazing asset and sometimes a stubborn and problematic dictator. Therefore, a few words on change processes are needed to round out this chapter's picture of some of the structural strands in the basic web of human psychology. If you haven't already, you are invited to learn about basic change theory,[44] including in relation to common rehabilitation topics such as exercise participation.[45]

The *transtheoretical model of change* (TMC) provides a foundation for understanding change. In basic form, TMC is presented linearly (Figure 6.4). In reality, change processes are non-linear and in continual flux. For a side trip, a simple overview that you can work with as a learning tool is found online (see Resources at the end of the chapter).

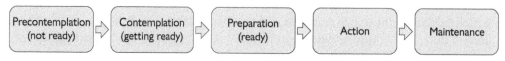

FIGURE 6.4: TRANSTHEORETICAL MODEL OF CHANGE

Finally, it is vital to connect personal values to any model of change. When committed action is informed by one's chosen values (more on this also in Chapter 17), our ability to transform patterns that are no longer working for us is enhanced. Principles of motivational interviewing (MI) may also assist us in bridging a common gap—the gap between idealism and realism in our lives. Bridging this gap assists us in preventing a common setup for the disappointment of perceived failure. Borrowing from a common teaching in recovery communities: "serenity is inversely proportional to…expectations."[46] This does not mean we abandon expectations; rather, we benefit from aiming for more realistic ones. We will have more on MI in Chapter 8; the reader is also pointed towards another side trip to explore MI if this approach is new to your practice (see Resources at the end of the chapter).

GOING DEEPER WITH SELF-REVIEW

Consistent self-review is part of a commitment to professional growth that IRP emphasizes because it supports mutual learning, quality of care, and a collectivist view of healthcare. What follows is a series of three tools to utilize as part of ongoing self-review. These tools build on understanding the normalcy of psychological processes in our lives and go further into personal psychospiritual development in support of those processes. Complete these in writing and continue to return to them as often as needed in practicing self-review.

Experiential pause: Tool 1: Identifying Values

Take some time to consider what is vital and meaningful to you in life. Consider what your highest aspirations are. In doing this, a starting point is to consider your present experience in life. What qualities and/or values, if embodied and enacted through your being, would serve you and your relationships with others? Courage, patience, gentleness, kindness? Forgiveness? Honesty? Gratitude? Contentment? It is important to find your own labels for the qualities and values. Write them down and consider them to be intentions, but also already part of your innate and whole being…just perhaps hidden, obscured, or as yet unrevealed. Now, focus on your bodily sensation(s) and be curious about how, if these qualities were fully embodied, it would feel. How would it affect your body language, posture, and movement habits? How would it have an impact on your listening to others? Your tone of voice?

Experiential pause: Tool 2: Confucius' Retrospective Review*

---

*   Author note: We believe this approach is attributed to Confucius; however, the exact source is unknown.

Every day I examine myself on these three points: in acting on behalf of others:

- Have I always been loyal to their interests?
- Have I always been true to my word?
- Have I failed to repeat the precepts that have been handed down to me?

Experiential pause: Tool 3: Pythagoras' Retrospective Writing[47]

1. Identify a recent challenging experience—preferably related to patient care, but any challenging relational experience that comes to mind.
2. Write out exactly what you remember happening with as much neutrality as possible, and particularly noting what feelings were evoked in the interaction. Include earlier parts of the day this event occurred to cultivate awareness of how the larger context of your experience entered into the situation. Be careful to not explain, judge, criticize, condemn, change, justify, or analyze yourself or the other person…be matter of fact.
3. Draw a line underneath this account and then rewrite the entire event, keeping everything the same except for your own responses, thoughts, feelings, and actions. Then revise your own part in the situation, changing yourself so that you act and think and feel according to the best and highest understanding conceivable to you.
4. Now, visualize this new version of the interaction in a mental rehearsal, engaging all your senses as vividly as possible in your imagination.

ORIENTING AND RESOURCING

Whether we are deliberately delivering an integrative model of care or not, we are human. We have struggles. We sometimes feel overwhelmed. Powerful emotions like anger, fear, shame, or grief may arise in us. Such emotions, whether they come up for us as practitioners or in our patients in treatment, can make us want to "escape" or "check out" of our present-moment experience. These emotions can more easily be dealt with if we have strategies that can help orient us (and our patients) back to a sense of strength, stability, and what is sometimes referred to as "centeredness," "rootedness," or "groundedness." One can imagine the earth/ground beneath as a reminder of a sense of stability and strength, a "constant" in the midst of a stressful and chaotic emotion or life experience.

In trauma-informed care (which is good care for all; see Appendix B), it is important to know when a person may benefit from guided orienting and resourcing skills for regulating and navigating through stormy waters. Beyond all else, your own presence, your capacity to regulate, and your comfort level with others' distress is vital. Specific strategies that may be helpful in the face of powerful emotions include enacting practices and asking questions such as those below that can aid in achieving focus, regulation, and comfort.

- To help maintain focus on the present moment, ask: "Can you share what is happening and what you are aware of right now? Does it help to remind yourself that you are here, now, in the present, and with me?"

- To facilitate co-regulation, make and/or invite increased eye contact,** attune to conscious breathing, and connect oneself to a strong sense of embodied presence. Then, invite empowerment through cues such as: "What do you need, if anything, right now?"

- To orient the patient, focus on senses. Ask: "What do you see, what do you hear, *right now*? Be specific, name what you can become aware of in your senses."

- Guide toward settling in the body and offer a reminder of the connection to the ground/earth beneath as/if needed. For example, ask: "Does it help to focus on slowing your breathing? What do you notice in your body? Can you focus on your hands and feet for a moment? Does it help to focus on the sensations of the chair against your seat and back? Would lying down help? Would it help if I placed my hand on your shoulder or back as you are experiencing this?" Remember that sometimes sensations in the body are not tolerated because they are experienced as overwhelming, so an external (instead of interoceptive) focus may be warranted/useful.

SUMMARIZING

In this chapter, we have looked over foundational concepts that support whole-person, psychologically informed, and integrated practice. As Joan Halifax said: "I believe that excluding any part of the larger landscape of our lives reduces the territory of our understanding."[48] This quotation underscores the importance of connecting dots across the various facets of human psychology and behavior.

Taking a strengths-based approach when exploring the unique psychological makeup that we and others carry is sage advice. Being mindful to not allow our shared tendency for negativity bias to rule our perceptions and our approach and instead striving to see the whole offers us a better lens. Additionally, when we understand that the foundations of psychology as presented in this chapter are shared amongst all people and grounded in our biology, the capacity to destigmatize and normalize our experiences is enhanced.

It is not our job to fix others. It is our job to be of service and to help remove barriers to their capacity to heal. This starts with presence and implicit acceptance. From there, we support the possibility of opening doorways that enable people to come to understand and define their own experience, to appraise and reappraise the experience, and to move in the direction of increased personal autonomy and connection along the way. For this reason, any exploration of the ways in which individual traits and characteristics might be influencing health is best done from a gentle, curious, and invitational stance—not an analytical or diagnostic one. The phrase "invitations into awareness and contemplation" reflects a solid stance for the recommended approach.

For any of this to develop and grow in ourselves, *self*-appraisal, -application, and -practice are needed. All efforts to deepen your own personal understanding of needs,

---

** Of note, in some cultures, such as some indigenous cultures, making eye contact is considered rude and inappropriate; this is an example of being aware of cultural differences and practicing flexibility as needed.

affect/feelings/emotions, communication, personality, coping, and cognitive-behavioral processes facilitate the possibility of transformational growth in others too. Understand and see yourself clearly by cultivating an accepting, compassionate, non-analyzing, and non-fixing relationship with yourself. Start there. Stay there. The rest will follow, and addressing psychological dynamics will become normal and natural—in the sense that it becomes second nature to offer whole-person support that needs no label...not even the integrative one.

Experiential pause: Having read this chapter, identify and write down at least one actionable item of interest to you. In doing so, consider ways in which applying the material first to yourself, and then to patients, might serve those who come to you for care.

RESOURCES

- For a self-study overview of personality traits see: www.colby.edu/psych/wp-content/uploads/sites/50/2018/03/Soto_2018.pdf.

- For an applied overview of the transtheoretical model of change see: www.embodyyourmind.com/wp-content/uploads/2020/02/Transtheoretical-Model.pdf.

- For a self-study guide to motivational interviewing see: www.nova.edu/gsc/forms/mi-techniques-skills.pdf.

- The Center for Nonviolent Communication offers free companion downloads of useful lists of needs (www.cnvc.org/training/resource/needs-inventory) and feelings (www.cnvc.org/training/resource/feelings-inventory) that we are more likely to experience when our needs are met versus those when our needs are not met. These can be a simple springboard for discussion.

- There are many variations on Plutchik's "Wheel of Emotions." These graphics can serve as a useful springboard to assist individuals in labeling their emotions. You can search the internet to find examples. A good overview of working with a fuller theory of emotion in relation to Plutchik's Wheel can be found here: https://positivepsychology.com/emotion-wheel.

CHAPTER 7

The Science of Integrative Practice

Daniel Winkle, MD and Matt Erb, PT

INQUIRING MINDS WANT TO KNOW

Science represents a rich backdrop to health care. Peer-reviewed science brings support and validation for health-care approaches, including integrative rehabilitation practice (IRP). Science is important, imperfect, and transforming. The vastness and steady expansion of references means we are only scratching the surface here and across the book. We encourage you to relate to the rapidly changing science by applying IRP principles to the science itself. For example, process orientation, complex thinking, and humility are necessary to best interact with the material in context. The ultimate aim of the science (and our relationship with the science) aims to support the reality of the person in front of us.

Most scientific pursuits are reductionistic. In relationship to clinical health care, integral thinking demands connecting dots and building bridges to pull us back up and out of excessive reduction; towards seeing the bigger picture of factors informing and influencing emergence. Further, integral thinking in relation to science is approached through the lens of understanding substrates of human experience. Human behavior includes implicit biological drives towards safety (security), nurturance (connection), and empowerment (autonomy). This lens helps us look for collaborative (instead of oppositional) understandings across different levels, and more importantly can drive the how and why of the care we offer our fellow human beings.

As we consider the relevance of multiple disciplines in offering up a foundational science, a solid starting point lies in the science of mind-body medicine (MBM). Why? MBM is already rooted in integral inquiry, including the complex field of psychoneuroendocrinoimmunology (PNEI). PNEI takes a transdisciplinary approach, connecting dots across: neuroscience, molecular biology, psychology, immunology, physiology, genetics, pharmacology, psychiatry, behavioral medicine, endocrinology, and more. PNEI and the MBM interventions that arise from PNEI have an increasing evidence base.[1]

MIND-BODY MEDICINE

Chapter 2 covered rationale for the foundations of mind-body medicine within IRP. Given that stress and allostatic load are relevant in some way to most experiences and forms of illness and disease (see Chapter 3), it follows that addressing the underpinnings of stress carries importance. An integral lens on stress reminds us that there are entry points for stress: physical, historical, environmental, mental, emotional, social/relational, financial, cultural, spiritual, and more. Across these, we must consider historical (remember adverse childhood experiences, ACEs, from Chapter 4?), present (e.g., loss of employment, relationship distress), and future (anticipated, worry, anxiety) patterns of stress. Effective patient support that is built on this integral construct of stress is often overlooked in our focus on "sick care." We miss roots. However, we can grow roots by further exploring the science and utility of MBM.

There are many changes that occur in the body in response to MBM interventions. Many changes are governed by changes in homeostasis and the stress response.[2] MBM skills can exert significant effects on central nervous system (CNS) neuroplasticity, the autonomic nervous system (ANS), hormones, the immune system, and even our DNA. Some people may have the perception that MBM is solely about relaxation. The relaxation response[3] is decidedly important, but as noted in Chapter 3, it is not a complete picture. MBM in context sees the use of these skills as part of the larger context of social determinants to health, processes of resilience, mature coping, and the cultivation of psychospiritual well-being. In this chapter, we explore how mind-body and integrative-oriented activities affect brain-body physiology, within the lens of an integrated body-mind-environment (BME).

A DELICATE DANCE

We are hardwired for survival. When real, potential, or perceived threat to bodily, psychological, or existential security is present, the integrated brain-body response ensues. The ANS is a critical system and consists of two divisions, the parasympathetic nervous system (PNS) and the sympathetic nervous system (SNS). The SNS mobilizes the body's resources to respond to demand. The PNS is geared towards returning the system back towards "rest and digest" states. These two synergistic divisions aim to support whole-organism homeostatic processes in response to continually changing BME conditions.

Defensive or excessive activation of the SNS is often referred to as the "fright, fight, or flight" response. On a need-based gradient, a sympathetic dominant response increases heart rate and blood pressure leading to: blood rushing to large muscles of the body; releases of neuroendocrine factors such as adrenaline; dilated pupils; increased respiratory rate; reduced blood flow to the gut; and increased blood glucose.[4] In optimal functioning, short periods of heightened sympathetic activity have no long-term consequences and are normal and healthy—"eustress" as coined by Hans Selye.[5] Think exercise.

For the PNS, excess activation is often referred to as the "freeze," faint, immobility, or collapse response. Extreme PNS activation reflects the biological basis of feigning death as well as dissociative states (loss of consciousness). These responses are best seen as occurring on an endless spectrum of combinations and variations in human experience.[6]

As described in the *polyvagal theory* (PVT), in optimal conditions the "highest" form of responsiveness to stress can occur through prosocial engagement, communal support, and higher cognitive processes.[7] PVT posits a mechanism for functional switching between stress response strategies, something that largely occurs outside of conscious awareness. PVT reminds us that we can develop awareness of these patterns and gain better conscious influence of them and that we carry a design for doing so in forums of mutual support. PVT will be presented in more detail and contexts across future chapters.

The doctrine of *autonomic* space suggests that autonomic function is dynamic, synchronous, and highly variable.[8] Numerous possible patterns of coactivation, co-inhibition, and reciprocal and independent activation/inhibition are possible.[9] Standard presentations of ANS function often miss the integral view of such variability, let alone a larger understanding of how the ANS is inseparable from the whole of the body's systems including the CNS,[10] the hypothalamic-pituitary-adrenal (HPA) neuroendocrine axis (see below), sensory modulation,[11] and more.

When the whole of integrated and distributed systems is functioning optimally, the activity within the ANS can be seen to effectively wax and wane in response to the endless flux of BME interactions. When this network loses capacity to optimally dance its waltz (aka *dysregulation*), negative impact on inflammation, mood, focus, neuromuscular tone, immune system function, and more may ensue.[12] While not absolute, dysregulated patterns of physiologic arousal/reactivity correlate to behavioral responses[13] and are increasingly associated with a wide range of conditions such as gastrointestinal disorders, pain conditions, cardiac conditions, and autism.[14]

Persistent dysregulation has implications within the whole of illness, injury, and disease states.[15] Figure 7.1 shows a simplified teaching construct to convey the concept of ANS dysregulation. As explored in Chapters 3 and 4, *allostasis* reflects the integrated processes for maintaining homeostasis through physiological and behavioral change. In some cases, increased "allostatic load" from unmitigated stress may exceed capacity and a host of physical, mental/emotional, and behavioral problems may arise.[16] The good news: many integrative therapies exert influence on the ANS,[17] carrying impact across the whole of integrated physiological systems. Consciously and actively participating in the creation of this influence comes with a reminder from Chapter 3's look at burnout in relation to stress: cultivating various types of conscious influence is considered part of cultivating resilience—the ability to "bounce back."[18]

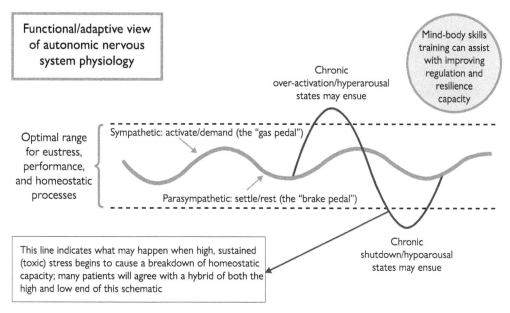

FIGURE 7.1: THEORETICAL PATTERNS OF AUTONOMIC REGULATION
Adapted from Ranjbar & Erb[19] (Under Creative Commons License: CC BY-NC-ND 4.0)

DYSREGULATION AS ADAPTIVE

Toxic stress (introduced in Chapter 4) ensues when stress is high, prolonged, and/or unmitigated. As initially covered in Chapter 4, the understanding that *early* stress may lead to pervasive dysregulation and impairment is well established in developmental science and informs models of toxic stress as seen in Figure 7.1. An evolutionary-developmental perspective on adaptations to stress proposes that stress, especially early in life, prompts the development of necessary, adaptive, yet potentially costly strategies that are unconsciously aimed at survival.[20] This perspective complements models of dysregulation and can be seen as consistent with models of maladaptive coping[21] and/or psychological inflexibility[22] as avenues of transmission for later biological influence that may ensue from early life adversity.[23] The evolutionary-developmental perspective includes a life-history framework[24] that considers individual differences that inform the uniqueness of BME interactions, underscoring the rationale for IRP's advocacy to approach historical factors as contextual considerations, without making direct or immediate assumptions as to relevance.

PREPARATORY-SET

Similar to PVT, the concept of the preparatory-set presents us with an additional integrative view of whole-organism responsiveness to physical, mental, or environmental stress that proves useful in clinical reasoning. *Preparatory-set* is defined as the: "unitary, largely subcortical organization of the organism in preparation for response to environmental conditions."[25] Five interwoven components are delineated: physical posture/muscle tone, visceral state/ANS, affective state, arousal/attention, and cognitive expectation. By affecting any component within the preparatory-set, associated shifts in the other components ensue as part of an integrated response to demand. Researchers have demonstrated associations between components of the preparatory-set. For example, changes in muscle tone or posture have been correlated with concomitant changes in ANS activity.[26] Movement and postural shifts, including those imagined, are correlated to emotional and affective states and can also be used to enhance emotion regulation.[27] Associations between ANS state and affective states have been observed between cardiorespiratory activity and heart rate variability and linked to emotions.[28]

A maladaptive preparatory-set reflects a model for increased allostatic load, while an adaptive one correlates with both regulation and the degree of resilience of the organism.[29] Therapeutic approaches designed for deliberate BME integration, such as yoga therapy, may be effective in cultivating regulation and resilience of the human system through these impacts on an integrated preparatory-set.[30] Preparatory-set reflects an evidence-extrapolated theory rooted in principles of interdependence within the whole. Preparatory-set and PVT both support cultivating whole-person inquiry and treatment approaches.

THE POTENTIAL FOR CONSCIOUS INFLUENCE

An integrated biobehavioral response to stress is necessary and useful for short durations. In animals, if threat passes, this intense activation is "discharged" (released) through a number of mechanisms, such as shaking, trembling, social engagement, changes in body temperature, and processes of elimination. In humans, this equally happens when BME conditions support it. However, the picture can look very different. Processes of memory and conditioning interact with each person's unique psychophysiological experience, setting a stage for the possibility of prolonged difficulty in returning to states of safety, rest, and balance.

Enter the potential for harnessing the power of the mind-body connection. MBM skills, which enhance conscious attention to one's unique blend of mental/cognitive states, bodily sensations, emotions, etc., allow us to willfully and actively contribute to the body's ability to restore balance. Our thoughts, beliefs, imagination, intentions, and use of skilled practices all can mitigate allostatic load, even in the presence of ongoing stress.[31]

While modern science is increasingly affirming the utility of MBM,[32] subjective reports of improvements from breathing and meditation have been passed down through centuries. These benefits may include stress reduction, reduced anxiety, decreased depression, improved memory, and increased efficiency. As authors of this chapter, we both have had the experience of practicing conscious, relaxed breathing over a long period of time. We have had the benefit of studying the neuroscience and physiology of this activity. Collectively, our breathwork and studies have led to finding ourselves thinking things like: "So this is what it feels like to have increased activity and neural connections in the prefrontal cortex and parasympathetic activity in my gut!"—all while noticing improved responsiveness to emotionally challenging events that might have significantly disturbed us in the past.

The use of MBM in self-care or clinical practice comes with a reminder: we are creatures of comfort and appreciate quick relief. Conveying the message that MBM is "powerful with patience," while encouraging its utilization from a place of innate valuation as opposed to expectation of or attachment to a quick fix, is sage advice.

NEUROENDOCRINE FUNCTION

Cortisol and adrenaline, the most well known of the body's primary stress hormones, are secreted in response to stress.[33] In healthy states, the release of adrenaline (shorter acting) and cortisol (longer acting) subsequently sets up an inhibitory feedback loop that can effectively shut the response down when the demand passes.

One of the well-known consequences of long-term dysregulation from toxic stress is a breakdown of the HPA axis, which manages the neuroendocrine component of the system.[34] However, such processes of breakdown are subject to many factors including individual variability.[35] The detection and perception of threat is one such variable (recall threat appraisal from Chapter 4).

Neuroception refers to the collective mechanisms that an organism uses to detect possible threat.[36] The traditional view of the link between neuroception and the HPA axis largely occurs in the hypothalamus. The hypothalamus is sometimes referred to as a master switching station for the ANS. As the brain processes senses/sensation and its link to thoughts and emotions, nerves in the hypothalamus are activated to signal the pituitary gland located just below the hypothalamus.[37] The pituitary gland then secretes hormones signaling systemic bodily processes. A primary site of action of signaling is in the adrenal glands located just above the kidneys—home to cortisol production. When corticocotropin releasing factor (CRF) stimulates the pituitary gland to make adrenocorticotropic hormone (ACTH), the adrenals ramp up cortisol production to prepare for demand.[38]

The science of the HPA neuroendocrine axis is foundational within PNEI research and our understanding of its importance is not immutable. In an important example of how established scientific understandings change as new discoveries are made, some recent research into the neuroendocrinology of stress lends us a hand. Researchers discovered that bony vertebrates are unable to muster the defensive responses to danger without the skeleton! The researchers found that, in both mice and humans, almost immediately after danger is detected the *skeleton* floods the bloodstream with the bone-derived hormone osteocalcin to turn on these protective responses. The researchers suggest that adrenaline is not necessarily needed to mobilize this facet of the fight/flight response and that osteocalcin may play a more vital role than adrenaline/cortisol. This explains why adrenal-insufficient patients can still mobilize this vital response. The research delineates how osteocalcin allows an acute stress response to unfold by signaling post-synaptic parasympathetic neurons to inhibit their activity. This leaves the action of sympathetic tone unopposed.[39]

What is the take home? First, it brings a reminder that our understandings, meanings, and beliefs are always evolving. We must be flexible! Second, this example offers us a glimpse into the idea that behavior, rooted in survival mechanisms, is best seen through an integral view of *whole-organism responsiveness*. For example, we tend to reduce to just the brain. While questions remain, the study suggests a rather instantaneous, whole-organism response to threat that may act independent of the classical view of HPA signaling. While the details of this science will continue to evolve, will the core understanding that at one level we are all driven by survival biology change? We can begin to see and support each individual's experiences through the larger lens of systemically distributed and coordinated responses—the whole depends on the parts.

> **Experiential pause:** Information overload? We spend much of our time absorbed in mental processes, aka thinking! Regular shifting of attention from the cognitive realm, to the body, is useful. Pause and see how this information is landing in your body. Improved focus/attention for learning is benefited by many things including relaxing tension as well as through movement. Would it help to take a quick movement break? Or to scan the body, attune to the breath, and relax body tension? Consider doing this frequently through the remainder of the chapter as well as across the book.

THIS IS STRESSING ME OUT

We've talked about stress both here and back in Chapter 3. Stopping to ask how stress is actually defined yields additional insight. For example, stress can imply a mental or emotional tension in response to certain conditions or circumstances: "I'm stressed out." But what does this mean at a scientific level? Given that "stress" is a highly subjective phenomenon, defining it can come in a variety of forms. Hans Selye, mentioned earlier, loosely defined stress as a non-specific response of the body to any demand for change.[40]

Stress can also be seen as the psychobiological response that ensues when an individual perceives that the demands placed on them exceed their capacity to cope, and therefore introduces threat to physical, psychological, and/or existential well-being.[41] A similar but simpler definition: stress is the body's response when the mind perceives a lack of resources. Here, we must ask a series of interrelated questions: Is our perception of the stressful conditions/situation accurate? If the answer is "no," how can our perception be reappraised to something more workable? If our answer is "yes," how can we take action that meets needs in relation to the conditions/situation; is this action an internal or external action? In working through this latter scenario, we must consider that "resources" applies to our earlier list of entry points—for example, if resources are absent at the physical, environmental, or nutritional level, is it possible to acquire or address those resources as part of mitigating stress? If not, do I return to an internal action? Most situations demand a hybrid of these strategies for responding to stress.

The most agreed-upon stressor is the imminent threat of physical/bodily harm. However, significant stress occurs when other aspects of our lives and identities are threatened. And, this includes the brand of stress that is not immediately addressable by the individual: stressors that are embedded in the social determinants of health such as employment/economic status, family dynamics, social status, and environmental/ecological conditions.[42]

In optimal conditions, when real or perceived threat ceases and a sense of safety is restored, the stress response "shuts off." Unfortunately, in humans the stress response can be maintained through various psychophysiological mechanisms such as:

- procedural (implicit or unconscious) memory and/or declarative memory (explicit memory of prior experience)[43]
- mechanisms of the imagination (more on this in Chapter 14)
- various facets of the psyche (perceptions, personality, beliefs, thoughts, emotions, etc.).[44]

Interestingly, even a belief that stress is bad for us can paradoxically add to or worsen the potentially deleterious effects of stress![45]

Experiential pause: What is one to do with the often-gloomy look at the impact of toxic stress in our lives? We tend to focus on deficits. Applying the IRP model assists. Many things, such as giving to others,[46] can ameliorate the effects of stress. IRP intends to understand and support the deficits while focusing on a strength-based approach: cultivating skills that support overall biobehavioral regulation capacity, resilience, relationship, and well-being in the context of all of these various "stress" constructs. Read the following examples, consider how they apply to working with the reality of stress in ourselves and with our patients, and write down your thoughts in your journal.

- What's right (with your body, your life, etc.)?
- It (any particular past or present stress pattern) may or may not be relevant— what do you feel? (person-centered)
- What's happening right now? (present moment)
- We have some tools that assist us in addressing the impact of stress in our health—would you like to experience some of these to see if they might support you? (person-centered, self-selected for choice/autonomy)

THE OFTEN-IGNORED SYMPTOMS

Individuals presenting with health challenges are usually met with a focus on "chief complaint." Fix-it efforts typically ensue. Inquiring into both the psychosocial context of the person's experience and the larger spectrum of possible accompanying symptoms may alert us to the relevance of stress and dysregulation as an underlying construct. Such symptoms[47] are shown in Figure 7.2. Many times our treatment methods address the end result of the impact of the stress response on component parts or symptoms, without attempting to address psycho-social-spiritual factors that tip the scale towards toxic stress. Furthermore, it is rare that attempts to address this construct aim to do so in an integral way. This creates a cycle: one symptom or problem is resolved and a new one arises because the underlying factors are either ignored or ineffectively addressed.

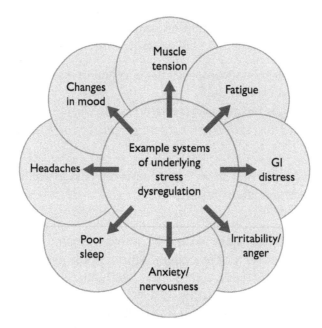

FIGURE 7.2: POTENTIAL STRESS IMPACTS

CONNECTING DOTS

As we move forward, there are additional and important topics to name. These include inflammation and immunity, the gut-brain and heart-brain connections, neuroplasticity and neurogenesis, and epigenetics. We'll touch on each before delving into the intersection of science, mind-body processes, theory, and philosophy. These topics have intricate connections taking us back to the basics of PNEI. In a reflection of the upside of scientific specialization, each topic warrants entire textbooks! Here however we present a short overview of each topic in support of connecting dots and encouraging integral thinking.

Inflammation and immunity

Toxic stress is linked to damage of the body's systems through immune and inflammatory responses. Inflammation plays a significant role in the etiology of disease across the lifespan.[48] There are many variables that contribute to inflammation, including the role that chronic stress plays.[49] When homeostasis is restored following acute stress reactions, cortisol and glucocorticoid hormones have an anti-inflammatory effect. This reflects a cycle of turning on and off inflammation for normal healing responses.

Prolonged physical or psychologic stress negatively impacts these processes. With prolonged elevation of cortisol and other glucocorticoid stress hormones, the body's reaction to the stress hormones changes from an anti-inflammatory response to a pro-inflammatory response. Chronically elevated pro-inflammatory immune responses have been linked to common diseases such as hypertension, atherosclerosis, diabetes, depression, Parkinson's disease, and cancer.[50]

In terms of immunity, stress equally takes a toll. The cells and organs of the immune system all have connections to the nervous system. Neuroendocrine receptors allow the integrated system to react and adjust to changes in the nervous system and/or hormonal activity in response to stress. Authors of a meta-analysis looked at chronically stressful situations, such as caring for a loved one with dementia, living with disability, and unemployment. In the chronically stressed, there were reductions in natural and specific immunity, decreased T cell proliferation in response to infection, and decreased antibody titers in response to vaccinations.[51]

Immune system changes may take place in the face of chronic stress in terms of how the immune system responds to stressful events. When faced with elevated cortisol, the immune system can either fall short (immunosuppression) or overreact (autoimmunity) in its efforts. An example is found in an altered ratio of neutrophil cells to lymphocytes, where an inability to make changes in these ratios in the presence of elevated cortisol has been correlated to susceptibility to developing cold symptoms when exposed to the rhinovirus.[52]

Inflammation and immunity do not occur in isolation from each other nor other processes such as tissue repair.[53] Even more importantly, they do not occur separately from the regulation of social behavior.[54] How does the whole of each person's unique BME experience across time show up in chronic inflammation, altered immunity, or…

The gut-brain connection

How often do we hear things like "What is your gut telling you?" or "I've got a gut feeling about this"? These phrases and metaphors are common and widespread across cultures and languages. Further, comorbidity between psychiatric disorders and functional gastrointestinal (GI) disorders is well documented; plausible models for the shared mechanisms that may promote and maintain both socioemotional and GI dysfunction exist.[55] Together, the commonality of mind-body metaphor in our culture and the prevalence of comorbidity point us back towards BME interdependence and a rich, growing science. All of the body's systems are intimately connected and communicating.

It follows that the stress response and gut are intimately linked, including in relationship to the body's microbiome. The introduction of processed foods in large quantities in the developed world has changed the gut microbiome.[56] Early-life factors can also negatively impact the condition of the gut microbiome in childhood. These include antibiotic exposure, lack of breastfeeding, birth by Caesarean section, infection, and stress exposure. This in turn can affect the body's stress physiology as well.[57] The gut, brain, and stress response are connected in part through the vagus nerve. They are also connected via the immune system, endocrine communication, and proteins/fatty acids that circulate through the bloodstream. Gut-brain communication is bidirectional. Prolonged activation of the body's stress response changes the microbiome, and changing the microbiome of the gut changes the body's response to stress.[58] Changes in the gut microbiome also are correlated to changes in serotonin responsible for changes in mood in the brain and gut motility in the digestive tract.[59]

The CNS and ANS communicate with the gut via cranial nerve X, the famous vagus! The vagus nerve is a primary route for both the efferent distribution of the PNS and bottom-up afferent communication. In essence, it is capable of turning the stress response up or down, even in the absence of changes in sympathetic activity.[60] Improved vagal nerve tone and its impact on mood has been studied using implanted vagal-nerve stimulators.[61] This is an example of a biomedical interpretation and approach to these connections and reflects advancements in technology and science. It also can be seen as reflecting a tendency to favor passive approaches to improving such physiological relationships. IRP encourages active participation even if/when such technology is deployed. Many things can improve vagal function including mind-body skills such as combinations of meditation,[62] conscious breathing,[63] exercise/movement,[64] body awareness,[65] and diet/ nutrition.[66] For the latter, beneficial and healthy gut bacteria can directly improve vagus nerve functioning.[67]

The heart-brain connection

Similarly, the CNS and ANS share the same intimate relationship with the heart and cardiovascular system that they do with the gut. How often do we hear things like "It's breaking my heart" or "Listen to your heart, not just your head"? The vagus nerve plays a vital role here as well. Heart rate variability (HRV) reflects slight variations in the time between heartbeats in relation to the breath cycle. HRV is governed by the ANS, and loss of heart variability has been associated with susceptibility to a wide range of health problems up to and including cardiac death.[68] HRV change in response to stress is increasingly considered a valid biomarker for measuring stress load in real time, and low levels of vagal activity are associated with loss of stress resilience.[69] Stay tuned for more on this interesting topic when we explore biofeedback in Chapter 10.

Neuroplasticity and neurogenesis

One of the primary ways the nervous system changes and adapts is through mechanisms of neuroplasticity. For example, neuroplasticity is one of the primary ways the brain recovers from injury. It is also how our nervous systems change and adapt through stages of the life cycle. *Neuroplasticity* reflects the nervous system's ability to form and reorganize synaptic connectivity, including in response to learning, sensory experience, or injury.[70]

Neuroplasticity is repetition driven. This underscores the pop phrase: "Nerves that fire together, wire together." Understanding this is important for several reasons. The first is a reminder that many important chronic health challenges that rehabilitation professionals work with, such as pain or anxiety, are embedded in neurophysiological patterns. The second is reflected in a need to emphasize repetition to influence neuroplasticity, which highlights the importance of perspective within a self-care supported approach to health care. There are no quick fixes. Patience is a virtue. Practice is necessary, whether we are working with stroke recovery or meditation for well-being.[71] Assisting patients in identifying values for implementing potentially beneficial activities is needed. This helps to support commitment and is often necessary for meaningful change.

There are many developing neuroscientific findings in regard to harnessing neuroplasticity.[72] One example study used fMRI to study neuroplasticity after a short four-week intervention with mindfulness training. The researchers showed changes of increased connectivity of the anterior cingulate cortex to other regions of the brain. The function of the anterior cingulate cortex has been implicated in the ability to resolve conflict and exercise control of cognition and emotion. This and similar studies indicate mindfulness training may have a beneficial impact on the rehabilitation process since these are common problems encountered during rehabilitation.[73] We will explore applications of meditation in Chapter 12.

A related topic that has changed early thinking around neuroplasticity is *neurogenesis*. Neurogenesis is the process by which new brain and nerve cells are generated from stem cells.[74] Previously, we believed that stem cells only produced new neurons in the CNS during childhood and adolescence. Early studies in rats[75] have been followed by contemporary human studies demonstrating that neurogenesis occurs as a continual process in the hippocampus of humans.[76] While many questions remain, recent research has shown that neurogenesis takes place in other regions of the brain, including those associated with executive function.[77] While particularly important for healthy brain development during childhood and adolescence, neuroplasticity and neurogenesis are shown to be active throughout our entire lives.[78] For some this may reflect a "neurobiology of hope" and the possibility of transformational change at any time and for any state or set of BME conditions.

Finally, the lessons from neuroplasticity and neurogenesis must not be isolated to the brain. Adaptability and plasticity as potential is best seen as applicable to the entire nervous system, the body's tissues, and the person as a whole. While we may get stuck in physical, mental, or emotional patterns, with support, we can enact shifts and changes across levels of our being.

Epigenetics

The field of epigenetics reflects inquiry into how DNA expression is altered based on experience and environment. Epigenetics highlights the potential for integrated BME interventions to affect our health. Epigenetic research examines changes in organisms caused by gene expression rather than alteration in the genetic code itself.[79] Whether a gene is expressed or not is primarily governed by DNA methylation. Some liken this to an on/off switching mechanism. In the IRP model, a multitude of BME conditions and interactions may include triggers for this switching mechanism. When the environment supports safety and allostasis, gene expression is positively influenced.

Consider the following research in light of IRP.

- Telomeres, which protectively "cap" the ends of chromosomes, are negatively impacted by various patterns of present, historical, or environmental stress.[80]
- Telomeres are positively impacted by various mind-body practices such as meditation, yoga, and Tai Chi.[81]

The study of epigenetics has potential to continue to steer us towards interventions capable of slowing or reversing the negative effects of stress. Epigenetics gives us clues as to some of the disease-preventing abilities of various integrative approaches. Epigenetics also helps us shift a paradigm of thinking from one of being powerless (genetic determinism) to empowerment, wherein we can contribute to concomitant changes in gene expression, when support across levels within the BME is enacted. Here we remind ourselves of holding self-care in context (Chapter 3), including in relation to the many "upstream" social determinants to health (Chapter 4). We have influence. And, there are larger interacting influences, and any notion of "responsibility" must be distributed and shared.

> **Experiential pause:** Information overload again? Shift, adjust, move, or otherwise regulate mind-brain-body tension. Take a minute or five and see how you might modulate your attention (if needed!) by shifting or moving your body-mind state!

PLACEBO, EXPECTATION, AND BELIEF

Placebo means "I shall please." Often the placebo response is defined as occurring when a person experiences improvement from the mechanisms underlying expectations and/ or conditioning: "rather than from the treatment itself."[82] There are identified problems with the phrase "placebo response" that the reader is encouraged to examine.[83] Taken in context, these arguments encourage the use of "meaning response, and its special application in medicine called the healing response,"[84] concepts that stand in support of integrative thinking. More on this in a bit.

It is generally agreed that placebo effects relate to expectations, as well as factors that bolster expectation. The placebo effect is represented by specific physiological correlates and is so well established that most scientific studies seek to rule out this phenomenon. Herein we have an interesting dynamic. For example, a majority of "placebo-controlled" trials cannot be replicated.[85] Second, the effect size above placebo effects in trials that have been reproduced is generally small, for example ~8% for cardiovascular medications.[86] The majority (75%) of overall treatment effect seen in randomized controlled trials for osteoarthritis treatment is attributable to contextual effects rather than the specific effect of treatments.[87] Even the impact from orthopedic joint injection reflects large and lasting impacts attributable to placebo over the "active" agent.[88] Perhaps placebo might be reframed as a key component of treatment itself and the effects of the "active" treatment as additive? Think "placebo plus" while simultaneously noting there are risks that come with this concept such as using placebo to support exaggerated claims and/or to suggest replacement of established and effective biomedical treatment options.[89]

With the preceding acknowledged, we can explore the ways in which expectations and beliefs interact at the cognitive level. The physiology of placebo is linked to the neurocognitive processes that represent both expectations and beliefs, returning us to core foundations within MBM. Beliefs exert powerful influences on biobehavioral patterns,[90] and play an important role in patient experience and outcomes in rehabilitation.[91]

Beliefs arise from a number of sources: individual, societal, and cultural. The current biomedical model has some difficulties with adapting to and honoring both the relevance of belief as well as various cultural approaches to health. For example, patients who choose to take vitamin supplements or utilize complementary and integrative health (CIH) modalities can be ridiculed. Due to this pervasive stigma, 47–71% of CIH users undergoing cancer treatment do not report their CIH usage to their health-care professionals.[92] We will continue to explore these dynamics from the lenses of person-centered care, phenomenology, evidence-based medicine, and philosophy across this book.

THE SCIENCE OF PLACEBO AND IRP

The use of opioid analgesia for pain control has demonstrated increased activity in the rostral anterior cingulate cortex measured using positron emission topography (PET) scan technology. This activity was reproduced in the same parts of the brain when given a placebo pill that the participant believed was a pain-relieving substance. The study demonstrated that the activity diminished both with placebo and opioid medication when given an antidote to opioids, naloxone.[93] This indicates that the mechanism of placebo utilizes some of the same physiological substrates of pain. In addition to mechanisms related to the endogenous opioid mechanism, placebo has been shown to act on/through via numerous other mechanisms. A few examples include:

- non-opioid analgesic mechanisms[94]
- endocrine/neuropeptide pathways[95]
- the immune system[96]
- central stress responses[97]
- motor control[98]
- cardiorespiratory centers.[99]

THE DARK SIDE OF PLACEBO

The placebo effect has been studied for decades and more recently attention has turned to the occurrence of the nocebo effect. *Nocebo* means "I shall harm" and reflects the same psychophysiological dynamics of placebo but in the opposite direction. Negative suggestions and expectations may arise in situ (individual mind-body dynamics) but can also be conveyed by direct verbal or non-verbal communication by the health-care professional.[100] Nocebo has come to the forefront in relation to informed consent. Nocebo is more difficult to study because aiming to have negative outcomes within a study is frowned upon. The nocebo effect was first observed when people in placebo-controlled drug trials were dropping out of studies due to reporting intolerable side effects whilst in the placebo group.[101] Consider the relevance of the following scientific findings in relation to placebo/nocebo and IRP.

- Personality has been linked to nocebo, particularly in persons with tendency to display aggressive, competitive, pessimistic, or perfectionistic qualities.[102]

- Cultural/social conditioning plays a role in placebo/nocebo. For example, certain pill colors, sizes, and perceived drug costs may have different effects.[103]

- Prior environmental exposures when receiving health care can influence future physiological responses.[104]

THE ELEPHANT IN THE ROOM

So, what exactly *is* going on with placebo/nocebo and our society's relationship to these mechanisms? Why do we exert so much time and energy to "rule out" placebo as a beneficial mechanism? Exploring these questions has implications for mind-body strategies in health care. In part, placebo reflects the biology of belief, expectation, hope, and even faith. The tendency to dismiss therapeutic impact as "just placebo"—as if it is a chance occurrence—displaces us from the power inherent in the mechanism. A perceived lack of specificity around the effect contributes to a failure of some to take particular therapies and treatment modalities seriously. This brings up the world of medical ethics. Recent peer-reviewed papers,[105] editorials,[106] and even entire conferences devoted to the topic of placebo promotion (and nocebo diminution) have shown up on the landscape.

For now, contemplate the following contextual definition:

[Placebo] is [the effect that arises in relation to] any substance, treatment, or modality that brings about healing [positive physiological change] based on either conscious or unconscious individual or collective [expectations and] beliefs. Placebo includes cultural context, represents the imaginal power base of the patient, is based on the inherent desire to relieve suffering, and—increasingly—has identifiable physiological correlates[107] [content added to clarify the definition and flow].

In this definition, it is important to recognize that "unconscious" reflects expectancies (anticipated future outcomes). When expectancies are accessible at the "conscious" level they are called expectations, which can be measured and are impacted by cognition and perception.[108]

Factors such as environmental cues, provider presence, ritual, and more reflect *contextual factors* that may facilitate expectation and thus placebo effects. Contextual factors are: "physical, psychological and social elements that characterize the therapeutic encounter with the patient."[109] The preceding definition of placebo/nocebo combined with an understanding of the many contextual factors that may facilitate or inhibit placebo/nocebo effects allows consideration of the type and nature of ingredients in patient care that may support tapping into the power of placebo (and diminishing nocebo!). Rossettini *et al.* delineate categories of interacting contextual factors:

- clinician features (e.g., professionalism, mindset, appearance)
- patient features (e.g., mindset, baseline)
- patient-clinician relationship (e.g., verbal and non-verbal communication)
- health-care setting features (e.g., positive distractions, supportive indications, comfort elements, and decorations)
- treatment features (e.g., therapeutic touch, technique characteristics, factors impacting posology).[110]

Each of these categories is deliberately considered in the formulation of IRP as a care approach inherently suited to enhance positive modification of health and well-being outcomes.

PLACEBO, BELIEF, AND ENACTIVISM

In this section, we aim to blend the science of placebo with integral, philosophical, and psychospiritual concepts. Similar to pain,[111] the topic of placebo lends itself well to this effort. This exploration aims to deepen understanding of how IRP supports patient experience and quality of care. Our investigation and presentation of placebo as a mind-body phenomenon also aims to name the risks of using the topic to support pseudoscientific treatment approaches.[112]

As suggested earlier, expectations, beliefs, and contextual factors are powerful mediators in our health.[113] This understanding must be approached regardless of personal opinion about the origins of "mind" or the nature of consciousness. To capture the understanding that placebo involves many contextual factors, the prior working definition brings insight. In the definition, we see the concept of *power base*.

Experiential pause: Take a moment, shift attention from the cognitive level to the body and breath. How are you interacting with this information? What comes up for you? Take a little time and acknowledge sensations, emotions, and your breath. When ready, contemplate the following questions.

- Where, ultimately, does power base (aka autonomy, agency, empowerment) lie in human experience?
- What internal or external resources support ownership of power?
- How does locus of control interact with or arise from other underpinnings such as the presence/absence of safety or nurturance?

- How does one's power interact with factors that are outside of one's conscious control?
- What does one's relationship to such factors look like?

These are questions that we encourage you to repeatedly contemplate around the why, what, and how of the care we offer to our fellow human beings.

If we consider placebo in relationship to the story that reflects each person's life experience, placebo represents relationships: "between culturally meaningful entities (such as treatments or therapies), our intentional relationship to the environment (such as implicit or explicit beliefs about a treatment's healing powers) and bodily effects (placebo responses)."[114] Here we see the BME construct—informed by living systems theory. The authors go on to explore why placebo appears puzzling to our existing scientific paradigm and suggest that it stems: "from a particular way of thinking (firmly and understandably entrenched in western culture) about the mind's relation to the body and the world, and a corollary view of the nature of medical science and treatment."[115] Placebo is not just puzzling, it also represents a *challenge* to the public, the scientist, and/ or the health-care professional's sense of safety and comfort in their work. Why?

Experiential pause: Take a moment, and once again become aware of the felt sense in your body, and your breathing. Invite a space of contemplation—a curious state of mind. Ask yourself this question: Why does the reality of placebo in our lives represent a potential challenge? To the public? To the scientist? To you and your own sense of comfort, familiarity, or safety in your day-to-day life or work? Jot down what comes up for you...

Now, on to *enactive*. What does this mean? *Enactivism* suggests that cognition can only arise through, and as a result of, complex BME interactions. Similar to the observer effect in quantum physics, enactivism claims that our environment is co-created. Co-creation implies that our environment is in an inseparable relationship with our presence and interactions within it. This occurs in and through consciousness. This implies that organisms do not just passively receive information from their environments, which is then translated into internal representations. Instead, natural cognitive systems (aka humans) participate in the emergence of meaning by engaging in transformational, and not just informational, interactions. In other words, humans enact the world.[116]

What on earth does this have to do with placebo? Enactivism presents us with a view or understanding that each organism is comprised of adaptive bodily processes, intention, and the properties of its environment—all as co-emergent aspects of a single, unified system. As such, enactivism provides us with a formal, singular word for our use of "BME relationships." Enactivism can be used to help explain the mysterious-looking world of placebo by suggesting that it is out of these unique interactions that such phenomena arise. This includes the way in which a patient and provider interact. Embedded within this is the notion of interdependence: human subjectivity is intersubjectivity.[117] This brings up a key question: How does your relationship with the patient and the environment that the relationship occurs in influence the patient's process; including the extent that placebo or nocebo effects emerge? Chapters 8 and 9 will support this question.

Finally, discussion and research exploring non-putative mechanisms underlying unpredictability, variability, and individuality in placebo and other reported and observed phenomena is occurring.[118] While the details of such discourse is beyond our scope, these topics underscore IRP's advocacy for beginner's mind, tolerance of uncertainty, supporting patient belief and choice, and more. Suffice to say there is much we do not know or understand.

SCIENCE IS NOT ABOUT CERTAINTY

Think back to the earlier examples of the systemic release of osteocalcin from bones as vital to the fight/flight response, or the view of the change potential of neuroplasticity and neurogenesis. This underscores a need to cultivate psychological flexibility within our relationship to science. As Italian physicist Carlo Rivelli reminds us: "Science is a process in which we keep exploring ways of thinking and keep changing our image of the world, our vision of the world, to find new visions that work a little bit better."[119]

Embedded within the values and concepts that have been used to define IRP is a call for cultivating greater tolerance of uncertainty. We must cultivate comfort with discomfort. We must look critically and compassionately. This requires addressing barriers to this goal for professionals, patients, and the health-care system alike. Addressing these barriers requires capacity for complex reasoning, the possibility of more than one right answer (both/and), and is rooted in the emphasis on each person's values, beliefs, and preferences.[120] For the latter, this sometimes comes in the face of opposition to our own belief system about what works and/or what is evidence based.

THAT'S (NOT) A WRAP

IRP demands scientific support equal to the biomedical care model. We must stay current on the evolution of science as it affords us an opportunity to develop greater flexibility and humility in our roles as health-care professionals. IRP consciously attempts to do so with a greater capacity for transdisciplinary integration. As such, IRP aims to increase capacity for approaching health challenges from multiple angles and integrated lenses.

As we close (aka open) our journey through this contextual view of a small portion of science, Rachel Naomi Remen, a physician and researcher at the University of California, San Francisco, offers wisdom: "Helping, fixing, and serving represent three different ways of seeing life. When you help, you see life as weak. When you fix, you see life as broken. When you serve, you see life as whole. Fixing and helping may be the work of the ego, and service the work of the soul."[121] What does this suggest? We must approach science as critical and valuable, and not the end game. We encourage holding meanings lightly, as all meanings evolve. Delivering care that is flexible and in a way that demonstrates humility, in service to the patient, is vital. This does not forgive us the responsibility to deliver grounded care. Instead, we argue that it *is part of* that responsibility to take this approach. We encourage continuously leaving space for the consideration that there are undetermined and, very likely, unknowable factors in our experiences of health and illness.

Experiential pause: Having read this chapter, identify and write down at least one actionable item of interest to you. In doing so, consider ways in which applying the material first to yourself, and then to patients, might serve those who come to you for care.

APPLICATIONS OF INTEGRATIVE REHABILITATION PRACTICE

The content of this section includes approaches that reflect skills that can act in support of well-being. Remember to apply them to yourself before rushing to deploy them in the clinic. Translating these approaches into *exploratory, non-fixing interventions* that reflect opportunities for the enhancement of health requires regular attention on the part of the clinician. Many of these approaches arise from various subtopics within the larger framework of mind-body medicine. While our choices are fairly inclusive, there are others not included that lend themselves well to the integrative rehabilitation practice (IRP) model.

Often, the question of dosing arises in health care. Here are a few tips to consider in relation to exploring mind-body integrated practices:[1]

1. **Dose matters**: Practice is important to yield adequate experiential learning as well as harness any potential therapeutic impact. The level of engagement, for example in mindfulness training, in part predicts physiological changes.
2. **Self-selection and realism matter**: From the person-centered lens, the best dose is self-paced and internally chosen. Any path towards transformation is best seen as a gradual process, and gaps between idealism and realism must be built. Patience is demanded.
3. **Individual characteristics and needs matter**: Some persons may be better suited for individualized approaches, and others for group-based interventions. The provision of choice via various offerings (not too many!) and a trial-and-error approach with regular feedback will guide the way.

A note for Section Two: Each chapter in this section starts with "A story." Our use of the word story is meant to convey honor and respect. While we will explore principles of narrative medicine and storytelling in more detail in Chapter 9, for now consider the difference between "case study" and "a story": we are not "cases" in need of study, rather we are rich, complex, and sacred beings having equally rich and complex experiences. Stories aim to be heard, validated, understood, and supported. Herein lies the intent for this format.

CHAPTER 8

From the Start

Shelly Prosko, PT, C-IAYT and Matt Erb, PT

A story: "Chayton" is a 41-year-old male referred for physical therapy for persistent thoracic pain and right leg pain. Chayton was told he has sciatica. He had an MRI of the thoracic and lumbar spine which was unremarkable except for some mild arthritis and questionable foraminal narrowing. The doctor told Chayton he probably has a pinched nerve. Chayton also underwent electromyography (EMG) and nerve conduction velocity (NCV) tests of the right leg which were normal. Chayton just relocated to the area for a new job and reports that he finds the presence of these symptoms a major irritant, impacting his ability to focus, but not really prohibiting him from completing physical activity: "I still do everything that I want, and sometimes it flares it up, but I'm not going to let it stop me." Chayton's physical therapist has 30 minutes for his first session and takes approximately seven minutes to record Chayton's symptoms, and gather pain ratings and a list of aggravating and ameliorating factors. "Did you do anything that caused this?" was one of the few questions asked before diving into a ten-minute objective evaluation which included: movement testing, a spinal/pelvic posture and alignment exam, palpation testing, core abdominal strength, and segmental spinal movement testing. The session concluded with manipulative therapy (high-velocity low-amplitude mobilizations) and two briefly prescribed core stabilization exercises to round out 27 minutes. Three minutes left for paperwork.

THE FIRST SESSION: INTERROGATION AND FIXING VERSUS COMPASSIONATE EXPLORATION AND CONTEXTUAL CONSIDERATIONS

Does Chayton's experience sound familiar? In looking at Chayton's story, we might question whether the skills that detect and support the depth of what patients are feeling and experiencing when they arrive for a health-care evaluation have been ignored or lost. A focus on learning and deploying evaluation and testing methods that aim to gather quantitative/objective data has replaced a focus on gathering information that supports a larger clinical picture of complexity. Without such a picture, avenues for supporting the whole person become harder to see or access. In this chapter, we present an integrative approach to the initial evaluation that supports patient experience and contextual considerations.

During medical evaluations, the average time it takes for a doctor to interrupt a patient is 11 seconds.[1] In general, clinicians elicit the patient's agenda in only 36% of encounters (49% in primary care, only 20% in specialty care).[2] What is going on here? The reasons are multifactorial and often include barriers beyond the clinician's control. High workloads and short appointment times pressure clinicians to rush. Time to explore the larger context is de-prioritized. Unfortunately, this misses the mark: symptoms do not occur in isolation. They occur in a life.

As clinicians, even if/when more time is available, we may:

- feel uncomfortable delving into the patient's life experience
- fear getting "off track" or lost in the story
- fear losing control of time
- be in our own state of overwhelm or distress, not fully present
- believe we can best help the person by relying on information and/or providing techniques more than hearing and supporting the person's lived experience
- feel confident that we have heard similar stories many times before and therefore believe we know the most effective way to treat "this condition"
- interrupt the patient to guide the interview towards the direction we believe is best.

Experiential pause: Imagine each of the preceding scenarios as both a clinician and a patient. Do any of the points feel familiar to you as a clinician? How do you feel the patient might experience them? How might the patient consciously or subconsciously interpret and relate to the interaction?

One hidden determinant to the preceding patterns lies in the fixer/fixee dynamic (Chapter 1) from which both the clinician and patient may be subconsciously operating. The result: swift entry into diagnosing, labeling, and "doing to" modes. Although usually well intentioned, premature or excessive emphasis on objective measures and/or rushing to offer something seemingly more tangible risks devaluing the person.

Physical therapists and educators Jacobs and Silvernail discuss the importance of the clinician's ability to look beyond specific techniques and become more of an *interactor* with the person and the environment, rather than being an operator who passively *does something to someone.*[3] Rapid deployment of fixing-oriented techniques may even add inadvertent harm by triggering the person's physiological defense mechanisms.[4] This physiological threatened state of defense in turn can perpetuate pain, fear, and anxiety, and negatively impact many aspects of recovery such as movement, function, and the therapeutic relationship.

In Chapter 5 we explored whole-person clinical reasoning. Data collection is a necessary process within clinical inquiry and reasoning. In our quest for data, we may forget that a thorough history or occupational profile is vital data.[5] Devaluation ensues when a person does not feel seen, heard, or understood—reflecting an interruption to their larger process of sense-making about their life and experience. Sense-making is an important part of healing, particularly in pain care.[6] Behavioral neuroscientist and psychologist Stephen Porges even emphasizes the value in: "respecting the individual's capacity to *experience* their own pain" [emphasis added].[7]

Building upon the foundations within preceding chapters, here we present an integrative approach to the initial evaluation that supports patient experience and contextual considerations. We offer guidelines and include the necessary conditions required for effective history taking and provide examples of questions and language that can be used and the rationale behind them. In the succeeding chapter we will deepen our look by expanding our understanding of phenomenological inquiry and narrative medicine within the whole of care and across time.

AN INTEGRATIVE-ORIENTED EVALUATION

Integrative care approaches require laying a foundation *from the start*. This assists in identifying existing expectations, followed by collaborative efforts towards meeting the patient's needs and bridging gaps. Examples of gaps include the patient's own lack of awareness or knowledge around the relevance of psychosocial factors and/or their own overly reduced belief in physical causality. Let's take a look at a possible framework for Chayton's evaluation visit:

> Chayton was sent a comprehensive packet of information prior to his appointment. The welcome letter stated:
>
>> Our clinic values every facet of your life. Modern medical science has shown that the factors influencing our health are varied, complex, and often build up over time. This reality means that a thorough look at your life history is important. We take a whole-person approach to care, and we will take time in your first session to get to know you. If possible, fill out these materials and send them in advance to allow your therapist to begin to understand your experience. If you are not able to do this in advance, no problem—we'll take time in your first session. Understanding your experience is vital to our ability to help guide and support you. As such, the majority of your first session will be devoted to this goal.
>
> In Chayton's packet was a health history form that, in addition to standard questions, included questions about social/family life, work history, perceived stress, and more. Chayton filled the forms out before arriving and brought them to his first appointment. To help prepare for the interview, the therapist thoroughly reviewed the material prior to asking Chayton questions.

How might the rest of Chayton's session look? How do we simultaneously gain an understanding of Chayton's condition from the biomedical lens (objective evaluation) and gain insight into the complexity that informs his condition? How do we see into what another person is experiencing, feeling, what they believe, what they perceive about their problem, how it's impacting them, how they make sense of it, and what they truly need (beyond our own biases as to what *we* think they need)? We'll come back to Chayton shortly. For now, consider that gleaning insight into the larger landscape takes time. We must not expect to achieve this all in the first visit. The first session lays a foundation, where we begin to glimpse into the vastness that informs Chayton's experience, and see it as an ongoing exploration and evaluative process. We emphasize that the integrative evaluation is significantly different from a traditional biomedical interview and evaluation. However, we also need to appreciate that traditional material may still be used, and then integrative methods further build upon and expand the traditional model.

STARTING WITH SELF

Before going further into skills for an integrative approach to evaluation, an important reminder: the integrative lens looks deeper. For some, this will not be familiar. It may or may not be comfortable or even desired. Integrative care must be an invitation. The effectiveness of this invitation is informed by the clinician's own capacity, presence, and comfort with the constructs.

To move beyond lip service, as clinicians we must address our own physiological state, behavior, cognitive processes, and emotions. Consider looking back at the general integrative rehabilitation practice (IRP) constructs and the invitations to know ourselves in prior chapters (e.g., the five broad traits of creative individuals in Chapter 2, the enactive model of compassion in Chapter 2, and the various experiential applications and self-review concepts in Chapter 6). In addition, consider the following principles adapted from a method of introspection[8] used in psychology and social sciences as clinician guidelines.

- Look for, examine, and challenge our own assumptions, opinions, especially implicit biases. Implicit racial bias is particularly worth exploring as this directly affects the treatment and care of patients with chronic pain.[9]
- Deploy "beginner's mind."
- Challenge yourself around fixed notions of "why"—i.e., why things work when they do.
- Reinforce complex clinical analysis and the concept of ongoing emergence.
- Encourage an understanding of process by demonstrating patience in ourselves and for/with others.
- Avoid "absolute anything"—i.e., avoid one-sidedness of representation and over-reduction of causation.
- Discover patterns of similarity such that seemingly dissimilar things are viewed via connecting dots within the whole.
- Look for errors that arise from dualistic thinking—i.e., avoid "either/or" thinking; consider "both/and" thinking.
- Be comfortable with uncertainty.

- Repeatedly, frequently, and consistently practice all of the above.

As noted earlier, a key tenet of IRP is rooted in the concept that if we are more aware of our own state, we will have a greater capacity to be more aware of another's state and needs.[10] Additionally, our own physiological state may influence another's state; self-regulation practices may assist with promoting resiliency and preventing professional burnout.[11]

What follows are principles that promote our own psychophysiological and spiritual health and development with the understanding that this is a vital, albeit often overlooked, facet of integrative rehabilitation. Table 8.1 offers an example of a *clinician manifesto* that serves as an inspiration for you to create your own personalized set of principles.

Table 8.1: Example Clinician Manifesto

Topic	Consider the following statements, personalize them, and include any additions you wish to make
Self-awareness	I am committed to finding healthy ways to express my emotions and to be aware of how they may affect those around me. I understand my skills, abilities, and limits.
Self-regulation	I am committed to practice to track, recognize, and regulate my biobehavioral state amidst continually changing BME (body-mind-environment) conditions.
Self-expression	I understand my beliefs and personal values and how they affect my decision making, commitments, and interactions with others.
Intrinsic motivation	I intrinsically value serving. I am in charge of my efforts and understand that outcomes are subject to complexity. I do my best with the conditions that are present, the resources available to me, and my current capacity and level of awareness.
Intention and values	I am clear in my intentions within each moment/interaction. I commit to acting in line with my values and to support the meaning and purpose for any given moment or situation.
Curiosity	I am committed to genuine curiosity towards myself, others, conditions, and experiences—particularly at times when I find it challenging to understand.
Compassion	I thoughtfully consider the views, values, perspectives, and feelings of others. I intend to connect with others through active listening, relatedness, and interpersonal attunement. I am motivated to take compassionate action and commit to service.
Self-compassion	I am committed to patience and kindness towards myself, including setting boundaries, forgiving myself for mistakes, and acting from a place of genuine care and concern for myself.
Humility	I cultivate self-confidence and self-respect with humility. I am dedicated to cultivating comfort with: discomfort and uncertainty; not being in control; and not having all the answers or solutions.
Communication	I am motivated to deepen my capacity for effective communication skills—both listening and sharing.
Mutual learning	I am motivated to respect and learn from those I serve including those who may not share the same views or values as me. I can find value in others and a sense of shared humanity.

Experiential pause: Take a page in your journal and draw out a similar table. Edit, add, or delete topics and statements so that it makes sense for you and is in your own words. Consider how you would feel if these were embodied in your life. Can you think of some specific examples on how each of these might be enacted? As you move through your day, remind yourself that you can find opportunities and moments where you can practice these concepts.

BUILDING THERAPEUTIC ALLIANCE

First impressions matter—a lot. Much of this is found in provider presence, body language, tone of voice, and facial expressivity. Sometimes these qualities are described as "soft skills"; however, it is best to see them as essential skills, rooted in presence.

There is a growing call in rehabilitation to deepen *therapeutic alliance*.[12] Interestingly, research in the field of psychotherapy supports that *therapist* variability in the therapeutic alliance predicts outcomes, whereas patient variability was unrelated to outcome.[13] Extrapolating this to integrative rehabilitation relationships reinforces the need for greater focus on supporting clinicians' ability to develop and monitor their contribution within the therapeutic alliance. Furthermore, there are associations between the quality of therapeutic alliance and clinical outcomes, treatment adherence, person-centered care, and patient satisfaction.[14] For example, it has been shown that therapeutic alliance seems to be as important as the therapy itself in pain modulation for people with persistent low back pain[15] and is a predictor of psychosocial and physical functioning outcomes in brain injury rehabilitation and low back pain respectively.[16] Part of cultivating therapeutic alliance involves a commitment to developing our capacity to provide: "personalized, responsive and fulfilling communication."[17] But *how* do we enact this?

The preceding manifesto provides a foundation. Integrative and transdisciplinary education and skills building, found across this book, take us further. For this chapter, a key aim is to establish a framework for whole-person support from the start. This calls for the creation of a *safe therapeutic container*. Miciak *et al.* (2018) identified and described necessary conditions of engagement to optimize a therapeutic relationship in physiotherapy: being *present, receptive, genuine,* and *committed*.[18] These conditions are established by the clinician and represent the intentions and attitudes of the clinician and the patient. They are ingredients in creating a perception of safety, a critical feature of any interaction, including the therapeutic relationship.[19] While the professional is not solely responsible for whether safety is established, if conditions that support the emergence of safety are absent in the first session, the opportunity to provide a sense of safety will be more challenging or may even be lost.

As noted earlier, enactive compassion is an important aspect of the therapeutic relationship. Some researchers suggest empathy and/or compassion may be taught in some capacity,[20] while others suggest it can only be primed to emerge as Halifax's model[21] outlines (see Chapter 2). Yet, we don't have conclusive evidence that states compassion training is *necessary*. Further, we must not put all blame and responsibility on the health provider for any apparent lack of demonstrated compassion, as there are broader systemic issues, medical culture, and organizational barriers that may influence one's ability to provide compassionate care.[22] In other words, the absence of compassion must not be seen as solely an individual issue.

At the same time, Gilbert and Mascaro explore the relevance of personal dynamics that may inhibit one's ability to provide compassionate care, many of which can be addressed by the individual.[23] For more on this topic, take a side trip into a book chapter that offers a valuable contribution, *Compassion in Pain Care*.[24]

THE RELATIONAL SPACE

As introduced in Chapter 6, effective communication is vital—not just in health care, but in all aspects of life. The formulation for effective communication occurs within each individual and in the space between individuals—aka the intersubjective space. Low's 2017 paper, as discussed in Chapter 3 in relation to a dispositional theory causation, also describes a conceptual model of the intersubjective space.[25]

Our adaptation of the *safe therapeutic container* and this *intersubjective space* is illustrated in Figure 8.1, where therapist and patient each enter the relationship with a unique body-mind-environment (BME) history and experience. Each person's BME experience includes complex factors including perceptions, expectations, thoughts, beliefs, past experiences, sociocultural factors, knowledge, ethics, values, environments, and more. When clinician and patient meet as equal human beings in the first session, two worlds combine—sometimes with ease, sometimes with friction, and in either case, alchemical potential. In each interaction, a new space is created, forming the backdrop wherein the introduced elements either support or detract from a trajectory that moves an individual towards well-being.

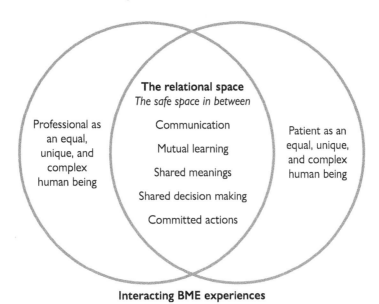

FIGURE 8.1: THE RELATIONAL SPACE

It is from this space that, together, the clinician and patient might co-create something new. Co-creation requires dialogue and the formulation of shared meanings. Physician and bioethicist Howard Brody uses the concept of *the joint construction narrative* to define the process that constructs and guides this dialogue and formulation of shared meanings; thus, the treatment plan.[26] This process is undoubtedly complex and calls the clinician to create and support the relational space in a way that enables the patient to be as fully engaged as is possible.

WHOLE-PERSON INQUIRY

Consistent with the keen practical sense of Socrates who believed that the easiest way to learn is by asking questions, a good starting point for any new interaction is with open-ended inquiry. Such inquiry affords opportunity for the person to share, and be seen, heard, validated, and believed. In doing so we begin to get a feel for the person and their communication style, area of focus, beliefs, contextual factors, etc. The content, language, underlying intention, and delivery of the question (body language, tone of voice), and the clinician's attunement/presence before, during, and after the questions have been asked, all matter. Rather than memorizing the words for "just the right questions" to ask, it is imperative that we gain a foundational understanding of the rationale behind the dialogue and focus on facilitating the individual's self-awareness and self-discovery that allows for choice and autonomy.

Table 8.2 was created in collaboration with Bronwyn Lennox Thompson, MSc(Hons), PhD(Cant), DipOccTh(CIT), and takes into consideration clinicians' expertise and best available evidence. The table provides a guideline for whole-person inquiry that includes fundamental domains, examples of questions to ask, rationale behind asking, and what to look for in the responses from the individual.

Table 8.2: Guidelines for Whole-Person Inquiry

Domain	What to ask (examples)	Why to ask (examples)	What to look for (examples)
History Narrative of how and why	Tell me about why you're coming to see me today. What's happened? When did it all start? What kinds of things have you already tried? Who have you seen? What effect did these treatments have? What have you learned thus far? What is your theory for why this is happening?	Helps us understand their concerns, beliefs, attitudes, what they've learned from seeing other professionals. Provides insight into response to treatment and the person's own theory about their health challenge.	Personal beliefs. Maladaptive beliefs/thoughts, nocebo language. Experiences with health care. Helpful or unhelpful information received. Degree of treatment seeking. Effectiveness/impact of treatment. Attitudes towards treatment (passive, active, self-efficacy). Understanding of health problems—health literacy.

Symptoms + relationship to symptoms	What are your symptoms? What is going through your mind when they happen? What leads up to them? What makes your symptoms worse? What helps? Have you found anything you can do to help? What else do you notice in your body? Any other symptoms?	Used for diagnosis. Helps us understand what the person's focus is and their specific concerns about the problem. Helps us understand contextual factors, such as antecedents, consequences, thoughts, and emotions, which help us understand the person's experiences and beliefs about their problem. Reviewing general systems can help connect dots towards a more integral picture and areas of focus.	Diagnostic information. Physiological arousal. Antecedents—triggers for symptom exacerbations and reductions. Consequences—actions the person takes, response to those actions. Beliefs. Attitudes. Self-efficacy.
Daily life experience	How do your symptoms affect your daily life? Can you take me through a 24-hour day from the time you wake? What are the most important activities you're having trouble with? What's going well? Are there any daily activities you're able to do with ease, you enjoy, and you hope to continue with?	Helps us understand the impact or disability arising from symptoms. Helps us understand the contexts in which the person lives, their routines, habits, and demands on their time/energy. Valuable info can be gleaned from what is going well during the day. All of above informs value-based goal setting and treatment planning.	Impact of symptoms on daily activities. Pattern of activity: consistent, irregular, boom/bust, overall activity level. Roles and demands. Areas in daily life consisting of positive experiences. What appears to be going well/working for the person? Note patterns or common factors.
Psychoemotional	With all this happening, how are you feeling in yourself? Would you be willing to share a bit about your experience with stress? What's going on with your sleep? Your appetite? Your "get up and go" or motivation? Your concentration and memory? Enjoyment in usual things? How is your mood? How are you dealing with the impact of these symptoms on you? What brings you joy these days? Hope? Pleasure? What lights you up and makes you feel alive?	Offers a gentle approach to inquiring about mood, anxiety; normalizes conversation about depression. Allows inquiry about symptoms commonly associated with low mood (loss of: appetite, motivation, enjoyment, sleep, concentration, memory). Provides opportunity to inquire about self-harm and suicidal thoughts. Extent of inquiry into these areas depends on clinician training; however, we have a responsibility to ensure safety of a person who may risk wanting to end their life. Develop a suicidal ideation response policy for your practice ahead of time. (You will not increase the risk of suicide by asking about it.) Identifying examples of what is going well or brings joy, etc., can inform goals and treatment planning.	Symptoms of depression, anxiety. Sleep patterns and disruption. General motivation and energy. Participation in daily life/withdrawal. Suicidal thoughts. Coping strategies. Sources of joy, hope, pleasure, confidence. Responses (verbal/non-verbal cues) during inquiries. Patterns of disorientation, disconnection/disassociation, difficulty with focus/concentration, memory recollection, or consistency with responses to your inquiries.

Domain	What to ask (examples)	Why to ask (examples)	What to look for (examples)
Social	Do you feel you have someone you can confide in and discuss your problems with? Someone you feel supports you? How are your friends and family managing things while you're dealing with your symptoms? How do they know you understand them? What do you think they notice, or don't notice? What do they do when they notice you dealing with your symptoms? Have your symptoms affected your relationship with your partner? Have your symptoms affected intimacy? How do you talk about your symptoms with your partner? Family? Friends? Work colleagues? How do they respond when you talk about things? What changes have you noticed over time?	Friends, family, and work colleagues provide social support and can shape what a person does about their symptoms. Understanding how the person demonstrates their symptoms to others provides insight into factors that may reinforce helpful or unhelpful coping strategies and illness behavior. Relationships are one of the strongest influences on health and treatment seeking: how partner or family members respond to the person's illness behavior can change over time from supportive to punitive. Helps us understand messages given from those around the person. Offers opportunity for the person to reflect on and be aware of support type available in their life: nourishing versus depleting. Can inform rehab program planning (person may benefit from support group).	Reinforcing behavior (resting, avoiding, seeking treatment, suppressing feelings and pushing through). Helpful or unhelpful responses. Social isolation. Loss of physical intimacy and partner support. Punitive or supportive responses to requests for help. Loss of social and recreational contact with others. Changes in role over time.
Work	What is your work environment like? What's happening at work? What is the impact of your health on your work? What does your immediate supervisor say? How do your work colleagues react? What tasks can you manage? What tasks are you having trouble with? What do you enjoy about your job? What do you value about your work? What parts of work are currently going well? What do you think will happen with work in the long run?	Work is one of the most important contexts in daily life and represents a large part of our self-concept. Understanding attitudes and demands of the workplace offers insight into the person's lived experience, and one that is often crucial in economic terms, but also affects social life and daily routine. Provides insight into the person's relationship to their work. The person's attitudes, beliefs and what they value about work can inform goals.	Responsiveness in the workplace: punitive or solicitous responses. Relationship to work: attitudes, beliefs, sense of value, meaning, purpose from work. Self-efficacy for work.

Goals, expectations	What are you hoping for from seeing me? What does a good outcome look like for you? How would you know things were better? If your symptoms were less of a problem for you, what would you be doing? What is your main concern today? What are your goals?	Clear identification of value-based, patient-centered treatment goals can be incorporated into treatment plan. Priorities can be identified for the initial and subsequent sessions. Above facilitates rehab process including therapeutic relationship, program adherence, and outcomes.	Expectations from treatment. Values, priorities. Saliency.
Meaning, purpose, values, existential	Is there anything you can think of that brings a sense of meaning or purpose in your life? When do you feel most connected to yourself, or most "like you"? When do you feel most at peace (what are you doing, where are you, who are you with)? How might your spirituality or religion influence how you deal with your problems? How might it influence the care I provide? Would you like it to be a part of your care? What matters most to you? What do you value most? What brings you joy or "lights you up"? Makes you smile?	Uncovers deeper beliefs to inform goals, plan, and therapeutic process. Helps us discover and incorporate meaning and purpose in treatment plan and facilitate patient-valued care. May provide value including adherence and outcomes. Spiritual beliefs can influence coping strategies, self-efficacy, outcomes, and treatment process.	Sense of connection or disconnection, wholeness, self-worth, purposelessness. Spiritual/existential beliefs and preferences. Potential barriers or facilitators to self-efficacy. Sense of agency: self-directed, partnership with divine, controlled by divine, feelings of being punished/deserving of problem, divinely abandoned or supported.

Experiential pause: As you review Table 8.2, notice and highlight the questions and areas that may already be included in a traditional rehabilitation approach and that are most familiar to you. Which areas are unique to the integrative approach and may you have less experience of exploring? What is your experience as you read about the areas that are less familiar to you?

It is important to emphasize that whole-person inquiry in IRP includes elements of the traditional interview. It is not to be viewed as an "either/or" situation, rather the IRP approach builds upon and further expands the traditional approach.

Let's go back to the second version of Chayton's story for a moment. When Chayton received his pre-visit packet he was surprised to see a question: "Would you like your spirituality discussed or considered in your care?" Chayton had taken note, left it blank, and subsequently forgotten about the question until the therapist asked about it. Chayton was pleasantly surprised to find himself sharing a little bit about his cultural and spiritual beliefs—revealing that: "Actually, this has been on my mind. I was raised in my indigenous culture, but have lost touch. Lately, with my health issues and stress levels, I think I'd like to reach out to one of the traditional healers in my community for insight." This was met by the therapist with: "That sounds like an important process for you. Is there anything else you'd like to say about that?" Chayton deferred, and the session continued.

ADDITIONAL CONSIDERATIONS
Weaving together therapeutic education and therapeutic dialogue from the start

Therapeutic education (TE) may carry beneficial neurocognitive and neurophysiological effects. We recommend a gentle exploratory approach to TE that meets the person where they are and offers invitations for understanding and reappraising the complexity of their experience. TE is a hot topic in rehabilitation and we will cover this in detail in Chapter 16. For now, be mindful to:

- consider moderation (there can be *too much of a good thing*). Particularly in the first session, a focus on creating relationship and connection, perhaps with just a few well-chosen pieces of information, helps to avoid cognitive overwhelm or aversion
- avoid making TE another modality where we are doing something "to" someone
- not rely on TE as our only way of providing psychosocial support to patients by telling them it is relevant but not offering experiential learning or substantial resources
- check for gaps in knowledge translation: "Would you be willing to share with me your interpretation of what I just explained?"
- provide choice and not make assumptions that the person wants to receive the education or even our questions. TE might be prefaced with: "Would it be OK to provide you with some information to consider?"

TE may be most effective when woven into the preceding guidelines for whole-person inquiry, which reflect a larger set of principles for *therapeutic dialogue* (TD). TD aims to facilitate each person's capacity to discover things for themselves and find better ways to understand and express their experience. TD assists patients to make their own choices, in a way that supports autonomy. In this regard, motivational interviewing (see below) can be woven in to enhance the effectiveness of our approach in the first session and onward.

Prefacing TD questions with brief educational comments can help the person understand why we are inquiring into various facets of their life experience. This is particularly helpful if they are not accustomed to this line of questioning in a traditional rehabilitation setting. Our earlier example with Chayton underscored this point. Another example might be: "Research has shown that past and present stressors have a profound impact on our bodies, though we certainly can't claim that any *one* thing caused our health challenge. I'm wondering if we might talk just a bit about any stress you are experiencing?"

Mind-body dialogue

Therapeutic dialogue includes "mind-body dialogue," which is rooted in mind-body medicine concepts and principles as in Chapter 3. All our preceding examples of interviewing questions and strategies reflect unforced invitations aimed at being friendly and non-threatening. When approaching the idea of building mind-body awareness through mind-body dialogue, it is once again critical that we do so from a stance of contextual curiosity and acausality. This maintains comfort and safety. If the patient demonstrates avoidance or even a simple lack of interest, we divert. Table 8.3, adapted from material presented by The Center for Mind-Body Medicine,[27] presents overlapping categories and examples.

Table 8.3: Examples of Facilitating Mind-Body Awareness[28]

Category: Clarifying and natural curiosity	Category: Present-moment attention and awareness
"Would you be willing to say more about that?"	"What's happening with the sensations in your back as you are talking about this right now?"
"Tell me more…"	"I'm wondering what you notice is happening in your body right now as you shared about that?"
"When you said 'X,' I'm curious if you can help me understand that further?"	"What are you noticing right now?"
"I'm curious if there is a feeling linked to that?"	"How does it feel to be sharing this story right now?"
Category: Explore before teaching/fixing	**Category: Affect awareness and labeling**
"What is your answer to that question?"	"I'm wondering if you could share more about how this experience is impacting you?"
"Well, with what you have discovered thus far, what do you think may be helpful?"	"I'm wondering what feelings this experience is bringing up for you?"
"What would you suggest to a close friend asking you this same question?"	"How does the presence of these unpleasant sensations in the body feel emotionally?"
"If you could hear something supportive right now, what would that be?"	"How are you feeling right now?"

Trauma history

There is growing attention to both trauma-informed care (TIC) and the public health topic of adverse childhood experiences (ACEs). Research supports correlations between ACE exposure and current health challenges.[29] It is important for therapists to consider these correlations, as they may impact the person's health processes and may not have been previously addressed or supported. There are various views on and strategies for exploring the topic that must be considered.[30] A full-text paper on the topic that includes a person-centered guide for rehabilitation professionals to use in clinical practice is available online at Archives of Rehabilitation Research and Clinical Translation.[31] Appendix B also offers a primer on TIC in the context of IRP.

Values-based goal setting

It is useful to begin the process of inquiring into a person's values in the first session, in a way that gets linked to the shared and ongoing development of realistic goals that are best seen as committed actions for living forward. Recalling the relational space (Figure 8.1), *shared decision making* is vital to a successful collaborative effort.[32]

Acceptance and Commitment Therapy (ACT) (Chapter 17) provides a valuable approach for this process. ACT includes the understanding that there is potential benefit to seeing that we are taking actions in our lives, not just for an expected outcome (aka "goal" which often implies an end of the unpleasant/difficult experience), but because we value something specific in life, regardless of outcome. We may value work, or family, or hold core values such as honesty, integrity, kindness, joy, or a sense of peace that is independent of the presence or absence of a problem. Helping to separate the attachment to outcome from the value can clarify and support motivational and change processes. Such an approach also supports the final component in the relational space: *committed actions* that the patient can take in service to their values.

Motivational interviewing

Motivational interviewing (MI) encourages individuals to engage in dialogue about doing something proactive, different, or new—in relationship to their problem or experience. The goal is to help the person discover their own need or reasons for taking committed actions, just as in ACT. Intrinsic to this is helping people connect with their own resources, personal strengths, and values, and then moving forward with those qualities regardless of whether there is immediate or significant resolution of their distressing symptoms. We recommend a free online resource of MI techniques and skills that offers opportunity for further home study of MI concepts.[33]

It is important to consider that frustrations, lack of confidence, or perceived "failures" can commonly arise in patients. ACT and MI may help the individual build confidence by identifying and focusing on examples of success and/or "what is right." To be clear, this is not contrived or forced—rather it is inviting awareness and recognition of any positive facets of themselves and their life, by seeing the larger picture and regaining a sense of being whole, despite the presence of challenges.

Contextual objective evaluations

In a traditional approach to evaluation, many clinicians will look for possible structural factors and/or pathology. This stance tends to launch into attempts to fix the perceived source of the problem, such as manual therapy techniques or corrective exercise. This happened in our opening version of Chayton's story.

Each of you reading this book arrive here from a multitude of different professional training backgrounds, credentials, and specialties. As such, you bring a set of objective evaluation skills with you. As mentioned in Chapter 1 you do not need to throw out what you've learned. However, in some cases, as we gain new skills, some things might fall away. It is vital that each clinician takes time to contemplate and discern how complexity and context (as opposed to over-reduction of causality) informs the objective measures we use and their relevance.

Additionally, as you continue reading, consider how the skills and approaches presented (especially across Section Two) may be converted into useful objective information for the record. Examples might include: new ways of understanding movement patterns; autonomic or neuromuscular function as seen in biofeedback measures; or breathing patterns.

Finally, when physical testing is warranted, be mindful that the message we convey to the patient may carry significant impact. We must choose our words wisely when presenting the rationale for testing, the findings, and, most importantly, our interpretation of those findings. The clinical reasoning and case formulation strategies presented in Chapter 5 can apply across professions.

Scales and measures

While scales can be of questionable value, they can sometimes provide insight into a person's experience as well as offer a quantifiable measure to gauge what is typically not objectively measurable—the psychosocial content of people's lives. Some outcomes include useful measures of the psychosocial facets related to the person's condition and experience; however, it is important to not rely solely on these. Nothing substitutes for the immense value gained from live interaction and an approach that seeks to compassionately and respectfully understand and honor another human being's experience. With that said, sometimes numerical scales can offer a different perspective of what the person is experiencing, allow for another way to communicate, and highlight areas requiring support. For example, for measuring a person's general perception of stress in their life, we could ask: "On a scale of 0–5, 0 being no distress and 5 being the worst possible, how distressing is this experience for you?" Or: "On a scale of 0–10, how much stress do you feel you are navigating presently?"

Psychosocial questionnaires that people fill out prior to the start of the narrative review can also act as screening tools and conversation starters and provide comfortable opportunities for further inquiry. For example: "On the Depression Anxiety Stress Scales, I noticed you marked a 3 on the statement *I felt I was not worth much as a person*. Would you be willing to share a bit more with me about that?" Or: "I noticed your response on the Self-Compassion Scale, *When I'm really struggling, I tend to feel like other people must be having an easier time of it.* Would you care to share more about this experience?"

Documentation

Yikes, we said it! Virtually all systems of health care require that we document our time and treatment efforts. The language found across this book provides you with a new language that is supported by the evidence and literature. Applying your creativity will be needed to carve out your own style. To give just one example here, consider the following: Neuromuscular re-education (a common code used in the US for physiotherapy): "Self-regulation training through a combination of therapeutic education, body awareness, breath awareness, and breath regulation training, to improve brain-body regulation of painful experience." See, that was easy!

A FINAL VISIT WITH CHAYTON

In the first session, when the therapist took time to acknowledge and validate the relevance of Chayton's stressors to his health, Chayton identified a clear pattern of symptom aggravation when under increased psychoemotional stress. Chayton self-identified a need for improved stress-management skills. Both his cross-country move and his new job had been exceptionally challenging. After some brief education about the possibility of including some mind-body regulation principles in his care, Chayton was asked if he would be interested. "Yeah, sounds good" was Chayton's reply.

Also in the first session, the therapist noted that certain movement provoked pain, and used that opportunity to emphasize that addressing this pain will include looking at the state of the tissues and how the brain and body are communicating. The therapist did not suggest a quick fix route with manipulation or corrective exercise. Instead, solutions were offered that involved many possibilities within the whole and it was explained that it may take a little exploring over time and that there would be things that Chayton would be able to do independently at home. The therapist also guided Chayton through a brief experiential practice that demonstrated that his pain experience could be influenced by many factors, such as mind-body tension or breathing. This experience helped reinforce the TE. The therapist also described pain from the lens of a protective response that may or may not be proportional to the degree of tissue damage and offered relevant examples that Chayton had experienced in his own life such as a headache (severe debilitating pain without tissue damage). This approach represents a more contextual view of traditional exam findings.

In the end, Chayton attended four one-hour sessions. When last seen, Chayton said that he was no longer concerned about the problem. He also shared that prompted by the first session when he had been asked about whether or not he wanted to include spirituality in his first session, he had thought further about the relevance of his traditional healing practices. He discovered that he felt he had: "gone off balance and was not fully aligned with his spirit." He had scheduled a trip to return home to visit family, and planned to meet with a traditional healer during that time.

CONCLUSION

Integrative care starts before the patient even arrives. It begins now with yourself, your efforts in reading this book, and enacting your version of the clinician manifesto. Our intention of this chapter was to present a model of care that reinforced the core needs of patient empowerment, safety, and support. Whole-person care advances with clinician self-care, the organization's values, policies, and materials (such as the inviting welcome letter and intake packet Chayton received), and a willingness to begin to offer opportunities to your patients for whole-person support. We encourage you to proceed in the spirit of *being* rather than solely *doing*—as this is an intervention unto itself.

Confidence and comfort level with any new venture take time and come with experience. With consistent practice, patience, self-compassion, and a genuine commitment to connect with, understand, and serve others, you will succeed.

Making mistakes in real time and learning from them is invaluable. If we approach integrative interviewing and evaluation strategies with hesitation or fear surrounding our scope or with uncertainty about our knowledge/skill/confidence level, it will be apparent. This is where adequate transdisciplinary training is critical. We need the skilled range of a generalist—and to knows its scope and limits. Seek additional support and mentoring, recruit colleagues, and continue to learn from those who have experience on this journey and are committed to ongoing learning with genuine curiosity.

> **Experiential pause:** Having read this chapter, identify and write down at least one actionable item of interest to you. In doing so, consider ways in which applying the material first to yourself, and then to patients, might serve those who come to you for care.

CHAPTER 9

Deepening the Narrative

Matt Erb, PT and Noshene Ranjbar, MD

STORYTELLING

There are potential hazards in health care that integrative rehabilitation practice (IRP) intends to address. These hazards include losing sight of the importance of subjectivity, the psychosocial realities of our lives, and the power of individual and collective beliefs. These aspects of human existence are often encapsulated, expressed, and transmitted via storytelling, including the stories we tell ourselves about ourselves. There is growing recognition of the importance and relevance of supporting the "story" of the patient in health care.[1] Others use these words or phrases: "narratives," "patient experience," "patient perspective," "fact sharing," "knowledge transfer," "lived experience," or "storytelling."[2] We can look past the labels to see valuable principles. *Narrative medicine* is a field built around these principles. Narrative medicine focuses on training the health-care professional to practice with "narrative competence": the capacity to enlist skills of empathic interviewing, reflective practice, narrative ethics, and self-awareness to create and sustain healing interactions (relationships) with patients and colleagues.[3]

"'Medicine,' most people believe, is about the real world of biology, physiology, disease, remedies and cures; and 'narrative' is about fictional or subjective worlds of literature, character, point of view, and plots."[4] As such, the worlds of medicine and narrative may appear to conflict. In an editorial in the *British Journal of Medicine*, several authors write: "Some narratives may challenge previously accepted norms, or force us to consider alternative perspectives. The diversity of narratives should therefore be embraced as opposed to being used as a justification for their exclusion."[5] The authors point out the need for developing a culture of value, acceptance, and transparency. This is foundational within IRP.

In a world driven by data and information, it is important to remember that narratives are also forms of knowing and evidence. Storytelling is a strength, a skill, and an important component of healing processes. Each story is a constructed version of reality, a reminder of experiences that leave lasting impressions. And yet, stories are malleable; they can be refashioned and retold to bear new meanings.

Storytelling can be seen as a vehicle for communication and mutual learning that is universal across culture and through all of known history.[6] Cognitive processes help us in making sense out of our experience. Storytelling is an effort to adapt to one's physical and social environment; to generate a sense of comfort and safety; to give order, coherence, and/or meaning to discrete facts, experiences, and feelings. Essentially, the mind must analyze and make meaning out of internal and external stimuli and attempt to solve problems for certain purposes, including in relation to physiological processes of self-regulation.[7] These interacting dynamics translate into the stories that we formulate and tell about our experiences, and ultimately into beliefs about ourselves, others, and the world around us.

PHENOMENOLOGY AND INTERSUBJECTIVITY

We have previously touched on the topic of *phenomenology*, which is both a philosophical study focused on the nature of conscious human experience and a qualitative action research approach to solving problems.[8]

> Phenomenology is consistent with the integral body-mind-environment (BME) concept in IRP:
>
> > For phenomenology...the individual in his/her unity is more than a simple sum of parts. Phenomenology sees a human being as an intending entity, in which body, mind, and the world are intertwined and constitute each other mutually, thus establishing the human being's integral functioning.[9]

Our use of phenomenology is also meant to reinforce the relevance and importance of first-person inquiry → supporting each person's unique experience and the story that reflects that experience. As seen in the preceding chapter on framing whole-person care from the start, the qualitative research lens implies a participatory and reflective process of addressing and solving problems together. Paraphrasing from R. D. Laing, the therapeutic process must be focused on the attempt to recover the wholeness of being human through the therapeutic relationship.[10] Telling and listening to stories is an *intersubjective* process from which recovery of wholeness can emerge, underscoring the importance of phenomenological participation, reflection, thought, and action.

For a person who is suffering, having their story heard and validated across the continuum of their care is empowering and supports healing processes.[11] As a person is heard and honored, trust forms. The intersubjective space becomes a space pregnant with potential for transformation. Within a trusting relationship, new skills and perspectives can be introduced, learned, and practiced. The capacity to reappraise and repattern appears in the physiological process of neuroplasticity/neurogenesis, in which new insights, approaches, and experiences actually change the neural structure of the brain and our habits of thought (Chapter 7). This process is an active "relational reformulation" and contextual reappraisal of one's story over time. The lived experience of transformation around even one facet of one's story can lead to enhanced resilience, wisdom, and capacity to meet present and future challenges with an enhanced sense of hope, wonder, courage, and resolve. Supporting each person's story can help them fully transform into the hero of their own journey.

THE LIVED EXPERIENCE OF THE BODY

Using a phenomenological heuristic as the framework for exploring experience means that the patient's subjective perspective must be considered with sacred respect. The subjective perspective arises out of each person's blend of perceptions, thoughts, memory, emotions, actions, social interactions, culture, and more. For many, this includes spiritual beliefs about the nature of their experience.

All this is found and experienced in and through the body, ground zero for our lived experience. In the contemporary science of mind-body medicine, and regardless of an ongoing neurophilosophical debate about the origins of consciousness, there is adequate evidence for mind-body inseparability.[12] For example, traumatic experiences are stored in somatic memory and expressed as changes in the biological stress response.[13] For this reason, IRP advocates for exploring the mind through the lens of the body and vice versa. When the physiological conditions that reflect psychological and emotional safety are established, the door opens to exploring a greater sense of one's physical reality—including the body—as an opportunity for learning.

HOW MEANING MAKING CONTRIBUTES TO HEALING

Cultivating fresh eyes and clearer sight around one's life experiences assists in the creation and re-creation, over time, of a story that provides a more unified and coherent view of those experiences. The process of creating such a story enables us to improve our relationship to our life experiences by making sense of them. As professionals, we must ask: "How does each person come to know and create a meaningful story about, and ultimately relate to, the whole of their experience?" This question matters...a lot. Each individual's experiences play a profound role in health and healing processes, including:

- preceding their medical care
- in the present, and including with their medical care across time
- in relation to their thoughts, feelings, beliefs, and perceptions, including anticipation and expectations of the future.

The relevance of many of these components of experience typically remains hidden or unaddressed, both in general and in therapeutic contexts. The focus of this chapter is to facilitate a deeper understanding of how important *meaning making* is in health care, and how supporting the lived and storied experience of the patient contributes to healing. What does this look like? More importantly, what does this *feel* like for the patient? We gain insight into this by listening closely to the stories that each person has to offer. This offering is a gift.

A STORY

Sheila's story provides some insight into how various elements affect the story the patient constructs around their health experiences and how that story is intertwined with the social and subjective facets of their existence.

A story: "Sheila," a 36-year-old transgender woman, arrives at the physiotherapy clinic. Despite having advised the clinic that they want their record to reflect that they wish to be called Sheila, Adam (their legal name) remains on their medical record to correlate with their insurance ID card and legal forms. The front desk advises them: "We don't have you on our schedule." In front of others in the crowded lobby, they explain that they wish for their record to reflect their name and pronoun preference. Subsequently, Jane (the physiotherapist), unaware of this, comes out and calls for her next patient: "Adam." Sheila gets up, comes to the hallway entrance, and explains again that they wish to be called Sheila. Their movements are slow, and their posture and body language express a mix of frustration and exhaustion. Once in the treatment area, which consists of numerous partially walled and partially curtained areas, Sheila asks: "Are there private treatment rooms?" Jane says: "No, I'm sorry, this is our only treatment area." Over the next 30 minutes, the time allotted to the appointment, Sheila attempts to describe their struggle with anxiety, fatigue, migraine headaches, lower back pain, and intermittent feelings of depression. Jane, however, knows she has another patient, is already behind by ten minutes, and has loads of paperwork. Jane rushes to screen for painful movement and offers a treatment: "I think it would help to do some mobilizations for your lumbar spine as well as a release for your neck muscles," and proceeds to deliver these treatments with more of an obligatory form of consent than an actual discussion and provision of choice. Jane ends the session by saying: "We need to see you two to three times per week for these treatments. In the meantime, it will help you to sit and stand up taller. I noticed you are slouching; correcting this will help your pain. We'll prescribe you some exercises next time." Sheila leaves feeling rushed, upset, and tenser than before arriving, wondering if "it's just me." This is their second attempt at receiving care for these symptoms.

THE CARE EXPERIENCE

Sheila's experience is not unique. We do not need to look far to hear stories of negative patient experiences. In 2018, Holopainen and colleagues published a phenomenographic analysis of interviews with individuals about their experiences of receiving care for back pain. These individuals' conceptions of their journey were categorized into themes of:

- **convincing care**: whether the patient felt convinced by the level and quality of the care they received, including the perception of the professional's presence and enactive demonstration of care and concern
- **lifestyle change**: the degree to which lifestyle factors were addressed
- **participation**: the degree to which the patient was invited to participate in their care
- **reciprocality**: how reciprocal the interactions were
- **ethicality of the encounters**: perceptions of the therapist's ethicality.[14]

The results showed a wide range of experiences from disturbing to empowering. A key finding was that improved quality of care correlated with the patient's perception of the degree of attentiveness of the health-care professional. This enabled the encounter to be perceived as supportive and compassionate. For this to be realized, it was critical that the professional gave the patient time to tell their story, even when it may have seemed unimportant to the professional. In this, we see a notable failure in Sheila's experience.

There are challenges to providing "space for the story" (Figure 9.1). System-wide advocacy is needed. And there remains a significant onus of responsibility on the healthcare professional to address these factors in the care they are providing. For example, a shift of values from a rush to offer a technique or perceived fix toward taking more time may need to occur. Deploying the principles found across this book acts in support of the discovery and co-creation of strategies for addressing the challenges in Figure 9.1.

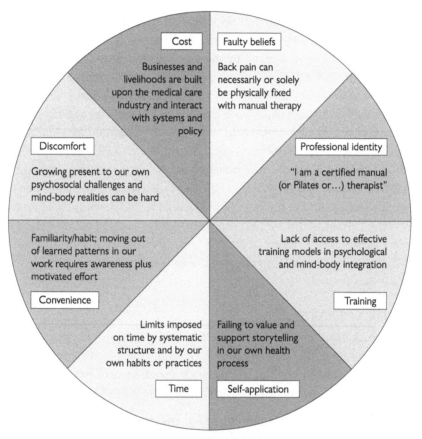

Each wedge reflects a category of possible barriers to creating the space and time needed for supporting the story. Within each wedge is a key example of the category.

FIGURE 9.1: CHALLENGES AND BARRIERS TO CREATING SPACE FOR NARRATIVE MEDICINE

During Sheila's first visit, Jane failed to ask an important question: "What do you believe is wrong?" Had this question been presented, Sheila would have had an opportunity to share a bit more about the many thoughts and feelings that were embedded in their experience of the many symptoms they described. A common response might be: "Well, they took a picture of the brain and of the back, and the brain looked OK, and they said we have some bulging discs and arthritis." This response comes from the structurally focused biomedical model. As we'll see in a bit, the ability to ask about each of the symptoms, not just the pain-focused ones, sets up exploring the larger landscape and potentially creating a map of previously disconnected or seemingly random dots.

ADDITIONAL PRINCIPLES FOR GUIDING A PHENOMENOLOGICAL APPROACH

In a paper presenting a framework for understanding and studying the integral nature of yoga therapy, Sullivan *et al.* discuss the relevance of phenomenology and the need to experience and explore things from unbiased, natural attitudes.[15] A natural attitude can be conceptualized as the neutral lens of a camera. This notion reflects the idea that each person's conscious experience is informed and influenced by an internal observer or witness. In mindfulness this is sometimes referred to as the "curious observer"; in Acceptance and Commitment Therapy (ACT) a similar concept is called "self as context." Such a larger perspective on one's sense of self creates space—space that is needed to appraise and reappraise our own storylines more clearly. Finally, Sullivan *et al.* note the work of Maura Dowling, who wrote that phenomenology was devised: "in order to hold subjective perspectives and theoretical constructs in abeyance and facilitate the essence of the phenomena to emerge."[16]

When looking from the professional's perspective versus the patient's at the construct of holding subjectivity in abeyance, we have what may look like a paradox. While IRP constructs must be applied to professional and patient equally, the timing and context of doing so may look different. Understanding these subtle differences is useful.

For the *professional* it is vital that we hold back our own subjectivity in favor of listening to the patient, with the goal of understanding. As Atul Gawande said in a commencement speech at the UCLA medical school:

> When people speak, they aren't just expressing their ideas; they are, even more, expressing their emotions. And it's the emotions that they really want heard. So I stopped listening to the man's words and tried to listen for the emotions.[17]

Listening in this way requires reservation of judgment, humility, and self-awareness of the subtle ways that our agenda can get in the way of the patient's needs—especially the need for validation. Being seen, feeling heard, and feeling cared for must be consciously embedded within the intersubjective space. This requires repeatedly stepping back for a fresh look at (or natural attitude towards) what is coming up for us in relation to the other's process. This fresh look is informed by ingredients from narrative medicine principles that combine with the other concepts within IRP. When viewing Table 9.1, consider that each section is not distinct, but overlapping and interacting. Also consider how this presentation overlaps and/or interacts with your clinician manifesto from the preceding chapter.

For the *patient*, the possibility for increased awareness, transformation of perspective, lifestyle change, and/or behavioral modification is supported by similar ingredients. However, for the patient these ingredients are *experienced*, as opposed to necessarily named, whereas for the professional they require conscious awareness and enacted intention. Professionals who create the space that supports the patient's subjectivity facilitate the emergence of the essence of phenomena (ongoing process), as discussed earlier.

Table 9.1: Ingredients for Narrative Medicine

Presence	Self-appraisal	Relationship	Space and safety
The embodied awareness, presence, and intention of the professional Enactive compassion The nature and intention behind the approach and tools deployed Enabling each person to come to know their own answers Cultivating and demonstrating comfort with discomfort Cultivating humility and patience Awareness of operating out of familiarity/ habit, including "fix-it" tendencies and dynamics	Beginner's mind Examining our own beliefs; reserving judgment Examining whether our actions arise from preconceived notions Holding meanings lightly in service to other Contemplating what is right action in any situation Examining attachments to outcome Cultivating humility and patience Recognizing/ addressing when we are over-extended, rushed, or dysregulated	Fundamentally relational care Safe container, mutual respect, seeing self/ other as interrelated processes of self-discovery Achievement and co-regulation Operating from a non-fixing, non-diagnosing, non-analyzing stance, even when working in a system that often demands some aspects of their opposites Inquiring into and supporting individual ethics and values Operating from the principle of mutual learning	Care environment Frequent invitations to awareness and expression Ample time for sharing that is an intervention unto itself Provision of choice, self-selection Experiential learning including experiences rooted in regulation— shifting physiological state away from defensive states Development of healthy attention to the body and what is right/working well— strength-based lens Recognizing power dynamics

RELATIONSHIP

Surveying the ingredients we have delineated thus far, we see further into the importance of relationship. The development of relationship is an act of service that helps increase the power base of the patient. When quality of relationship (or the intersubjective space) is supported, it sets up increased potential for exploring, reappraising, and contextualizing the many facets of one's life that may have an impact on health experience. Ultimately, this must occur in a natural and unforced way. It is not something you *do* per se.

When the intersubjective space is consciously fed, the improvement of relationship extends from the clinician-patient relationship to other levels such as *within* (body, any part of one's experience, and the whole of self) and *with* (other individuals in one's life, one's environment, etc.).

STEPPING IN OR STEPPING BACK: THE NON-FIXING STANCE

When does the professional step in to offer specific frameworks for reappraising what is not working without coming across as invasive or fixing? We all carry habitual patterns—

conditioned reactions, behaviors, thoughts, emotions, beliefs, and perceptions—that contribute to our challenges and inform our experiences of suffering. Awareness of this seeming dilemma offers two routes that can be loosely described as inaction and action.

- Being present, accepting, and experiencing things as they are.
- Interacting with the experience in proactive ways.

However, note that both ultimately reflect empowerment. Both are important and vital components in the development of a mature relationship with our experience of life.

So how do we enact this delicate balance of action versus inaction?

> **Experiential pause:** While being aware of your body and breath, read the following passage from the ancient text of the *Tao Te Ching* slowly. Consider your own meaning and interpretation of the words, and if any insights come to you, jot them down in your journal.
>
> *Do you have the patience to wait*
> *till your mud settles and the water is clear?*
> *Can you remain unmoving*
> *till the right action arises by itself?*
> *The Master doesn't seek fulfillment.*
> *Not seeking, not expecting,*
> *she is present, and can welcome all things.*[18]

How might we translate the concept implied in this poem into health-care practice? In early chapters we discussed the intersection of living systems theory with the study of emergent processes. We noted that there are endless possible paths and courses that any individual's BME experience might take. When we enter into a therapeutic relationship with those who come to us for support, the IRP approach is served by a reminder that we are in charge of our efforts, but not fully of the outcome. This adage does not release us from offering quality, evidence-based care and tracking the quality of care and outcomes that aim to improve health-care delivery. Consider that healthy therapeutic alliance has a positive impact on outcomes.[19] Consistently and consciously supporting the relational space (Chapter 8) over time includes the ability to allow others to have the vital experience of consciously navigating their own emergent process. Putting forth best efforts and intentions combines with letting things take their own course—a combination that acts in support of caring, empowering, quality care. What we do (the content of the health care we deliver) and how we deliver that care both interact and matter in this recipe. Seeking feedback across the care process may enhance patient experience and outcomes, and the reader is invited to learn about feedback-informed treatment as an added consideration.[20]

POWER STRUGGLES

Giving power back to another, and even taking back our own power, has never been quick or easy. As providers and therapists, our education and training give us a sense of power and agency, one we had to step into, claiming it for ourselves. That process took courage for each of us and involved at least some level of stress, fear, and overwhelm at some point along the way. Processes of taking back power are a necessary part of growing into mature, autonomous adulthood for every human.

For a patient who has felt disempowered by their illness or prior experiences with care or authority, receiving or taking back one's power can paradoxically feel threatening or overwhelming. One may run into the error of swinging too far towards a self-authoritarian view of health. In this paradox, the provider and/or patient can fall into the trap of believing that we can just "change our mind," "think our way out of this," or worse, believe we are to blame because we do not have the right thoughts, attitudes, or behavior patterns. In other words, we misinterpret what power actually is. Is it positive thinking? The "manifest your destiny" and "law of attraction" movements, for example, are fraught with reductionism that loses sight of the larger socioeconomic, geopolitical, and psychospiritual contexts.

We can approach giving and taking back power in our lives as a gradual process. Some (much?) of this power is found in our narratives. The creation of a safe container, aka the "relational space" (recall Chapter 8), allows for the possibility of enhanced appraisal and reappraisal processes within the therapeutic encounter. With support and patience, we can transform our relationship to any part of our experience—towards greater empowerment.

Taking back power is best seen as a delicate process and potentially an unnerving one to us as individuals, as well as to larger living systems (i.e., organizations, societies). Each of us experiences different states, conditions, and capacities around the notion of embodied ownership of our experience. Supporting patients in building the capacity to "experience their experience" in the most mature and healthy ways possible is an important function of health-care provision. This support must include understanding of the complexity within and across layers of BME interactions, as well as the many social determinants of health and how they thread into principles of collective interdependence.

BELIEFS

Beliefs are embedded in our narratives and stories. Do we see them? In ourselves? In others? As a professional you might initially see another person's beliefs as wrong, maladaptive, or "not evidence-based." It is best, however, to approach them as an important part of each individual's process. Gentle guidance and support may allow for an eventual shift in beliefs that are not serving the person well. Instead of an attempt to "fix" another's beliefs, we can practice creating an experience that allows each person to speak, hear, write, and rewrite their own story. As you develop capacity for this in yourself, how to support the same in others becomes clearer.

Power is taken away if we suggest that another's story, and any beliefs embedded in that story, are wrong or maladaptive. Even when we might see a larger or relative process or truth, there is no need to suggest this out of the gate. While skilled education presents opportunities to reframe, this education occurs within the intersubjective space. The professional's relationship with the patient is the foundation on which self-reappraisal can be built for both.

We must remain mindful to deliver practices rooted in the best-available evidence whenever possible, and to do so in a way that does not violate patient beliefs, values, culture, or experience. We must also do so in a way that aims to maintain a balance of clinician-patient personal power. The benefit to the patient of taking a person-centered approach to evidence-based care includes cultivation of their sense of empowerment as well as validation of their uniqueness in their lived experience. Professional agendas and/ or inflexible beliefs have potential to get in the way of this goal.

For the provider, the benefit of committing time and space to listen and engage the patient's narrative lies in bringing individualization, greater depth, and creativity into clinical work (remember Chapter 2?). We argue that doing so reduces the tendency for professional burnout (remember Chapter 3?) through reducing the burden that the provider carries when they hold all the power in the clinical dynamic. Drs. Rita Charon and Peter Wyer, physician leaders in delineating the relevance of narrative medicine, suggest:

> Medical practice is poised astride insoluble tensions between the known and the unknown (or at least the knowable and the unknowable), the universal and the particular, and the body and the self. Nested, these tensions beget and amplify one another. The unwary physician, caught in the headlights of one of them, usually succumbs to the paralyzing effects of all three.[21]

BELIEFS WITHOUT EVIDENCE?

It has been argued that: "belief without evidence is always morally wrong."[22] This concept is useful when it underscores the notion of the professional "believing responsibly." In other words, we approach our work with "beginner's mind"—a willingness to build our own reappraisal capacity. This must include, when appropriate, admission of if/when we are wrong in our own approach in providing care. In this, we evolve with flexibility as we learn and grow. However, we must be exceptionally mindful to not imply that a patient's beliefs are "wrong."

Beginner's mind is important here, as we all may be carrying unhelpful or faulty beliefs that unconsciously limit us. If we hold our meanings rigidly, we are led into blindness and potential harm. For the professional this could represent *cognitive fusion* with the notion that the scientific model is the sole deciding factor in care strategy, usurping the patient's beliefs, preferences, and subjective experiences. In the context of evidence-based medicine as relates to patient experience, we are at risk of losing the contexts of phenomenology, philosophy, metaphysics, and spirituality. Consider the idea of *holding one's meanings lightly* as part of psychological flexibility. In ACT, this is known as *cognitive defusion.* Consider what cognitive defusion implies, looks, and feels like in practice—*for you, the professional, and not just as taught to the patient.*

Finally, in addition to understanding that we all, at any given time, are carrying faulty or unhelpful beliefs, we need to know that our narratives, storylines, and beliefs are likely serving a larger purpose. This larger purpose might include:

- efforts at coping
- efforts towards autonomy
- a form of hope
- a valued part of cultural or spiritual context
- a doorway into the innate healing mechanism of placebo.

OUTCOMES?

As touched on earlier, outcomes are an important part of health care. And outcomes, like people's lived stories, are subject to countless individual and collective determinants. Ultimately, outcomes are part of a larger life story. If an outcome is "bad," what (and who) determines this? How do we know that it is bad? IRP encourages us into a deeper understanding of both *process* (everything is part of a larger process) and *emergence* (uncertainty as to what will manifest next) as a fundamental reality of human lives. This demands repeated exercise of humility.

Humility is part of psychological flexibility. We can hold space for many possibilities. If we fuse into a belief that there is always going to be a *reproducible* or *reducible* way revealed to us, we lose flexibility. We may also lose sight of complexity, context, creativity, and other facets of the art of medicine. This includes the possibility that there are multiple ways of knowing. All these ingredients can come together and interact to inform each individual's unique attempt to recover wholeness.

TELLING A NEW STORY

Let's piece all this together and take a different look at how Sheila's experience might go under new conditions.

"Sheila," a 36-year-old transgender woman, arrives at a physiotherapy clinic, referred to them by an integrative-medicine-trained family physician. Prior to arriving Sheila discovered that a close friend had been to the same clinic and had a positive experience. Sheila arrived expectant. The first thing they noted was a sign: "All are welcome here," with the word "welcome" printed in multiple languages. This felt comforting. The receptionist, having documented their preference to be called Sheila, recognized this upon their check-in process. Shortly thereafter, Jane (the physiotherapist) arrives in the lobby, calling for "Sheila." After a warm "Welcome, we'll be heading back to room 4 today. Let me know if there is anything that might make you more comfortable with your visit," they go together to a private room. Upon arrival, Sheila notices the quiet feel of the space, with natural and/or incandescent lighting, and nature photography on the walls.

The first thing Jane says once they are seated in the room is: "Again, welcome. I'd like to start our session today by hearing about your experience and what you are seeking support around." Sheila, remembering their last experience at another clinic, is apprehensive about how much time they have to share and asks: "How long is our session today?" Jane lets them know that each appointment is scheduled for 55 minutes and says: "Today is only a start of our seeking to understand your experience and how to best support you. Take as much time as you need to tell me about what you have been experiencing." Sheila begins sharing about their pain, fatigue, and headaches. They were not interrupted in this process. Several times Sheila paused and received this response: "Is there more?"

At the time, Sheila was not conscious of the position of Jane in the room, nor her body language, but later contemplated how comfortable they felt in sharing. Sheila was surprised to subsequently be asked about their stress levels (including past stress), sleep, other symptoms like indigestion, and any history of accidents, injuries, or any type of trauma or overwhelm. This last question came with a preface that the questions may or may not hold relevance to their experience, but: "these questions help me get a glimpse of the complexity of possible factors that could be impacting your health." As Sheila was sharing about their stressors, Jane also asked: "As you're sharing about this, do you notice anything in your body?" Sheila was surprised to notice increased tension in their shoulders, face, and jaw and increased lower back pain, as well as fidgeting and shifting more.

Sheila didn't notice, but 20 minutes had passed before Jane explained a little bit about the model of care that this clinic offered. They were also surprised that Jane advised: "There often is not going to be any quick fix, including not a purely 'physical' one, but there is definitely support and potential, and if it feels right to you after our first session, we can begin to offer some experiences and skills that might help. These include…[a few examples were offered]…and we will want your feedback at each step of the way as to what is resonating and what is not well suited to your current experience. Do you have any questions so far?"

In this first session, the only "treatment" was to become aware of their breathing pattern with brief education on the autonomic nervous system, which relates to the stress response in the body. The presentation of this made so much sense to Sheila: "The nervous system is always helping us ask 'Am I safe?' and other areas of the brain and body are asking, 'Do I belong? Am I loved?' Without these basic needs addressed, our ability to move into a greater sense of understanding or even meaning about our experience is more limited, because we are wired for these things—survival and connection."

By the time this experience was done, Jane and Sheila had about 20 minutes left, and Jane asked if they would be open to a movement exam and asked if it would be OK to touch certain parts of their body. "Sure, that would be OK." After the movement screen, Sheila was invited to lie down and Jane advised: "I'm going to gently touch those areas we mentioned, let me know if anything is uncomfortable, and if anything feels stressful or upsetting, we will immediately switch course." Jane's approach was not rooted in a drive to fix these areas, but rather to bring awareness. Her intention was not to diagnose misalignment, though in the backdrop of her medical screening knowledge, she remained alert to red flags or signs of tissue pathology. There were none.

Jane proceeded by contacting these areas gently and in the process asked Sheila: "What do you notice?" Jane even asked Sheila: "What do you think your back is thinking or feeling today?"—which was one of Sheila's biggest somatic concerns on that day. Sheila, in response to the question, felt a surge of emotion and a few tears moved into expression as they considered the question. Jane noticed their response and asked if they wished to share. Sheila responded: "My back told me it is sad and tired."

Jane subsequently asked if Sheila wanted to try an experiment that might feel supportive. "Sure," Sheila responded. Jane continued: "As you notice my touch, see if you might send a welcoming message to the area of the body being touched, such as 'Soften, settle.'" Jane invited awareness of their breathing and their "whole-body sense." Jane added: "Sometimes, when we are stressed and our needs are not being met, we unconsciously protect...we guard...or hold our bodies in tension. This includes our breathing. You might pay attention after you leave today, to notice your breathing from time to time. You might also notice the places in the body that are sore, with some gentle attention, and an intention to soften or support those areas if possible, and only if it feels helpful for you to do so."

Sheila felt different after their first session, and at the second session reported: "You know, when I left here, I felt a sense of hope. I'm not sure why, but I appreciated the time you took to hear about my difficulties. Thank you." This began Sheila's journey through a care experience that included plenty of opportunities to share, choose treatment experiences, and discover their own answers and solutions to their difficulties. It was a gentle approach, and an experience of support. Sheila experienced biofeedback training (Chapter 10), which they found helpful in gaining understanding about what was happening in the body; and guided imagery (Chapter 14), which brought not only a sense of spiritual connection and meaning (Chapter 18), but also deeper experiences of relaxation than they had ever remembered consciously experiencing. They experienced a form of "manual therapy" (Chapter 23) that was rooted in a combination of lighter touch and assisted movement and that was combined with training in "mind-body skills" that offered them a new sense of and relationship to their body. They began to listen more deeply to and trust the wisdom and signals of their body. Sheila gradually learned to apply principles of ACT. Over four months, and a total of twelve one-hour sessions, Sheila still had some of the original challenges; however, they were lessened in severity and impact. More importantly, Sheila reported: "I'm much more in balance. These things are still a part of my experience, but they aren't as big of a focus to my attention anymore. I now know how to get unstuck and shift what is happening when it feels limiting or disturbing. I also have a renewed commitment to why I am here and what my purpose is in this life. I feel reconnected."

Experiential pause: After reading the preceding story, contemplate what you have learned thus far on your journey of exploring IRP. What ingredients are reflected? Write down what these are, and then return to Table 9.1 and compare. Add to the table as you create from this base.

CONCLUSION

IRP sees individuals as embedded in multiple levels and types of relationship. Relationship inspires the way in which we make sense of ourselves, others, and the world around us. Stories are how we make meaning out of experience, and structuring care within a backdrop of narrative medicine provides support for the story. This includes deepening our understanding of ingredients that enhance intersubjectivity. Creating a safe space for the patient to share is of paramount importance. Borrowing words that may have been falsely attributed to Aristotle, we tap into an important principle: "Educating the mind without educating the heart is no education at all."[23] A heart-centered approach to the story informs the safety of the space.

As noted in our opening, hazards exist in the delivery of health care. One of the biggest hazards is losing sight of the profound relevance of subjectivity. Creating the conditions for Sheila's experience to be a positive one does not come without challenges. Narrative medicine recognizes the larger processes playing out in our life experiences and helps us navigate this hazard. Focusing time, energy, and attention towards the narrative, which really means *deliberately focusing on the larger landscape and the whole of this sacred person that is here with me now*, is much more than: "fictional worlds of literature, character, point of view, and plots."[24]

When we see ourselves as interconnected with the individuals and systems that we work with/in, we are supported in our commitment to move forward with co-creating enhanced ways of delivering health care. As we progress through Chapters 10–23, we present many example strategies that demonstrate experiential learning of IRP principles. Along the way, we will meet others and see how their experiences can be enriched. Come along as we see the principles of narrative medicine play out in their stories too…

Experiential pause: Having read this chapter, identify and write down at least one actionable item of interest to you. In doing so, consider ways in which applying the material first to yourself, and then to patients, might serve those who come to you for care.

CHAPTER 10

Exploring Biofeedback

Geoff Sittler, OTR/L, BCN

A story: "Caleb" is 47 years old and has a complex history. Caleb first presented to occupational therapy (OT) through a primary care setting that primarily served clients experiencing a combination of challenges with poverty, chronic disease, addiction, and homelessness. Through referral, Caleb started attending groups that the clinic offered on mind-body skills, nutrition, and leisure activities. His health history included substance abuse, bipolar disorder, neurodiversity (autism spectrum disorder), frequent headaches, persistent back pain, and high blood pressure. In the six months prior to attending groups, he had been to the emergency room and/or admitted to the hospital 16 times. During the mind-body skills group, Caleb experienced thermal biofeedback which focuses on autonomic regulation of peripheral vasculature. His hand temperature increased by nine degrees, allowing Caleb to have a lived experience of the mind-body connection. After attending groups for a number of months, where Caleb's overall mind-body health had improved, he expressed interest in trying additional biofeedback strategies in individual OT. His heart rate variability (HRV) evaluation showed overall low variability, a finding associated with many of his health challenges. Over several more months of integrative therapy that included biofeedback and other mind-body skills training, his HRV improved in both quality (respiratory sinus arrhythmia) and the amount of variability. In addition to biofeedback training, time was spent exploring Caleb's values and goals and how to use practically the skills he was learning to support each step on his journey. Treatment included support around the social determinants that were impacting his health, including work with both a social worker and a vocational rehabilitation professional. Over six months, Caleb achieved a number of profound goals including:

- acquiring and maintaining stable housing and sobriety for the "longest time that I can remember in my adult life!"
- no ER visits/hospital admissions
- joining a gym and exercising three to four times a week
- enrolling in NAMI (National Alliance on Mental Illness) peer-to-peer training and starting in a peer-support role
- volunteering to be a peer-support group facilitator at the clinic.

Often, when asked to define biofeedback, responses range from "I don't know," to "That's an energy therapy from the 70s, right?" Very few realize that they may have used biofeedback multiple times already during their day, albeit unconsciously. If you looked in a mirror today to make an adjustment in your appearance or noticed and responded to clothing feeling tighter or looser after lifestyle changes, then you have used biofeedback. A simple definition of biofeedback is when you receive useful information about yourself and then make personal changes based on that feedback.

In 2007, a formal definition for biofeedback was created by a task force established by the Association for Applied Psychophysiology and Biofeedback (AAPB), the International Society for Neuroregulation and Research (ISNR), and the Biofeedback Certification Institute of America (BCIA, now known as the Biofeedback Certification International Alliance):

> Biofeedback is a process that enables an individual to learn how to change physiological activity for the purposes of improving health and performance. Precise instruments measure physiological activity such as brainwaves, heart function, breathing, muscle activity and skin temperature. These instruments rapidly and accurately "feed back" information to the user. The presentation of this information—often in conjunction with changes in thinking, emotions, and behavior—supports physiological changes. Over time, these changes can endure without continued use of an instrument.[1]

Biofeedback allows people to gain insights that they may not otherwise access. Anyone working in the helping professions can implement biofeedback to assist their clients to actively contribute to their health. Regardless of whether you are a health coach encouraging a client to explore the connection between nutrition and sleep, a counselor helping someone explore how their thoughts are connected to their behaviors, or a surgeon educating about the importance of exercise after a major procedure, biofeedback can be a valuable addition to your overall approach.

As explored in earlier chapters, a foundational tenet of mind-body medicine lies in the understanding that we can actively impact our own physiology. This includes biological processes that are typically assumed to be outside of conscious influence. There is high potential for applying principles of self-regulation in ways that impact our health. However, the capacity to regulate our biology is not seen as absolute nor sustainable. We must return to principles of body-mind-environment (BME) complexity. Aiming to support greater psychophysiological flexibility to ride the waves of BME changes reflects a good lens. Remaining mindful to not suggest that any "tool" guarantees a "fix" to the unpleasant facets of our experience is also in play. Instead, we seek to take positive action as a valued intention. Taking an active role in our health is always a wise choice, regardless of outcome.

In Caleb's case, his transformation had many "ingredients," including an early and profound experience of biofeedback that was combined with facilitation of the relaxation response.[2] This and other experiential activities occurred in a group setting of mutual support that included simple, functional education on the science of hypervigilance and autonomic dysregulation. The relaxation response was facilitated through evidence-based techniques such as autogenic training (AT).

AT is a form of mind-body regulation training where a series of simple, suggestive phrases are repeated. This technique can facilitate systemic mind-body regulation effects. Literature supports AT use for a number of the conditions Caleb was experiencing, including anxiety and persistent pain.[3] After the AT experience, where Caleb's hand temperature increased nine degrees in 15 minutes, he exclaimed: "This is the most relaxed I can recall feeling in a long time, perhaps ever." This experience holds value independent of the recorded physiological response.

AN OCCUPATIONAL THERAPIST'S EXPERIENCE

When I was 27 years old, I experienced a panic attack for the first time in my life. My heart was racing, my breathing was rapid, and I started to notice that my hands were feeling numb. I subsequently learned the importance of having someone I trust help me understand what was happening with my body. I had been engaged for about five months, and had been experiencing somatic symptoms due to anxiety for weeks before experiencing a full panic attack. In looking back, I can see that my body had been trying to tell me what my head did not want to believe: I was not ready to get married. Throughout the ordeal I had been confiding in my mother, who had patiently supported me while I navigated the process of realizing what I needed to do. She didn't try to fix it. During the panic attack I was talking with her on the phone as the fear escalated. When I started to struggle to hold the phone due to the numbness in my hands, this "feedback" became a negative reinforcer, exacerbating the feeling of panic. She calmly and reassuringly guided me through a diaphragmatic breathing exercise as she simultaneously explained in simple terms that the rapid breathing was causing the numbness. This experience helped me understand the power of the mind-body connection and was a turning point in my personal and professional life.

Before this crisis, exercise had been a regular part of my life as a tool for self-regulation, although at the time I don't think I realized the value of it for my mental health. After the panic attack, it was apparent to me that I needed to expand my skill set to manage the challenges of life. I started exploring yoga and learning about meditation and energy work. Mindfulness and meditation were extremely challenging for me during these years of exploration. I was fortunate to make several friends who regularly practiced meditation. Their support and guidance kept me motivated not to give up. Eventually, I came across biofeedback, which was an effective approach to guide my mind and body into a meditative state. I also realized biofeedback could be an effective modality to integrate into my work, as biofeedback bridges a gap that exists for some: understanding the scientific basis of the mind-body relationship.

My early days in the profession of occupational therapy were challenging, as I struggled to define my role. Was I there to educate, support, care for, or fix? It felt as if I wore many different hats and I struggled at times to define what OT was for me. I was discussing this challenge with a fellow OT who defined our role as a "guide." He said that OTs can provide the direction and support to assist those individuals we care for, and that ultimately the other person needs to navigate their experience in process. This helped me better understand my job and how we might best serve those who come to us for help.

A GUIDING TOOL

If we contemplate what a guide does, we see they provide direction and support using knowledge, wisdom, and tools. In the past, explorers utilized topography, celestial bodies, and other cues to navigate the world. As technology advanced, the compass made traversing our environment more accessible. Now, anyone with access to a smartphone has GPS technology with step-by-step directions at their fingertips.

Biofeedback and the other tools laid out in this book may be seen as analogous to these way-finding tools. Instead of telling people how to find places in the external world, biofeedback provides support for *exploring and guiding* ourselves. Part of the power of biofeedback is that it allows clients to experience and influence parts of their physiology which they:

- would otherwise not have access to
- do not understand in relevance
- believe may have been lost permanently to injury, disease, or time.

Biofeedback reflects psychophysiological (mind-body) interactions and in context is seen as a synergy between self-awareness and physiological regulation. At least partially, biofeedback operates from principles of classical and operant conditioning.[4] Both classical and operant conditioning reflect processes of learning. Classical conditioning involves the involuntary pairing of two stimuli, while operant conditioning pairs stimuli with voluntary behavior and response.

Applied biofeedback is best seen as active therapeutic learning, as opposed to a thing you do to another. Through relational and experiential feedback and without assumptions, we seek to understand what the client's experience is like at all stages, with an approach designed to support the individual through the lens of larger processes.

Clients who are suffering from a disease, especially those with a major stress component, can benefit from biofeedback. As covered in Chapter 3, stress plays a varying role in most chronic disease and influences the course of illness or injury regardless of causality.[5] Thus, biofeedback principles carry widespread applicability as part of a care approach. In addition to the management of stress, the efficacy of biofeedback is supported with strong evidence for many conditions including: headache, persistent pain, Raynaud's disease, incontinence, anxiety, and hypertension. Numerous other conditions have various levels of evidence (Table 10.1) to support the consideration of biofeedback as part of an integrative treatment plan.[6]

Table 10.1: Evidence for Biofeedback: Efficacy ratings for biofeedback training on various medical conditions

Level 5 (efficacious and specific) / Level 4 (efficacious)	Level 3 (probably efficacious)	Level 2 (possibly efficacious) / Level 1 (not empirically supported)
Level 5 (efficacious and specific) ADHD **Level 4 (efficacious)** Anxiety, anxiety disorders Chronic pain* Constipation (adult) Depressive disorders Diabetes—glycemic control Erectile dysfunction Epilepsy Fecal incontinence Headache (adult) Irritable bowel syndrome Preeclampsia Raynaud's disease Temporomandibular disorders	Alcoholism/substance abuse Arthritis Asthma Autism Chronic pain** Diabetes—diabetic ulcers Facial palsy Insomnia Motion sickness Performance enhancement Post-traumatic stress disorder Tinnitus (biofeedback) Traumatic brain injury Urinary incontinence (children, females, and males)	**Level 2 (possibly efficacious)** Cerebral palsy Chemo-brain Chronic obstructive pulmonary disease Chronic pain*** Coronary artery disease Diabetes—intermittent claudication Hyperhidrosis Immune function Repetitive strain injury Stroke Tinnitus (neurofeedback) Vasovagal syncope **Level 1 (not empirically supported)** Chronic pain****

*Muscle-related orofacial, non-cardiac chest, posture-related

**Muscle-related low back, phantom limb, pelvic floor, patellofemoral, cancer-related, fibromyalgia

***Carpal tunnel, myofascial pain syndrome/"trigger point," whiplash, PMS, muscle spasm, functional/recurrent abdominal

****Pain/spasticity due to not taking breaks among repetitive movement professions, reflex sympathetic dystrophy, trigeminal neuralgia

Compiled from Tan et al.[7] with permission from The Association for Applied Psychophysiology and Biofeedback, Inc.

Biofeedback is most effective when delivered by a professional trained in the biofeedback intervention and does not necessarily require advanced certifications to include in a care plan. Basic biofeedback principles assist others in understanding how to attune to information in their bodies, and understand what this physiological data represents and how to subsequently access positive influence within complex BME interactions.

THE "BIOFEEDBACK RELATIONSHIP"

A key component of success for the use of biofeedback lies in the relationship between the client and their "guide" (i.e., therapist, teacher, coach, etc.). In looking at the story of Caleb's experience, we see that the support received from both the therapist and the group were important ingredients in combination with therapeutic education (Chapter 16) and biofeedback experiences. Having the support of a trusted guide was also true in the case of this author's experience of moving through a panic attack with the wisdom and support of a family member.

Trust, faith, and/or belief in the guide and/or the approach being deployed supports the capacity to move through a challenging experience. This trust/faith dynamic is inherent in our understanding of placebo effects. The importance of establishing rapport in relation to placebo is increasingly emphasized,[8] yet we may not fully realize the extent to which the supportive, attuned relationship supports placebo effects.

You can be extremely competent with the use of biofeedback technology, but if the person you are working with does not feel comfortable with or trust you, no amount of technical expertise will allow this person to experience optimal benefit from utilizing biofeedback.

TYPES OF BIOFEEDBACK

There are multiple biofeedback systems and approaches used in clinical, educational, and research settings. The physiological information that is used in clinical biofeedback comes in various forms, often called channels. The most common types include:

- peripheral temperature, covered in more detail below
- HRV, covered in more detail below
- surface electromyography (SEMG): recording muscular electrical activity from the surface of the skin; an example of a specialized area of SEMG is training pelvic muscle dysfunction, typically to treat incontinence
- galvanic skin response (GSA)/skin conductance activity (SCA): measurement of sweat gland activity in the hands via the amount of electrical activity the skin will allow to pass; this is often used as a sensitive measure of changes in emotional activation and arousal[9]
- respiration: used to measure respiration rate, diaphragmatic breathing, CO_2 (capnometer) feedback, and volumetric feedback
- electroencephalography (EEG) biofeedback/neurofeedback: measuring and displaying the electrical activity of the brain and displaying it in a visual and/or auditory format to allow for retraining brainwave patterns.[10]

The client's goals/health challenges, equipment options, clinical setting, diagnosis, and potential number of sessions for training all have an impact on which form of biofeedback to include. Complex multimodal biofeedback systems are available and include monitoring, feedback, and recording across different channels. As noted above, however, you do not need to undertake this route or degree of investment to successfully apply biofeedback in practice.

SUPPORTING REGULATION AND RESILIENCE: BIOFEEDBACK AS PROCESS

As defined earlier, biofeedback is best seen as a process (contributing to the regulation of specific physiological "channels") within larger processes (the context of the therapeutic relationship, other facets of care, and larger spheres of the person's life experience and conditions). In biofeedback, once a client can "see" physiological channels or patterns of biological function, the therapist can then assist with further steps in the learning process: how to positively influence what is being shown to them. When a client, such as Caleb, experiences the temperature on their fingers increase after participating in a guided meditation, they have activated the parasympathetic branch of their autonomic nervous system (ANS).

Autonomic comes from the concept of autonomous or "self-governing." In medical context, autonomic has been used to denote the concept of automatic, involuntary, and non-conscious. Until the work of Elmer Green and associates at the Menninger Foundation in the late 1960s, it was largely believed that humans had no ability to sense nor control this part of the nervous system.[11] The work of the Menninger Foundation started a paradigm shift from the concept of self-governing to self-regulating—moving from a non-conscious process to a conscious and intentional one. The ability to proactively contribute to the body's regulation processes is a core concept embedded in the work of mind-body medicine and is one of the foundational components of integrative rehabilitation practice (IRP).

As mentioned earlier, one facet of the learning processes that allow a person to develop volitional control over their ANS and its impact within systemic physiology is operant conditioning (instrumental conditioning). Operant conditioning, defined by American psychologist B. F. Skinner, is a process that occurs through rewards and punishments for behavior. Through operant conditioning, an individual makes an association between a particular behavior and a consequence.[12] Skinner's early focus was on observable, measurable physiological responses and less on the related impact of the mind, thoughts, and emotions due to limitations in quantifying these areas. The underpinnings of how biofeedback works, consistent with the integrative call to embrace complexity, are more than solely through processes of conditioning. Along this line, Schwartz and Andrasik note:

> Although it is helpful to view biofeedback primarily as instrumental conditioning of visceral responses, this model is limiting in that some professionals believe that human learning includes major cognitive dimensions as well as environmental reinforcers, for example, thinking, expectation, visualization and imagery, foresight and planning, and problem-solving strategies.[13]

Additionally, biofeedback may be more effective when combining its embedded operant conditioning principles with the concurrent training of other mind-body skills: this combines modes of learning. Examples include combining breath awareness and regulation skills, body awareness and neuromuscular relaxation training, mental imagery, meditation, and/or AT as described earlier. Ultimately, the biofeedback process must include translation "into the world" where the client gains real-time capacity to respond more effectively to stress in daily living.

GETTING STARTED: KEEP IT SIMPLE

A brief exploration of the various books, websites, training courses, computer systems, and other devices for biofeedback can be overwhelming for anyone interested in learning about biofeedback. A recommendation for learning about the utility of biofeedback is to start simple and to explore using these techniques with yourself first. If you haven't used biofeedback with yourself, it will be challenging to explain this approach to your clients.

Experiential pause: A simple form of biofeedback that most of us can try is taking our pulse. For those with motor control and sensory feedback in their hands, start with finding the carotid artery on your neck or your wrist and get a sense of the length of time between each heartbeat. Now, take a fuller, deeper breath, hold for two to three counts, and then exhale through pursed lips, taking longer than it took you to inhale. See if you can feel the lengthening/slowing between heartbeats that occurs in concert with the exhalation phase. This is self-monitoring of heart rate variability and reflects the fact that during an inhale, tonic vagal efferent activity on the heart is withdrawn, allowing sympathetic activity to effectively accelerate your heart. Then, during exhale, parasympathetic flow through the vagus effectively slows the heart. Voila! You have just discovered the very basis of HRV feedback.

INTRODUCING BIOFEEDBACK TO CLIENTS

For clinicians and educators, graduating our clients and students so they no longer need our services is the ultimate goal. When the role of biofeedback is explained, it can be helpful to use the analogy of learning to ride a bike with training wheels. Ask the client if they have experienced feeling balanced on a bike before and if they can define it. The response to this question is usually challenging to articulate. Some will state: "I guess it is just a feeling and you know it when you feel it." Others with a less-developed feeling element might even state: "I guess I hadn't thought of it as a feeling."

The role of biofeedback is analogous to training wheels in that it helps individuals view and feel their nervous system in a different way. Eventually, felt experiences of "balance" can be achieved. Remember that we are not built to stay in perfect balance all of the time, but to be able to assist in returning to balance when demand has passed: think resilience and adaptability. A longer-term functional goal lies in developing a generalized set of skills that are easily exercised in daily life to improve responsiveness to demanding BME conditions when they arise. Eventually, the assistance of monitored feedback is replaced with capacity to detect shifts and assist in regulation independently. This is analogous to removing the training wheels from the bike and advancing innate capacity.

TEMPERATURE REGULATION

Already introduced in Caleb's story, measuring body temperature is one of the simplest and most accessible options for exploring biofeedback. Thermal biofeedback is rooted in a well-known aspect of our physiology that can be easily accessed through any thermometer. Almost all of us have had our body temperature taken to evaluate our health. The standard method of measuring temperature to evaluate for an ailment like the flu is done sublingually or at the forehead to obtain approximate measures of core temperature. With thermal biofeedback however, we focus on the distribution of peripheral body temperature, which is gauged at the fingers or toes to assess ANS control of circulation.

A key indicator of sympathetic dominance is colder hand and foot temperatures relative to the core body temperature. This reflects a vasoconstrictive gradient controlled by sympathetic efferent activity. Activation of survival-oriented musculature through changes in blood flow and neuromuscular tone are just a few of the outcomes caused by these integrated responses. Redirection of energy and resources towards large muscles and the core causes decreased circulation at the surface of our skin and on the aforementioned peripheral gradient.

Conversely, balance in the ANS is reflected by higher temperatures in our extremities from the vasodilatory effects of increased systemic parasympathetic activity. This is typically present in low-demand, low-threat conditions—states of safety or "rest and digest." The presence of historical, high, or prolonged states of activation may lead to limitations in achieving such capacity. Individuals like Caleb often have experienced chronically dysregulated states for months or even years; when an experience of relative balance is achieved, it is often met with pleasant surprise.

Biofeedback and many of the other tools that will be explored in this book can facilitate decreased sympathetic and/or increased parasympathetic activity. This has implications across many other aspects of physiology, such as central nervous system (CNS) function, and inflammatory and immune processes. In the case of simple thermal regulation, the response is evidenced by an increase in the temperature of the fingers. Other measures can be taken to reflect beneficial shifts in physiological state. Such shifts can positively impact allostatic load.[14]

Experiential pause: Thermal biofeedback exercise

1. Gather materials to measure your peripheral body temperature. You can use a thermistor, kitchen/home digital thermometer, or "Stress Square/biodot."
2. If available, affix a temperature measuring device to the pad of one of your fingers. You can use medical tape, a band-aid, etc. to affix the device (Figure 10.1). Be careful to not over tighten when placing the device with tape or a band-aid since this will decrease blood flow and compromise the exercise. Note: If you do not have a device, you can still appreciate a sense of the temperature and any change that occurs. To help, you might lightly touch your fingers to the warmest part(s) of your body and get a feel for the current temperature.

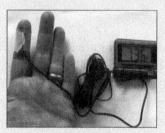
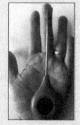
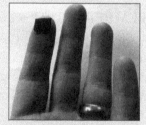

Thermistor   Kitchen thermometer   "Stress Square"

FIGURE 10.1: SIMPLE TEMPERATURE BIOFEEDBACK

3. Make a note of how you are feeling currently. You might even rate how you feel and then use the same rating scale to indicate any changes after the exercise.

4. Complete a mind-body technique designed to promote ANS regulation effects. Some examples include using AT or guided imagery. For AT, you can repeat (slowly, silently) (or listen; see Resources at the end of the chapter) each of the following phrases four to six times each, imagining that you are feeling the words happening in your body:
   - My arms are feeling relaxed, heavy, and warm…
   - My legs are feeling relaxed, heavy, and warm…
   - My heartbeat is feeling calm, yet strong…
   - My forehead is feeling relaxed and pleasantly cool…
   - My breathing is feeling calm, smooth, and relaxed…
   - My belly is feeling relaxed, and radiating warmth…

5. After completing the activity, note any change in the biofeedback device used in Step 2 and assess any perceived change using your self-rating scale from Step 3. If you obtain "Stress Squares," the following guide, Figure 10.2, gives a general indication of the level of tension in the ANS:

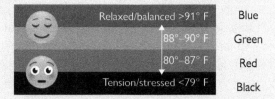

FIGURE 10.2: RELATIVE PERIPHERAL TEMPERATURE RANGES

6. If you are working with a client, discuss whether the biofeedback reading aligns with their perception. In general, gaining conscious influence over the ANS is a slow process. One's mind-body state, and response to training, is a process and must be explored gently and patiently. Ultimately, warmer temperatures indicate greater ANS balance in non-demand conditions. Also, for some, lowering arousal level through parasympathetic activation can lead to feelings of unease. For example, individuals who equate maintaining vigilance to safety may feel "less relaxed" when in a state of lower arousal.

7. Additional discussion with your client may follow regarding the functional implications of using biofeedback to promote improved regulation. Some examples include improving sleep patterns, management of anxiety to avoid isolation, or engagement in community activities such as shopping or leisure.

SYSTEMS THEORY AND BIOFEEDBACK

Several general keys for working with each person in relationship to biofeedback include:

- discovering the unique patterns of mind-body interactions that are present
- transforming embodied stress responses by targeting biofeedback processes
- remembering that not all stress is bad.

Towards the latter point, applying systems theory (Chapter 1) to biofeedback is important. There is a complexity to the naturally occurring and fluctuating physiological patterns, reflecting the presence of multiple feedback mechanisms within BME patterns. In other words, many mechanisms operate simultaneously to control a system: they are related and interdependent. An unstable (dysregulated) system is associated with poorer health and reduced resilience capacity. Stressors can arise from various "entry points" or levels within the living system, causing disturbance. When optimized, stress and demand activate integrated control mechanisms to achieve allostasis. As such, our non-dual lens reminds us that positive, as well as negative, experiences are important for system function and stability. In integrative care, we must also apply such thinking to social dynamics, and even organizations as living systems. While decidedly a complicated question, we must ask ourselves: What do the principles of biofeedback look like in therapeutic relationships, in organizational structure, and the physical environment/ecosystems?

Another story: Juliette was a 53-year-old female receiving care in a skilled nursing facility. Among a number of health issues and comorbidities, Juliette was experiencing severe Raynaud's disease. This condition causes some areas of the body—such as the fingers and toes—to feel cold/numb in response to cold temperatures and/or stress. In working with her OT, Juliette observed that Raynaud's presented a significant challenge for her due to severe pain in her fingers. No medical professional had ever suggested a mechanism, nor the possibility of treatment. She had resigned herself to the condition. Her primary method to manage the discomfort was using gloves to keep her hands warm, but this created added challenges with daily activities such as being able to hold utensils or attempting to turn pages in a book.

Juliette identified her finger pains as the primary area of concern and she expressed a desire to discontinue use of the gloves if that was ever possible. Due to the fast-paced and demanding environment of the skilled nursing facility (SNF), the OT had limited time. However, it was enough to explain the condition and for Juliette to express interest in exploring mind-body strategies. She felt hopeful just from hearing the explanation and that there was research supporting the fact that the condition was amenable to change. Thermal biofeedback was instructed using real-time guidance combined with music. She identified classical music as the most relaxing genre for her. Each session started with diaphragmatic breathing (Chapter 11) and basic guided imagery (Chapter 14), followed by a thermal biofeedback protocol (see above). After just five sessions, Juliette no longer needed the gloves to manage her pain. A simple recorded technique afforded her the option to practice at home, paired with an inexpensive portable biofeedback device which was offered in her final session before discharge.

IS BIOFEEDBACK THE RIGHT MODALITY FOR YOUR CLIENT?

As you consider to what degree you may wish to pursue the various forms of biofeedback in your practice, we must remember the possibility of gaps between idealism and realism.

We must bridge these gaps to deploy biofeedback and the larger scope of IRP successfully. We must also consider and emphasize an approach that offers the benefits of relative simplicity in the face of complexity.

At a minimum, the core message of mind-body medicine can be conveyed and explored in the foundations of integrative practice: we can have positive influence over processes of health and we can learn to track and monitor BME interactions throughout the day. The simplest forms of biofeedback that we present are accessible to nearly anyone and reflect the minimum starting point. In doing so, even with a single experience, like the thermistor feedback that Caleb experienced in a group, we can leave individuals with the understanding and ability to "track" mind-body patterns. Training ourselves to notice when the stress response is showing up in bodily measures as we move through various conditions, experiences, and environments is a vital skill. In other words, pay attention and exercise the ability to become aware, regulate, and rebalance throughout the day. If interest and motivation exist, some may move on to more complicated forms of biofeedback, which require various levels of training and equipment expense.

For a more structured approach, and to promote increased likelihood of longer-term changes, biofeedback benefits from consistent practice and reinforcement. This is true with most forms of mind-body medicine (MBM), where the "slow but powerful medicine" reminder comes into play. Patience is thus a valuable trait to accompany biofeedback and other mind-body skills training.

Finally, we must become capable of assisting clients in the development of committed actions that are rooted in their values. As such, principles of motivational interviewing (introduced in Chapter 6) or Acceptance and Commitment Therapy (introduced in Chapter 17) may further assist in identifying the best avenues for exploration as well as individual goals that are applicable to and attainable for each person. For now, a reminder: we must not make assumptions that, simply because there is evidence and/or that we have found clinical value in the approach, it is the right path for any given person at any given time.

HEART RATE VARIABILITY

Due to an expanding evidence base, HRV assessment and training is encouraged as an important part of IRP. HRV is a known indicator of our body's ability to manage allostatic load.[15] HRV reflects a step up in complexity compared with simple temperature feedback as it requires some degree of further training. HRV is a solid candidate for measuring both physiological resilience/stress capacity and objective improvement over time, which may otherwise be hard to demonstrate clinically. This is especially true when the presenting challenges are more mind-body (biobehavioral, psychophysiological, quality of life, etc.) and/or chronic (such as persistent pain) in nature. As such, a closer look is warranted.

HRV is a measure of the heart rate's beat-to-beat interval and in part reflects the state of the ANS's action on the heart's intrinsic system. It is also reflective of blood pressure (BP), gas exchange, and gut, heart, and vascular tone.[16] Higher HRV reflects consistently variable time differences between each heartbeat and in general reflects healthier states and higher physiological capacity to respond to demand. If there is minimal time difference between heartbeats, we have lower HRV. This reflects lower physiological capacity when faced with varying life circumstances. In Caleb's story, through the use of biofeedback and mind-body skills training as part of his larger IRP experience, he demonstrated increased HRV over time. Given that HRV has been correlated with improved top-down regulation (such as prefrontal inhibitory control over threat-defensive responses, emotion regulation, and social behavior),[17] increases in HRV may reflect such positive overall shifts within Caleb's experience.

As discussed in earlier chapters, the physiology of the ANS is integral to survival and health processes. HRV gives us a glimpse into the status of the ANS, and is considered an effective way to measure this important facet of the larger integrated psychophysiological matrix. HRV reflects capacity for how our systems manage the varying demands of life, through our nervous system's ability to seamlessly shift between the sympathetic and the parasympathetic divisions of the ANS.[18]

TRAINING RESILIENCE THROUGH HRV

How adaptable are you when faced with stressful situations? The possibility of positively impacting HRV has implications for numerous physical and behavioral health conditions.[19] Further, evidence links constructs of resilience to HRV.[20] HRV training can be used in conjunction with any of the other physiological markers (multimodal training) or as a standalone approach. The most accurate method used to measure HRV is through an electrocardiograph (ECG) sensor that collects the electrical signals of the heart. This is often combined with a respiration monitor to look at patterns of synchrony between HRV and the respiratory rate, and together defines the larger phenomena of respiratory sinus arrhythmia. A simpler option is to evaluate HRV through the use of a photoplethysmography (PPG) sensor.

The PPG measures changes in blood volume pulse in arteries and capillaries that correspond to changes in heart rate. Heart-rate changes are detected through the use of an infrared light (usually by a light-emitting diode, or LED) typically attached to the finger, wrist, or ear.[21] Most commercially available options for HRV devices utilize PPG technology; however, most research-grade equipment will use ECG and respiration together. Cost can vary from <$100, into the thousands, based on quality, portability, and purpose (e.g., personal/home options versus research grade).

If you would like to further explore HRV biofeedback, additional training beyond this chapter will be needed. Learning to complete resonant frequency analysis (RFA) is a good place to start. An RFA can be used to determine a person's optimal breathing rate/pattern. Each person has a unique RFA breathing rate, typically between 4.5 and 7.0 breaths/min.[22] This has high potential to increase vagal-nerve parasympathetic action on the heart alongside decreased baseline sympathetic action.[23]

As you will learn in Chapter 12, bringing awareness/attention to the breath before necessarily manipulating its parameters is a useful idea. Once awareness is established, conscious control using an RFA breathing rate (or other self-selected approach) can assist individuals in enhanced mind-body regulation. Visual tools such as breath pacers may be useful for some and problematic for others.

RFA can be used to support the creation of breathing patterns designed to optimize the potential for the emergence of ANS balance and its impact on systemic psychophysiological states. A common word used to denote balance from a biobehavioral lens is "coherence," wherein the physiological state optimizes one's ability to think and feel simultaneously. In a sense, this reflects capacity to be awake, alert, and even active, yet physiologically relaxed at the same time. Another way of viewing this is through the lens of arousal and the cultivation of optimal states of arousal. In models of mind-body dysregulation, training individuals into the "window of arousal" or "zone of tolerance" are phrases often used to denote this. HRV is currently the most common physiological measure used to correlate to the idea of an optimal state of arousal, including scientific constructs of resilience.[24]

WEARABLE BIOFEEDBACK AND FUTURE TRENDS

Biofeedback training has traditionally been offered through a professional in a clinic or office. This is done using expensive computers and specialized equipment. Advances in technology in the last few decades have allowed companies to develop standalone devices, smart-device apps, and/or computer games. This has dramatically increased accessibility to biofeedback. These devices are guided by everything from HRV to brain-wave (EEG) data and provide personalized guidance on mind-body habits. Through the use of haptic feedback, some wearable devices signal users to move, adjust posture, or breathe more deeply through vibrational cues and do not require additional technology such as a smartphone. Working collaboratively with those we serve can help identify whether acquiring such technology is feasible and accessible.

BIOFEEDBACK IN CONTEXT

Personal responsibility is known to play a vital role in health. Conveying the message that we have influence within the whole of our health experience is important. Biofeedback provides a visible and practical language in support of this. As we navigate the topic, we must also remind ourselves of even larger contexts—such as the reality that social determinants (Chapter 4) play a significant role in health. The choices that people make are subject to the choices available to them.[25] Similarly, the clinical care we provide may account for only a small fraction of the impact on each person's health experience.[26] As such, how we utilize the time we have with each individual matters greatly. Biofeedback, delivered in context, and self-selected as part of a treatment approach, can deliver in this regard.

CONCLUSION

Biofeedback is an evidence-based modality and is the first of numerous empowering tools presented in this section of the book. Biofeedback can range from simple to complex. In some cases, access to formal biofeedback training can be limited. However, simplified and accessible versions exist that carry similar weight and message as more expensive/complicated approaches. The value of biofeedback is underscored by examining the relevance and importance of exploring mind-body processes within the larger framework of IRP. Supporting the power of regulation processes through the mind-body connection assists us in mitigating allostatic load. Biofeedback reflects the potential we have to actively and consciously contribute to physiological processes, acting in support of resilience and general well-being. In other words, it can benefit everyone!

Experiential pause: Having read this chapter, identify and write down at least one actionable item of interest to you. In doing so, consider ways in which applying the material first to yourself, and then to patients, might serve those who come to you for care.

RESOURCES

The goal for this chapter was to provide an overview of applied biofeedback. If you would like to further explore this modality, the resources listed below are good options to begin with.

- For the temperature biofeedback experiential, which is the same technique that was mentioned in both Caleb's and Juliette's stories, go here for a sample: https://oregonmindbody.com/meditations/autogenic-training.mp3.
- Books:
  » *Biofeedback Mastery—An Experiential Teaching and Self-Training Manual* (2008) by Peper, E., Tylova, H., Gibney, K., Harvey, R., and Combatalade, D.
  » *Biofeedback: A Practitioner's Guide* (Fourth edition) edited by Schwartz, M. and Andrasik, F.
- Professional organization and certification in biofeedback:
  » Biofeedback Certification International Alliance (BCIA): www.bcia.org.
- Professional training:
  » Stens Corporation (www.stens-biofeedback.com) offers equipment as well as in-person and online training in biofeedback. Historically, they have offered a useful "Everything You Wanted to Know About Heart Rate Variability" distance-learning program.
  » HeartMath offers a unique approach to HRV training, which includes various meditation concepts, and offers a professional certification program (www.heartmath.com/hmct).
  » Embody Your Mind (www.embodyyourmind.com) offers online learning in various facets of mind-body and integrative medicine, including clinical applications of biofeedback. *Disclosure: Matt Erb, PT, co-editor of this book, is*

founder/owner of Embody Your Mind, and thus discloses a financial relationship to this listed resource.

» The Center for Mind-Body Medicine (CMBM) (www.cmbm.org) offers training in a broad set of mind-body medicine skills including the simple/ accessible temperature biofeedback presented in the chapter. The CMBM approach emphasizes using a small-group model (see Chapter 25).

– Temperature biofeedback supplies: If you are interested in purchasing lower cost equipment for thermal biofeedback, you can find options by searching online:

» Affordable options to start with include "biodots" and/or "Stress Squares," which are liquid-crystal stickers that use color to reflect body temperature.

» Various thermistors provide real-time visual readouts. One of the most popular and affordable is the "Stress Thermometer."

CHAPTER 11

Exploring the Breath

Kellie Finn, MS, C-IAYT, ERYT-500

A story: "Raffi," 48, is sitting in a chair when I enter the room. He is hesitant for company. He has just eaten food for the first time in a week. He tells that me if he digests it well, he'll be released. I let him know that we can simply chat, that he can ask me to leave at any time. He tells me that he was admitted for accidentally drinking bleach. He explains how it happened. I ask how his body is feeling; he responds: "Uncomfortable, all mixed up." He's tired of the hospital. I ask questions and he talks about his wife, two boys, love of cooking for them. He talks of his job, coworkers, and love of working out, which has fallen away this past year: "You should have seen me! I was all muscle, double my size." His body looks lean, stoic, lifted, clenched. His arms are engaged though they rest on the chair. In a pause, I ask if he's open to trying a breathing technique that might help with discomfort and digestion. As he closes his eyes, I invite him to soften back into the chair, to let it hold him. I offer cues for watching and feeling the breath. I notice his arms and face soften; his chest appears less gripped. Eventually, I invite him to place his hands on his abdomen and use them to invite breath there, adding in various cues to support focus. He stays for only a few breaths, then opens his eyes and says he doesn't want to do it anymore, it's uncomfortable. I tell him that's fine and ask him how his body feels now. He reports: "not great." Without prompting, he begins to talk about his sons again, and then his father and his childhood. He talks about his father's sudden death a few years back, and the impact on the family. He shares detailed memories of his dad working on cars in the yard where, as a child, he would help. "He could fix anything." Tears roll down his cheeks, but he keeps talking. Multiple times he says: "I don't know why I'm telling you all of this." He shares more stories, getting out of his chair to show me pictures on his phone of his father, sons, mom, himself when he was weightlifting, his wife. He comes back to his sons, saying how important it is to him that he is as good a dad to them as his dad was to him. He can't wait to get home to cook for them. I ask him again how his body is feeling, and he says, somewhat surprised: "It feels fine." He reports that the discomfort is fading.

Breath sustains all forms of life without bias, for a time determined beyond the will of the entity. It is the only involuntary physiological process that can easily be directed consciously. Does this mean we have the power to participate with the quantity or quality of our life? What is the gain of giving breath more attention? How dependent is the quality of our living experience—physically, emotionally, psychologically—on the quality and quantity of this curious current? In this chapter, we will touch on the enigma that is our breath while glimpsing the growing body of research supporting interventions through various breathing practices for nervous system regulation and symptom management. We will:

- examine why knowing specific applications of breath is relevant
- examine the importance of this force in practitioner self-care
- have an opportunity to experience the potency of our own breath
- explore avenues for enhancing breath awareness with clients.

A YOGA THERAPIST'S EXPERIENCE

Most of the work I do as a yoga therapist is on two hospital acute-care units. Physical, mental, and/or emotional pain are common and woven into fear, confusion, self-doubt, mistrust, and life assessment. Breath, for its accessibility and versatility, is my go-to. Beyond recognizing its health benefits, reflection on breath as a companion and a revealing force for connection never fails to awe me. Every moment, without effort and for as long as it deems fit, this circular rhythm weaves its way through our body carrying responsibilities that affect every cell and sensation of human aliveness. It is a constant gesture of sustenance, embrace, and possibility. Even its shape of movement strikes me. Our breath is a constant circle of give and take, of one thing perpetually leading to another. What a beautiful mirror of how breath works with our body and life: the quality of our breathing affects the quality of our health and, in turn, the quality of health reflects the quality of our living. Arriving full circle, the quality of our living affects the movement of our breath.

As a child with severe asthma, and now as a dedicated yogi, I can't remember a time when I wasn't aware of my breath and its relationship to my aliveness. The breathless panic episodes of youth that triggered shame, limited activities, and necessitated multiple visits to the intensive-care unit forced me to learn mental and physical relaxation techniques, to relax and let myself be breathed. Today, breath is a salve. I seek it out for company, emotional regulation, revelation, remembrance of the bigger picture, decision clarification, and overall health, and to cultivate therapeutic presence in my work.

In Raffi's case, breath awareness was offered as an aid to support physical digestion and help alleviate discomfort, but breath also has the synthesizing power to pull forth that which needs attention beyond the conscious eye. In response to Raffi's hesitation for company, I also made a point of consciously deepening my own breath to support therapeutic presence, not knowing where the session might go or that there were things needing digestion beyond the food he'd eaten. Where the breath took us surprised us both, such is the wonder of this remarkable mechanism of life.

A UNIVERSAL LANGUAGE

Some languages try to capture the larger meaning and relevance of breath in a word. In Hebrew, *ruach* translates as wind or breath, and also references the vital principle that resides in and animates the body, an apparition, the soul. In Greek medicine, *pneuma* is the form of circulating air necessary for the systemic functioning of vital organs, as well as the material that sustains consciousness in a body. *Chi* in Chinese philosophy is life force, the substance for which all existing phenomena are constituted. It is associated with breath, life, and health. Cultivating healthy chi is seen as honoring and sustaining the divine within the body.

In Sanskrit, the word *prana* is associated with the breath. Prana represents "vital force." It is seen in humans as the energy that drives every action—conscious or unconscious—every thought, inspiration, and emotion, as well as the force that fuels every living cell. It is believed that we are born with a certain quantum of prana and we maintain, increase, or decrease it through our lifestyle choices. Breath is seen as a primary influence on prana, and *pranayamas* are intentional breathing patterns intended to support vitality, prevent or manage disease symptoms, control mind activity, regulate the nervous system, and ultimately align us with consciousness itself. Many of the breathing practices used in modern integrative healing methods are based on pranayamas, with an increasing amount of research (covered below) confirming that breathing in specific ways offers potentially positive health effects. This complements what has long been stated: that exploring and supporting breath is universal to life and healing.

SUBCONSCIOUS REGULATION

In exploring breath as an intervention for health, it's useful to understand its operation in the body. Respiration is reflexive and includes external respiration (breathing mechanics of gas exchange), internal respiration (biochemistry of gas distribution to/from tissues), and cellular respiration (utilization by mitochondria/cells).[1]

The medulla oblongata, a stem-like structure located in the brainstem, controls breath rate (as well as heart rate and blood pressure), which is intimately woven into the sympathetic (SNS) and parasympathetic (PNS) portions of the integrated autonomic nervous system (ANS) (see Chapter 7). Inspiration is accompanied by increased sympathetic response: bronchi dilate, oxygen transfers to the bloodstream, and the heartbeat increases.[2] In the absence of a need to respond to specific demands, the increased sympathetic effects are seen as an "allowing" of sympathetic action as the braking effects of the parasympathetic system are temporarily withdrawn. This mechanism reflects a controlled response to demand by the vagal nerve system, without a need to increase baseline sympathetic activity. Subsequently, during expiration, increased parasympathetic activity ensues: bronchi constrict, CO_2 transfers out of the blood, and the heartbeat decreases.[3] Through baroreception, as well as peripheral and central chemoreception, pressure and chemical levels are also registered, reflecting a larger picture of respiration.[4]

The hypothalamus, sometimes called the master switching station for the ANS, exerts a powerful influence on breathing.[5] It, along with higher cortical centers, links into many other facets of an integrated whole-organism responsiveness, including information about our emotions and any action demands. These networks of information influence the parameters and qualities of respiration, as well as the neuromotor control of specific muscle groups responsible for respiration (diaphragm, intercostals, abdominals, and accessory muscles).

RESPIRATION, GAS EXCHANGE, AND THE INTEGRATIVE LENS

Nasal inhalation is beneficial for a variety of reasons, including filtering (cilia, shape) and conditioning to body temperature (warming, humidifying), thereby protecting the lungs from pollutants and dryness. Nasal inhalations also stimulate nitric-oxide production and absorption. While nitric oxide is produced via other means, the greatest site is in the paranasal sinuses.[6] Nitric oxide is antiviral and antibacterial, as well as a potent bronchodilator and vasodilator, helping to lower blood pressure and increase the lungs' gas-exchange capacity.[7] Nose breathing also regulates (slows) breath flow and optimizes movement of the diaphragm.[8]

The diaphragm, the main muscle of respiration, is responsible for ~75% of all respiratory effort, influencing rate and depth of respiration.[9] The diaphragm separates the thoracic and abdominal cavities, with three openings for necessary communication and passage between the upper and lower body (esophagus, aorta, thoracic duct, vena cava, vagus nerve). Its size, shape, and movement: influence correct posture and locomotion; stimulate venous and lymphatic return and digestion; permit quality and pitch in speech and non-verbal expressions (sighing, yawning, coughing, emotional animation); and promote defecation, expectoration, urination, and vomiting.[10] Sounds important!

Optimum respiration influences and is influenced by everything from how food is digested and metabolized, to emotional and psychological well-being, to the ability to both concentrate and fall asleep at night. The body's health is reliant on the central-autonomic connectivity cuing the length, rate, and ratio of our respiration to support alertness and engagement in equal measure to relaxation, assimilation, and surrender, and the body responding to these cues.

THE VAGUS NERVE, REGULATION, AND CONNECTION

In addition to carrying "rest and digest" (parasympathetic) messages to the viscera, the vagus nerve is also responsible for such varied tasks as heart rate, gastrointestinal peristalsis, sound filtering from the environment, control of speech, and keeping the larynx open for breath control.[11] Further, cardiac vagal tone is part of the shared physiological basis of breathing and emotion. Vagal tone is influenced by breathing and impacts emotional regulation, psychological adaptation, emotional reactivity and expression, empathic responses, and attachment.[12] Vagal activation is suggested to increase the prosocial hormones: oxytocin, vasopressin, and prolactin, associated contributors to the increase in feelings of love and bonding that can lead to community building: a recognized necessity for well-being.[13] Optimal vagal nerve physiology, as reflected in heart rate variability, can arise from the active effort of conscious breathing and occurs when the breath paces at about five to seven breaths per minute, a breath pace that optimizes PNS outflow[14] (see Chapter 10).

ESTABLISHING A BASE

Having said the preceding, there is no set ideal on how bodies (and the unique people that inhabit them!) should breathe. Dr. Erik Peper at San Francisco State University states: "any set breathing pattern is by definition pathological and does not reflect the dynamics of the system."[15] Throughout the day, breath dynamics automatically shift in response to: food choice, circadian rhythm alignment, emotions (present and stored), thought structure, anatomical patterning (current and chronic), sensory perceptions, environment, and more. Using the breath as a skill for enhanced regulation of the nervous system is reliant on building kinship with it. Bottom-up regulation ensues from feeling into the breath, making breathwork an excellent resource for increasing proprioception, interoception, and exteroception. Practicing watching the breath can support top-down regulation, even in the absence of conscious manipulation of breath pattern.[16]

> **Experiential pause:** In exploring the breath, start by discovering your own. Soften judgment and befriend curiosity, and begin to observe and follow the rhythm of the breath as it is. Attune to qualities such as the temperature or the sensations along the pathways that air moves. As breath enters the torso, notice the movement of the breath: what part(s) of your body expand first? Where does it go from there? Can you feel the breath in the back body? The ribcage? Describe the qualities of the inhale. Is it smooth? Shy? Choppy? Hesitant? Does the inhale feel thorough? At the end, does it pause? When your body exhales, what do you notice? Does the movement of breath feel relaxed? Rushed? Long? As the breath continues to breathe you, become aware of places in the body where breath doesn't move, pockets that feel remote, or hesitant. Does your attention shift how your breath moves? Does focusing on your breath calm or agitate your mind? What do you notice in your body? Can you feel your blood pulse, heartbeat? What else?

CONSCIOUS REGULATION

Breathing carries both unconscious and conscious dynamics. As a learned behavior subject to the same principles of mutual learning as any other behavior, an integrative look at breathing includes the role of motivation, intention, emotion, attention, perception, and memory.

Breath rhythm can either be in *reaction* to living (ANS dictated, reflecting chronic stress pattern or defeating behavior/structure alignment), or in *action* for living (intentionally companioned, consciously directed to balance inner/outer circumstances).

Here, breath becomes a form of agency. One could even argue that we choose how much we're going to feel by unconsciously or consciously adjusting the depth of our breath. Through exploring companionship with the breath, we cultivate it as both a guide and a skill that can help us navigate the minutiae of being human, while also connecting us back to the universal wonder of aliveness.

Finding agency means we are sensitive to our body's respiratory rhythms in response to external and internal influences (think body-mind-environment (BME) applied to breathing). Building this affinity takes commitment. A recommended starting point is non-directive attention to the breath. Such attention supports the cultivation of awareness, concentration, inner witnessing, and conscious regulation of the nervous system.[17] We can then, if deemed useful, interact with the breath in more directive ways—for example, lengthening, or changing the depth, the physical pattern, and/or qualities. Such directive efforts towards influencing the breath can be tailored in ways that support vitality of mind (e.g., emotional regulation, cognition, narrative), body (e.g., alignment, metabolism), and spirit (e.g., assimilation of life experiences, wonder/grace).

Changes in breathing patterns alter interoceptive messages, primarily those traveling through vagus nerves. Sensors throughout the respiratory system (nose, throat, thorax, bronchia, diaphragm, lungs) stimulate the brain, which heightens attention, subjective experience, emotion regulation, and behavior. Vagal pathways that branch to the central PNS also branch to the anterior cingulate which is involved in decision making, fear extinction, evaluation, emotion regulation, and amygdala reactivity.[18] By consciously slowing breath rate, we can, for example, perceive a threat and stay calm while working to investigate circumstances. This is particularly relevant for individuals with post-traumatic stress disorder (PTSD) or other states of hypervigilance where imminent threat is not present but the feeling of it is.[19] As such, connecting the breath to interoception training (more in Chapter 13) reflects IRP's theme of connecting dots within the whole.

Studies also reveal how breathing practices are useful interventions for reduction in anxiety, depression, disorders of attention, stress, and stress-related medical conditions.[20] We can use breath to modulate heart rate variability (HRV), vigilance, central nervous system (CNS) excitation, neuroendocrine function, ANS function, chemoreflex, and baroreflex sensitivity.[21] Conscious breath applications thereby become a non-pharmacological intervention toward emotional and physical enhancement. All in all, the integrative view of how breathing interacts as a unifying feature within the BME matrix of functioning is stunning.

GOING DEEPER IN APPLICATION

We can offer breathing practices to others in a way that inspires curiosity and commitment by continually cultivating knowledge of, confidence with, and personal insight into our own breath patterns and capacities. Building relationship with our own breath allows the breath to be a component of a care session. For example, longer, relaxed breaths can support safe space, build mutual presence, and have a mirroring aspect. The ability to relax our breath and body has potential to influence others' physiological state.[22] This is illustrated in how individuals tend to breathe slower and deeper when with others who are relaxed.[23] Mirroring also happens when a facilitator notices shifts in their own breathing, such as shortening or holding. This recognition can be a window into what is being experienced with a client at a subtle level, or perhaps is highlighting an area that the facilitator needs to look at for their own process.

When talking with clients, bringing dual attention to the alignment and animation of the client's body and their vocal prosody, as much as to their narrative, will yield insights into the subtler levels of experience. The relationship between breathing and emotion is bidirectional, and threads into our living lens and formulation of narrative. Quality of voice, speed of words, reactions, and physical mannerisms all provide insights and help stimulate questions. Does the movement and quality of the client's breath appear fluid? When and where does it pause? What is the person's relationship with their present-moment experience? How does what is noticed in their body tie into what they're saying? At certain points it may be useful to interject attention on the breath. Examples include:

- "I am wondering if it might be OK to pause for a moment and take a few breaths together?"
- "What do you notice in your breath right now?"
- "It looks like your breath may have stopped when you said that—did you experience that?"

Such pauses reflect invitations into greater awareness (Chapter 8) in relation to the breath and can be incredibly potent in the larger process of becoming aware of and transforming dysfunctional psychophysiological/biobehavioral patterns that are linked into health processes.

Taking note of other facets of the breath is important. This may include observations of rate, depth, ratio of inspiration to expiration, sequences of chest-wall movement during respiration, symmetry of breath, and accessory muscle use. Is the client's posture affecting breath flow? Is yours? These observations help to clarify which approaches to breath awareness and training to explore. Such patterns may reflect self-defeating, reactive, or learned breathing habits that are arising from and/or influencing disease processes.[24] Common patterns to look for include the following.

Shallow chest breathing

When we are frightened or startled, the abdomen contracts in and up, shortening range of motion in the diaphragm. Shallow, short inspirations ensue. When we breathe in a shallow or restricted way, the body remains in a cyclical state of stress. Breath exchange becomes reliant on overexertion in upper accessory respiration muscles (neck, shoulders) contributing to jaw, neck, and shoulder tension. It's worth noting that this pattern may associate with other factors like work duties/environment or generalized high-stress living. Shallow or restricted patterns may be associated with digestive problems, impacts on immunity, various anxiety disorders, depression, exhaustion, pulmonary disease including edema, panic attacks, and hyperventilation.[25]

Hyperventilation

Also known as over-breathing, this pattern may overlap with chronic chest breathing and is a symptom of the body falling into hypocapnia (decreased arterial CO_2). Hypocapnia may be clinical or subclinical (meaning within or outside of developed standard biomedical measures). Hypocapnia may be tied to psychoemotional imbalance such as that found in persons experiencing PTSD, stress, panic, and affect dysregulation.[26] Hypocapnia may also be representative of specific disease processes: infection (pneumonia), lung disease (asthma, chronic obstructive pulmonary disease), traumatic brain injury, diabetes (diabetic ketoacidosis), or digestive disorders such as irritable bowel syndrome.[27] Often, as discussed throughout this book, such physical and psychoemotional dynamics are interlinked and not mutually exclusive. The physical environment may also trigger this pattern (high elevation).[28] Compounding symptoms may include headaches, seizures, dizziness, feeling breathless, cold hands and feet, chronic muscle tension, inflammation, and emotional dysregulation.

Breath holding/frozen breath

Here the whole body contracts, suppressing the natural undulations of action that respiration expresses in the body. The body is stiff and lacks animation, and the individual may appear smaller than they are. This posturing is often seen in individuals with history of toxic stress, trauma exposures, and high protection/defensive states in the face of distressing sensations, symptoms, or experiences. It may be linked to patterns of experiential avoidance. With any form of trauma history, cultivating a safe physical and relational environment is essential. Breath awareness is used to re-establish safety in the body as much as to connect to inner and outer resources of inspiration.

Throat holding

In this pattern the voice quality is strained, whispery, and/or childlike with a visible holding of tension in the jaw, neck, and facial muscles. An individual may describe feeling like they can't fully swallow, or that they have a "knot" in their throat. Adding sound to breath, especially lower tones, encourages release (see Chapter 20).

Breath grabbing

This pattern often has a psychomotor basis, showing up as physical agitation with quick, constant, interruptive speech, and/or a fast-paced breath with minimal pausing. The physical body may present with a leaning forward or lifted quality, physical tics of agitation, and challenges with silence or allowing a shared pause in speech.

Paradoxical/reverse breathing

With this pattern the abdomen moves in and up on the inspiration, and down and out on the expiration. This can be a compensatory pattern associated with advanced lung disease or a learned behavior associated with chronic tension in the upper body, heartburn, digestion problems, or mental confusion.

Collapsed chest breathing

This is similar to frozen breath with a shallow, lifeless quality in respiration; however, in this pattern the shoulders are hunched, the chest appears deflated/concave, and the abdomen protrudes out. This posture may reflect a pattern of mind-body discord, such as with states of dissociation, shame, depression, grief, and/or the general sense of life as a burden.

Emotional mirroring

Patterns of emotion will be exhibited in breathing patterns. Dennis Lewis lists common breath expressions and examples of commonly associated emotional states.[29] Recognizing a physical pattern and inquiring about emotions associated with that pattern can be particularly useful in working with individuals who struggle to identify emotions in themselves or others (aka alexithymia—recall Chapter 6; Chapter 13 explores alexithymia in relation to body awareness as well). Noting IRP's call for a heuristic approach that invites others to discover and name things for themselves, the following examples are provided to stimulate your attention to somatoemotional breathing dynamics.

- **Anger**: Shallow inhalations, strong exhalations, physical tension.
- **Fear**: Quick, shallow, and irregular breaths, feeling of a knot in the belly.
- **Grief**: Spasmodic, sobbing, jerky inhalations, long-sigh exhalation, feeling of emptiness in the belly.
- **Depression**: Shallow, lifeless inhalations and long sighing exhalations, sensations of thickness, fatigue, and dullness.
- **Impatience**: Short, uncoordinated breaths, feeling of tension in front of the chest.
- **Guilt**: Often arises with restricted, suffocating breath and sensation of oppressive heaviness.
- **Boredom**: Shallow, lifeless breath, little sensation at all.
- **Positive feelings, such as love, compassion, kindness**: Deep, comfortable, and energizing breathing, affirming and enthusiastic feeling throughout the body.[30]

The principles found in Chapter 8 provide the backdrop to safely invite others to explore such relationships. Overall, it's important to remember that breathing behaviors are a convergence of, and contributor toward, dysfunctional health patterns. Learning to identify relationships between symptoms and respiratory patterns and exploring how they may be linked to other levels (cognitive, emotional, spiritual) is important for both the clinician and the patient. While there are prescriptive breathing practices for particular conditions, it is important to maintain inquiry and an attitude of experimentation, such that care plans honor the dynamic assembly of each unique person. Offering breathing interventions and healing explorations with emphasis on introspection goes a long way in fostering compassion, insight, and sustainability in establishing healthier patterns.

PRESCRIPTION VERSUS EXPLORATION

Breathing practices are mobile and can be applied anywhere at any time. However, recommending breathing practices must be approached with context, especially when using breath *prescriptively* beyond observation within a care session. In exploring what best addresses an individual's needs, inquiry is necessary.

- Overall, is SNS or PNS currently presenting as dominant?
- How is the client's current environment affecting them?
- What do you know about their history and current life circumstances?
- What is their relationship to their inner world of feelings and emotional expression?
- What are the client's intentions for health?
- How much time and consistency is a client willing/able to successfully apply to explore techniques beyond the session?
- Why am *I* prescribing this? Am I trying to fix, or support?

For many, the notion of "less done consistently" may reflect movements toward sustainable transformation in the long term. Some may approach it from the *p.r.n.*—as needed—approach; however, education and support around values-based committed action can inform the context of this strategy. Others might approach breathwork with rigor, but do so with an attachment to a perceived outcome and/or as a form of experiential avoidance. These ideas reflect the cultivation of context if/when "prescribing." IRP advocates the need to address the tendency to take concepts or techniques and deploy them from a "this-is-the-solution" paradigm, effectively missing the integrative lenses of complexity and process orientation.

CLINICAL APPLICATIONS

As explored earlier, the first step in working with clients is building breath awareness. This awareness benefits from including the relation of breathing to physical posturing and the larger link to overall mind-body patterns. Once breath sensitivity is established, numerous breathing practices exist. Yoga offers the greatest depth of options, but many other traditions and contemporary approaches also offer breathing techniques to experiment with. If the client demonstrates interest in exploring various established breathing practices, options from this chapter can be useful experiments.

Experiential pause: Find a comfortable sitting or lying position. Bring awareness to the body and the current state of the breath. Shining the light of awareness on the breath will often naturally change it; however, start with the stance of curiously observing. Then, gradually begin to lengthen each breath. An increase in the total volume of each breath may accompany this, but go slow and do not aim for maximum. Eventually, see if you can reach a 1:2 inhale/exhale ratio where the exhale is about twice as long as the inhale. How does this act on your body-mind state? Is this practice then more about "taking" or receiving? Giving or releasing? Consider using your journal to document your experience and thoughts.

The preceding breathing practice is consistent with resonant frequency analysis breathing as explored in Chapter 10 on biofeedback and reflects breathwork to increase the length of the exhalation that is generally accessible for most individuals. The ~1:2 ratio embedded in this technique brings about increased systemic parasympathetic activity.[31] In one study, adding a short hold showed a 52% increase in oxygen consumption and metabolic rate, which supports multilevel digestion and encourages overall vitality.[32]

Another potentially useful breathing exploration is known as three-part breath (see next experiential pause). This technique builds upon traditional diaphragmatic breathing and can help to: slow the rate of breath, lengthen the exhalation, improve HRV, tone muscles involved in breathing, support digestion (both by increasing PNS and from the mechanical action of the diaphragm which "massages" the organs of digestion), influence body metabolic rate, and stimulate venous and lymphatic return.[33]

Experiential pause: Three-part breath

1. Find a relaxed seated or supine position. Place both hands on the lower abdomen below the navel. Feel into the weight of your hands through your breath. Gradually direct the breath into this area as if the breath could be poured solely into the lower portion of the torso, like water filling the base of a glass. Breathe here for three to five cycles.
2. Taking a relaxed, non-direct breath, shift your hands to the solar plexus area. Now invite three to five cycles of breath to fill this area of the torso, each expanding out evenly on all sides.
3. Again, take a relaxed, non-directed cycle of breath as you place your hands under the clavicles. Easefully invite breath to evenly fill this upper portion of the torso, as if you could fill just the upper lobes of your lungs. Stay for three to five cycles.
4. Eventually, one hand should slide back to the lower belly while the other remains on the sternum. Following the inhale, direct the breath to fill from bottom, to middle, to top—with each breath expanding the torso circumferentially. Each exhalation is relaxing. Aim for six to ten smooth breaths like this. Eventually release the pattern and scan through your body. What do you notice?

As part of continually clarifying the clinician's intention for breathing practices, some additional concepts and examples are useful. If the client's health condition is pervasive and linked to stress dynamics (of which many chronic illnesses and diseases are), any breathing practices that promote ANS balance and flexibility may be useful. Slow breathing that builds elongated expiration (like the earlier experiential pause) reduces psychophysiological arousal in anxiety-provoking but non-dangerous situations/conditions.[34] This approach resupplies inner reserves and can offer spiritual resourcing for individuals who are unable to avoid demanding circumstances (high-stress working environment, caregiving, repercussions of treating chronic illness).

Purposeful resistance breathing is another commonly taught strategy. Ujjayi from yoga is an example. Here a slight contraction of laryngeal muscles and partial closing of the glottis cultivates an even lengthening of both inspiratory and expiratory phases while creating a subtle ocean-wave sound in the back of the throat. This sound is focusing for the mind, and together the contractions, vibrations, and breath control stimulate vagal pathways, inducing increased PNS and decreased SNS activity (e.g., effect: slowing heart rate).[35] Slowing the heart rate conserves energy and allows replenishment of energy reserves, while also shifting focus away from reaction and toward reflection. Other forms of resistance breathing (straw breathing, pursed lips) are encouraged practices for persons with pulmonary diseases (asthma, chronic obstructive pulmonary disease—COPD, chronic bronchitis, emphysema). Posturing interacts with ventilation/perfusion dynamics and so positioning (arms/chest open) may combine with breathing strategy to optimize physiological impact.

BUILDING RESILIENCE

An approach from yoga known as *bhastrika* underscores another important point: we do not want to convey that resilience is solely about relaxation/quieting, as we must learn to regulate under demand. This conveys the idea of training the relationship between the SNS and the PNS—the ways in which these components of the integrated ANS relate and interact. In bhastrika, both the inhalation and exhalation are propelled with force through the nose using strong abdominal contractions. Bhastrika has been shown to increase SNS and CNS excitation—seen as a form of arousal/demand. However, this is used in controlled settings/by invitation and is combined with the PNS-regulating effects of breathing, along with mind-body intention, body awareness, and other facets of yoga practice.

Theoretically, bhastrika may train (enhance) overall ANS flexibility/capacity, and thus resilience. This can be likened to the effects of other forms of exercise that require SNS activation but carry a moderating/regulating effect to counteract the stasis of prolonged SNS activation in states of toxic stress.[36] Also of note, the systematic pressuring action of the diaphragm, particularly with forced breaths, moves the brain mass and influences the movement of cerebrospinal fluid (CSF). CSF is the substance protecting the functions of the CNS (it brings in nutrients and collects metabolic cellular waste). Though the heart moves CSF quicker, the diaphragm moves a larger quantity of it. The diaphragm's influence on blood, arterial, venous, and lymphatic circulation also impacts intracranial pressure, affecting motor performance (coordination and strength) and cognitive functions (memory, attention, sensory perception, language skills, and problem-solving).[37]

The bhastrika technique is also similar to "chaotic breathing"—a rapid nasal breathing-based meditation technique taught by The Center for Mind-Body Medicine. Over time, as you discover these and other techniques, look to develop an ability to interpret the technique through various lenses as to the how/why it may impact the whole of each person's experience, not just the neurophysiological.

BREATHING AND PAIN

Attention to breathing is vital in pain management. Recall that *pain* is conceptualized across levels—not just physical but also mental (anguish, despair), emotional (depression, anxiety), and spiritual/existential (grief/purpose).

Pain triggers stress (SNS), and long-term unmanaged pain tends to breed reaction (more pain, fear, anxiety). Pain and breathing interact bidirectionally in both negative and potentially positive directions.[38] In clinical care, depression, hopelessness, and disassociation are commonly present with unmanaged pain.[39] Yet pain can also be an incredible doorway toward deepening faith, compassion, and spiritual resourcing.[40]

With physical pain, sometimes using a longer, fuller, directive breath to go into pain helps with redefining the experience. This approach is often used in guided imagery (see Chapter 14) for pain. One can imagine gathering up the tension at the end of the inhale, and breathing it out.[41] Short holds after inspiration are associated with raising somatic pain thresholds and decreasing pain perception.[42]

Using the imagination to "body breathe" can also be useful. Here, encouraging an individual to breathe into areas where pain isn't present (inhale in and out through hands, feet, skull, or any combination of parts) encourages softening and recognition of the whole of self. This redistributes attention into awareness that pain is one sensation, or one part of their experience, amongst many.

With emotional pain, is there a place in the body associated with emotions?[43] [44] Are there associative sensations? What is it like to breathe and experience the emotion, instead of bracing against it? Is space possible with the sensations? Can the breath create containment (rage, anxiety) or allow emotions to expand and wash through (grief, fear, doubt)? In the process of any of these techniques, attention to words, shapes, colors, textures, images, or other associations adds depth.

LESSONS LEARNED

Working with the breath from a person-centered approach requires adaptability and flexibility in meeting whatever is present and whatever might emerge. Approaching breathing from the lens of experimentation and mutual learning is wise and encourages client curiosity and a team approach toward health. Other avenues to consider with breathwork are as follows.

- If the client's body presents with patterning prohibitive to ease in breathing, the inclusion of simple and gentle stretching that softens and lengthens the torso while cuing in breath to explore sensation and sensitivity is a helpful approach.
- If working with someone who presents as an over-thinker, consider offering well-chosen (relatable, applicable) education (see Chapter 16) about respiration, the nervous system, and research on the practices being explored.
- If working with dissociative tendencies or low affect, consider using props (straps, blocks, bolsters, blankets) to increase supportive attention on the body from which to build breath awareness. Use of questions and a feedback-informed approach encourages continual investigation and supports present-moment being.
- A calm, steady voice with focus on one's own breath while watching the client's body goes a long way in supporting a rhythm that is honoring and foundational, and breeds expanse.
- Recognize that changes in breathing may bring up psychoemotional content/ states. For example, both slow and rapid/forceful breathing practices could trigger symptoms in individuals with panic/anxiety disorders. Similarly:
  - manic episodes in bipolar disorder could be triggered by rapid/forceful breathing, as it can increase lithium secretions, causing a drop in serum level
  - flashbacks could be triggered with PTSD
  - altered states of consciousness or psychotic episodes could be activated in individuals with a tenuous sense of reality.[45]
- The cuing of breathing practices for individuals experiencing altered states/schizo-typy should be mindful to not combine breath practice with overt stimulation of the imagination. Instead, an approach that remains focused on clear recognition/ articulation of current circumstances/conditions encourages stability.
- The Resources section in Chapter 6 serves as a useful guide if difficult cognitive-emotional-behavioral dynamics arise, which may occur even when following suggested precautions. This is not necessarily "bad" and these rare situations can be approached as an opportunity for mutual learning instead of through the lens of error or pathology.

CONCLUSION

While breathing practices might serve as a primary intervention, as reflected in Raffi's story, breath is most powerful when companioned with other parts of the integrative care approach. For example, breath can be a foundation for physical movement (Chapter 15) to encourage proprioception and interoception while alleviating tension in the body during movement. Breath awareness can support curiosity and a safe physical base with dissociative tendencies (building inner resource). Other examples include the use of breath as a foundation for exploring meditation (Chapter 12) or within spiritual inquiry (Chapter 18).

In closing, consider a final breath practice that may be useful when feeling out-weighted by life, or even as part of daily centering:

Close your eyes and feel into how your breath is moving in your body. Stay with this until the feeling of the breath softens and anchors a sense of weighting. Then in this quieter place, internally recite: "One body, one mind, one heart, and no idea when my expiration date is, what is it that I want to do in life?"

This practice, like others, can "weed-whack" a disheveled mind and body toward what is most important. Breathing practices can also awaken wonder, curiosity, determination, or clarity of action. These practices can stimulate a deeper recognition of agency, accountability, and limitation. "I will not be in the current configuration forever, but while I am still being breathed, what feels necessary?" As you move forward, see if you can work with your breath to re-enliven the mystery of life, stimulate solace and love, and carry you forth from memories of earlier contemplations—where they have led from and what they are leading you towards.

Experiential pause: Having read this chapter, identify and write down at least one actionable item of interest to you. In doing so, consider ways in which applying the material first to yourself, and then to patients, might serve those who come to you for care.

CHAPTER 12

Exploring Meditation

Betsy Shandalov, OTR/L, C-IAYT

A story: "Hal" is a 55-year-old male with three years of persistent low back pain due to a work-related injury. He had two failed spinal surgeries. He received traditional occupational therapy (OT) and physical therapy (PT) at the time of the injury, and PT after both surgeries, but failed to improve significantly. He completes his basic self-care and daily hygiene; however, he cannot drive, walk long distances, nor stand for long periods. He has been out of work since the onset of his injury.

Hal was referred to work with me, a holistic OT and yoga therapist, with the goal of improving his independence and function throughout the day. Hal is a recovering alcoholic and used to attend Alcoholics Anonymous (AA) meetings, but now it is too painful to drive there or sit in a meeting. Hal is married and has one child in college and one child still at home. I met Hal in his home; he was lying on his couch. His wife was present for our session. Hal described severe pain. "It is taking over my life. I can't even walk outside anymore." With a look of despair, he added: "You are my last hope, can you help me?" Hal had been in so much pain that it had taken over his life. He struggled to shift his focus in his mind from the pain cycle to finding function in life. He stated that he felt like it was: "completely debilitating, mentally and physically." The goal of our treatment was to bring calm to his mind and body and help shift his pain perception and increase his daily activity.

After the customary introductions, ample space to hear Hal's story, and my experience with clinical decision-making process in partnership with the patient (Chapter 8), we agreed to start with a meditation experience. Hal preferred to stay lying down. With invitation, Hal chose to use a soft weighted eye pillow (relaxes ocular tension) and a small bean bag on his belly (increases body awareness) that I had brought to the session. Also through invitation and choice, I covered him with a blanket (supports feelings of comfort). These props support the possibility of an overall relaxation response. We proceeded with a simple meditative body scan. Hal naturally focused on where he had the most pain. He rated his pain as an 8. To assist Hal in shifting his awareness, I asked him to find something that was relatively "loose, neutral, open, or comfortable" in his body. It took a bit, but Hal found a few areas that were calmer. This was new. He stated: "I guess I never noticed places in my body that did not hurt."

I then assisted Hal in identifying an intention. He chose an intention of peacefulness for his session, and while it was hard for Hal to do, I invited him to imagine feeling sensations of peacefulness in his body. We then proceeded with a simple imagery of white light surrounding his body to symbolize peace, safety, and protection. I encouraged Hal to envision the white light traveling through each and every cell of his body, with special attention on areas of pain.

Using simple instructions, I guided Hal to become aware of the sensations of his breath. This was followed by another "experiment": gradually slowing his breathing into an approximate 1:2 inhale/exhale ratio. Hal settled on ~3 seconds in/6 seconds out as "just right." The guided breathing included cues to notice and soften the belly with each breath.

I asked Hal if it was OK if I placed my hands on his shoulders so we could breathe in unison (see Chapter 11). We breathed together. I also asked his wife if she needed some relaxation and self-care. She stated that she would love to find a way to not be so anxious and worried. I asked her if she would like a blanket around her shoulders, and she accepted. She sat in a chair at the nearby kitchen table, and we all continued to breathe together. Providing a healing environment can help create that mind-body shift even before we begin the treatment. Hal was willing to breathe in unison with me with the support of the props above. Hal's wife felt relaxation at the same time.

This led us into an ~15-minute guided meditation practice. The practice was also made accessible to him by recording it on his phone. This practice included principles of mindfulness and acceptance applied to discomfort and pain. When it was complete, Hal repeated a body scan and stated that, on the 1–10 scale, his pain was a 5. He reported: "I feel the best I have felt in a very long time." His wife reported feeling better as well. Hal felt well enough to sit up on the edge of the couch with his feet grounded on the floor. We discussed how he could build these breathing and meditation practices into his daily routine. When Hal had pain throughout the day, he would stop and breathe with a focus on fuller inhalations and slowing his exhalations. Hal and his wife also mutually agreed to start the day with a guided meditation.

I checked in a week later and Hal was walking around his house more. He stated that he loved the meditation that was recorded on his phone and had downloaded a meditation app too. "I can't get over how much focusing on my breath is helping me with the pain." In the next session, we explored his life values and areas he wished to take committed action towards. These included:

- get out of the house more, including to walk down the street
- improve his mood and feel more positive about his life
- if possible, cut back on his depression medication
- attend AA meetings again
- discover more activities that he and his wife could do individually and together
- consider a return to part-time consulting work.

Hal and his wife and I met for seven one-hour sessions. We began each session with a guided 15-minute meditation. We discussed how the loss of community hurt his heart and made him sad. We made a daily and weekly schedule that included meditation, rest, getting outdoors, and heart-opening and core seated yoga poses as moving meditation, and included a time for daily phone contact with friends and family. After those seven sessions, Hal was able to walk down the street, and with his wife's support, he returned to his first AA meeting in a long while. He expressed that he realized that meetings were vital for him, even if he had some pain. He noted that the presence of his AA friends reminded him of his spirituality, and that meditation was actually a part of the program, but he had never really grasped it until now. In his final session Hal stated: "I have come back to the land of the living." He declared that he was committed to using meditation practices for the rest of his life.

MEDITATION AS MEDICINE

As we just saw in Hal's story, finding a meditative practice can be effective treatment. Hal struggled with pain and motivation to be active with his life. The meditation for coming inward assists in shifting attention out of habitual patterns. The visualization of sending light into the body introduces the possibility of positive relationship (caring, comforting), reflecting principles of self-care and self-compassion. Certain conscious breathing practices carry potential to impact the stress response by subduing the flight/fight response and facilitating the relaxation response.[1] The inclusion of mindfulness-based cognitive techniques ("I am more than this," principles of observing, and acceptance) affords for a shift in attention from the challenge and into a larger context. Such shifts reflect the possibility of reappraisal of one's experience. In neuroscience, these skills are often described as reflecting "top-down" neurocognitive processes—capable of altering brain-body communication patterns.[2] For Hal, it was only by experiencing a beneficial impact that the utility became self-evident.

Hal's wife was included in the experience, and together they realized that they had never had a self-care routine. They had worked so hard throughout life and did not (yet) understand the benefits of purposely supporting the regulation processes in their bodies. After discovering this together, Hal experienced decreased pain and his wife reported a sense of relief around feeling helpless in relationship to Hal's distress. Over time, they expanded to include movement meditation: walking in nature together. Hal was reconnecting with his wife and this opened the door to returning to his AA community where members also performed meditation techniques together.

In this chapter, we will explore the utility of meditation and mindfulness principles and techniques within integrative rehabilitation practice (IRP). These topics have a growing body of evidence that supports health processes. As with all of our topics, we will approach meditation in context. And, in one sense, meditation *is* context in that conscious awareness is the backdrop to our lived experiences of body-mind-environment (BME). Meditation and mindfulness enhance and support the nature and quality of our awareness, perceptions, and relationship to our experience. In this lens, the concept of meditation supports IRP's phenomenological heuristic: care for each person's capacity to come to know and define their own experience.[3]

AN OCCUPATIONAL THERAPIST'S PERSPECTIVE

I have always been excited to try new things. During my second pregnancy, I was worried and anxious about how I would care for two children who were less than two years apart. The job of taking care of one child and being pregnant with a second child was already stressful. I began attending a weekly 90-minute guided meditation class to find some quiet and create space for healing. I had never formally meditated before. I loved experiencing this feeling of quiet. My body felt like it was floating as I left every Thursday night. I was calmer, could think more clearly, slept better, and felt "centered."

When my first daughter was born, it was a very difficult birth. I had to have an unexpected C-section because she was breach. Subsequently, the birth of my second daughter was my first vaginal birth. She was nearly two weeks late, and my body needed to do a lot of healing from the trauma of her birth. I then had a third daughter less than two years later. Her birth was not as traumatic, but having three children under the age of four challenged my capacity in ways for which I was not prepared. I stayed at home to take care of our three girls.

When my middle daughter was around five years old, we noticed challenges. She experienced sensory sensitivity. Any noise in her environment or clothing on her skin disrupted her nervous system. On many days she had uncontrollable tantrums. Her body and mind were calling out for help and I had no tool in my toolkit to assist her. I searched for answers. While on our family vacation in Hawaii, I met with an Ayurvedic practitioner. This changed my life. After meeting for four hours, she suggested that I study yoga. As synchronicity would have it, the following week I began a 200-hour Iyengar yoga training, and the following year I completed a year-long *YogaKids* training. Similar to my early meditation experiences, I noticed that my mind and body felt more balanced. I had tapped into ways to transform my experience. When I meditated, I saw instant benefits. I spoke more calmly and mindfully with my daughter, and her behavior began to change too. Eventually, we practiced breathing and grounding exercises together.

I began supporting my clients by including these and other integrative approaches and had positive results. I realized that when I quieted my mind and body with meditation and yoga, I was preparing my body to help others. When I guide someone through a breath practice, I connect with my breath as well, and it feels as if we are breathing and healing together.

I also incorporate mini meditations throughout my workday. I inhale for a count of five and exhale for a count of five while I focus attention through the body and down to my feet, before and after I see every client. By midday, as I am getting tired, I sit down and do a technique called palming: I rub my hands together and then fingertip tap on the top of my head, eyes, and cheeks to awaken and refresh my body and mind. I realized that these frequent check-ins on how I am feeling benefit both myself and my client.

In both Hal's and my own experiences, understanding what our body needs is important. Meditation affords us the ability to create space and embodied presence. Meditation brings us into present-moment awareness. For some of my clients, a structured approach for practicing is needed and valuable. For others, these skills develop functionally through learning to exercise real-time checks, pauses, body awareness, and breathing.

Experiential pause: Preparing the body for focus

- Sit with your feet flat on the ground. Sit in a way that feels upright, yet fully supported and relaxed at the same time.
- Feel your bottom on the chair. Notice your legs. Notice your belly, then your chest and your heart. Notice your arms, neck, and head. Rub your hands together a bit, creating warmth from your hands.
- Place your warm palms on your eyes, and think the word "soft."
- Take a deep breath in through your nose and exhale through your mouth.
- Gently remove your palms from your eyes. What do you notice with this short routine?

MEDITATION AND MINDFULNESS: DEFINITIONS

Meditation denotes practices used to focus or train the attention of the conscious mind. Many meditation practices aim towards a particular goal such as achieving mental clarity, promoting an emotionally calm state, or advancing intentions rooted in one's spirituality. Mindfulness is "the awareness that emerges through paying attention on purpose, in the present moment, and nonjudgmentally to the unfolding of experience moment by moment."[4]

"Meditation" and "medicine" are derived from the same root word that means to "take the measure of" and "to care for." These words come from the Latin word *meditari*: "to ponder." This implies that any act, form, or state of meditation is rooted in a notion of contemplative presence, as well as caring gestures of attention.

Sometimes, meditation is focused on breathing. Sometimes, meditation is active. And other times, it is a general intention for a quieter state of mind. "Mindfulness" is often used singularly, paired with meditation, or used interchangeably with meditation. We'll explore various aspects of mindfulness and meditation shortly, but for now consider the idea that they can be seen as an active form of *presence*—an embodied demonstration of a strong yet quiet potential within the mind-body relationship. Mindfulness as a practice reflects approaches to cultivating this notion of presence, in relationship to one's experience of BME.

MEDITATION AND MINDFULNESS: A BRIEF HISTORY

In our ever-changing world of technology and innovation, more people than ever before have taken to meditation and mindfulness practices.[5] According to the National Center for Complementary and Integrative Health:

Meditation is a mind and body practice that has a long history of use for increasing calmness and physical relaxation, improving psychological balance, coping with illness, and enhancing overall health and well-being. Mind and body practices focus on the interactions among the brain, mind, body, and behavior.[6]

From an anthropological perspective, constructs of meditation appear to have evolved across a variety of populations and geographically distinct regions of the world. Meditation practices are found in cultural and religious traditions (examples: Buddhism, Christianity, Islam, and Judaism), non-religious settings (examples: yoga, indigenous populations), and a growing number of contemporary, secular forms.

In the 1950s and 1960s, researchers began focusing on the effects of meditation on health.[7] This movement arose out of Westerners' curiosity about reports of extraordinary feats of bodily control by Eastern meditation practitioners. This scientific look at meditation has since moved on to produce a vast number of studies. Dr. Herbert Benson and colleagues at Harvard Medical School were among the early researchers of meditation and coined the phrase *relaxation response* in the 1970s.[8]

In 1979 Jon Kabat-Zinn founded the Mindfulness-Based Stress Reduction (MBSR) Clinic at the University of Massachusetts Medical Center. MBSR uses a combination of mindfulness meditation, body awareness, yoga, and exploration of patterns of behavior, thinking, feeling, and action. It is an eight-week evidence-based program that offers secular, intensive mindfulness training to assist people with stress, anxiety, depression, and pain management.[9]

MBSR is a practical approach capable of enabling individuals to have more choices and take wise action in their lives. Kabat-Zinn defined mindfulness as: "the non-judgmental acceptance and open-hearted investigation of present experience, including body sensations, internal mental states, thoughts, emotions, impulses and memories, in order to reduce suffering or distress and to increase well-being."[10] Twenty years later, The Center for Mindfulness in Medicine, Health Care, and Society at the University of Massachusetts Medical School was formed and it continues to support the successful growth and implementation of MBSR in health care worldwide.

Kabat-Zinn's work has assisted in bringing meditation practices, as part of the larger lens of evidence-based integrative medicine, into mainstream health care. Such efforts continue to bridge the gap between *medicine* and *meditation* as two words with the same origin. As we continue, we will take an overview of a few of the profound advancements in meditation science and contemplate its role in the modern health-care system.

MEDITATION AS AWARENESS: A BACKDROP IN IRP

Meditation and mindfulness are impacting the future of science, health care, and well-being. We have already established the need to explore mind-body processes as an important function within IRP. Meditation or mindfulness call us back to the important and foundational base of awareness. In a sense, awareness, as rooted in conscious subjective experiencing, underscores everything. Thus, the nature and quality of awareness is of utmost importance as an IRP topic.

Self-awareness is the first step in taking an active role in our own health care. It is only through self-awareness that we can establish an understanding of the connections and relationships within the BME, including our own personal beliefs and spirituality. Developing your own unique version of these connections and relationships enhances your ability to share effectively the utility of meditation practices with others in a therapeutic context.

MEDITATION IN A FAST-MOVING WORLD

It is easy to get caught up in the busyness of the world. We may lose connection with one another and ourselves. For many, stress and anxiety are at an all-time high in our modern world. The pace of life and our digital lifestyle bring chaos to our minds and bodies. For example, researchers show that increasing sound/noise and light pollution can negatively impact health.[11] These examples of environmental stress can be seen as independent of but interacting with individual psychosocial stress patterns. As a result, many folks stay in a heightened state of stress, activation, and arousal.

If such patterns are left unaddressed, they gradually impact allostatic load, health processes, and well-being. The growing field of *contemplative science* (a current term for the collective fields that study meditation constructs) is providing new understandings and solutions to post-normal times, and mindfulness is warranting entire issues of peer-reviewed journals.[12]

"Living mindfulness" is a concept that understands the nature of contemporary life and intends to embed the construct of mindfulness/meditation into daily living. It is something you *become* more than something you do. While practice is needed and encouraged, not everyone needs nor is going to commit to a formal sitting meditation practice. While the practice is not always named, we have already been exploring simple, accessible ways to embody the principles of mindfulness/meditation throughout this book. This and subsequent chapters aim to deepen and expand upon living mindfulness as a foundation of mind-body medicine, as embedded in IRP.

TYPES OF MEDITATION

According to The Center for Mind-Body Medicine, there are three main categories or types of meditation: concentrative, mindfulness-based, and expressive/dynamic.[13] In reality, most forms of meditation weave together various aspects from each of these categories. For example, awareness of the breath is frequently used as an anchor within meditation practices. Breath awareness and/or breath regulation can help focus the mind/body back into the reality of the present moment. Ultimately, and regardless of type/form, meditation can:

- assist us in improving our relationship to any aspect of our experience
- help us build or transform the quality of our awareness
- support our ability to shift out of habitual patterns
- explore existential truths or psychospiritual teachings such as the nature of impermanence and/or defining what matters most to us in our lives.

With these general principles in mind, let's look at the three categories of meditation: concentrative, mindfulness, and expressive/dynamic.

Concentrative meditation is a focused awareness on a particular object. This might include sustained attention on an image, a physical sensation or point on the body, a word, or a sound. A common example is choosing two words, one for your inhalation and one for your exhalation, such as: inhaling "gentle," exhaling "calm." Researchers demonstrated positive effects in, for example, treatment for post-traumatic stress disorder, from practicing concentrative attention by silently repeating a personalized (self-selected) *mantram*, a word or phrase with a spiritual meaning.[14]

Experiential pause: Concentrative meditation 1

Take a moment, choose two words that carry a meaning and intention that you have for yourself, and see what it is like to repeat them slowly to yourself. You might also "breathe them" (pairing your words with breathing in…breathing out…). Spend a few minutes exploring this experience and consider trying on different words to see if/how the experience changes.

This example combines conscious breathing with a meaningful mental intention. Many individuals will say: "I can't do that, my mind is too busy." A good response is: "The point is not necessarily to change the fact that your mind is busy. In fact, one could argue that you can't stop or change thinking. Instead, you notice that your attention wandered into a stream of continuous thoughts. You then choose to consciously, repeatedly return attention to the present moment. In doing so, you provide the conscious mind an alternative point of focus—something other than those thoughts!"

Experiential pause: Concentrative meditation 2

Choose one point on your body associated with the sensations of breathing, such as the nostrils, or throat, or somewhere on the chest/belly. Focus your attention here, watching the sensations of the breath at this body point. See how long you maintain your attention before you notice that the mind has drifted away from the task. Repeat…many times.

Mindfulness meditation involves being aware of whatever arises into the field of conscious attention from a "curious-observer" stance. Mindfulness practices often focus on the idea of meta-awareness. Meta-awareness, also called meta-cognition, relates to processes considered central to the therapeutic effects of mindfulness training. These include shifting one's experiential perspective onto an experience itself (decentering) and meta-cognitive insight (cognitive defusion, e.g., experiencing thoughts by looking *at* them rather than *through* them).[15]

Said another way, a mindfulness metaphor describes watching things: "like the neutral eye of the camera."[16] However, our cameras have filters—some that improve the picture and others that distort it. If we become aware of something inside or outside of ourselves and the filter habitually says "Yuck, bad, criticize, reject, etc.," we may experience suffering.

In contrast, the mindfulness filter, as described by Kabat-Zinn, supports the development of a non-judgmental view.[17] Dr. Dan Siegel adds a filter to the lens—COAL: **c**uriosity, **o**penness, **a**cceptance, and **l**oving-kindness.[18] The mindfulness concept of meditation is what many people typically think of when the word "meditation" is mentioned. This concept might evoke notions of long periods of sitting doing nothing, which for some might evoke anticipation of long periods of dis-ease! However, with education, support, and practice, becoming mindfully aware of the nature of thoughts, beliefs, perceptions, sensations, emotions, and habitual reactions can occur anywhere, anytime. We'll cover some of the current science of mindfulness practice shortly.

> **Experiential pause:** Mindfulness meditation
>
> Take a few minutes, adjust your posture for comfort if needed, and simply sit and watch whatever arises. Watch thoughts, bodily sensations, or other senses. Watch emotions/feelings arise and dissolve. Watch the breath. Remain as neutral as possible to whatever is being experienced, like the neutral lens of a camera.

Expressive/dynamic meditation includes active techniques, such as chanting, dancing, moving, or vigorous forms of breathing. Movement engages the mind-body state in a different way than when the body is still. Meditative movement, which can also be called active, expressive, or dynamic meditation, uses movement in conjunction with a meditative intention. Certain aspects of yoga, Qigong, or Tai Chi fit in this category of meditation. Praying a rosary (Catholicism), counting prayer beads (many religions), or making prayer ties (a practice of North American indigenous populations) can be seen as dynamic meditations. They are active and involve movement and/or "doing." Mindfulwalking and walking a labyrinth (path system) are also dynamic meditations. In mindful walking, you apply the principles of mindfulness to the often-unconscious act of walking.

> **Experiential pause:** Active meditation
>
> After reading this, set down the book. Choose to walk slowly...either indoors or outdoors. Experience the act of walking in a new way. Feel every facet of the sensory experience. You might even label things neutrally; for example: "Noticing the foot contacting the ground, noticing weight shifting to the left, noticing bird chirping in the tree, isn't that curious..." Continue for as long as you would like, walking mindfully, and noticing.
>
> Note: If you have physical limitations to walking, you might choose movements that you routinely are able to do, but complete them slowly, noticing how this feels.

You could even just use your finger and mindfully trace a pattern on a desk or a table. Purposeful slowness of any movement increases awareness. If movement is not possible, use your imagination. As you will see in Chapter 14, the brain/body does not know the difference between what is real and what is imagined!

MIND WANDERING

Many people experience the mind as being constantly full of idle chatter. The phrase "monkey mind" is used to describe the tendency of the mind to jump rapidly from one thing to the next. Sometimes it can seem difficult to redirect the mind.

Separate from the sometimes-busy cognitive level of mind, *mind wandering* is defined as a state of perceptual decoupling, or disengagement of attention from perception.[19] In meditation research, the idea of mind wandering is considered a normal phenomenon. Some research suggests that humans spend nearly half of the time in thinking states that are decoupled from conscious attention to their present sensory environment; however, the mechanisms underlying this process may be altered in persons experiencing persistent pain.[20]

There is a resting state of brain activity that is associated with mind wandering. This *default mode network* (DMN) is sometimes called a "task-negative" network but this does not imply that it is a "bad" thing. The DMN is a large-scale brain network connecting various regions of the brain. The DMN was discovered accidentally in resting test subjects, because this area is very active at rest! The DMN has been shown to be involved in daydreaming, thinking of the future, planning, ruminating, or an unconscious "autopilot" state of mind.[21] We can call this mind-*wondering*!

DMN changes have been associated with conditions and states such as persistent pain and depression.[22] For example, patterns of activity in the DMN are related to the extent to which a person has negative self-evaluation. The presence of this aspect of DMN is so strong that it can predict relapse in depression.[23] Additionally, when we have negatively appraised physical experiences, DMN patterns in relationship to sensory, cognitive, and emotional correlate(s) of that experience may become altered, potentially reinforcing a negative pattern.[24]

Individuals differ in how often their minds spontaneously wander away from pain. These differences are linked to the disruptive effect of pain on cognitive performance, and brain-behavior relationships have been shown to underscore individual differences. When people's minds wander away from pain, certain associated patterns of DMN activity have been demonstrated.[25] Simplified: neurophysiological patterns of attention, tracking, and/or searching for painful sensations may lead to more pain.[26] It follows that modifying existing patterns of attention to various sensations, such as pain, may be useful.

Researchers have shown that during cycles of *focused attention → mind wandering → becoming aware → shifting back to focused attention*, there are specific sequences of neural activation in the brain (Figure 12.1).[27] The good news: these neural patterns can change with practice, supporting a host of potentially beneficial effects.[28]

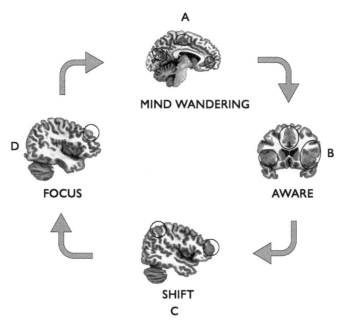

FIGURE 12.1: PATTERNS OF BRAIN ACTIVATION DURING MEDITATION PRACTICE
A) ✦ *activity in ventromedial pre-frontal cortex and bilateral posterior*
cingulate cortex, parts of the default network
B) ✦ *activity in dorsal anterior cingulate cortex and bilateral anterior insula*
C) ✦ *activity in right dorsolateral pre-frontal cortex and*
right posterior parietal lobule and over time with practice
D) ✦ *activity in right dorsolateral pre-frontal cortex*
Adapted from Wendy Hasenkamp[29]

MIND-*WONDERING* AND "GROUNDING"

While acknowledging that mind wandering is normal, the monkey-mind concept, approached from a meditation stance, brings us the notion of mind-wondering. Monkey mind is experienced as being disheveled, chaotic, and/or disturbing. Someone who is *in* a monkey-mind state may constantly feel restless or not grounded. Often, such agitation is due to the interaction of emotion and thoughts, a core principle of Cognitive Behavioral Therapy.

A shift towards a meditative relationship in and to the busy cognitive level of mind allows us to *wonder*: "Hmm, isn't that curious, I wonder why the mind is producing this thought?" Hint: The mind is working to create a sense of coherence, order, understanding, or control. This effort often runs amuck.

In *The Mind Illuminated,* the book's authors state the importance of "grounding" exercises[30] to assist in meditation efforts. These exercises bring awareness more deeply or fully into the body (aka "ground") and assist transitioning out of disheveled states. *Grounding* intends to convey strategies to center or orient people more fully to the body in the present moment. Grounding techniques may include basic body scans, building capacity for attending to unpleasant sensations, evoking whole-body awareness, relaxing body tension, and/or becoming aware of other senses like sights, smells, or sounds. This latter part of becoming aware of the senses is linked to *orienting* one's attention to its relationship to the physical environment. Orienting is important because it connects the conscious mind to sensory-processing regions of the brain, as well as being a reminder that there is a physical connection of the body with one's immediate environment. Both grounding and orienting are essential concepts in meditation and are built on pulling attention more fully into the present-moment experience. Often, we are pulled into the past or the future. It is vital to come back to *what is happening right now*.

> **Experiential pause:** Grounding and orienting
>
> Become aware of the sensations of your eyes. Look around you. Name three things you see, such as: "red painting, wall clock, and open window." Next, become aware of your nose and sense of smell. Next, attune to your ears. Name any sounds you can detect. Bring your awareness to your head and envision a string attached to the crown of the head, going all the way to the sky. Become aware of your feet, and imagine roots growing out of the bottom of your feet, deep down into the earth below. Search for a sense of connection, sensation, or flow through the bottom, from top to bottom, or bottom to top, whichever you prefer.

MEDITATION AND INTENTION

Intention or purpose can support meditation. Intention can be used as a premeditation ritual to stabilize attention, define a purpose or value for the practice, and promote motivation. Intention provides a map or direction. Not setting an intention is like getting in a car and not knowing where you are going.

Setting intention may help with mind wandering and monkey mind. It is estimated that for 47% of the time we are thinking about things that are unrelated to what we are actually doing, and while this is considered normal, it can become problematic: this tendency is associated with the perception of unhappiness.[31] The use of self-affirmation statements may enhance intention; however, research to date has not supported that self-affirmation is sufficient to engage behavior change.[32] Combining the practices of intention and meditation may bring about positive changes in support of enhanced well-being,[33] and as you will see in Chapter 17, combining mindfulness, affirmation, and intention constructs together within Cognitive Behavioral Therapy approaches may yield even greater impact.

> **Experiential pause:** Sit or lie comfortably. Briefly scan your body, offering a gentle invitation to soften and settle. Envision your body as being light like a cloud. Next, contemplate and choose a valued quality you wish to embody more of in your life. This will become your intention. Examples might include gentleness, kindness, bravery, patience, love, courage, or gratitude. Imagine finding your valued quality as

a felt sense in the body: How would this quality impact your body language, posture, movement, voice, and larger presence? How would it feel? When you've finished, write down your response to this experience. Consider how your response might change from day to day and over time with regular practice.

SCIENCE AND MEDITATION

Science changes constantly, and with that change comes a need to continuously transform our views and approaches to health care. The science of meditation is no exception. At one point, scientists thought our brains did not change after childhood. Now we have a better understanding of the potential for both neuroplasticity and neurogenesis as overviewed in Chapter 7. Take all present findings with a grain of salt!

Meditation and mindfulness research support that we can actively contribute to beneficial brain-body changes over time. In a 2007 science-review book, Sharon Begley defines the importance of conscious attention and how that attention is empirically observed to transform the brain.[34] In particular, the conscious attention exercised through meditation and mindfulness changes the human nervous system in multiple ways, including:

- decreased stress reactivity
- enhanced self-awareness and self-regulation
- enhanced attention/focus
- improved emotion regulation
- enhanced body awareness
- improved memory processes. [35]

Dr. Sara Lazar and her team at Harvard University are one of many pioneering groups conducting studies of the brain before, during, and after meditation practices. In one study, Lazar compared long-term meditators with an inexperienced control group. The long-term meditators demonstrated notably increased gray matter in regions of the prefrontal cortex and sensory and auditory regions, as well as measures of working memory and decision making.[36] In another study, Lazar and her team demonstrated that decreased stress perception following participation in the MBSR eight-week program yielded decreased gray-matter density in the amygdala, a structure that has been shown to be hyperactive when under high stress.[37] In another study by Lazar's team, people who have never meditated were divided into a control group and an active group. Following participants' completion of the same MBSR program, the researchers found increased gray-matter concentration in the active group participants in the following brain regions:

- the posterior cingulate (involved in mind wandering and self-relevance)
- the temporoparietal junction (associated with perspective taking, empathy, and compassion)
- the left hippocampus (involved in learning, cognition, memory, and emotion regulation)

- the pons, where many regulatory neurotransmitters are produced.[38]

Many other researchers have examined various physiological effects that may arise from engaging in meditation practices. A sampling of these studies broken into subtopics includes:

- improvements in neurocardiac function, such as reduced blood pressure, reduced cardiovascular risk, and improved heart rate variability[39]
- potentially beneficial changes in electroencephalography (EEG) patterns[40]
- positive epigenetic influences[41]
- enhanced immunity and reduced inflammation[42]
- reduced anxiety/depression[43]
- improved pain management[44]
- increased empathy, compassion, and improved relationships[45]
- enhanced memory, learning processes, attention, and cognition[46]
- enhanced neuroendocrine function.[47]

PRECAUTIONS, CONTRAINDICATIONS, AND CHALLENGES

Meditation and mindfulness practices are helpful for many people but not for everyone. Precautions and/or contraindications exist. For example, while mindfulness practices can transform the symptoms of toxic stress and/or of trauma history, it is important to choose practices that fit the learning style, regulation capacity, and general comfort/tolerance levels of the client. Sitting quietly, and focusing on the breath and/or interoceptive body awareness, especially for longer periods of time, can be unsettling for some. Start with short periods of practice. Offer choices with permission to shift attention when needed. Benefit can be derived from only a few minutes of noticing the breath or bodily sensation.

Additional considerations include the following.

- When training awareness, we sometimes see a double-edged sword. What if becoming aware is met with a filter of self-judgment, criticism, or aversion? Here is where *quality* of awareness matters. For example, research into self-compassion and loving-kindness meditations demonstrates that the quality or "filter" on awareness matters.[48] It is often said that there is a space between any stimulus and our relationship or response to that stimulus. It is in this space where the facilitation of awareness can include additional support for transforming filters and relationships that are not optimized for enhanced relationship with self, one's experience, or others.
- If a person has a history of altered states (hallucinations, schizotypy, psychosis) or other unmanaged or uncontrolled mind-body states (severe affect dysregulation), caution or avoidance is needed. Teaching grounding practices for these folks is an important consideration.
- Meditation and mindfulness may evoke strong emotions, including prior emotional associations that are not therapeutic for the client. These individuals need

additional care to assure experiences are in a *window of arousal* (psychophysiological tolerance).[49]

- For some, meditation and mindfulness could appear to interfere with their religious beliefs. The individual's perception/belief system is always the deciding factor if such an association or expression is disclosed. Often, self-selected practices that arise out of the person's religion or culture is the answer.
- For an unsure client, it may be helpful to start with a short trial of focusing attention on the breath and/or their bodily sensations.
- For people in pain, there may be a need to stand, walk, and/or move often. This was definitely true in the case study with Hal at the beginning of this chapter.
- For everyone, we must distinguish between discomfort rooted in novelty or unfamiliarity and the discomfort rooted in past trauma or emotional conditioning.
- For everyone, we must be aware of not using meditation to "check out" of our experience or avoid discomfort.
- It is important to call out context: meditation does not "fix" anything. Despite our uniform desire to fix what ails us, IRP reminds us that many things are not imminently nor easily fixable per se. If something persists, we might be better served by seeking to improve our relationship to the experience. It follows that, as professionals, we seek to offer an approach that foundationally aims to support the possibility of increased well-being. The earlier references on meditation and pain reflect a good example of this in action: reduced pain levels may not be significant, but quality of life across other measures can be realized.
- In the end, some individuals will find meditation practices to be unhelpful, ineffective, uninteresting, or uncomfortable.[50] Our job as therapists is to assist the client to develop a mind-body program that works best for them, regardless of whether it includes meditation and mindfulness practices.

SOCIETY, EDUCATION, AND THE FUTURE OF MEDITATION

Meditation is a mind-body practice that shares space with many integrative health practices and disciplines. As noted in Chapter 1, for many years, most mind-body practices like meditation were considered to be "alternative." However, in 2014 after a comprehensive review of the evidence base for the growing academic and clinical dissemination of integrative medicine, the US Congress renamed National Institutes of Health's subdivision on this topic to the National Center for Complementary and Integrative Health (NCCIH).[51] This move validated a "both/and" view of biomedical/integrative care approaches in support of improving quality in health care.

NCCIH began conducting a five-yearly National Health Interview Survey in 2002.[52] The results are overwhelming: according to the survey, 4.1% of adults practiced meditation in 2012, but this tripled to an estimated 14.2% of adults in 2017.[53] The rise in meditation practice is partially linked to research demonstrating enhanced pain management, lowered blood pressure, decreased anxiety, improved brain function, stress reduction, decreased inflammation, increased cell-mediated immunity, and biological markers for aging.[54]

WRAPPING UP

There is growing support for embedding meditation into medicine (health care). Applying principles of meditation/mindfulness to yourself supports your well-being and potentially the care you offer to others.[55] Imagine the impact if every rehabilitation professional spent time breathing, meditating, and *being* with their clients!

In summary, meditation and mindfulness:

- are evidence-based mind-body practices that focus on the interactions within the whole of mind, brain, body, environment, and behavior
- represent tools (non-fixing) that assist in creating a calmer, quieter presence in relationship to the many fluctuations within our BME experiences
- help enhance physical relaxation, improve psychological balance, assist in coping with illness, and enhance overall health and well-being
- must continue to be studied in order to develop optimized therapeutic approaches for offering safe and effective meditation/mindfulness experiences in rehabilitation.

We are in challenging but exciting times. Researchers are revealing that our body systems have substantial plasticity and continue to change across our lifespan. Meditation and mindfulness studies are revealing that we can transform our brains and bodies for many things, such as better memory and focus, reduced stress response, and even extended life expectancy. Clinical implications are far-reaching across the many intersections of physical, mental, emotional, and spiritual health.

Science will continue to reveal how meditation and mindfulness will evolve to assist overall health. While meditation and mindfulness do not fix everything, and carry noted precautions, the principles reflected are rooted in enhancing contextual awareness in our lives. These practices offer support for transforming individual and collective well-being. May we all uncover deeper presence throughout our days as we establish a personal practice ourselves and perform these practices with our clients. May it contribute to the expansion of quality living for generations to come.

Experiential pause: Having read this chapter, identify and write down at least one actionable item of interest to you. In doing so, consider ways in which applying the material first to yourself, and then to patients, might serve those who come to you for care.

RESOURCES

Meditation apps:

- There are many! Find your favorite. A few common examples include: Insight Timer, Calm, Buddhify, and Headspace.

- Free, meditation-based mind-body self-care lessons: https://cmbm.org/ thetransformation/resources.

CHAPTER 13

Exploring Sensation

Peggy Ninow, OTR/L, SEP, CHTP

A story: "Seren" arrived at the hospital on a cold December night. When she was brought into the emergency department (ED) she was in a catatonic state and appeared to be having a seizure. After she was stabilized medically, she was transferred to the inpatient mental health unit for further evaluation and care. Every day, the staff had more questions than they had answers. Seren had an expired driver's license from another state but no recollection of her past, where she lived, nor how she had come to be there. Through further investigation it appeared that Seren had lost her parents at a young age in a boating accident. It also appeared that she lived through a major hurricane and may have been a victim of sex trafficking. Anytime Seren heard a loud sound, a deeper voice, or any unexpected sound, she would fall into some level of dissociation; she would present with collapsing, fainting, or seizure-like shaking. Sometimes she would begin to gag or vomit. Not only did Seren have amnesia and severe dissociation, she also experienced: severe pain in the back, arms, neck, and legs; electric-shock sensations throughout her body; unusual skin lesions; and what appeared to be a vague autoimmune condition. Seren's care demanded a mind-body integrated understanding. Very slowly, over several months, with support that included gradual reconnection with her body, Seren's system began to regulate and Seren began to re-emerge…

Rehabilitation professionals work with sensation in a variety of ways, ranging from painful sensations, to altered sensations (paresthesias), to the role of individual sense modalities in recovery following injury. In this chapter, we move deeper into how we view and work with sensation. Seren's and others' stories will illuminate the importance of exploring the role that sensation and body awareness play in processes of regulation and resilience.[1]

AN OCCUPATIONAL THERAPIST'S EXPERIENCE

For over 25 years, I have been on a journey to help clients and their families better understand the complex nature of pain and trauma in the human condition. My work has traversed the areas of industrial rehabilitation, persistent pain, and acute mental health.

In 1995, I joined a large rehabilitation clinic in Minneapolis, Minnesota. Most of my patients presented with persistent pain. I saw individuals experiencing mixtures of spinal pain, fibromyalgia, chronic fatigue, migraines, and trauma. Many had comorbid mental health challenges. Initially, my goal was simply to help clients better manage their symptoms. As an occupational therapist, I focused on problem-solving, modifying daily activities, and teaching techniques and skills that would decrease the impact of pain and other symptoms on day-to-day life. As a result, I observed my clients' worlds getting smaller as they reduced or altogether avoided any activity that might "flare up" their symptoms.

I felt there had to be a better way. I believed that people could become whole again. This is where my quest began. I started to incorporate a variety of integrative techniques into my practice, including Qigong, biofeedback, guided imagery, healing touch, and other somatic techniques. I had varying degrees of success. Some people would quickly return to health, others would find little or no relief, and others experienced increased symptoms. After years of frustration, I began to see a pattern. People who could describe healthy home lives and strong relationships, past and present, seemed to have better and quicker results in their rehabilitation and quality of life. This underscored the relevance of psychosocial environment and historical factors. With further study, I came across a body of knowledge encompassing work by Stephen Porges, Karen Moore, Peter Levine, Bessel van der Kolk, and Kathy Kain. The authors discussed groundbreaking research, including the relevance of adverse childhood experiences (ACEs) (see Chapter 4) that rocked my world.

Pieces started to fall into place. Many patients who were experiencing persistent pain conditions were more likely to have a history of trauma, adverse experiences, or other forms of toxic stress. Kathy Kain, an expert in both mental and physical health-care models, explains that when we experience support and safety in early childhood our nervous system's capacity for states of safety and pleasure is enhanced.[2] When people experience high stress or trauma, especially early in life, they may be "wired" differently. The neural platforms that develop in response to healthy nurturing can be thwarted, leaving the adaptive responses necessary for survival in command. The understanding that these clients' experiences and behaviors could be rooted in heightened activity within threat appraisal systems was helpful context. Their systems were either in a constant state of activation/over-arousal or shutting down into states of overwhelm or exhaustion. To "relax" or "regulate" was foreign to their systems.

Because these patients had primarily functioned in a survival state, they had never fully experienced biological states of safety. I had to find a new and better way to interact. I needed a new language, one that could not only penetrate the neocortical "thinking brain," but also connect with and inhibit the primitive survival brain. I found this language from a host of sources, including Somatic Experiencing (SE)—a therapeutic approach to stress, trauma, and mind-body health.

I began my study of SE in 2012. SE is an approach that utilizes gentle strategies focused on sensory awareness and processing to assist the nervous system out of maladaptive patterns. This new avenue opened my eyes to an entirely new layer that I had been missing with most of my clients: their history! It was amazing how working together with my clients with this understanding brought forth an entirely new layer of awareness and understanding.

RECONNECTING WITH SENSATION

Sensation is crucial; the brain needs sensory function to operate. Without sensory input, our brain cannot function optimally. It is peculiar that the use of the word sensation peaked in the late 1800s and then has steadily declined.[3] Did we collectively "check out" of our bodies? Are we in need of rediscovering the rich landscape of sensation? Consider that *sensation* is from the medieval Latin *sēnsātiō* meaning understanding, knowledge, intelligence.[4]

According to Winnie Dunn, an occupational therapist whose work focuses on sensory processing: "Sensation *is* the brain's source of information" [emphasis added].[5] Information from our senses allows us to understand the world and respond effectively to the continuous flux of body-mind-environment (BME) interactions and stress patterns. We integrate our sensations and sensory responses with cognitive and emotional responses to know ourselves better. While efforts to define patterns and sub-types of sensory processing exist,[6] the ways in which sensory integration to cognitive-emotional levels are explored must be unique to each person. Having conscious connection to and understanding of our sensory system allows us to track the world both around and within us and supports every facet of daily functioning.

Karen Moore, another occupational therapist, recognized that our senses can help us relax, make us more alert, and assist us in feeling more capable and "organized": they are a guide, and our relationship to them matters. The focus of Karen's work encompasses the *whole* of sensation, as presented earlier. According to Moore: "We can use sensory input to help with self-regulation. Sensory input helps fine-tune our nervous system and helps make it more resistant to stress."[7]

Sensory awareness and processing are increasingly linked to:

- mental health conditions
- cognition, learning, and memory
- one's ability to recognize others' affect in the context of empathy and compassion.[8]

There are a number of subtopics that relate to sensation, including exteroception, proprioception, and interoception. These words have been given a variety of definitions and meanings. For our purposes, *exteroception* reflects the monitoring of information originating outside the body, as found in the five primary senses: sight, smell, sound, taste, and the sensation that can arise in relation to the skin as a sensory organ (touch, temperature, pressure, vibration, etc.). *Proprioception* is typically defined as the conscious perception or awareness of the position and movement of the body in space. *Interoception* traditionally has defined conscious awareness of the subtler internal levels of bodily function such as visceral state.

Increased support in relationship to sensation can create meaningful changes for ourselves and our patients equally. In doing so, the principle of "not too little, not too much" presents an important context. Hyper- and/or hypo-attention to sensory processing, especially when it carries a negative valence, is associated with conditions such as pain, anxiety, and depression.[9] Some people have more or less innate mindfulness in how they experience their body and this also impacts psychological well-being.[10] Understanding the importance of these principles, followed by the development of relevant awareness in ourselves, is a starting point. This flow is followed by translating these principles into simplified clinical practice.

"FEELING"

Have you ever wondered why the word *feeling* applies equally to the physical and emotional realms? This link is found in definitions of pain, which include both physical sensation and emotion as inseparable components of pain. Unfortunately, these are often split. However, integral thinking and research both support that they are not mutually exclusive or modifiable in isolation.[11] The dual meaning inherent in the word feeling underscores a vital point: sensation is an interface, a connecting point between the body and other realms of our experience.[12] For example, tracking sensation interacts with tracking feelings at the emotional level. How often do we hear the intelligence of the body in our language? "I've got a gut feeling about this," or "I feel it in my bones." Remember the earlier meaning of the word's origin? Research attempting to sort through relationships between emotional and physical symptoms has demonstrated common/ shared as well as unique/individual patterns,[13] underscoring the need for a person-centered approach to exploring relevance.

FROM AN EXPANDING DEFINITION OF INTEROCEPTION TO BODY AWARENESS

Building on the preceding dual meaning of feeling, the conceptualization and clinical meaning of interoception is expanding from just the sense of internal bodily processes, to a term that refers to multiple interacting components of sensing that reflects complex neurophysiological correlates and implications.[14] According to this model, the concept of interoception is broader and includes:

- emotional experience stimuli[15]
- visceral monitoring[16]
- *neuroception*—the monitoring of the physical/social environment for danger versus safety[17]
- social-emotional skills[18]
- a felt sense of insight, intuition, inner knowing, and decision making.[19]

This expanded definition of interoception combines with exteroception and proprioception to encompass a more complete view of sensation. Subsequently, *body awareness* defines the personal, active, and conscious experience and interpretation of the whole of sensory experiencing. Body awareness reflects various types and qualities of attention on the body, including of BME relationships, and in context of the development of body management. Enhancing how we attend to sensation is rooted in the intention to support and deepen each individual's understanding of and relationship to their multisensory experience.

Poor body awareness and/or distorted body image have been linked to alexithymia, carrying relevance to numerous conditions such as depression, anxiety, and persistent pain.[20] *Alexithymia* is difficulty in identifying and describing one's emotions and sometimes correlates with externally oriented thinking and a general difficulty with the regulation of one's emotions.[21] These links underscore the need to understand and address body awareness training in support of changes in function (mood, symptom management, social engagement, leisure, work, etc.).

Body awareness training can enhance one's sense of self, including in relation to posture, mood, movement, body language, communication skills, and more. While further research on various approaches to training body awareness is needed, enhancing body awareness can support the treatment of numerous conditions commonly treated by rehabilitation professionals.[22] Body-awareness-enhancing therapies support embodiment processes that may have been disrupted at some point. Such therapies tap into the integrity of the whole self, the innate wisdom of the body, and/or an inner resource or guide.[23]

Experiential pause: Was Seren able to label her feelings and how was that connected to body awareness? How did the staff working with Seren create safe space for emotional awareness and expression? Take a moment and reread Seren's story. As you do so, see if you can concurrently:

1. imagine what Seren's felt sense must have been like; imagine how she was experiencing her inner world, her body, and the external (including social) environment
2. attend to the felt sense in your own body as you imagine working with Seren. What do you notice?

THE IMPACT OF PERSONAL HISTORY ON SENSORY PROCESSING

We each have unique ways of processing and *making sense of sensation*, depending on various developmental factors, medical events, or traumatic experiences. For some clients, an acute traumatic event, such as a car accident or surgery, could be a "key" to understanding their present health experience. For others, it could be early childhood adversity such as illness/medical care, being born prematurely, sexual or physical abuse, or growing up with parents who were not present physically, mentally, or emotionally.[24] Some of these experiences may arise out of connections or patterns that are rooted in the parents' own trauma histories.[25]

When working from the lens of supporting the neurobiological correlates of safety and comfort through sensing, we are often able to realize changes in symptomology. When survival-oriented regions of the nervous system settle and threat response loops are regulated, many individuals can make sustainable progress in their rehabilitation process. However, this does not always come easily for clients with complex chronic health, comorbid, and/or pain concerns.

Kathy Kain, mentioned earlier, explains that most people seeking health care benefit from cultivating a deeper awareness of the body. This is especially true for those who may have ACEs, high stress, and/or developmental trauma in their history.[26] In her 40 years of study/practice of mind-body approaches for helping patients with pain, she uncovered something consistent with the findings of the ACE research. Kain found that many individuals are not aware that their experience is impacted by physiological patterns that arose from relational, attachment-based, and/or otherwise complex facets of development trauma. Such clients may believe that the way they feel (tense, anxious, shameful, etc.) is "normal" because they have always felt this way. In these cases, the impact that set up the pervasive dysregulated biobehavioral patterns may have occurred very early in life, during times when the senses are creating conditioned somatic patterns.

Researchers such as Bowlby[27] and Schore[28] note that if early nurturing does not occur optimally, a person is more vulnerable to illness, injury, and psychological wounding in their adult life. As covered in Chapter 4, the influence of early-life attachment patterns may reflect a backdrop to many health conditions. It is an error to assume that interoception and neuroception automatically develop and can be relied upon to work correctly across the lifespan. The patterns within these regulatory systems deeply impact how a person experiences themselves, others, and the world around them. In contemporary mind-body therapy models, these narratives are not as easily accessed by the neocortex or by speech, but instead are uncovered through attention on the subtle, felt sense of the body.

As such, the use of somatic awareness training and/or touch-based therapy models are fundamental when working with patients with complex histories and clinical presentations. Once again, while emphasizing that these principles are particularly relevant in relationship to high stress/trauma history, the principles are useful on a spectrum for *all* clients. The cultivation of positive sensory relationships within the mind-body connection stands in support of regulation, resilience, and cultivation of well-being.

Regardless of the presence of such past experiences, approaches that support the biological underpinnings of human behavior such as safety, nurturance, and autonomy provide a language and approach for therapeutic interactions. This is the language of the nervous system. Exploring and improving one's awareness, understanding of, and relationship to sensation is vital. Such an approach can assist in taking the common dynamic of blame/shame out of the client's experience and their treatment sessions. Clients become able to recognize how survival patterns and adaptive strategies, driven by impersonal drives in the nervous system, present an unaddressed barrier to freeing up greater capacity for healing. Imagine having a part of the brain that wakes up every day saying: "Well, you didn't die yesterday, so let's just repeat those same patterns." For many, this can be a reality. Without a felt sense of safety, the wear and tear on the physical body can increase exponentially. The good news: when the nervous system experiences safety, social engagement and increased connections with our environment can emerge. In essence, safety supports improved homeostatic processes throughout our entire system.[29]

CLINICAL APPLICATION

Sensation, arousal, and safety

When first approaching a client, an immediate priority is to ask yourself: "How do I create safety?" *This looks different with every nervous system.* Some people feel safest in solitude with a great distance between their body and another person. Others feel safe in a room filled with people. In a sense, the practitioner needs to be a sleuth and discern what works for each individual through experiential learning—lots of feedback, choices, and experiences.

Remember Seren? Treatment sessions with Seren were slow and deliberate. Initially, the primary goal focused on providing her with experiences that had potential to support a sense of safety. It often took 20 minutes of sitting with Seren, slowly moving closer and talking quietly with her, before her nervous system would settle enough to engage. Some days, eye contact and getting closer than six feet was too much for her nervous system. Other days, she was more able to interact, reflecting changes in her physiological state.

The terms *arousal* and *activation* are used to denote levels of regulation as described in biobehavioral theories and approaches such as polyvagal theory (PVT),[30] neurovisceral integration theory,[31] SE,[32] or sensorimotor psychotherapy.[33] These models are built upon foundations of mind-body integrated science translated into clinical support. These models remind us that the range of behaviors accessible to an individual are directly impacted by physiological state. Understanding how to work with an individual within a "window of tolerance" or "zone of arousal" is vital.[34] See Figure 13.1, which emphasizes the concept in relation to trauma history, noting that the concept is clinically useful outside of the relevance of trauma.

For Seren, it was imperative to discover and then reinforce how feeling safe in her body actually felt. While Seren's case may reflect an extreme history, and while IRP acknowledges larger contexts beyond individual stress/trauma history in examining causality, addressing sensation and body awareness when working with the mind-body relationship remains uniformly important. These principles underpin mind-body medicine skills training in general.

Awareness and appraisal of one's sensory experience is vital. Sensations of safety are something that many may not consciously be aware of, such as relaxed muscles or a calm stomach. The healing effects of creating and sensing safety in the body can be profound. For Seren, these were totally new sensations. Seren began to tolerate being out of her room. She became more tolerant of interacting with staff and peers, and began to express her emotions, as well as to enjoy baking and craft activities. Over time, her blank stare shifted and she became a warm, smiling person who enjoyed interacting with others. Her physical pain symptoms decreased, but would flare when her stress response increased. There is growing evidence that pain processes are linked to autonomic nervous system dysregulation, processes of dissociation, toxic stress, and trauma history.[35] Seren's experience demonstrates some of these relationships and physiological patterns.

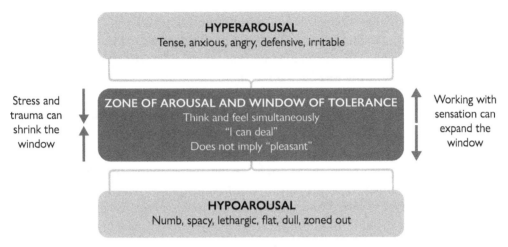

FIGURE 13.1: ZONE OF AROUSAL/WINDOW OF TOLERANCE
Adapted from the National Institute for the Clinical Application of Behavioral Medicine[36]

Another story: "Carlie" was a 38-year-old nurse who presented with debilitating migraines and post-concussion syndrome. Carlie had fainted and hit her head while shopping. She remembered that she had started to feel dizzy, fell backwards, and hit her head on the corner of a shelf. Carlie's initial report of symptoms included dizziness, nausea, headaches, difficulty concentrating, "brain fog," cognitive difficulties, and feeling unstable when walking. She was easily overwhelmed by external stimuli and experienced: tension in her neck, shoulders, and jaw; no appetite; poor sleep with nightmares; and increased anxiety. She noted that since her fall, migraine headaches had become more intense. Carlie was unable to work, drive, or exercise. Everything was stressful: "I feel like my brain is overloaded." Carlie had other medical issues that appeared to contribute to her current issues, including asthma, history of gastric bypass surgery, and a history of falling down the stairs at age three.

Experiential pause: With what you've learned thus far, jot down questions that you are wondering about in relation to Carlie and her experience. How might you begin to address the relevance of sensation and body awareness in working with Carlie?

Going deeper—working with sensation

When Carlie arrived for her first session, she exhibited tension throughout her entire body—"global high intensity activation." Anxiety, coupled with her physical symptoms, comprised the perfect storm to inhibit higher cortical function. This is sometimes described as an "offline" state, which is a simplified way of describing decreased distribution of resources to higher cognitive processes due to the survival circuits prioritizing threat detection and defense.[37]

Carlie stated: "It seems like I don't remember what people tell me. I can't focus long enough to read, and tasks that used to seem simple feel impossible and overwhelming." The use of sensory modalities to calm the state of her nervous system was one component of what proved effective. Instead of automatically continuing with the initial interview in a sitting position, Carlie was offered the choice to lie down if that would feel more comfortable. She chose to lie down on the treatment table. Through the presentation of additional options, a weighted blanket was placed over her to provide deep pressure proprioception that often supports physiological quieting. Pillows and pads created extra sensations of support. Carlie was encouraged to take time to focus on the sensations of the blanket and supports. She was invited to say whether anything was feeling different. After about ten minutes, Carlie's entire system began to settle. Visible tension drained from her face and she reported: "My headache is less intense. I can feel my jaw relaxing. I can think more clearly now. This is the first time in three months that I have felt anything close to being relaxed."

In order to interact with and benefit from these therapeutic approaches, Carlie's system needed to have the experience of slowing down—the relaxation response.[38] Use of the weighted blanket was an effective, simple, passive tool to assist the process. Over the course of ten sessions, Carlie experienced a variety of simple techniques, including enhanced body awareness and movement practices. These treatments created openings for her to comprehend and gently progress with more demanding treatment approaches, including:

- therapeutic education (see Chapter 16) on what a concussion entails (increases understanding and normalizes the seemingly random symptoms that are common with concussion as being linked to a dysregulated nervous system[39])
- consideration and support around the way in which trauma affects implicit memory and the state of the nervous system (impact injuries, physical boundary breach, renegotiating the fall, grounding, and supporting the parasympathetic nervous system)
- gentle bodywork to improve neuromuscular regulation (decrease tone and increase awareness of holding patterns) and to enhance brain-body communication including autonomic regulation to viscera, organs, and joints
- cognitive skills such as mindfulness-based practices.

The importance of co-regulation

As rehabilitation professionals, we need to understand the importance of self-regulation and be responsible for the state of our own nervous system. Both our and our clients' systems are constantly assessing the environment. In some cases, especially for those with a trauma history, individuals may have heightened attention to certain stimuli.[40]

As introduced earlier, the term *neuroception* is used when defining the components and processes of sensing that are linked to mechanisms of threat detection. This is a vital facet of PVT as taught by Stephen Porges. Porges explains neuroception as the way in which our nervous system determines danger versus safety. Neuroception happens continuously without awareness—it is running in the background at all times. It takes cues from inside the body and from both the physical and social environment.

We all are capable of picking up on stress or dysregulation in others—including the state of our health-care provider and/or the larger environment where care is provided. Sensitive individuals may experience an amplification of normal neuroceptive processes. When the professional is dysregulated, the client's system will interpret this as a signal of danger and even, possibly, that the client is doing something wrong, at fault, or to blame. Even seemingly benign choices that we make may alarm our clients. For example, clients may misinterpret a neutral face as threatening. We need to consciously extend cues of safety to our clients through facial expression, voice, awareness of safety through appropriate physical proximity, intent with any touch utilized, and environmental choices. We have to learn how all of this applies to our own nervous system to be able to work optimally with our clients. All of this becomes possible through processes of self-awareness. In the context of this chapter, this self-awareness is directed to emphasize attention on the sensory landscape of the body.

The construct of co-regulation (first introduced in Chapter 1) is rooted in the understanding that one person's physiological state (reflected in body language, tone of voice, facial expressivity, and movement patterns) has a profound physiological effect on others.[41] Sometimes a client's system is so disorganized that the only way we can effect change is through the supportive interaction of our own system. The presence that our "system" conveys can be powerful. The development of body awareness in both the professional and the patient is viewed as potentially supportive of co-regulation, and thus physiological states of safety.

When the physiological state of safety is present, the possibility of improved mind-body organization increases markedly. Safety is not a thinking thing; it is an embodied state. In the language of PVT, this is labeled a "ventral vagal experience"—a simplification reflecting the relevance of the parasympathetic outflow from the myelinated ventral division of the vagus nerve. It is best, however, to see this as a systemic, integrated brain-body state interacting with the physical and social environment.

When we are stressed or experiencing overwhelming events, our system may shift away from "ventral vagal safety" and move into greater sympathetic responses and/or into "dorsal vagal dominance"—more of a freeze/immobility/braking pattern. This latter concept is equally a reduction—used to convey the relevance of these central nervous system correlates to the organism's overall integrated threat-response patterns. These contextually "primitive" responses may disrupt our awareness of bodily sensation, the environment, and/or others. When this ensues, it can move us towards greater defensiveness. In other cases, it may facilitate isolating/immobility behaviors and coping patterns.

These types of behavioral responses can also be seen as somatoemotional states that are deeply embedded in biological (and thus sensory) processes. These states are often conceptualized as reflecting autonomic dysregulation and are marked by unpleasant sensory experience.

A few clinically translated examples[42] include:

- depression (dorsal vagal prevalence)
- anxiety or rage (fight/sympathetic prevalence)
- withdrawal/isolation (flight/sympathetic or combination if successful fleeing has occurred)
- fainting (dorsal vagal dominance placing the physiological state into preservation/ conservation mode)
- irritable bowel syndrome (alternating overactivity between sympathetic and parasympathetic states).

Additional clinical considerations

In addition to persistent pain conditions, underlying patterns of dysregulation are increasingly linked to other clinical conditions, such as gastrointestinal disorders and cardiac problems.[43] Patterns of dysregulation influence mind-body relationships such as those found in interoceptive processes.[44] Exploring and addressing the somatic roots of these patterns requires the practitioner's capacity to safely inquire, educate, and address the relevance of each person's unique history, its possible impact on their present health experience, and how that is found in the present sensory landscape of the body.

De Jong *et al.* looked at the impact of mindfulness-based cognitive therapy that included body awareness training for persons with comorbid persistent pain and depression.[45] Such approaches must be navigated with the reminder to never minimize a person's self-report of and beliefs around their experience. It is possible that reports of possibly relevant factors may not be complete or accurate, especially if the impact was caused by early life experience. It is also possible that historical factors get overemphasized out of context by either the professional or the client.

Having said that, clinical experience supports the understanding that many individuals' systems become sensitized. Response to sensory stimuli may become overly reactive or disproportionate. This overactivity may set up a situation where an individual perceives typically benign objects and occurrences as threatening. This misinterpretation can include situations where even normal sensations from physiological processes in the body are categorized as aversive or harmful. This type of dynamic may get woven into patterns of emotional awareness, sensation, pain, anxiety, and/or depression.[46] In these cases, individuals' systems will process, interpret, and/or experience sensation (both external and internal) differently. By gradually facilitating increased awareness and interpretation of, and ultimately comfort with, sensation, a practitioner can help such clients to transform limiting patterns.

When appropriate and self-selected by the client, providing safe and supportive touch therapy can promote new experiences of sensation. Touch therapy can increase awareness of the body in general by addressing unconscious and sustained guarding/protection patterns. This operates via sensory-motor paths in favor of regulating neuromuscular tone and increasing capacity to experience the relaxation response. Care must be taken as to the amount/depth and type of touch. For example, excessively light touch may be more activating than the provision of firmer touch.[47] Continual feedback from the client is vital to determine value and impact. Ultimately, the clinical motivation lies in restoring experiences of the body as a safe place, as opposed to the traditional view of manual therapy as fixing the tissue itself (see Chapter 23). This must occur in the context of an attuned relationship—supporting the biological underpinnings of social engagement. For some, such experiences can be the first that their nervous system has had of the biological underpinnings of safety and nurturance.

PRACTICAL APPLICATIONS AND EXPERIENTIAL LEARNING

The experiential learning that follows reflects techniques accessible to any practitioner, regardless of their skill level in addressing topics such as past trauma. If the past is impacting a person, that impact is found in what is happening in the present. As emphasized in Chapter 6, building capacity does not imply regressive analysis of childhood, psychological content, or the approaches that a specialized psychologist might deploy. When we return to principles of choice, present-moment awareness, experiential learning, and self-expression, we can offer a lot by enhancing attention on the sensorial realm of the body.

There are many avenues to exploring sensation. The following techniques reflect a sampling designed to build core skills. These techniques reflect various capacity. They are for you to learn and experience first and eventually apply clinically. Keep in mind that clients will also have various capacities. For some, these techniques are advanced. If you work with persons with high sensitivity, trauma history, etc., remember that starting slow, and providing repeated choices and regular opportunities for feedback, supports safety through graded development.

> **Experiential pauses**
>
> 1. "What do you notice is happening in your body right now?" This is a safe, simple way to direct attention to the body—for the therapist or the client. It allows self-selection.
> 2. Directed/focused body-awareness training can be useful for some. The following is a shortened example of a body scan practice.
>   a. **Choice and resourcing**: You may choose to do this with your eyes open or closed. At any time, if the experience feels overwhelming, choose an exit strategy such as opening the eyes, looking around the room, shifting or moving the body, or having something to eat or drink…whatever helps you regroup.
>   b. **The technique**: Become aware of your experience of breathing—the sensations of air moving in…of air moving out. See if you can simply notice

these sensations—the body breathing itself. What is this like? Now, rotate your attention through the body sequentially—noticing the sensations at each point. Remember that the mind will like to categorize everything into good/bad, pleasant/unpleasant, novel/normal, right/wrong—so if possible, see if you can meet whatever you notice with curiosity and a quality of "no praise, no blame." Move from top to bottom and back and forth, left…right… What do you discover? Along the way, did you notice that by coming into awareness, you had feelings come up? Or perhaps that you were able to relax a part of you that felt sore, tense, or tight?

3. Use quick checks on yourself and teach this to your clients.
   a. Stop, take three breaths.
   b. Become mindful/present in the moment.
   c. Connect with your own senses: "What do I see, hear, feel, smell?" (Remember: all senses are vital to any construct of sensing/sensation. Present-moment attention to the full landscape is important. The "organ" that makes things real for us is the collective organ of sensation. Often, the busyness of our world leaves little room for this type of attention.)
   d. Connect with your body: "What do I sense?"
   e. Set an intention: "I am fully present with this experience."

4. Link sensation to emotion. For some, this can take time. Go slow. The following is an example of how to begin to work with this.
   a. As you notice the sensations of the body, what emotion(s) are reflected in those sensations? How do the physical feelings link to the emotional feelings, your mood, or the state of the mind?

LESSONS LEARNED

It is important to remember that, initially, some individuals may not be able to tolerate high or sustained attention on their body, nor be able to remain in an optimally regulated state for long periods. This is especially true when first accessing these potentially positive experiences of the body. Building capacity is a process that takes time, choice, ongoing support, regular feedback, and patience on the part of both the therapist and the client.

Here are some lessons learned:

- The goldilocks principle: We need to become skilled in knowing what is too much, what is not enough, and what is just right for a client's system and their awareness of that system. We are all at risk of putting too little or too much attention on the sensations of the body.
- When/if orienting attention to the body is not successful and leads to dysregulation, resourcing and reorienting to the outer/physical environment and/or action/movement is often a better choice (revisit Chapter 6).
- We need to remember that these parameters change from day to day as BME dynamics are continually in flux. The client's experience interacts with our own

process and state, as well. We can see our systems as "moving targets." This is why awareness of sensation is crucial. A model of "co-tracking" sensory experience is an important way to tailor our care. This approach improves functional moment-to-moment capacity for optimizing regulation, relationship, and coping strategy.

- A general goal is to give our clients the skills to know *when* they are dysregulated and to know *how* to smoothly return to balance. The goal here is not perfection, rather greater flexibility.
- Sensation is best explored in the context of developing appraisal and reappraisal capacity. This capacity stands in support of: enhanced understanding and relating to our sensory experience; decreased aversion; increased "comfort with discomfort"; and, ultimately, the possibility for positive experiences of the body.
- When dysregulated, connection and curiosity are compromised. By bringing ourselves and our clients comfortably back into the rich landscape of bodily sensation, we enable curiosity and connection—with ourselves, others, and the larger world.

SENSING YOUR WAY FORWARD

Sensation can be seen as a foundation within the lived experience of the body. Sensation brings our experiences and our world to life. When sensation is supported through body awareness training, we can move into a fuller sense of being.

Recognizing that it is often unpleasant and aversive sensations that bring individuals into rehabilitation care settings, we have touched on a number of important foundations in advocacy for distributing resources into exploring, training, and supporting the complexity of sensation in ourselves and those we work with. Body awareness is embedded within many of our other skills such as mindfulness, imagery, and movement training. You will gain increased capacity to weave together these topics and techniques. Consider what it means to *sense* your way forward...

> **Experiential pause:** Having read this chapter, identify and write down at least one actionable item of interest to you. In doing so, consider ways in which applying the material first to yourself, and then to patients, might serve those who come to you for care.

RESOURCES

SE is a therapeutic model that numerous health-care professionals (mental health, physical medicine, social work, and many rehabilitation therapy professions) are training in and integrating into their clinical practice. It is built on much of what has been overviewed in this chapter. Go to https://traumahealing.org to learn more.

CHAPTER 14

Exploring Imagery

Leslie Davenport, MA, MS, LMFT

A story: If he brought an expectation of healing to our initial appointment, it was from the hurry-up-and-get-on-with-it school of life—a stoic and earnest desire for a quick solution to the recent medical distractions that had gotten in the way of significant momentum in his career in finance. "Daniel" has suffered a heart attack at the age of 51.

In our first encounter, it was easy to see several facets of Daniel. We often think of ourselves as having a genuine, unified self. And yet the fluid nature of life evokes a broad spectrum of responses within us, and these different reactions, or selves, are layered within our personality and emerge in different situations. With Daniel, there were several distinct faces that could shift as easily as the tilt of a kaleidoscope.

When he first arrived in the office, ten minutes early, he took advantage of that extra time in the waiting room to work on his laptop. His crisp, tailored appearance expressed his success and professionalism. Although he seemed friendly and engaging, I think it was mostly the subtle slump in his upper back, a fatigue around his eyes, and a weight that rested in his voice that showed his face of sadness not far below the surface. And yet in certain moments, especially when he later described walks in the botanical gardens not far from his house, it was easy to see a youthful face expressing all the delights of a seven-year-old boy eager for an adventure.

Daniel was not familiar with guided imagery, but he came on the recommendation of his physician, who prescribed imagery as a useful stress-management technique during cardiac rehabilitation. In the first few sessions, we focused on some practical skills around his goals, such as reducing muscular tension by learning progressive relaxation and breathwork. We also brainstormed some tips for ending his work focus at the end of the day in a more mindful way.

Daniel now asks whether there is a way we could address the pain in his chest. Although the surgical procedure, which had implanted a stent in an artery to increase the blood flow to his heart, had healed well, there is still lingering pain.

Trusting the success of our work together so far, he agrees to try guided imagery and to "visit his heart" as a way to discover more about the pain.

"Close your eyes," I begin, "and take those long, full breaths you've been practicing."

I watch Daniel fill his abdomen with breath, then expand the breath into his ribcage, continuing until the breath rises up under his collar bones. The out breath is just as complete, and his body softens a little more fully with each exhalation. We take time for several breath cycles to deepen his relaxation.

"Now that you are more relaxed, bring your attention inside your chest and sense your heart. Invite an image, which may be literal or symbolic, to arise for your heart. Whatever appears, describe aloud what you become aware of."

An image arises easily, and Daniel describes his heart as: "tender and bruised with blue, purple, and pink patches." He says his heart feels battered. This makes sense to him as he considers his recent surgery and heart attack. He also describes his heart as having a weightiness to it, as if there is something heavy caught at the bottom. I suspect this is related to the heaviness I have heard in his voice.

I encourage him to continue exploring and ask: "If your heart had a voice, or some way of expressing itself, what would it want you to know right now?"

There is a pause, and then emotions flash across his face—eyebrows rising in surprise and then downturned lips.

He speaks with the gentle voice of his heart: "I've been waiting a long time for you to come back."

Although he can't say why he feels tearful or even know quite what the message means, he is deeply moved and curious.

Over the next few weeks, he tells me the story of how his family had moved to this country from Eastern Europe when he was three years old. His father, who had died four years earlier, was very committed to the family and had been a hardworking man, a shopkeeper by trade. Making ends meet had not come easily in those days. When his father finally found the means to move his family to America, fueled by the strong purpose of fulfilling the dream of a better life for his children, it was a momentous event.

With some gentle sorting out over the next several sessions, it becomes clear to Daniel that he is living his father's dream, his father's heart's desire, and not his own. He had learned early that it broke a strong family rule to voice his own view if it deviated from the family values. Although Daniel had proven to be quite capable in the business world, he had silenced his own call to landscape gardening as a young man because it did not fit the family legacy's picture of success.

"How would you like to respond to your heart's message?" I asked him during another imagery session a few weeks later.

His response arises immediately with a clear and strong voice: "I want to give my father's dream back to him so that there is more room for my own."

Over time, it becomes clear to Daniel that he wants to anchor his life in the strong, clear voice of his heart that has championed his own dreams.

The intention for such deep change can be accelerated when it is made visible. This is evident in the rituals and ceremonies that arise within all cultures and mark transitions. For example, a wedding ceremony makes visible the intention and reality of a relationship that has evolved into a life partnership. The ritual of clapping at the end of a musical performance is a ritual of appreciation and marks the transition of the theatrical experience. I encourage Daniel to consider whether there is a way to honor his significant transition to reclaim his heart's desire through a symbol or ritual.

Not long after, Daniel arrives at our appointment and has barely taken his seat when he fishes a small round stone out of his pocket. He had found it on one of his walks at the botanical gardens in his neighborhood. He rests it in the upturned palm of his left hand.

"I'm not really a religious man," he says as he curls his fingers over the stone, "but I feel like I've been praying all week, sending thanks to my father for what he's given me. I've been imagining that the parts of my father's life I've been carrying have seeped into this stone in my pocket."

He opens his hand, showing me the stone, now infused with his father's dreams. He announces his plan to visit his father's grave next month and respectfully place the stone there.

When we conclude our work together, it is not clear whether Daniel is going to remain in the finance business or make a significant career shift. It is clear, however, that he is now making his choices, on a daily basis, in a way that is more responsive to his own heart. The last time I saw him, I could recognize it in the ease of his walk and hear it through the new clarity in his voice. He had placed his fingers on the pulse of his own life and discovered the life rhythms that have heart and meaning for him.

Daniel's story, like most examples of healing journeys, is multilayered. We know that we can no longer simply treat symptoms, attempting to isolate a health concern away from the rich emotional, belief-based, cultural, and historical facets of a person's life. As part of the imagery approach, Daniel learned progressive relaxation and breathwork, preparatory practices to transition into an imagistic state of mind. He learned to tune in somatically, becoming more aware of cues and messages from his physical state and stress levels. He developed the capacity to sort through family influences and recover lost parts of himself. And perhaps most key in his healing, he learned that his heart could speak to him through imagery, providing a map for authenticity, fulfillment, and a healthier lifestyle. As a result, Daniel participated in a much more comprehensive approach to his cardiac rehabilitation and was progressing beautifully with his medical goals on the completion of our treatment series.

Imagery is a healing mechanism found in virtually all world cultures and is an integral part of many ancient, indigenous, and wisdom traditions across time. It is an implicit language of mind, brain, and body together and in concert with the environment(s) being navigated. In this context, it can be seen as a vital form of communication within the integral view of body-mind-environment (BME).

Imagery reflects a way in which our minds code, store, and process energy and information. There are many types of and ways of working with imagery, such as guided imagery and motor imagery, as well as the presence and role of spontaneous and undirected imagery in our lives. This chapter will explore the amazing, creative, and therapeutic power of imagery, with a predominant focus on guided imagery: a form of deliberate, directed use of one's imaginal faculties for therapeutic purposes and processes.

GUIDED IMAGERY
The power of imagery

Guided imagery is like a Rosetta Stone that decodes and translates the deep mind-body undercurrents that run through our lives. When we open to the clarity that emerges naturally through imagery practice, there is a growing experience of well-being, a visceral wisdom that surpasses ordinary logic. We experience wholeness regardless of the circumstances of our lives, and we often discover fresh and surprising ways to improve the conditions we're experiencing. We naturally begin to live in a qualitatively different way: more present and responsive to the moment-by-moment gifts and challenges of daily life. Guided imagery increases the opportunity for organically leaning toward health-wise choices.

Some of the most frequently asked questions by clients and clinicians alike are: What is the most effective type of guided imagery? Should guided imagery be scripted or spontaneous? Should it be accompanied by music or an approach that emphasizes the somatic or visualization aspects? Should the client recline or sit upright? What about particular breathing techniques to prepare for the imagery session? The list of possible guided imagery technique refinements is a long one, and the queries are most often fueled by a genuine motivation to maximize the transformational benefits of the imagery experience. The answer to nearly all of these queries is "Yes!" There is considerable research that endorses the efficacy of many different styles of guided imagery. The most appropriate applications depend on both the needs of the client, and the training and theoretical orientation of the practitioner.

The spectrum of guided imagery approaches can be broadly divided into two primary camps: scripted and non-scripted. In receptive, or non-scripted, imagery, like the kind used with Daniel, the practitioner supports an exploration and dialogue with whatever symbols appear, facilitating the client's discovery of their own healing path.

Scripted guided imagery

Both scripted and non-scripted guided imagery approaches have inherent strengths. The theory that favors a scripted imagery style maintains that a trained practitioner can effectively "install" a reparative physical and/or emotional system into the client using a very detailed and carefully shaped imagery script. A healthy body or mind may have been derailed through trauma, family or cultural conditioning, or a genetic malfunction, and the scripted imagery recalibrates the person's system to once again thrive.

For example, this excerpt from *Rituals of Healing: Using Imagery for Health and Wellness* is frequently used to help cancer patients integrate a new template of a healthy immune system: "Imagine the macrophages…as the warning of an invader sounds, they swell up, becoming large and powerful, connecting with each other, moving in a flank. Watch as they approach an invader, reach out, lasso it with their armlike extensions, and inject it with potent enzymes."[1]

This type of scripted approach has yielded excellent results in improving patients' medical and psychological conditions. Perhaps the most cited and influential research on scripted imagery consists of two hallmark studies out of the Cleveland Clinic. In the initial study, scripted imagery that provided guidance for imagining and "rehearsing" a successful surgical procedure and outcome was used in preparation for major colorectal surgery. The results showed 75% overall patient satisfaction, a 65% decrease in pain and anxiety, and 33% fewer side effects compared with the patients who did not receive the imagery support.[2] A second study was conducted that provided imagery preparation to patients undergoing cardiothoracic surgery, with virtually identical results.[3]

Non-scripted guided imagery

Non-scripted or receptive imagery recognizes that each person's symbolic imagery is infused with unique meanings, and the intuition of the client is entrusted to discover the most effective images for their own healing. For example, a scripted imagery session may direct the listener to imagine walking on a beach for a relaxing stress-reducing experience. But if the person listening to the script almost drowned in the ocean as a child, imagining the sounds of the waves could trigger unintended panic. Or if someone was raised in the Midwest and finds their greatest comfort by a river or meadow, the invitation to the beachside may not be as soothing.

A non-scripted stress-reduction session would invite an image to form from within the person that depicts a relaxing, safe environment that appeals to the client. A non-scripted session is still therapeutically guided with an infrastructure, but instead of recommending specific images, an invitation is made for them to arise spontaneously. The practitioner would facilitate a full vivification, exploration, and deepening of the client's imagery with an interactive infrastructure. Depending on the person, the imagined peaceful place could be anything—a mountaintop, an ancient temple, or their own backyard. This receptive imagery approach can also be applied to a wide range of medical, psychological, and psychospiritual concerns.

The word *receptivity* comes from the Latin root *re-capere*, meaning "to take back." It suggests that imagery can help us reclaim parts of ourselves that may have been covered over, forgotten, or disowned, making them available to us again.

It is more challenging to research the effectiveness of non-scripted receptive imagery than scripted guided imagery because of the increased variability that comes with the open-ended nature of the process. A study out of California Pacific Medical Center in San Francisco tested a non-scripted, interactive style of imagery. The researchers found that the imagery sessions increased relaxation, provided patients with insight into the nature of their health problems, and assisted patients in discovering and cultivating healing intentions.[4]

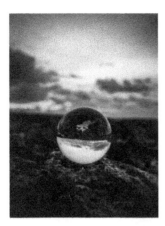

Tips and reminders for working with guided imagery:

- A quiet environment with low external sensory input, as well as permissive and relaxed conditions.
- Patience—like other forms of mind-body medicine, imagery is best seen as slow but powerful medicine. Be sure to allow pauses within the imagery for the patient to engage with their experience.
- Confidence and proficiency increase with practice, practice, practice.
- Engage all senses including interoception, proprioception, and the whole-body sense.
- Imagery content needs to be congruent with the values of your patients—stay with the provision of options and choices and always remind patients that they can exit any imagery experience at any time.
- Refrain from interrupting the images that can arise for a patient. It provides a greater therapeutic value to explore the particular and unique meaning that the images have for the patient.

FIGURE 14.1: WORKING WITH GUIDED IMAGERY
Image source: Louis Maniquet @ Unsplash

AWARENESS AND RELAXATION: FOUNDATIONS FOR WORKING WITH IMAGERY

When introducing guided imagery, begin with relaxation exercises, such as muscle relaxation and awareness of the breath, to support the shift from the cognitive thinking into receptive imagistic experience. The relaxation practices initially need to be paired with imagery that encourages emotional resiliency, such as inviting and exploring a special or safe place. A patient's ability to enjoy a safe-place imagery experience establishes that they have access to the emotional stability needed when applying imagery for more clinically charged themes, such as an active illness or revisiting a traumatic event.

Because imagery softens a person's familiar mental filters and defense mechanisms, the feelings and perspectives that arise in a session are often surprising to the client. This is an important consideration for those with a traumatic history, as there is a risk of emotional flooding if the past trauma surfaces unexpectedly during guided imagery. Helping a client establish familiarity with their own inner resourcefulness and feelings of wholeness creates a clinical safety for more advanced and in-depth work. For a review of principles of care that support safety, see "Orienting and resourcing" in Chapter 6, as well as Appendix B on trauma-informed care.

I invite you to experience this simple, relaxing imagery experience. Since it is done with the eyes closed or lowered, you could have a trusted friend read it to you slowly or pre-record it for yourself. Anytime you see three dots (…), let there be a brief pause. You'll want to set aside 20 minutes in a comfortable place where you are free from interruptions.

Experiential pause: Safe Place Imagery

Sit or recline in a comfortable position, letting your body be well supported, and let your body release into the support. Invite your body to soften as much as it wants to, allowing a sense of relaxation to begin to emerge… Now, turn your thoughts for just a moment toward the last several hours—the activities, conversations, and things you have experienced... Take a snapshot of that time; although it was recent, recognize it as part of your past. Let the snapshot drift away from you, and make more room for this moment, now... Turn your thoughts for just a moment to the things you anticipate doing later today or tonight... Take a snapshot of that time; recognize it as part of your future. Now, let the picture drift away from you, and make more room for simply being present—here, now... As you breathe out, release your focus from anything that doesn't require your attention in this moment...

This moment, which is fresh and uncluttered, has never been lived before. Take a moment to recognize the arrival of this new moment... Begin to let the qualities of peace and spaciousness that are a natural part of this moment ride on your breath. As you take a full breath in, silently say the word "clarity." When you breathe out, silently say the word "peace" and continue to relax even more deeply. Breathe in "clarity," breathe out "peace." In "clarity," out "peace"...

On the next in breath, let the fresh, clear feeling rise up to the top of your head. As you breathe out, let peacefulness, in the felt sense of softening or opening sensations, flow over your scalp and forehead... Now breathe clarity into your mind. As you breathe out, feel the peace in your mind that is always present beyond thoughts... Breathe fresh clarity into your eyes, and your face. As you exhale, let your eyes rest, and your face relax... Notice your jaw, allowing it to be slack and loose as you exhale...

Let the next breath bring fresh energy into your throat, open and clear. On the out breath, feel ease flowing into your neck, shoulders, and upper back... Feel the relaxation seeping into your muscles and allow them to soften in response... Let the flow of relaxation travel into your arms, hands, and fingers. Notice the subtle sensations that arise. Do they feel warm, or tingling, or light? Just notice...

Now bring your awareness and breath into your torso. Breathe freshness and clarity into your heart and discover the peacefulness that resides there as you breathe out... Breathe fresh energy into all the vital organs, allowing them to feel natural, comfortable, and relaxed as you breathe out. Breathe in clarity; breathe out...and continue relaxing...

Let your breath and awareness continue into your hips. Feel your belly receiving your breath, rising on the inhalation, and settling on the exhalation—fresh and peaceful... Let the fresh energy and peaceful feelings flow into your legs, all the way to your feet and toes. Feel the soles of your feet relaxing, the way they might feel on warm sand, soft grass, or a smooth river stone... Feel your whole body, a three-dimensional sensation, vibrant and relaxed. Breathing in, your whole body clear. Breathing out, your whole body comfortable. Breathing in, your whole being clear. Breathing out, your whole being peaceful...

Now invite an image to form for a place, an environment, that would support these relaxing feelings—it may even deepen them. This place could be indoors or outdoors, familiar or even imaginary, a place where, right now, you could feel comfortable and safe. And when it begins to take shape, even if it surprises you, begin to notice the colors...the textures... What's the temperature like?... How about sounds or a particular quality of silence?… Scents?… What time of day is it?… How about the season?… Notice how it feels to be here… What qualities do you experience?… If there is anything you want or need to feel even more relaxed, go ahead and make those changes now…

Find specifically where and how you would enjoy this place the most—it could be sitting, reclining, walking… Take a moment to really enjoy these relaxing feelings, noticing how it feels in your body, in your mind, in your emotions…

If this place had a voice, or some way of expressing itself to you, what would it want you to know right now?…

In a moment, we'll be bringing this to a close. Before we do, is there anything else wanting to be known or expressed?…

In the same way that you can carry a glass of water from one room to another, you can carry the feelings from this place into your daily life. So keeping with you anything you find valuable, gently let the images fade, knowing that you can always return there at another time in a similar way… Begin to sense the room you are in, noticing again the support beneath you, the light, the sounds… And when you feel ready, taking the time you need, open your eyes again.

You may now wish to take a few minutes to write, or even draw, your experience as a way to integrate it more fully.

HOW IMAGERY SUPPORTS HEALING

Although the term guided imagery is used synonymously with visualization, mental rehearsal, and mental imagery, these terms can be misleading. As you just experienced, guided imagery involves all the senses, not just the visual one. With some people, the cognitive mind dominates, even when engaging in a guided imagery experience. In other words, some will think their way through an imagery experience and have difficulty accessing their senses in the form of imagination, sensing, and feeling. So often I hear: "You know, I tried guided imagery in a workshop, but I just can't visualize any picture in my mind." However, seeing pictures is not the goal of imagery! Although most people do have a visual orientation when it comes to internal sense perceptions, there are also kinesthetic impressions, auditory responses, olfactory memories, and more—all of which are valid portals for the full expression of internal guidance. We may just sense something, and it is accompanied by a feeling that rings true. All of these internal impressions are the language of imagery, and most people have a combination of inner senses that are engaged during the imagery process.

There are also misconceptions about what it means to "see" internally. Try this one-minute exercise to become more acquainted with your innate imagery skills.

Experiential pause: The Doors Experiment

Pause for one minute and answer this question: How many doors, including closet doors, do you have in your home? (Find your answer before continuing.)

Unless you recently remodeled, you probably didn't have a number quickly jump to mind. I expect that you took a tour of your home, mentally walking into each room and looking around. It may not have been a clear Technicolor movie, but you likely retrieved the information you were after. This is what is important in imagery—having ways to accurately access the information through your internal senses, and it may or may not come through a visual form. When we facilitate an imagery session for a healing exploration, all the internal senses are encouraged to become engaged.

Now try this brief experiment to explore an even stronger sense of the mind-body connection.

Experiential pause: The Juicy Lemon

You can read through this exercise, imaging as you go, or it can be even more powerful to have someone read it to you.

Find a comfortable place to sit and take three full breaths, bringing your attention to the letting-go quality of each exhalation. Each time you breathe out, allow yourself to relax a little more fully, letting go of the day's activities for a few minutes.

Now let yourself imagine that in front of you is a bowl full of bright yellow, ripe lemons—the kind that are a little soft to the touch, bursting with juice and citrus flavor. Go ahead and pick up one that looks like it is at the peak of ripeness and feel the weight of it in your hand, with its cool, smooth, and dimpled yellow skin. Now carefully slice the lemon open and cut it into four wedges, inhaling the fresh lemony scent that fills the room. Notice the pale, juicy pulp on the cutting board.

Now, put one of the lemon slices in your mouth, noticing the textures, and bite down, letting the juice run over and under your tongue, and tasting the familiar, tangy, sour, and sweet lemon flavor.

What did you notice? Did you have any physiological response in your body? Consider writing or drawing in your journal anything else that happened for you during this experience.

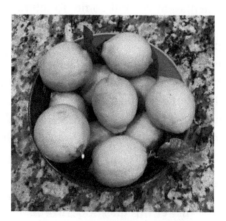

FIGURE 14.2: BOWL OF LEMONS

A version of the lemon exercise was part of a study with 131 college students. Perhaps not surprisingly, 94% reported an increase in salivation, which is a parasympathetic nervous system response.[5] Images are the natural language of communication between our mind/emotions and our body's autonomic nervous system. If we just told ourselves "Start salivating now," we would not have had the same results. Our everyday use of imagery and the mind-body connection is also evident when we worry. For example, you may have faced the anticipation of a difficult conversation with a neighbor or friend. It's common to imagine the familiar surrounding with the ambient sounds, scents, and feel of the setting where the talk will occur. We run through imagery scenarios of what may happen and anticipate seeing a tense face and hearing an angry tone of voice. If we had the right medical equipment, we could measure changes in blood chemistry, muscular tension, and blood pressure. Maybe you'd feel a flush, a racing heart, shallow breathing, or sweaty palms. Learning to *skillfully* navigate this inherent mind-emotion matrix to cultivate healing options is at the heart of guided imagery work.

THE SCIENCE OF IMAGERY

While the use of imagery is as old as humanity, with the growth of research, including the advent of fMRI studies, we have learned that imagery processes draw on many of the same neural structures used in real-time life experiences.[6] Essentially, the brain registers full sensory imagined experiences very similarly to our lived experiences. Using guided imagery to consciously influence mind-brain-body networks opens the door for corrective and intentional healing experiences.

Consistent with the integral lens on mind-body science from Chapter 7, Figure 14.3 (adapted from Hadjibalassi[7]) reflects a compilation of general understandings from psychoneuroimmunology and mind-body medicine as relates to imagery. Here, we see the translation of processes of mental imagery into central neurophysiological correlates, influencing the limbic regions of the brain (strong associations and influence on emotion[8]), and the influence of these regions over the autonomic nervous system. This in turn can either reduce or add to allostatic load, impacting numerous other systems and systemic processes. An important point is that imagery reflects an approach that can been seen as potentially beneficial for constructs of general well-being.

Researchers have demonstrated that beyond expected patterns of sensory region activation, there appears to be a "core imagery network" involved in the brain. Specifically, the "default mode network" (DMN) was identified and seen as operating independent of the specific sensory modalities.[9] This would suggest a higher-level cognitive process that is mediated by a network that is outside the sensory cortices, yet interacting with them. The authors of this study suggested that the DMN likely supports all types of mental imagery and relates to the demands of retrieving necessary stored information to support mental imagery. The study also confirmed that imagery shares the same neuroanatomical pathways as direct sensory processing (e.g., activity in auditory or visual *association* cortices) but that, interestingly, the *primary* sensory cortices are deactivated during imagery. It is interpreted that this may be to allow the generation of internally generated images and sounds by blocking out the associative sensory regions from external input that would normally be processed by primary regions.[10]

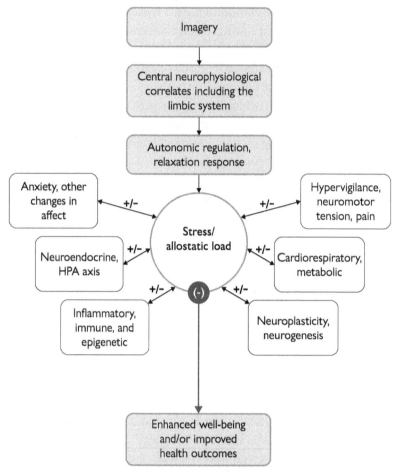

FIGURE 14.3: BIOLOGICAL UNDERPINNINGS OF IMAGERY
Adapted from Hadjibalassi[11]

The effectiveness of guided imagery on health, healing, and recovery is supported by numerous studies. In addition to the earlier-mentioned studies related to surgery, a sampling of the many lines of inquiry includes relevance to pain management of various conditions,[12] immune function,[13] inflammation,[14] sleep,[15] dreaming,[16] eating disorders,[17] cancer care,[18] cardiac care,[19] injury recovery,[20] joint replacement,[21] post-traumatic stress disorder,[22] depression,[23] health-related anxiety,[24] and general health behavior.[25]

According to the Veterans Administration's Evidence Synthesis Program, there is variable quality of evidence for the use of imagery in various conditions. The highest quality of evidence was recorded from studies into rheumatic disease and cancer. Lower overall quality of evidence was analyzed for stroke, Parkinson's disease, menstrual disorders, fibromyalgia, critical illness/use in ICU care, and cardiac surgery. Areas where imagery is often utilized, but the research is unclear or insufficient, include musculoskeletal pain, insomnia, headaches, anxiety, and depression.[26]

GOING DEEPER: USING IMAGERY FOR DECISION MAKING AND CULTIVATING INTUITION

Guided imagery can be used to support greater clarity regarding a health or life situation. This kind of imagery helps us dip down below our usual problem-solving methods, and often brings fresh insights to a situation. One particular practice refers to the source of insight as your own heart, but the source of more intuitive knowing can be understood in any number of ways. The wording can be changed to best match your or your client's orientation. For example, some may call it a higher self, wisdom, intuition, essence, spirit, mystery, or "right-brain knowing." The primary characteristic is that guidance arises from a different part of the mind than our cognitive, problem-solving linear way of reasoning.

Experiential pause: Journey to the Wisdom of Your Heart

Please go to the Resources section at the end of this chapter for a link to a pre-recorded version of this exercise. You are encouraged to take the time to do this and document your experience in your process journal before moving on with the remainder of the chapter.

IMPORTANT TOPICS AND CONSIDERATIONS

Before wrapping up this chapter, there are some topics related to imagery that carry significant importance in rehabilitation. These include negative health imagery, motor imagery, and precautions.

Negative health imagery

In imagery studies, it is sometimes said that the body does not know the difference between what is real and what is imagined. This statement reminds us of the earlier science overview: there are direct and specific physiological responses to imaginal processes. Just as positively constructed imagery can yield beneficial physiological effects, negative health imagery reflects the presence of common but overlooked and generally negative dynamics in our healthcare environment. Think of the common image of a bulging or herniated disc. Anatomical drawings of discs typically convey a red-hot, pulsing, and inflamed area. Through mind-body processes and linked to nocebo biology, this often reinforces fear, movement avoidance, and neuromotor protection patterns. It is vital to develop awareness of how thoughts/beliefs and emotions/feelings about one's body and health condition exist as inseparable from processes of imagery. Simultaneously, the rehabilitation professional must: assist in building capacity to reframe and reappraise these dynamics (principles of Cognitive Behavioral Therapy, Chapter 17); work with the principles of therapeutic education (Chapter 16); and deploy integrative movement retraining (Chapter 15).

Motor imagery

In rehabilitation research and clinical practice, motor imagery is a hot topic.[27] For example, the usefulness of motor imagery in stroke recovery continues to be examined, including with/without the use of virtual reality and other technology.[28] This research will continue to expand as technology and research advance. While beyond the scope of this chapter, principles for working with graded motor imagery, sensory discrimination, and mirror therapy have been delineated.[29] For now, consider the understanding that visual feedback (e.g., seeing oneself in a mirror) is rooted in biofeedback principles (Chapter 10) as well as processes of imagery, and can aid motor learning for posture and motor/movement learning. Similarly, demonstration of a skill, mental rehearsal of that skill, followed by completion, can equally enhance learning processes.[30] Be creative as you deepen your understanding of the many facets of imagery.

Precautions

Consider each of the following points.

- As with all techniques and approaches, do not over-reduce imagery's effects: nothing is a "cure all/fix all." There is potential that some may minimize the seriousness of symptoms and/or resort to using imagery in place of necessary medical care. Imagery pairs well with other forms of medicine and healing.
- In some cases, the use of imagery and relaxation can become an avoidance mechanism from experiencing/feeling distress, discomfort, difficult sensations; experiential avoidance is covered further in Chapter 17.
- It is important to understand the concept of resourcing. Imagery has strong associations to both emotion and memory processes. As such, the use of explanation, invitation, choice, and consent are foundational. Building individual resource skills, such as preferred exit strategies if overwhelming emotion arises, building capacity to tolerate unpleasant sensation/emotion, and self-regulation skills, is valuable in the context of imagery.
- Patients with a history of psychosis or other mental illness who have difficulty differentiating the internal world of imagery from the external world need to be treated with expertise.
- Patients with dissociative disorders from traumatic etiology need to be treated by skilled practitioners who understand guided imagery in relation to trauma.
- Patients with anxiety, panic disorder, and/or traumatic backgrounds may become anxious with relaxation or closing their eyes. This is addressed through

the provision of choice and continual feedback if imagery is utilized in the care approach.

- Because imagery can lower blood pressure, if you are working with a patient where low blood pressure is being treated medically, their blood pressure needs to be monitored.
- If you are working with pregnant women, any "letting go" language during the relaxation should be replaced with terms like "comfort" and "ease," and include acknowledging containment and presence of the growing child within during a body scan.

CONCLUSION

Imagery, used appropriately, is an indispensable ally for many rehabilitative needs. It is a doorway to internal clarity, provides access to a natural healing matrix, and adds buoyance to our emotional well-being.

Our contemporary Western medical culture highly prizes achievement and logical analysis, and while we certainly wouldn't want to be without it, imagery sheds light on aspects of life that are inaccessible to the logical mind. The rational and intuitive parts of the mind are like two legs that keep us moving forward—so why would we set out on a healing journey with one leg becoming excessively muscle bound and the other atrophying? We can strengthen and utilize everything we're made of.

And yet imagery is not only about accessing our different ways of knowing. As we increasingly gain skill in navigating our inner mind/emotions-body matrix, a deep congruence develops—an integration of perspective and experiences that can infuse our lives with balance and well-being.

Because imagery is a natural way that we process experiences, it is available to everyone and is very low risk. Sometimes it takes getting past our own misconceptions of imagery to feel comfortable, but it is an inherent capacity. Like anything of value, it takes practice to increase skill in navigating the many facets. While we come to the end of this chapter, you are only at the beginning of the support, deep relaxation, and discovery available to you through guided imagery. Imagine that!

Experiential pause: Having read this chapter, identify and write down at least one actionable item of interest to you. In doing so, consider ways in which applying the material first to yourself, and then to patients, might serve those who come to you for care.

RESOURCES

- For the experiential pause referenced earlier in the chapter, go to http://lesliedavenport.com/audio and scroll down to the "Support for your healing and transformation" section to the "Journey to the wisdom of your heart" recording.

You will need a piece of paper and pen, and 20–30 minutes of undisturbed time. Steps 1, 7, and 8 are done with your eyes open, and 2–6 are the meditative imagery experience with the eyes fully or partially closed. It's suggested that you fill in your answer on Step 1, and then complete the rest of the worksheet after Step 7 as a way to record, reflect on, and further integrate your experiences. A written version of this exercise is also found on pages 49–53 of the author's book *Healing and Transformation Through Self-Guided Imagery.*

– For other free audio recordings of guided imagery by the author, see http://lesliedavenport.com/audio.

– There is an excellent overview of recent guided imagery research compiled by Martin L. Rossman and Dean Shrock in Chapter 6 of *Transformative Imagery*, entitled "Medical Applications of Guided Imagery."

– Belleruth Naparstek's website has a collection of articles called "Hot research" under the "Blog" tab: www.healthjourneys.com.

– Martin Rossman's website has a downloadable PDF of guided imagery research: www.thehealingmind.org.

– Guided imagery training programs:
  » The California Institute of Integral Studies offers a certification in guided imagery with Leslie Davenport every Fall. It is offered through the master's program in Integrative Health, but you do not need to be a student at the school to enroll. It is a hybrid course with a one-day retreat, live webinars, and self-paced online learning modules: www.ciis.edu/academics/course-descriptions/transformative-imagery.
  » The Academy for Guided Imagery offers a certification, and it can be found at: www.acadgi.com/certification.
  » Imagery International is a professional organization for those interested in the use of imagery. It has tele-workshops, an annual conference, and a calendar and directory of trained imagery practitioners and programs: https://imageryinternational.wildapricot.org.

REFERENCES

Reader note: Portions of this chapter contain excerpts from three publications, and have been included and revised with permission.

Davenport, L. (2009). *Healing and Transformation Through Self-Guided Imagery*. Berkeley, CA: Celestial Arts.
Davenport, L. (Ed.) (2016). *Transformative Imagery: Cultivating the Imagination for Healing, Change and Growth*. London: Jessica Kingsley Publishers.
Davenport, L. (2017). *Emotional Resiliency in the Era of Climate Change: A Clinician's Guide*. London: Jessica Kingsley Publishers.

CHAPTER 15

Exploring Movement

Rachelle Palnick Tsachor, MA, CMA, RSMT
and Irena Paiuk, MscPT, BPT, CMA

A story: "Tiny," a 12-year-old girl, walked into the clinic in a crouched gait with her mum. She seemed to be suffering. As she progressed slowly along the room, her mum asked her to hurry up and do her best, even though she was in severe pain. Tiny's voice could hardly be heard.

Her mum presented Tiny's medical history, which was supported by medical notes, and then the focus of the interview turned to Tiny as she slowly whispered her perceptions of illness. Tiny reported severe bilateral knee pain with persistent intensity of 8/10 and persistent low back pain of 4/10. Her pain was aggravated by any activities dealing with gravity, such as walking, standing, sitting, and transitioning from sit-to-stand; her pain was eased slightly by lying down. She mentioned a constant sense of severe weakness and avoidance from attending school and meeting friends (due to pain and walking distance). A new symptom, constipation, recently appeared. While watching Tiny's movement, her physiotherapist wondered how her whole being was affected.

Note: In place of patient/client, we will sometimes use the label "mover" to emphasize an integrative view of movement and the importance of supporting individuals as active agents. The professional is equally a mover. Thus, "movers in relationship" supports one of the core backdrops within integrative rehabilitation practice.

In integrative rehabilitation practice (IRP), movement is not only a subject of rehabilitation, it is also a lens through which to perceive action and interaction. A traditional rehabilitation approach assesses and analyzes movement capacity through the lens of function, using quantitative tests to describe movement as forces, distances, velocities, pressures. Movement is categorized as normal or abnormal, controlled or uncontrolled. This approach is typically followed by prescriptive exercise and/or manual techniques with the purpose of restoring joint mobility, soft tissue flexibility, neuro-dynamics, etc. Exercise, however, is only one aspect of movement. While any movement performed is considered physical activity, exercise is planned, structured, repetitive, and intentional, intended to improve or maintain physical function. We know that exercise indirectly influences the whole mind/body,[1] yet rethinking movement as a larger concept is useful because movement can imply other levels beyond the purely biomechanical: Intention? Attention? Relationship? Energy? Beliefs about ourselves? Transformation? Individual versus collective process? Emotion? Movement can be a way to perceive and address what is out of balance, or stuck.

In traditional rehabilitation terminology, the categorization of a patient, therapist, or even department as "orthopedic" or "neurological" might narrow the scope of movement observation, analysis, and treatment. Too often, this can increase our tendency to delineate impairments and address them as pieces of a person. An example of this is seeing flexibility or strength only locally, rather than their inter-relatedness throughout the whole of the living body and the larger scope of the individual's lived experience of the body. When assessing neuromotor control, do we wonder how the mover might feel about loss of control and offer another movement parameter, such as spatial intent, to restore sense of control via aim rather than tensing? When addressing the construct of core stability, can we wonder how it might reflect instability or stability and a larger sense of personal agency as larger themes in life? Addressing parts may be useful; however, reconnecting and integrating parts into the whole person is better supported by frequent back and forth between:

- delineation and integration
- mobility and stability
- relating changes in the distal parts to movement in the core.

MOVEMENT ACTS AS A SOCIO-PSYCHO-BIOLOGICAL REGULATOR

Movement is often a path into and the goal of rehabilitation. Integral thinking challenges us to consider movement as not just physical, but also as movements of the mind, emotions, and more. "Movement" is essential to life. The world is built upon continuously arising and dissolving movement. In physical terms, much of what we do is accomplished through movement: from activities of daily living to sports, arts, work, love, and play.[2] Whether volitional or passive, physical or energetic, we move.

Beyond the functional role of physical movement in rehabilitation and injury prevention, movement influences, and is influenced by, learning, thinking, emotions, and physiology.[3] Our earliest years are in great part devoted to learning to move and discovery through movement. Until language emerges in the second year, movement serves nearly every purpose—it is our first language of communication, relationship, and autonomy. Our need to plan movement is theorized to have given rise to our capacity to think abstractly.[4] Daniel Wolpert suggests that the reason we have brains is to direct movement, so we can meet our survival needs.[5] Emotions are considered to exist to tell us our needs and drive our movement to meet them.[6] The word emotion itself derives from "to move" and can be conceptualized as e-motion—energy in motion/moving. Examples of emotion described in terms of movement include:

- valence (how emotion drives us to move towards or away, forward/backward)
- arousal (activation or deactivation, related to awareness and attention, particularly in our horizontal plane)
- dominance (social relationship, which might change our body's shape vertically, literally rising or sinking).[7]

Not surprisingly, our movement not only reflects our emotions[8] but also influences them.[9] As science discerns that our mind itself is based in our capacity to embody action, movement can no longer be siloed according to function or expression. Living/general systems theory (see Chapter 1) reminds us that anatomy is not movement, rather movement is the response of anatomy to fulfill our socio-psycho-biological needs. In other words, movement is a vehicle via which the body/mind navigate and interact with environment (body-mind-environment—BME). For example, how I bend to pick something up can reflect my feelings about the task, my social beliefs about who in society picks things up, or my thoughts about what I will do with the object I pick up. Likewise, movement affects our anatomy, as is frequently quoted: "form follows function."[10]

Movement is also innately social. We engage with others through posture and gesture. We respond to our social environment with our bodies. We watch others' movement to understand their feelings, and match aspects of their movement(s) to relate and respond to them. In essence, movement is a primary way in which we navigate and cope with our environment.[11]

When movement is impaired, one's interdependent experiences of self, environment, and life (contemplate BME again) are intimately impacted. Movement is therefore an act of integration serving to organize separate things in the complexity of each whole person: a movement emerges through convergence of body parts, space, and energy in relationship to many contextual levels. From a macro perspective, voluntary movement is relational, intentional, dynamic, and richly associated with neuromuscular-skeletal systems. Its relational components can be categorized as *intra-relational* (moving to support one's personal needs such as coughing to clean the airways or touching a painful body part to relieve pain), or *inter-relational* (retreating from a bee or shaking a friend's hand). Whether the movement is intra- or inter-relational, it can be intentional (reaching towards a glass of water) or non-intentional (reflexive), and it is a consequence of integrated activity of neural, skeletal, and muscular systems.

TINY

So how does the preceding introduction to movement as a socio-psycho-biological regulator relate to Tiny? Just months earlier, Tiny was a 12-year-old attending seventh grade without any chronic medical condition or allergy. A month prior to her physiotherapy (PT) referral, she was diagnosed with a severe respiratory infection. She was treated with antibiotics; however, her pulmonary condition was exacerbated and she was admitted to the hospital. While hospitalized she complained of widespread pain and difficulty keeping upright. The pain worsened during the hospitalization and concentrated mostly in her legs and knees. Eventually, she wasn't able to stand independently and started to use a walker. In addition, she gradually became aphonic.

Upon discharge from the hospital, chest X-ray and clinical examination indicated her pneumonia had fully resolved. Subsequent rheumatological, neurological, orthopedic, and otolaryngological examinations were negative and didn't correlate with her clinical presentation. She was finally given an unspecific diagnosis—arthralgia with fatigue—and referred to PT. In Tiny's case, most aspects of her life were impacted, including: speaking, ingestion and digestion, participation in school, and emotion regulation. With her movement clearly compromised, her physiotherapist wondered: How might this all affect her personal agency—her sense of ability and capacity to act and interact effectively in the world?

In working with Tiny, her physiotherapist wondered: What is Tiny's movement expressing? What dots might be connected in observing interconnections between her absence of voice, widespread shortening of muscles, and patterns of pulling into herself and out of the world? Did the coughing shorten her muscles, pulling her into collapse? As her posture shrank, did her reduced breath movement diminish her sense of safety, confidence, and presence? Tiny's physiotherapist began contemplating how to gently and respectfully support and explore this expression of a difficult, contracted, and withdrawn place that Tiny was in.

AN INTEGRAL LENS ON THE SCIENCE OF MOVEMENT

Through the lens of systems theory, changes in one system affect other systems and the whole of the integrated BME experience. This was true in Tiny's case. How does this occur at the physiological level? Recall the foundations of Chapter 7, viewed through the lens of movement. Consider how voluntary movement affects blood pressure, cardiovascular health, arousal, digestion, processes of restoration, and more.[12] In turn, these physiological parameters are affected by and affect neurotransmitters, social interactions, and emotions—all of which interact in response to stress/demand.[13]

Voluntary muscles are not the only movement generators in the human body. Non-intentional movement, as perceived through the expanded lens as movement, is present in all body systems: blood flow, lymph flow, cerebrospinal fluid (CSF) flow, peristalsis, visceral movements, and even cell migration (cellular movement). Each of these examples of movement is in turn influenced by, and affects, voluntary movement.[14] Therefore, voluntary movement can be an interface with all other systems, one that is responsive to the mover's intent—we can, with awareness, refine how we move, indirectly using voluntary movement to influence parts and the whole.

With this understanding that voluntary movement can influence so many aspects of health, we can now dive deeper into the concept introduced earlier, of movement as a socio-psycho-biological regulator. As an under-recognized single lifestyle factor with potential to impact all aspects of health,[15] it is critical for rehabilitation therapists to grow their understanding of the depth that movement reflects. In this section, we'll glimpse the science of how movement relates to a variety of topics, as well as some introductory clinical considerations. As you read each subsection, consider how you might apply each topic to yourself as a mover in this world, and then to other movers in your professional work.

Mind-body integration

Mind-brain-body exist in an inseparable relationship, including relationship to movement, neuroplasticity, neurogenesis, and the relationships between physical and mental experience.[16] When addressing movement in rehabilitation, the therapist has potential to influence and support well-being at all levels, micro and macro.

Embodied cognition

Building on mind-body, consider how movement interacts with thinking and intention. We now understand that the capacity to move underlies our capacity to think. Cognitive science views cognition as embodied, skillful, ongoing interaction with our external world—a framework of science that stands in support of the integral BME construct.[17] Thinking often relates to intention and action in space, underscoring the inseparability of mind and body in relation to movement.

Sociocultural considerations

In infancy, movement is our first language of communication. Movements help us connect to our caregivers, including in ways aimed at meeting survival needs. (Recall the information in Chapter 4 on attachment and threat appraisal processes.) Synchronizing movement increases interpersonal synchrony as well as bonding between groups: matching aspects of body language helps us relate.[18] In part, movement is socially and culturally determined, with some aspects of movement regulated by position in society (e.g., Western women were once taught to keep their knees together). Social status, dominance, or confidence are often communicated through movement and posture. Access and utilization of space may be affected by self-perception of gender, definitions that are in great part shaped by society and culture. For example, strength is often praised in those identified as boys, while those identified as girls have often been encouraged to be gentle, giving them socially sanctioned access to gentleness or light touch in movement that may be discouraged in boys. These types of cultural expectations affect perception of one's status and reinforce limited movement options.[19]

Enactive compassion

Known as *kinesthetic empathy* within movement therapy professions, enactive compassion (discussed in Chapters 2 and 3) can be described as the experience of *being moved by* and then *moving to support* another's experience. For example, even in just reading a description of Tiny walking "in a crouched gait," we are affected because our capacity to see and envision movement in others can activate empathy. Others' emotions are recognized from the briefest glimpses of whole-body movement,[20] which means that changes to our movement can affect the empathy we experience and arouse in others. Therapists can take advantage of the many ways in which movement facilitates co-regulation, because socially relevant movement stimuli are quickly perceived by the motor system. This suggests to therapists that our interactions prompt modulation of the sensorimotor system during interactions.[21] When movement is restricted, how does it affect the mover's relationships? How does the practitioner's movement affect the mover?

Emotion

Introduced earlier, emotion reflects an integrative, bidirectional relationship with movement. Movement doesn't only express our emotions—feedback from our body also plays a crucial role in our feelings.[22] Through the bidirectional, interactive role that movement plays in integrating expression and function, therapists have the opportunity to explore and use movement to support integration processes of the mover. As therapists, can we consider how immobility (e.g., after traumatic brain injury, stroke, Parkinson's disease, or other movement-limiting conditions) might affect the capacity of those we treat to experience and express emotions? And recognize how emotions affect motivation to persist?[23] A deeper understanding of the interconnected nature of movement in its functional and emotional aspects may contribute to a better understanding of the whole health picture of individuals we treat.[24] As therapists, when we expand our awareness to notice how emotions are expressed through movement and are affected by it, we can better relate to these movement aspects during the treatment process. Because movement influences emotion, therapists can work with movement dynamics and the changing shape of the body's core to indirectly help movers become unstuck from overly set patterns that are limiting both function and expression.[25]

Touch as communication

Effective communication has been explored in prior chapters, and the general relevance and impact of touch will be discussed further in Chapter 23. Here, we reflect that touch may take place through invitation during movement. Touch supports patient-therapist relationships and interpersonal communication, and increases adherence to treatment.[26] Touch can be demarcated as procedural/task-oriented or expressive (caring);[27] however, providing a procedure such as exercise training still has a strong relational component. Examples to offer new movement experiences in relationship include: purposeful touch to provide sensorimotor cues for new coordination when moving a limb; using tactile manipulatives, such as manually rolling a toy truck to awaken spatial intent and subtle shape adaptation of the hand and wrist. Communication through touch can be conveyed to the entire system quickly and deeply, in some cases bypassing the need for verbal conveyance. Ultimately, touch as a guidepost to explore movement must be approached as a relational interaction of care, regulation, wholeness, and even sacredness.

Sensorimotor integration

In essence, movement training supports ongoing refinement of links between sensation and movement.[28] Movement results when brain-body processes of prediction meet sensory information in the moment.[29] The smoothness of prediction and action can be disrupted by injury, leading to a misalignment between intention to move and movement coordination. Contemplative or somatic approaches facilitate slowing down movement, breaking it down into smaller parts to allow the mover to perceive and integrate more nuanced perception and coordination, without exiting the feedback loop. Examples of sensorimotor integration include:

- using contact statements[30] such as: "I noticed you are leaning back—what is that like for you?"
- using therapeutic dialogue (Chapter 8) that draws the mover into kinesthetic awareness in relation to other domains (thoughts, feelings), such as: "What's happening for you during this movement?"
- invitations to experiment: "What would it be like as you bend forward if you move more slowly and breathe more smoothly and purposely?"
- providing experiences of pleasant sensation; this helps to increase potential to transform sensory feedback loops and relationships
- zooming out—learning to focus on whole-body activity → whole-person function. As movers become familiar with reframing their relationship to the presence of painful sensations, they can zoom out to larger inputs.[31]

Imagery

Building on the topic of embodied cognition (the intertwining of movement and cognition), movement and thinking are equally embedded into processes of mental imagery. For example: "Across a motor to mental gradient of skill learning, there is now compelling evidence that motor imagery contributes to enhance motor skill learning and motor performance."[32] The functional plasticity occurring during the incremental acquisition of a motor sequence is also reflected during motor imagery.[33] The functional equivalence between motor imagery and motor performance is supported by the functional plasticity that occurs during mental practice, which closely mimics that observed after physical practice of the same motor skill.[34] Movers respond to behavior observed in videos as if the situation was real for them. Audiovisual stimuli presented to movers appear to induce a psychophysiological response in which individuals respond as if they are in the story presented in the video: Pleasant stimuli improve fatigue-related symptoms while reducing physiological stress during exercise, while unpleasant stimuli globally increase activity in the autonomic nervous system, increasing exertional responses more than the pleasant stimuli.[35]

Autonomy and control

Our first locus of autonomy develops in our body in relationship to the mastery of movement, and remains vital to empowerment in relation to our environment (physical and social). Injury and illness, therefore, can adversely affect the mover's sense of empowerment and self-efficacy, and can sometimes create a loss of trust in oneself and one's body. This can be compounded when therapists are too authoritative over a patient's knowledge of themselves: we risk subtly sending them signals not to trust their bodies. As therapists, we are more effective when we recognize how working on ourselves can indirectly affect our work with each person.

Beliefs and expectations

It can be useful to shift the focus of our movement work from constructs of diagnoses and pathology (something the person "has") to a larger view of movement as an active response to any moment (something the person does, chooses to undo, or do differently). How do beliefs, expectations, and other facets of individual psychology (see Chapter 6 and Chapter 17 for more) interact with movement? Beliefs can restrict what movement is perceived to be possible. For example, if I don't believe I can do it, I probably won't try, or if I believe it isn't worth my time, I won't bother. Emotions such as fear (see the following section) are often at work in relationship to these beliefs and are reflected in the body. Inviting awareness—a curious exploration—around one's beliefs and/or expectations about their body and movement may open doorways that were previously closed.

Protection and defense

Kinesiophobia (pain-related fear of movement due to anticipating pain or reinjury) plays a role in the development of chronic symptoms and their perception.[36] A greater degree of kinesiophobia:

- changes muscle activity and motor behavior towards defense, hypervigilance, and avoidance
- predicts greater levels of pain, poorer prognosis, increased disability, and reduced adherence to treatment
- can lead to more sedentary behavior,[37] functional disability, and physical deconditioning.[38]

Kinesiophobia research addresses fear as a psychological event,[39] dividing clinical interventions for kinesiophobia into two separate domains. First, psychological, by implementing Cognitive Behavioral Therapy, therapeutic education, mindfulness, and/or Acceptance and Commitment Therapy strategies. Second, physical, expanding movement and functional capacity, as well as increasing baseline tolerance levels to painful movements. Are these separate domains of kinesiophobia?

Addressing kinesiophobia is often approached through the use of graded exposure training.[40] Regulation of emotions in general, and addressing the fear of movement in particular, through integrated approaches, are not yet routine interventions for people suffering from kinesiophobia.[41] Contemplative movement-based practices such as yoga, Tai Chi, Qigong, the Alexander Technique, and dance movement therapy may also be useful in the integrative management of pain and other health challenges.[42]

A movement-based approach explores dynamic qualities of movement holistically: What qualitive components shifted the mover out of effective action? Fear can drive movers to restrain movement quality (over-tensing) and variability, reducing their spatial intent as the coordinator of their movement. Simple attention on *where the movement is going* can reduce the tension involved in fear, and radically shift the negative feedback loop. For example, while fear of falling can activate equilibrium responses such as protective extension (exacerbating the sense of falling or tension), orienting attention upward in space can activate righting reflexes, leading the mover into easier uprightness.

Mental health

In the bidirectional relationship of mind and movement, state of mind directly affects coordination and ease of movement. "Simply put, disequilibrium in the mind, such as the states associated with cognitive distress, is accompanied with disharmony in the body…"[43] In bidirectional relationship, movement affects mood, depression, anxiety, stress, and more.[44] Systematic reviews about yoga provide some of the strongest evidence that somatic (mind-body awareness) movement practices are effective adjunctive treatment for depression, anxiety, and stress.[45] More on yoga in Chapter 24.

Trauma

Trauma is described as any experience that overwhelms our capacity to feel and process those feelings.[46] In trauma, events happen faster than the body can sort out, yet are experienced in deep non-verbal ways, which the fast pace of verbal processing often leaves behind. Trauma response intimately impacts integrated movement systems and can lead to long-term influences. Movement provides opportunity to expand our capacity to physically repattern any latent impact of prior trauma exposure, including support for the restoration of the sense of personal power, efficacy, and body agency.

Presence in sensation during movement develops awareness of subtle bodily experience during action, raising awareness in the mover of responses to stimuli (from within and without) as they happen.[47] If loss of power is an essential injury in trauma,[48] attention to sensation in movement supports empowerment because one is more aware during physiological responses to triggers; thus can respond with nuanced choices to breathing, to space, and/or to shift weight away without dissociating. Clients learn skills to prevent being overwhelmed by sensations so new meaning and responses can emerge.

Memory

Movement is integral to memory. It affects our capacity to remember and create meaningful associations because we generate stronger memories when moving.[49] Gesturing improves our ability to problem-solve, decreasing load on working memory by conveying information through a second, image-based, modality,[50] and even watching others' gestures improves memory, as compared with listening without observing gestures.[51] The same neurons in our hippocampus (place cells, grid cells, and border cells) that navigate our movement in space are responsible for encoding memory (which later consolidates during resting).[52] Locomotion, such as running, has been linked to increases in brain-derived neurotrophic factor (BDNF)[53] and is thought to promote brain health, cell regeneration, and neurogenesis in the hippocampus, the seat of memory formation.[54] Complex movement increases neuroplasticity,[55] and acquisition of new motor skills is strongly linked to neuronal plasticity at cortical and subcortical levels, evolving over time to engage different spatially distributed interconnected brain regions.[56] The effects of exercise on memory therefore play a role in recovery and combating memory loss in Alzheimer's and Parkinson's disease.[57]

Attitude, relationship, and quality

When working with polio patients in the 1950s, Irmgard Bartenieff, a dancer, PT, and a founder of Dance/Movement Therapy (DMT), had a motto: Activate and Motivate. Motivation (intent of the movement) coordinates the mind-body, driving people to move. More recent studies confirm that attitude matters: those who view exercise in a positive light got more unplanned physical activity during the day than those with a negative view, and physical activity includes things like fidgeting, pacing, and choosing stairs over elevators.[58] Motivation also predicts moderate behavioral change[59] and exercise intensity,[60] and even unconscious motivational processes affect engagement in physical activity.[61]

Studies attest to the general physical and mental health outcomes of physical activity.[62] It therefore makes sense to focus not only on restoring function to a non-pathological state, but also to attend to both one's relationship to movement and/or exercise, and the quality of experience while moving. Movement that is pleasurable and rewarding for its own sake will be less stressful and help regulate emotions as well as physiology. Lifestyle factors significantly impact health, especially chronic conditions, with even small bouts of movement improving health.[63] Discovering ease and pleasure in moving has potential to impact physiology from cardiovascular health to brain function.[64]

Experiential pause: Take a few minutes and recall Tiny's story. Now contemplate how any of the preceding topics might be interacting in Tiny's experience and how you as a clinician might begin to explore and support the complexity embedded within that experience. You might also bring to mind a current or past mover with whom you are working. Contemplate the same topics in relation to that person. Using self-reflection, do the same in relation to yourself.

CONTEMPLATIVE MOVEMENT PRACTICES AND SYSTEMS OF MOVEMENT ANALYSIS

Contemplative or somatic practices that develop awareness during movement enhance recognition of sensation, coordination, emotion, and meaning in movement. Such integration is critical for personal growth and transformation. Entering into movement with awareness of inner experience permits movers to gradually integrate their inward perception with the outward attention, so they have choice in reaching out into space to proactively meet their needs, making choices towards balancing phases of exertion and recuperation.[65]

The extent to which movement can be explored at these deeper levels is vast. Entire systems such as the Laban/Bartenieff Movement System (LBMS), Alexander Technique, Feldenkrais, Yoga, Tai Chi, and/or Qigong require hours and even years of study. To gain an appreciation for the depth that these movement studies reflect, Table 15.1 provides a summary of core LBMS concepts.

Table 15.1: Overview of Laban Efforts: Descriptors of qualitative aspects of movement

Effort factor	"Fighting pole" ←——————→ "Indulging pole" A *spectrum* of characteristics and qualities		Function/ developmental task
Time (attitude towards when to move)	Sudden/abrupt: accelerating, rushing, hurried, urgent/fast, "now!"	Sustained/gradual: decelerating, hesitating, deliberating, lingering	Decision/timing, intuition
Space (attitude towards where to move)	Direct, single focus, or single aim: linearity, precision	Indirect/multiplicity of focus: flexible, adaptable attention	Thinking/attending
Weight (attitude towards the movement's force or impact)	Strong/powerful: increasing pressure, firm touch	Light/delicate/soft: decreasing pressure, fine touch, gentle	Asserting/intention
Flow (attitude towards the movement's progression)	Bound/constrained: controlled, stiff, rigid, restrained, or precise	Free/unconstrained: releasing, outflowing, abandoning, decreased control	Feeling/affect regulation, autonomy

The Laban Effort system, sometimes referred to as "dynamics," relates interior state and intention to subtle motion characteristics. Laban describes these efforts as the "how" of motion/movement. There are many ways to walk towards something, but the combination of the Efforts displayed during that path indicate something about the mover's inner state. There are four "Effort Factors"—Time, Weight, Space, and Flow—which may scale between "fighting" and "indulging" polarities.

Experiential pause: Carefully evaluate Table 15.1. Consider writing down your answers to the following reflections: How does this presentation compare to and relate to the way in which you currently view and interact with movement? What can you reveal by exploring self-awareness of your movement tendencies? How might these qualitative dynamics assist you in more deeply understanding others, including your patients?

Therapists trained in these integrative movement systems and approaches are able to observe posture and movement on a continuum from stability to mobility, inner to outer, exertion to recuperation. Informed by a person-centered approach, therapists can work with patients to identify patterns and meaning, teach experiential anatomy, and support the gaining of new movement patterns to support homeostasis, co-regulation, and neuroplasticity. The reader is steered towards further learning opportunities and experientials in Resources at the end of the chapter.

Experiential pause

Purpose: Grounding and centering by freeing tension or holding ("bracing strategy"), expanding inward perception of voluminous "container" (the body) from periphery to core, and balancing between exertion and recuperation through oscillatory movement. Can serve as a preparatory exercise in rehabilitation session.

Action: Position yourself comfortably in supine position, with your legs extended on the floor and slightly apart. Grasp your hands, and place them at chest level (sternum), facing the elbows sideways. Gently press the palms together, and move your arms from side to side, initiating movement from your elbows. Gradually increase the frequency of this movement to shake the whole body, and, at the same time, gradually lower your hands until they are in front of your navel. Allow the movement to resonate into your breath, pelvis, chest, and legs. Allow your jaw to follow the pull of gravity and your voice to emerge.

Experience: Sense the rich mobility of your "voluminous container" through freeing any binding in your muscles and joints. Find greater support from the floor by riding the sensation of the lateral rocking movement. When the sense of exertion is identified, allow yourself to stop and release the weight of the body parts into the floor. Observe how the stillness and calmness in your muscles increases the awareness of inner rhythms and volumes of your heartbeat and breath, and through the breath to yourself and your available inner space.

Note: This activity is just one of many that can begin to bring new light to movement and exercise. In the Resources section, there is a link to videos that explore a series of similar guided experiences to take you further.

MOVEMENT AND THE RELATIONAL SPACE

Recall from Chapter 8 the relational space. How does movement factor into the therapeutic relationship and the larger concepts embedded in IRP? Movement can be approached as an exploration and process of mutual learning. How can you support yourself and the patient as equal movers in exploring the purpose and meaning of movement(s) from the lens of BME interactions? Beyond gross/obvious movement, remember that mutual relationship exists at the non-verbal movement level. The clinician's presence, movement choices, and expressions such as tonicity, vocal tone, and speed all convey movement qualities that affect rehabilitation itself.[66]

Early in Tiny's rehabilitation process, she did not yet have integrated awareness nor the language to express her interior. The physiotherapist's capacity to develop the *relational space* (Chapter 8) combined with the physiotherapist's integral skills to support the whole of Tiny's process. Recall that the relational space is informed by the principles of mutual learning and co-regulation. Co-regulation is not static, but dynamic, expressive, and receptive. Co-regulation involves movers in relationship—being together versus doing to. What does this feel like? Research supports the concept that attunement through movement and embodiment activates co-regulation.[67] Beyond our skill set in working with others, attending to our own movements (in numerous contexts) can co-regulate the mover through our own self-regulation.

INTEGRATIVE MOVEMENT ASSESSMENT

The development of relationship informs "assessment." What does "objective" movement evaluation look like in the IRP approach? How do we attend to the many facets embedded within a person's experience of movement? Current models of clinical thinking and decision making foreground a pattern-recognition process, relying upon physical and non-physical assessments to test the therapist's establishment of a correct diagnosis. Of note, the importance of clinical intuition in the medical community is now acknowledged.[68] Movement is an emergent process, greater than the properties of any single irreducible aspect of it, thus we need to attend to how the mover's intention and expression influence the number and quality of their functional movements. Consistent with earlier material in this book, we must acknowledge the importance of patient-therapist interaction, implicit acceptance of their experience and process, active listening, openness, and empathizing for establishing an attuned connection.[69]

As we gain more knowledge of the larger scope of movement, we begin to observe discrete details. We notice the interaction of body parts during action, unfolding in ever-changing movement phrases (units of discrete actions, each with a beginning/preparatory movement, middle/main action, and end/follow-through), responsive to intent. We observe not only range of motion or joint angles, but also the qualitative, dynamic movement phrasing: When does the movement modulate from stronger to gentler? Faster to slower? How does this movement sequence (phrase) result in spatial organization (near/far reach; high/low; forward/back)? How does the changing shape of the body (growing/shrinking; bulging/hollowing) adapt to purpose of the movement?

Intention and expression influence the number and quality of functional movements, patterning the brain-body relationship, and ultimately reflecting how we wish to be in and influence our world. Assessment that listens for intention and observes expression lays the groundwork for integrative intervention. Thus, the processes of clinical reasoning and case formulation (see Chapter 5) in relationship to movement must include possible biopsychosocial effects, rather than solely the bio-physiological components.[70]

Since movement varies in response to intention, we can see movement's context when we observe and analyze with the purpose of identifying patterns of behavior. Diversity of movement analysis approaches can be valuable because movement is unique to each individual.[71] Observing movement through several lenses expands the clinician's scope of perception, including in relationship to "Body Story-Telling" and the co-creation of new meanings.

Tiny's case is an example of how analyzing the same mover through different lenses (e.g., PT and LBMS) may induct therapists' clinical reasoning and influence the defining of the cause-affect-effect route. For example, to support homeostasis, or self-regulation, LBMS looks at:

- the capacity of the mover to move adeptly between dualities, such as flexion/extension, exertion/recuperation

- coordinated affinities among the body parts and their dynamics during movement, such as the descent of the diaphragm during inhale, coordinated with freeing of muscular tension in the rest of the body and sense of safety and/or coordinated release of flexion during extending movements across body segments.

In Tiny's case, limitations in activities and body functions (joint mobility, voice, muscle strength, balance, etc.), as usually defined in PT, were examined as a thematic duality of *inner-outer/self-other*. Disintegrated/unbalanced interplay between Tiny's Inner-Outer worlds can be described by aphonia, constipation, paradoxical abdominal breathing, being shaped by gravity forces in vertical (slouched posture), and crouched gait.

Stability-mobility is another thematic duality to observe in Tiny's movement. Unsupportive strategies of core bracing/holding, binding in joints and muscles, fragmented internal rhythms of breath, and/or peristalsis eventually challenge Tiny's mobility and restrict the fluid balance between stability and mobility. This uncoordinated neuromuscular control may contribute to exertion and fatigue. Contemplating movement patterns through these and other broader perspectives, such as relationships and access to space, rather than only within the mechanical body itself, can be transformational for movers.

MORE OF TINY'S STORY

In Tiny's case, slouched posture, with flexed and internally rotated arms and legs, along with her reduced extensor muscle strength, slow movement, and paradoxical diaphragmatic breath, seemed to express withdrawing behavior consistent with the biobehavioral basis of defensive collapse or freezing response.[72] Emotions of fear and anxiety can be significant factors affecting therapeutic compliance, motivation, and the quality of coping strategy.[73] Thus, prior to focusing on function, it seemed helpful to initiate treatment by playing with different dynamic movement qualities to promote a shift in the mover's emotional state and decrease/relieve the level of fear (kinesiophobia).

To assist in this exploration, modeling clay was used. It served to initiate connection and safe self-expression, and promote openness and shape changes by facilitating three-dimensional movement in her arms. There was a confidence in moving the clay as a representation of her body (Figure 15.1), which gave her the confidence to envision changing her movement.

Playing with the clay promoted: directness in space, attention to time component (working quickly or continually), and activation of muscle and joints in relation to the material (clay); and assisted in renewal of her inner-outer relationship. Using the clay enabled Tiny to create forms and shapes, consciously or subconsciously. These forms and shapes carry meaning and potential to reflect currently invisible somatic processes towards change.

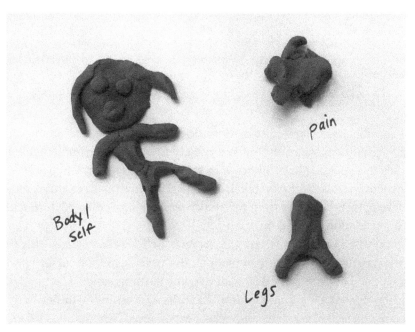

FIGURE 15.1: BODY REPRESENTATIONS: EXAMPLES OF CLAY MODELING
Note: Pain and body/self were both created in the first session and legs was created in the fourth session.

Moving on to working the clay over painful body parts (Figure 15.2) expanded Tiny's scope of sensory input from these body areas, allowing different stimuli from pain to be processed. Additionally, working with the clay in this way supported new relationships with both self and others to emerge. These experiences with the clay deeply affected Tiny's perception of her body, which consequently influenced her ability to move and locomote.

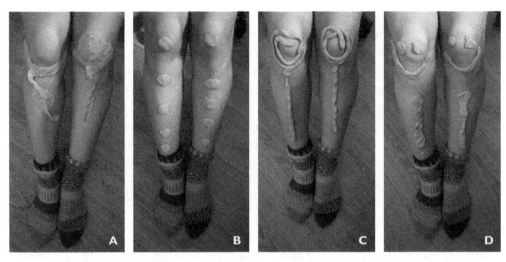

Image A: Example of clay modeling of pain, sensations, and movement, second session.
Image B: Clay shapes created at the third session. Here, imagery related to a supportive axis of length appeared. The clay use is more gathered than scattered.
Image C: Clay shapes created at the fourth session. These shapes focused on spatial intent, and dynamic and rotational movement qualities. Modeling the clay in a spiral shape may symbolize an unconsciously internalized new movement pattern of rotations.
Image D: Clay shapes from after the fifth session. The clay appears to express embodying three-dimensional volume/space as well as emotion. While abstract, direct parallels to the patient's rehabilitation process were observed.

FIGURE 15.2: USE OF CLAY MODELING FOR SENSORIMOTOR PROCESSING

Tiny's work with clay integrated sensorimotor experience, body autonomy, and the use of imagery. Gradually, touch and movement experientials were implemented through choice—key to respecting her withdrawal state and the presence of hyperalgesia. Touch and movement were used for pain relief, expansion of movement potential, repatterning, and the development of relationship. Self-touch was also implemented during movement to affect body relationship and ownership.[74]

Tiny progressed through therapy and achieved self-set rehab goals. This movement journey was intertwined with contemplations, discoveries, mutual curiosity, welcoming the unknown, and respecting the pace of developmental progression. Her physiotherapist's observation was that Tiny found a lot of curiosity in working with her body through these avenues. Instead of a dictated movement experience, Tiny was afforded experiences of movement from a place of what felt right for her, not what the physiotherapist felt was the correct movement or progression.

BEGINNING APPLICATIONS

There are entry points for all rehabilitation professionals to work with integrative-oriented movement practices. Increasing awareness of how movement interacts with thoughts, feelings, intentions, and levels of body and breath awareness reflects a good starting point.

Experiential pause

Part 1: Identify a basic movement to work with, such as raising your arms. You will now repeat the movement several times in a row following these instructions, noting that you can substitute any motion in place of raising the arms.

1. Raise the arms (no other cues).
2. Raise the arms a second time and notice any thoughts that accompany the movement. Any emotions/feelings? Beliefs? Memories, images, or associations?
3. Now, raise the arms a little more slowly and with just the right amount of movement for you right now.
4. Next, raise the arms using the least amount of effort needed; allow it to happen in a light, gentle, smooth, natural, or effortless way.
5. Next, raise the arms noticing what is happening everywhere else in the body.
6. Next, raise the arms noticing what is happening in your breathing pattern.
7. Next, identify a value, quality, or intention (such as patience, strength, gentleness, or courage) that you wish to embody more of. Raise your arms with this in mind and see how it influences your movement.
8. Finally, repeat one last time, putting all of the preceding together in your awareness as best you can. How do these levels of awareness change the movement and your experience of the movement?

Part 2: If you currently have a painful movement pattern in your body, we will apply these principles to that movement. If you do not have an active issue, you might imagine a recent time when there was pain or simply imagine putting yourself in the shoes of a mover with whom you have worked. Before completing the movement, imagine completing it and see if you notice any tension arise. If there is tension from approaching the movement, it is important to identify a cognitive-emotional strategy of reassurance. Working in a "zone of tolerance"—not too little, not too much—is important. In painful conditions, you must find an acceptable challenge point for the range of movement utilized. Now, use the principles from Part 1, and repeat with the painful movement.

(Used with permission, courtesy of Matt Erb, PT and Embody Your Mind.)

MOVING AHEAD WITH A LARGER VIEW

Movement is a complex and multifaceted phenomenon that is beyond body, biomechanics, and physicality. It is an intra-personal interaction where a change in the part can represent a change in the whole. Movement is also inter-relational (self-other) as well as relational to space (inner-outer), as space embraces/contains the movement. Addressing relational components assists in cuing the movement, analyzing it, and perceiving it.

Although people may show up with a physical complaint, changing movement can indirectly affect many other levels of a person's being—mental, emotional, spiritual, social. For example, someone who is slouched or stooped may be able to breathe better once supported in uprightness by their spine, and as their chest and shoulders open up, they may interact differently with others or feel different about themselves and/or the issues and challenges they are facing.

Therefore, we must be able to ask whether our purpose is simply to repair a perceived dysfunction to some previous or desired level of function. Although pathology may bring a person into the clinic, such as movement restriction or pain, as people improve, they may rightfully change their rehabilitative goals to match emerging beliefs about perception of wholeness. The goal of rehabilitation might begin as relief from pain or dysfunction, then, as standards rise, the mover may hope for coordination, agility, high performance, energy, well-being, wholeness, peacefulness, and insight. Change itself is a developmental process[75]—one that is supportive of larger processes. Our approach must be designed to meet people where they are without making assumptions—acting in support of the potential for the emergence of well-being.

> **Experiential pause:** Having read this chapter, identify and write down at least one actionable item of interest to you. In doing so, consider ways in which applying the material first to yourself, and then to patients, might serve those who come to you for care.

RESOURCES

The goal for this chapter was to provide an overview of the integrative nature of movement. If you would like to further explore the facilitation of awareness through movement as taught in the Laban/Bartenieff Movement System, go to https://vimeo.com/showcase/7118023 for some example lessons.

CHAPTER 16

Exploring Therapeutic Education

Molly J. Lahn, PT, DPT, PhD

A story: "I'm at the end of my rope." "Juan," 57, sat slumped in the chair, leaning away from his painful right lower back and hip, after he had slowly walked into the treatment room. Juan has experienced persistent low back pain since being rear ended in a motor-vehicle collision 30 years ago. After a number of failed treatments, he ultimately underwent an L5-S1 fusion. Things got worse, not better. The pain is now moderate to severe on a constant basis, and has spread from primarily the right side to the left. No longer able to work, he has been on disability insurance for six years. He has not been able to play golf, go fishing, or even work around the house for long. "I've been in pain for 30 years," he said, "and it was recommended I try this therapy but I don't see how this is going to help. I've tried everything."

Similar to the research on the effects of mindfulness and mind-body practices,[1] the field of health education suggests that medical and scientific information, if applicable and translatable, can influence positive biobehavioral change through "top-down" (brain-body) neurocognitive mechanisms.[2] *Pain neuroscience education* (PNE) is an example that has gained much attention from both clinicians and researchers, and is sometimes considered a therapeutic intervention unto itself. This chapter is about safely and effectively harnessing the power of education within a therapeutic container, uniquely tailored to each individual's experience. In the integrative framework, PNE is offered as an opportunity for cognitive appraisal and reappraisal, and not from the pervasive "fix-it" lens.

In this chapter, we will overview PNE and discuss how the lessons that come from PNE extend to other topics. We call this broader application *therapeutic education* (TE). In addition to PNE as a key example of TE, mind-body medicine offers another example. The provision of accessible TE around mind-body science such as autonomic nervous system regulation in relation to psychosocial stress assists in normalizing the reality of mind-body processes in our lives.

THE PROBLEM OF PAIN

Juan is not alone, and his scenario is seen every day in therapy offices worldwide. Persistent pain is an: "urgent global public health concern."[3] Around 20% of the world's population suffers from pain lasting longer than three months.[4] Pain is a complex issue that involves more than just physical symptoms. It often coexists with mental health comorbidities such as anxiety and depression, restricts daily activity and mobility, and reduces quality of life.[5] Pain conditions are more disabling than any other chronic health condition, including stroke, cancer, diabetes, and heart disease.[6] For example, lower back pain is the most common cause of years lost to disability.[7] In addition, pain has a large impact on health-care costs and utilization.[8]

Despite epidemic-level prevalence and high costs of pain, traditional treatments employed for persistent pain are, for the most part, not effective. While the prescription of rest, imaging, medications, spinal injections, and surgery are being inappropriately used around the world, evidence-based first-line treatments are underutilized.[9]

Among the most pressing concerns is the current US opioid epidemic. Even though prescribing rates have increased since the 1990s, reported levels of pain are not proportionately decreasing.[10] Even more, opioid use carries high risk of adverse events. The Centers for Disease Control and Prevention's (CDC) latest data show that 46 Americans die every day from prescription opioids. Other significant adverse effects include depression,[11] opiate-induced androgen deficiency,[12] suppression of the hypothalamic-pituitary-adrenal axis,[13] and dysregulation of emotion and social behavior.[14] Perhaps most significant in the discussion of persistent pain states, long-term use of opioids can actually cause opioid-induced hyperalgesia.[15] In weighing the risk-benefit ratio, opioids are a poor solution for persistent pain. Furthermore, there is evidence that despite using opioids, there is minimal impact on disability associated with their use.[16]

The Institute of Medicine calls for nothing short of a cultural transformation in how we treat pain, emphasizing the need for a more integrative-minded approach rooted in the backdrop of a biopsychosocial model.[17] Moreover, the first rung of the ladder in pain care should be self-care and active approaches.[18] According to *The Lancet*'s high-value care recommendations for pain, a critically important part of establishing self-care is education about the condition.[19] Similarly, the International Association for the Study of Pain (IASP) states that education should be considered as first-line care[20] and a central component of pain care globally.[21] Indeed, the IASP made education the focus of its outreach efforts in its 2018 Global Year for Excellence in Pain Education.[22] Before examining current approaches to pain education in more depth, it is important to examine the evolution of our understanding of pain itself.

CURRENT CONCEPT OF PAIN

Pain is frequently defined as: "an unpleasant sensory and emotional experience associated with actual or potential tissue damage, or described in terms of tissue damage, or both."[23] There are some useful points within this definition. The first is found in the understanding that pain is both a sensation and a subjective experience that involves a number of dimensions. These dimensions include: affective-motivational, cognitive-evaluative, sensorimotor, and even sociocultural elements. For example, anxiety, catastrophizing, and fear-avoidance of movement increase the risk for developing persistent pain states, whereas optimism and self-efficacy positively predict recovery from injury.[24] Further, as opposed to a single transmission line for pain, nor a single "pain center" in the brain, current scientific investigation suggests that the neurophysiological correlates of pain involve complex brain-body and whole-person dynamics.

A second interesting point from the IASP's current definition is that pain is an experience that exists in relationship to real or *potential* tissue damage. One author stated it this way: pain is a "highly complex, subjective human experience that is felt in the tissues but interpreted by the mind as a response to perceived threat."[25]

Significant debate around defining pain remains.[26] Despite ongoing challenges in adequately defining pain, there are facets of the IASP definition that support both a flexible approach to defining pain and ultimately the integrative construct.

Noting the widespread and cross-culturally observed use of "pain," the term pain is frequently used to refer not just to physical sensations of pain, but equally to mental anguish, emotional distress, and even spiritual dilemmas.

From a Cartesian dualist perspective, pain occurs somewhere "out there"—in an immaterial mind. From a reductionist lens, pain is often considered to be solely in the brain. The biopsychosocial (BPS) conceptualization is increasingly advocated to combat these problematic views, and there is a growing awareness for the treatment of pain to adopt the BPS approach, despite the fact that the approach was brought forward as early as the 1980s.[27]

While the linguistic and philosophical debates will continue, integrative rehabilitation practice (IRP) intends to address these challenges in working with pain. IRP supports flexibility by reminding us to not overly reify any definition of pain, nor see pain as caused by any one single issue. Further, IRP features concepts such as "both/and," complexity, and person-centered support that focuses on the lived experience of the patient. Ultimately, pain is somewhat of a mystery that may defy linguistic definition.[28]

PAIN PARADIGMS: AN EVOLUTION

Theories describing the perception of pain date back many centuries or even millennia.[29] The current prevailing approach to pain is based on theories of pain that emphasize "pain pathways" from the periphery to the spinal cord and brain, such as the gate theory and specificity theory.[30] This concept, along with the emergence of the allopathic medical model and imaging techniques, such as MRI and X-ray, contributed to an approach that has focused on identifying and treating pathoanatomical structures. In other words, pain has been approached from a "find-it-and-fix-it" perspective. The "find-it-and-fix-it" approach is sometimes effective in acute pain states that are clearly associated with tissue damage or pathology. In the case of persistent pain conditions, however, extensive evidence indicates that there is actually little correlation between pain and pathoanatomical findings.[31] For example, most low back pain is not related to any specific spinal abnormalities,[32] nor do baseline MRI findings predict future low back pain.[33] The search for such explanations (and treatments based on those explanations) has not made any appreciable impact and may in fact add burden.[34]

Similar to medical approaches that target pathoanatomical structures, patient education in the therapy setting has often focused on explaining anatomical or biomechanical views of pain causality. In persistent pain conditions, however, this approach can increase patient stress and fears about their condition, and result in negative outcomes.[35] Even the widely used terminology that describes pathoanatomy, such as "degenerative disc disease," "bulging discs," or "bone-on-bone," contributes to an expectation of pain and heightened fear and anxiety.[36] Darlow *et al.* explored the perceptions of people diagnosed with knee osteoarthritis and demonstrated that participants were strongly influenced by the language used by their health-care providers.[37] No matter how advanced the arthritis, the study participants believed their condition was progressive and that joint replacement surgery was inevitable. These negative expectations were strongly influenced by clinicians' language and explanations. The authors concluded that the adoption of a biomedical model limited participation in activities, increased fear and negative expectations for the future, and forced the study participants to make decisions and sacrifices that were unnecessary.[38]

In addition, education focused on pathoanatomy does not explain phenomena such as pain that lasts beyond tissue healing time, spreading pain, hyperalgesia and allodynia, pain in the absence of known injury or pathology, the responses of the immune system, and how stress is connected to pain. Perhaps more importantly, people experiencing persistent pain are more interested in learning about their pain, not anatomy or biomechanics.[39]

In contrast, other patients may experience negative outcomes due to the *lack* of imaging findings that can explain their pain. These are the patients who are led to believe that their pain is "all in their head."

While the biomedical model is appropriate and helpful in many circumstances, such as acute pain conditions and in ruling out sinister causes for persistent pain, in many cases clinicians and patients alike are often left frustrated and at a loss for answers. The prevailing model generally does not explore or address many possible contributing ingredients to the emergence of pain. This reinforces the call to explore the much larger context of people's lives in which pain occurs.

Fortunately, in the last 40 years, advances in neuroscience, cellular biology, and molecular medicine have contributed to this much broader and integrative understanding of pain as a whole,[40] including the functional and structural changes that occur in the central nervous system in persistent pain states.[41] This also includes the role of emotion in the chronification of pain[42] and the fact that pain may carry benefits such as the facilitation of self-regulation, pleasure seeking, and social engagement.[43] All of this has profound implications in pain care, contributes to the context of PNE, and supports the advancement of integrative efforts.

Experiential pause: What is your "elevator speech" about the nature of persistent pain? Write it down as you formulate it. If you had only about one or two minutes to explain to a patient or a colleague about the physiology behind persistent pain, what would you say? Take some time and speak it out loud. You are also encouraged to present it to someone and seek their feedback.

PNE

Clinical pain management has featured education about pain mechanisms and behavioral approaches since at least the early 1980s.[44] There are now multiple terms for pain education, including therapeutic neuroscience education, explain pain, pain biology education, and others. At its core, rather than education focusing on coping strategies, PNE is about what pain is, what function it serves, and its biological underpinnings.[45] PNE attempts to convey an understanding of the biological and physiological processes involved, such as altered peripheral and central neurophysiology, neuroplasticity, immunological and endocrine changes, and neurological facilitation and inhibition. More importantly, it reduces focus on pathology associated solely with anatomical structures[46] and includes consideration of body-mind-environment interactions and historical factors.

SEVEN KEY CONCEPTS OF PNE

As described above, pain is a complex topic, but a few key concepts are deemed important to convey when educating patients. These are known as the seven Target Concepts in Pain Education.[47]

- **Pain is a protector**: The human organism is hardwired for survival, and pain is one of the most powerful means of defending the organism. Essentially, pain functions like a highly sophisticated alarm system.[48]
- **Pain includes a brain output**: Potentially threatening stimuli from the body's tissues, activated by inflammatory chemicals and mechanical input, are registered by sensory afferent nerves (type C and A-delta fibers) that synapse with second-order neurons in the dorsal horn of the spinal cord and then to the brain. This is known as nociception.

    In turn, the brain assists in continual processing of sensory information from the environment and the body, comparing it with previous experiences and assessing the level of potential threat. Sensory inputs are processed by the brain, and based on experience, novelty, and/or perceived threat level, the brain contributes to the overall determination of response.[49] In describing nociception to patients, it is taught that the body's tissues do not simply send "pain" messages to the brain, nor are there "pain nerves"; rather tissues may communicate sensory messages that are experienced in a much larger context, and include multiple interpretive processes within the whole of the organism. From an integrative perspective, we must examine the implications of neurocentrism, as nociception alone is insufficient for a pain experience. Similarly, while the brain is necessary, it is also not sufficient for pain.[50]

- **The physiological processes underpinning pain can become overprotective/overactive**: In persistent pain states, the networks associated with pain may undergo neuroplastic changes, such as up-regulation of neural signaling. Such changes have been shown throughout the nervous system, including the spinal cord and brain (brainstem, thalamus, limbic system, and cerebral cortex),[51] resulting in heightened processing of nociceptive stimuli and/or other heightened physiological responses.[52] Multiple processes contribute to up-regulation, including increased synaptic excitability, lowered thresholds of activation, expansion of nociceptive neurons' receptive fields,[53] and neuroinflammation.[54]

  Other factors involved in persistent pain mechanisms may include loss of spinal cord inhibitory inter-neurons and increased facilitation and/or reduction of inhibitory descending modulation from the brain. There is also altered cortical processing of nociceptive inputs, as well as cognitive-affective mechanisms that facilitate pain.[55] At a cellular level, there is dysfunctional synapsing mechanisms, neuronal death, changes in neurotransmitters and ion channels in the brain and spinal cord, and loss of gray matter.[56]

  This state, often referred to as *nociplastic* pain, is most strongly predicted by the clinical hallmarks of: disproportionate, non-mechanical, unpredictable patterns of pain in response to non-specific aggravating and easing factors; pain that is disproportionate to the level of injury; diffuse tenderness to palpation; and the presence of psychological factors such as strong emotions, poor self-efficacy, overprotective beliefs and pain behaviors, and difficulty with family/work/social life.[57]

- **There are many contributors to pain**: As stated previously, pain reflects an integral experience. It is modulated by somatic, psychological, and social influences.[58] Many factors influence the sensitivity level of pain processes, including tissue damage if present, and integrated peripheral/central changes such as autonomic, immune, and/or inflammatory changes.[59] Influences coming from outside of the body altogether (such as physical and social environment), as well as "inside" the individual (such as memories, expectations, beliefs, emotions, perceptions, personality, and stress levels), influence pain processes.[60] Researchers suggest that psychosocial factors are actually more effective predictors of pain and disability levels than pathoanatomical issues.[61] In rehabilitation, especially physical therapy, psychosocial factors have sometimes been framed as "yellow flags."[62] If taken out of context, these factors can add to stigmatization as opposed to normalization of such factors in our lives (see Chapter 6). Skilled PNE/TE within IRP explores the larger landscapes of people's lives without pathologizing or reducing causality.

- **Pain is not always an accurate marker of tissue state**: Because there are many factors involved in the emergence of any pain experience, including perception of perceived threat, pain is not always directly related to what is occurring in the tissues. Tissue damage can occur without pain (such as the common experience of having a bruise and not recalling how it occurred), and pain can occur without tissue damage. As noted above, multiple studies have demonstrated a lack of correlation between tissue damage found on MRI and back pain. For example, degenerative changes of disc signal loss and loss of disc height were seen in 90% of asymptomatic individuals age 60 and over. In addition, there is no significant relationship between imaging findings and surgical outcomes.[63]

- **We are all bioplastic**: This element of pain education highlights the nervous system and body's ability to change. Neurophysiological networks can and do change over time. A multimodal, active approach to pain rehabilitation, of which PNE is a helpful component, is encouraged.

- **Pain education is treatment**: The modern definition of pain features how cognitive state can influence the pain experience, known as neurocognitive modulation.[64] PNE is hypothesized to directly affect these cognitive-affective mechanisms about pain and its perception.[65]

Researchers have explored multiple aspects of how PNE can be helpful in the clinical setting. Tailored education about pain helps to shift mindset away from passive treatments.[66] Level 1 evidence demonstrates that PNE also improves participation in rehab programs, reduces kinesiophobia and catastrophizing, and can reduce pain and disability itself.[67] A 2016 systematic review indicated that PNE can improve behaviors associated with pain, fear-avoidance, health-care utilization, and movement.[68]

CLINICAL APPLICATIONS: SETTING THE FOUNDATION FOR TE

There are a few key elements to consider in applying TE in the clinical setting, whether for pain education or other applications. The evaluation process, including a thorough history, review of systems, and physical exam, is a critical first step.

The exam process is where the foundation of biomedical care plays a significant role.

Setting a foundation of success starts immediately upon meeting the patient. The history and interview portion of the exam is covered in Chapters 8 and 9. Specific to this chapter, throughout the exam and subsequent sessions the clinician should listen carefully and ask direct questions. This provides important background that can affect the treatment plan and how TE is best approached. Some good questions to ask are: "What do you think is going on with your pain? Why do you think you hurt? What do you think should be done for your pain?"[69] Listen especially for fear-related words such as "crumbling discs" or "pinched nerves." It is helpful to use reflective listening and, as clearly as possible, restate and summarize what you are hearing. "So, what I hear you saying is, you believe you have crumbling discs in your back; is that correct?" Often, when patients hear their perceptions reflected back to them, they feel validated and know that they are clearly being heard, and it also affords an opportunity for greater self-awareness. Once the clinician knows more about the patient's perceptions, unhelpful or inaccurate mental models can be challenged.[70]

As such, the clinician should attempt to get a sense of all elements of the patient's experience besides the physical symptoms, such as any anxiety, depression, confusion, or other affective elements, and any other pertinent psychosocial stressors.

The clinician should identify functional impairments related to pain as specifically as possible. Oftentimes, more in-depth questioning can reveal other factors that interfere with function, such as fatigue, deconditioning, or mental health factors. The clinician should also inquire about the patient's functional priorities and goals. With that information and other cues from the history, the clinician gets a sense for how in depth any TE should be and any specific perceptions or patient fears that should be addressed.

The patient should then have a thorough evaluation based on the applicable rehabilitation profession, including screening for medical red flags. Overall, the history and evaluation are critical in establishing therapeutic alliance, an element that cannot be underestimated. Spending time with the patient, physical touch, and empathic listening are all highly desired by patients experiencing pain.[71] The patient has to trust that the clinician has a clear clinical impression and has ruled out serious medical issues. Because TE often significantly challenges their beliefs,[72] patients need to trust that the clinician knows their pain is real. They also have to trust that rehabilitation will not make their pain worse.

The first relationship-building experience with the patient, the history and evaluation, are the most fruitful opportunity to establish this level of trust and form the foundation for effective TE of any kind. Establishing safety, trust, validation, and rapport also opens the door for the possibility of an even larger inquiry into contextual psychosocial factors when appropriate and needed. This may include the need to address psychosocial factors within scope of practice,[73] as well as the possible relevance of past stress exposure and adverse childhood experiences.[74]

CUSTOMIZE THE PLAN

In synthesizing the history and clinical exam, a clearer picture of the patient's pain experience, and the many possible contributing ingredients to it, can emerge. Both the treatment and the educational message may be influenced by the relative impression of nociceptive, peripheral neuropathic, or nociplastic influence, as well as the extent to which psychosocial factors may need to be addressed.[75] It is important to gain as clear a clinical impression as possible to deliver PNE messages that are specific to the patient's individual concerns so that it is as relevant for each person as it can be. Such clarity is not achieved in one session and is best seen as evolving in relationship over time. PNE, as a process, provides guidance for when the care plan may need to dive deeper into the provision of additional support for addressing emotional and other psychosocial factors.[76] Figure 16.1 demonstrates a model of integrative care that fits such a theoretical flow. Note that this is a guideline only, acknowledging the importance of adequate transdisciplinary training, clinician experience, scope of practice, and, ultimately, creativity and wisdom (Chapter 2).

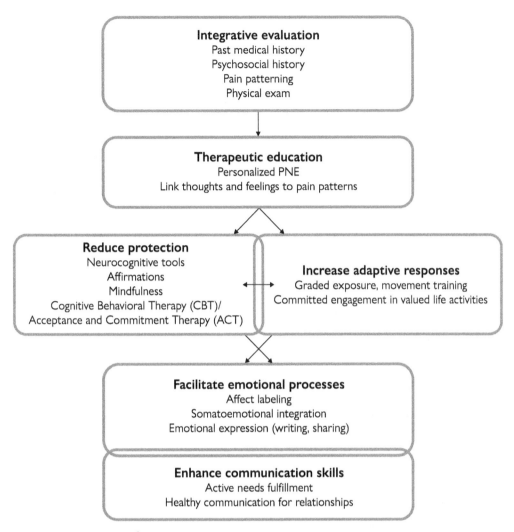

FIGURE 16.1: EXAMPLE ALGORITHM FOR CARE PLAN DEVELOPMENT
Adapted from Lumley and Schubiner[77]

Individuals who tend to respond well to the inclusion of PNE are those with higher levels of fear and catastrophizing, more chronic than acute symptoms, and centrally mediated pain rather than nociceptive pain, and those who are more motivated to know why they are experiencing their pain.[78] Getting a sense of readiness for PNE helps to "dose" accordingly.[79] If the patient appears to be a good candidate for PNE, it is recommended to first ask permission to teach about their pain.[80] This is another way of establishing a partnership with the patient and establishing level of readiness.

In designing a care plan, rehabilitation professionals should also consider other ways to address psychosocial content. As the algorithm in Figure 16.1 demonstrates, PNE alone may be insufficient, as multiple factors play a role in the overall success of the plan. For example, self-efficacy[81] has been shown to be more important than kinesiophobia in mediating the relationship between pain and disability.[82] Similar to any other form of patient education, PNE is not as effective as a standalone treatment and is rather designed to be used in conjunction with other rehabilitation strategies.[83] Clinicians must not assume that cognitive restructuring, behavioral changes, nor increased self-efficacy will ensue with the provision of only PNE.

When exploring the context in which PNE is delivered, it is important that new information is enhanced through actual practice.[84] For example, cognitive concepts from PNE such as "sore but safe" are more apt to become lived experience by repetition of self-regulation skills, graded movement training,[85] and/or cognitive-behavioral approaches (see Chapter 17) under the guidance of the clinician. Further, effective learning must be self-evident,[86] such as in one's ability to teach the same material to others.[87] For PNE, this starts in the clinic by inviting the patient to listen in a way that allows the patient to explain the material back. For example: "Can you share back what you just heard?" This form of dialogue reinforces learning and also allows the clinician to check for gaps in perception.

JUAN'S FIRST SESSION

Juan's scenario illustrates a few of these concepts. His history revealed multiple other areas of pain besides the lower back, poor sleep quality, a number of current psychosocial stressors, and challenges in early life. He also endorsed "boom-bust" cycles of activity in which he was hardly able to function for a few days after a day of increased activity. A recent lumbar MRI showed moderate degenerative disc height loss and mild bulging, moderate facet arthropathy at multiple levels, and facet arthropathy at L3-4 with a stable fusion site.

Juan had tried numerous previous treatments, and prior physical therapy (PT) worsened his pain. When asked what functional goals he had, he was unable to come up with anything other than: "I just want this pain to go away."

Throughout the session, he used pathoanatomically focused language, such as: "I was told I have flattened discs and severe arthritis. If I keep going this way I don't know what'll happen."

Juan's physical exam was notable for a negative red-flag screen, reduced range of motion in all planes, pain behaviors, signs of kinesiophobia, diffuse tenderness to palpation, and impaired endurance.

During this first visit, therapeutic alliance was already being established. The clinician explained Juan's exam findings and provided reassurance that there was nothing indicative of a sinister pathology. The clinician also addressed his fears right away about disc degeneration and arthritis, explaining this as a normal process associated with aging that is found in many asymptomatic people.

On reviewing his history, imaging findings, and exam, Juan presented with features of nociplastic pain among the other findings. This, along with fear-avoidance, inaccurate beliefs about pathoanatomy, and catastrophic thoughts, made him a good candidate for including PNE in his treatment approach.

With permission, Juan was introduced to the idea of pain as an alarm system and how multiple domains of one's life can contribute sensitivity to the alarm system. He was offered additional educational resources for between visits. He was also encouraged to start tracking daily steps to get a baseline of physical activity and to write down two to three functional goals to bring to the next session.

In the first session, despite Juan's initial concerns, some degree of therapeutic alliance was established. His final statements upon leaving the office were that nobody had previously done such a thorough exam or really listened to him, and he felt some degree of optimism. The foundation for further TE and therapeutic intervention was already built.

IMPLEMENTING PNE

Once the foundation for PNE is in place, the specifics of how to deliver it can be considered. The first, and often overlooked, step in implementing PNE is usually "de-education" prior to "re-education."[88] As noted above, modern pain science represents a fundamental paradigm shift that can sharply contrast to purely pathoanatomical models. For some, simply providing education on normative data found in imaging studies can greatly reduce fear-avoidance and catastrophization.[89]

One of the main goals of PNE is to reconceptualize pain. Congruent with this, PNE has been shown to be most effective when presented as metaphors or stories that can help shift mental models.[90] One of the most widely used metaphors is comparing the nervous system to an alarm system, as noted in Juan's scenario above. Much of PNE can be done in short sessions of five to ten minutes, and/or woven throughout a session in parallel with other clinical interventions, such as manual therapy or therapeutic exercise. Establishing the "dose" of PNE should always depend on individual patient presentation and can be as little as a few sentences, such as "You have a sensitive alarm system and you can make it less sensitive," to a multi-hour curriculum as part of a comprehensive rehabilitation program.

PNE can be presented both in a group format and during individual rehabilitation sessions.[91] Clinicians can use online videos, drawings, simple verbal descriptions of the metaphors, books, and patient handouts, among others. Even more effective is to use anecdotes and examples from patients' own lives.

PNE can be an important adjunct to active rehabilitation, particularly exercise and movement,[92] as it shifts perceptions about physical activity. While changes in beliefs do not have to precede behavior change,[93] for some, PNE can be a precursor and important part of behavior change in other areas of self-care. Furthermore, PNE explains how the sensitivity of the alarm system can be reduced through key areas of self-care including: sleep hygiene, goal setting, graded functional progression of movement and graded exposure, mind-body skills to self-regulate the stress response, and time-contingent (as opposed to pain-contingent) pacing. The focus is on achievements, functional levels, and progress, not pain.

> **Experiential pause:** Imagine Juan is sitting in your office. He describes his "degenerative disc disease" and pinched nerves. Write down two or three key things you could say to establish an empathic connection while helping to provide less fearful, more accurate information. Include awareness of your body language, facial expressions, and tone of voice as you imagine a mutual interaction with Juan.

WORKING WITH CHALLENGES

There are a few challenges that commonly surface when introducing PNE. One of the most pressing is the patient's concern: "You're telling me my pain is all in my head." (Recall Chapters 3 and 6 for background on this topic.) A helpful way of addressing this before it is even an issue is to present basic information about pain arising physiologically from many components. A soup analogy, where possible "ingredients" are listed, is useful. The patient must be reminded that there is a biological basis to their pain. The idea of integrated and interpretive processes between brain and body can be introduced after other fundamental PNE concepts have been covered, thus establishing more buy-in at the outset.[94]

For some, it may also be helpful to normalize psychology as represented by biological underpinnings: "All pain occurs in context, meaning that our stress levels, environment, past experiences, and our thoughts and feelings all contribute to the biology of pain." If these steps are taken and this common dynamic still surfaces, it is important to convey that all pain is real and none of it is imagined or "all in your head" in the figurative sense. The patient can be reassured that even though the feeling of pain is real, it does not necessarily reflect the degree of tissue damage, relevance to imaging findings, poor posture, and so on. In addition, even though the brain is believed to be involved in the generation of pain, it does not imply that people can simply "think pain away" or that it is their fault.

Another challenge that often presents in the clinic is the patient who still feels that "something must be fixed," despite hearing the PNE messages about normal findings on imaging, the lack of correlation between pain and physical damage, and so on. Reviewing normative data and even repeating parts of the clinical exam can be helpful in providing reassurance. The clinician can also simply ask the patient what they perceive needs to be done (such as imaging, having an injection, or surgery), and then have the PNE discussion around that topic so that it is specific to the patient's concerns.

In some cases, patient concerns are not explicitly stated, but can manifest as various forms of aversion or lack of buy-in to the PNE and/or active rehab approach. With reflective listening and careful dialogue, the clinician can sometimes bring these issues to light and thus be able to discuss them directly. It is important to express empathy, validation, and support for the patient's perspective and reflect the oftentimes strong messages that the patient has gotten in the past, as well as affirm that it can be difficult to embrace a new way of approaching pain. The patient can then be reassured that therapy will "meet you where you are" and work according to patient readiness and preferences.

Despite even the best efforts of the clinician, the clearest communication, and optimized therapeutic rapport, some patients may not wish to embrace PNE, nor the larger paradigm of self-care. It is best to work with whatever therapeutic interventions the patient is ready to embrace. The use of *motivational interviewing* and awareness of readiness for change is very helpful here. (See Chapter 6 including the recommended learning resource on this topic.) In some cases, establishing rapport in this way opens the door for improved engagement with mind-body integration and/or lifestyle medicine.[95]

On a related note, PNE and much of pain rehabilitation encourages self-empowerment, but there is a risk of the reverse interpretation if a patient does not improve: "If I can do so much to help myself, then have I somehow failed if I'm still in pain?" It is very important that pain is not categorized as any kind of personal or moral failure. (Note: You may wish to review Chapters 3–6 for further reinforcement.)

Finally, PNE is still evolving, and has not been found to be effective in all situations. One review, for example, suggested short-term but not long-term impact[96] from the intervention, and that delivering intensive PNE in an acute setting was not effective.[97]

TE as a whole, PNE included, is also not without potential pitfalls. Any education that inadvertently infantilizes, preaches, fails to support emotional well-being, lacks experiential translation, or fails to account for systemic and structural factors in health will fall short of a truly integrative perspective.[98]

Finally, as models of thought evolve, the BPS model itself is being called out as having limitations. This includes a tendency to deploy it in a fragmented way that lacks whole-person, caring support.[99] The critical point is that any model applied to patient care, whether it be PNE, TE as a whole, or even the larger BPS model, needs be delivered in the context of solid clinical skills, empathic connection with the patient, and consideration of each patient's individual needs. This is congruent with several core tenets of IRP: complexity and context matter, health is a process, and care must be personalized.

JUAN'S PROGRESS

At his second PT session, Juan was able to articulate a few simple functional goals, such as increasing standing tolerance in order to promote working in the yard, and he had started to record his daily steps.

The second session's PNE featured an introduction to nociception or "danger" messages, and how multiple factors can influence how the brain processes the information coming from the tissues. His fears about exercise and movement were addressed prior to initiating therapeutic exercise, and he was educated about a graded walking program.

This session also introduced the "good news" about pain: just as the alarm system can become sensitized, the system can also become less sensitive with all of the skills he would be continuing to learn in therapy.

Subsequent sessions introduced how other life stressors can influence the pain experience, the basics of sleep hygiene, and autonomic self-regulation or mind-body skills with education on the chronic stress response and how this affects pain. He was also instructed further in how to implement proactive pacing. Treatment included a few sessions of manual therapy (see Chapter 23) as his symptoms became less irritable.

At his final PT session, Juan reported that he did initially have difficulty buying in to this approach but had realized significant gains. He was starting to gradually incorporate a few working hours per week and had tried golfing. He still had moderate pain levels but was less fearful about the future. He was no longer using any pathoanatomically focused language, and kinesiophobia was greatly reduced. Objectively, his gait had improved cadence and speed, trunk range of motion had improved, and he was less tender with palpation and joint glides. Juan did not conclude therapy pain-free, but he had gained a diverse skill set for self-care, felt much more confident in resuming important activities in his life, and was making tangible functional gains. His trajectory had shifted towards greater well-being (see Figure 3.6).

FINAL THOUGHTS: WORDS AS MEDICINE

"Like drugs, words have an ability to change the way another person thinks and feels."[100] As discussed in Chapter 9, narrative medicine—and the broad construct of a phenomenological model—is important in defining integrative care approaches. To take this further, we might consider that each and every word in bidirectional relationships matter. Keep this in mind throughout every facet of the time you spend with your patients.

An important part of rehabilitation professionals' role is to communicate with patients so as to rebuild self-efficacy and resilience.[101] Language can have a strong influence on sociocultural and other psychophysiological factors involved in health processes.[102] Health-care professionals can teach patients about pain and promote self-efficacy outside of formal TE by simply changing the "everyday" clinical language so that it reflects what is now understood about pain, disease, mind-body, and health processes. Terms such as "normal age-related changes," "sensitive nerves," and "sore and stiff, but intact" are less alarming and yet accurately convey clinical findings. On a fundamental level, words can soothe and bring comfort, ultimately serving healing processes.

An additional point when considering the use of language within the health-care team is that TE/PNE is not just for the persistent-pain or chronic-disease settings. Ideally, these sorts of messages are incorporated right away in the acute or even emergency-department setting to reduce the risk of catastrophization and fear-avoidance that can lead to chronicity and high rates of health-care utilization. For example, patients presenting with acute to sub-acute lower back pain who received an in-office 15-minute verbal, one-on-one PNE session demonstrated clinically significant improvements in active trunk flexion, modest reductions in pain, and improvements in straight leg raise range of motion immediately after the session.[103]

CONCLUSION

PNE is part of a cultural revolution in how health care is approaching the worldwide epidemic of persistent pain, and it reflects the significant advances that have been made in understanding the nature of pain. Fundamentally, it is critical to understand pain because it changes the way people respond to it.[104] In the author's clinical experience, many patients say PNE is the most helpful part of their entire rehabilitation process.

Person-centered education sets the foundation for the rest of the rehabilitation program, especially active movement and exercise. PNE is simple to combine with other approaches, requires no equipment, and is cost effective.[105] As part of a multimodal rehabilitation approach, PNE delivers an empowering and hopeful message and sets the foundation for allowing real and lasting change.

Finally, it is imperative that we take the lessons learned from PNE into the larger landscape of TE as a whole. As such, the reader is encouraged to extrapolate these constructs to any of the topics included in the larger IRP approach described in this book.

Experiential pause: Having read this chapter, identify and write down at least one actionable item of interest to you. In doing so, consider ways in which applying the material first to yourself, and then to patients, might serve those who come to you for care.

CHAPTER 17

Cognitive-Behavioral Integration

Margaret Gavian, PhD and Matt Erb, PT

A story: "Mikel" appears unsettled, his right leg continuously moving, and he is frequently shifting, with distressed facial expressions. He has just undergone a second surgery for persistent lower back pain, has a history of depression, has a mild traumatic brain injury (TBI), and is unable to work. Due to substance use and "difficulty with relationships," he is newly divorced and has supervised visitation with his two children on Saturdays. A former marathon runner, he can no longer jog, and increasingly is spending long periods of time in states of inactivity and social isolation. Professionally, Mikel is a retired Marine, educated as an engineer, and employed with an aerospace company. However, he has been on medical leave for four months, recently transitioned to 60% of his normal salary under a long-term disability insurance policy, and is under pressure to return to work or lose the security of his position. His primary care doctor referred him for "mind-body therapy," and he expresses, with an irritated tone: "This is not all in my head, my back is trashed, and they keep messing up the surgeries." His therapist listens patiently, attuned to his voice, facial expressions, and body language. The therapist notes a familiar desire arise—to be able to help; to have the solution that Mikel is seeking. Mikel asks: "Can you really help me?" The therapist responds: "I certainly hope I can be of help to you, and I am glad you came in today. Tell me more about what this experience is like…"

WHAT IS COGNITIVE BEHAVIORAL THERAPY?

Cognitive Behavioral Therapy (CBT) is a form of treatment that focuses on examining the relationships between thoughts, feelings, and behaviors. CBT has many evolving principles and models. Collectively, CBT approaches have been found to be an effective form of support for a wide variety of patient challenges such as pain, depression, anxiety, and substance use.[1] As mentioned in our earlier exploration of core psychological constructs (Chapter 6), CBT approaches emphasize a look into how thoughts inter-relate with other facets of human experience including: needs, feelings, personality, personal history, relationships, and communication. Exploring cognitive-behavioral constructs—

how we appraise and respond to our health experiences—enhances the mind-body integrated capacity of rehabilitation practice.

Drawing from CBT, functional cognitive-behavioral integration is advancing in various ways within rehabilitation practice. Functional cognitive-behavioral integration reflects a variety of approaches that can be integrated within the scope of practice of rehabilitation professionals. These strategies are aimed at safely exploring the many ways in which one's thoughts, feelings, perceptions, and prior experiences impact one's present (including physical) experience; and vice versa—the ways in which one's physical state influences how one thinks, feels, and behaves. Opportunities for exploring these patterns is vital to whole-person care. In this chapter, we explore how cognitive-behavioral approaches enhance integrative rehabilitation practice (IRP).

MIKEL'S HEALTH EXPERIENCE

Looking at Mikel's experience, we once again see pain as a common component for which people seek care. Mikel's experience helps us explore how the domains of thoughts, feelings, and connected behaviors affect his experience of pain and, bidirectionally, how pain affects those domains. However, in doing so, we invite the reader to proceed with the understanding that the inclusion of cognitive-behavioral constructs is applicable across all populations—to any health challenge or life experience.

In considering Mikel's story, we discover a belief that his "back is trashed." Such a belief implies a perceived fixed state of being. Similarly, a person with depression may consciously or unconsciously believe: "I am worthless." A person with anxiety may believe: "I am in danger." When Mikel's thoughts connect to a sense of brokenness, his thoughts may feed into feelings of worthlessness or sadness; this may lead to increased isolation from others (the resulting behavior). Often, a person in distress like Mikel is unaware of how their thoughts are interacting within their overall emotional and physical experience, influencing how they behave and interact with their world. These thoughts often influence how they relate to their problem (e.g., making poor nutritional choices, failing to take committed actions that serve well-being).

With gentle guidance, individuals can become more aware of underlying beliefs that are operating. From this place of awareness, one might then learn to identify, reframe, and/or "unhook from" maladaptive thought patterns. Relating differently to thoughts/beliefs can influence both feeling states and behaviors/actions. Changes in behaviors (including physical, such as postural or movement patterns) can equally change how we think and feel. Through thoughtful exploration of these dynamics, patients can become more empowered with skills to positively influence their physical and emotional experiences.

A LOOK BACK AT THREAT APPRAISAL IN THE CONTEXT OF COGNITIVE-BEHAVIORAL PROCESSES

Threat appraisal (see Chapter 4) is hardwired to help support survival, safety, and overall health. Our mind-body network is sensitive to threat across many domains. In looking at the pain component of Mikel's health experience, we are reminded that pain is currently understood as an integrated biobehavioral response and experience. This includes understanding that pain processes are embedded into the stress response in the body. Ultimately, the body's integrated stress/pain response is responding to a sense of threat—either real or perceived—and rooted in defense, protection, and survival.

Mikel's story is a common reminder of how complex an individual's health experience can be. Mikel is struggling, and with more than just a physical symptom—he is also struggling with surgeries, divorce, separation from his children, late effects from a concussion sustained in active military duty, and an inability to work at his previous level of functioning. Linking various domains of one's pain experience[2] to cognition, consider how the following relate to Mikel's experience:

- psychological (e.g., "The doctors are messing up my surgeries")
- environmental (e.g., "I've had to move to a low-rent apartment with hardly any of my belongings")
- social (e.g., "I don't have a wife anymore and rarely see my children")
- existential (e.g., "Who have I become?"; "There's nothing to live for"; or "Will I always be this way?")
- physical/body (e.g., "I can barely get out of bed some days, let alone exercise")
- financial (e.g., "How will I make ends meet without being able to work?").

Cognition is embedded within brain-body physiology. Each of the preceding examples carry *neurocognitive* influence. Thoughts, beliefs, and expectations can be "threat generators," influencing integrated physiological cascades. The psychophysiological threat appraisal system is modulated by an array of changes across numerous physiological processes, including: inflammatory, neuroendocrine, immune, sensorimotor, and other systems (see Chapter 7). Threat appraisal processes are also influenced by developmental and social determinants (see Chapter 4). Ultimately, the body does not differentiate between types of threat (e.g., financial and existential), and these domains cannot be decoupled from each other. Mikel's appraisal of his financial threat is related to his existential threat of his life purpose and is experienced similarly in his body.[3] As we've encouraged across this book, the tendency to bypass parts of each person's whole, including their cognitive processes, falls short.

COGNITIVE-BEHAVIORAL INTEGRATION IN REHABILITATION

Mikel is not alone. Fifty-two percent of persons with pain also experience symptoms of depression[4] and these individuals often have twice as much sick leave from work as those without depression.[5] Many other patterns of body-mind-environment (BME) interactions exist, as covered across earlier chapters.

If we listen closely to patients' narratives, we will often hear a number of interwoven cognitive-emotional-behavioral dynamics, even without using purposeful psychosocial-oriented interviewing as presented in Chapter 8. As such, the question is not so much *if* but *how*, *when*, and *to what extent* to engage in this type of exploration. With education followed by the development of clinical skills, this answer becomes clearer over time.

Various principles, strategies, and techniques derived from cognitive-behavioral models can be included to support the whole of each person within rehabilitation. While there are a handful of pioneers in the integration of behavioral psychology and transdisciplinary neuroscience within rehabilitation professions, the effective use of cognitive-behavioral constructs is lagging behind the call for such integration.[6]

For many in rehabilitation, the extent to which these dynamics are explored, if at all, is through intake forms, brief past medical history, and outcome tools such as the Fear-Avoidance Beliefs Questionnaire (FABQ) that give a glimpse into psychological factors. Reliance on such tools is insufficient if one wants to explore the whole of Mikel's experience and provide safe, non-stigmatizing support. With a deeper dive into the history of Mikel's pain, we learn that he heard he had a bone spur on X-ray in his lumbar spine very early on. When a patient hears such information, what do they think? What conclusions do they make about themselves or the medical system? What are the effects of these conclusions? One conclusion may be a *belief* that they have "a bad back" and the linked *emotional* response of fear. How does this response then impact Mikel's daily choices and behaviors? Drawing upon whole-person case formulation (Chapter 5), we must be equipped to go deeper in exploring the following questions as they relate to cognitive-behavioral dynamics.

- Why is this person presenting to me in this way, at this time, and what is maintaining their predicament?
- What can be done to reduce this person's distress and disability?

Linton and Shaw suggest that assessing and supporting patient beliefs and emotions may be more important than reaching a definitive diagnosis.[7] Further, they suggest that when a symptom is chronic and medical red flags have been ruled out, further medicalization (e.g., conducting additional diagnostic tests) may add harm as it reinforces a patient's misdirected efforts to find a cure/fix. This precludes the shift towards exploring and addressing the functional/behavioral challenges wrapped up in the experience. Increasingly, this shift of focus is called out as being needed in rehabilitation, especially for pain care.[8]

Exploring and applying cognitive-behavioral constructs to our own lives may enhance our effectiveness in supporting our patients in doing the same. Integrating cognitive-behavioral approaches for rehabilitation professionals may come with various degrees of discomfort or challenge that need support (such as adequate training and supervision).[9] While research is needed to examine IRP's theory that self-application enhances clinical translation and quality of care, we suggest this route in support of principles of interdependence and mutual learning.

APPLICATIONS

There are specific CBT-related models that can assist rehabilitation professionals in exploring beliefs and emotional experiences in relation to pain and other health challenges. Examples include Acceptance and Commitment Therapy (ACT),[10] Cognitive Functional Therapy (CFT),[11] Mindfulness-Based Cognitive-Behavioral Therapy (MBCBT),[12] and Emotional Awareness and Expression Therapy (EAET).[13] These and similar approaches require some degree of study, training, and/or mentoring to employ effectively. These models are generally accessible within the scope of practice of most rehabilitation professionals (see Chapters 1 and 6), and each professional must determine their own training needs, skill level, professional boundaries, and comfort in that regard.

In the sections that follow, we highlight ACT as an example of a growing cognitive-behavioral integrated model utilized within rehabilitation professions. We encourage the reader to further explore this and other valuable approaches to discover what is best suited for their individual practice (see Resources at the end of the chapter).

ACT

ACT reflects a "third wave" evolution of cognitive-behavioral approaches[14] and integrates principles of mindfulness as introduced in Chapter 12. ACT is built upon an experimental analysis of human language and cognition known as relational frame theory (RFT).[15] ACT is also built upon *functional contextualism*, a philosophy of science that focuses on human behavior in relation to each individual's historical and situational contexts[16]—a concept that is consistent with BME and other IRP concepts in that it supports foregoing overly reductive explanations of human problems.

ACT addresses important psychophysiological dynamics present in persistent pain and other health conditions and is highlighted due to the evidence base and its utility.[17] In fact, the dynamics that ACT addresses can be seen as universal tendencies. As such, ACT can be helpful in promoting and sustaining lifestyle and behavior change in general, including in relation to obesity, physical inactivity, and substance use/addiction.[18]

ACT is predicated on accepting, not fixing, "problematic" reactions, as well as focusing on action that individuals can take that reflect their own values. Key components of ACT are found in a sub-acronym: **A**ccept your reactions and be present; **C**hoose a valued direction; **T**ake action. Another central component of ACT is found in the acronym FEAR. FEAR is often responsible for contributing to one's distress. In this representation, the following cognitive-behavioral processes are explored and addressed: **F**usion with thoughts; **E**valuation (negative) of one's experience; **A**voidance of the experience; **R**eason-giving for chosen behaviors. Moving from FEAR to ACT(ion) is a valued concept embedded within the ACT model.

Figure 17.1, known in ACT as the "hexaflex" model, illustrates six key challenges that are considered common within human experience. ACT posits that these challenges inform *psychological inflexibility*; they often interact with one another synergistically to create distress for an individual. These challenges represent targets for consciously enacting "pivots" that can be applied to one's experience in support of well-being and valued living. For example, when we notice ourselves in a pattern of experiential avoidance, we can pivot back and come into a fuller experience of the present moment by learning how to be with the discomfort that is happening.

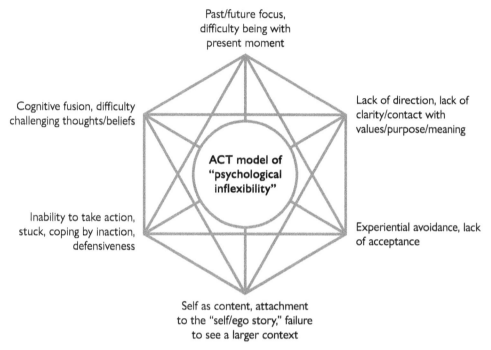

FIGURE 17.1: ACT MODEL—SIX CHALLENGES THAT UNDERSCORE PSYCHOLOGICAL INFLEXIBILITY

ACT in relation to IRP language encourages us to consider how these areas of inflexibility may be embedded and represented within the whole of one's BME patterning, including how one can "fuse" with thoughts and/or maladaptive beliefs about one's diagnosis, symptom, and/or body (part). For example, Mikel may have difficulty being with the present moment in his thoughts and feelings about his past relationship, and by focusing on the past may not engage in creating new purposeful or meaningful relationships in the present.

COMBINING ACT AND MIND-BODY MEDICINE IN IRP

As noted, the ACT model is typically framed as a model of psychological flexibility/inflexibility. We underscore the efforts of this book with a backdrop of mind-body integration, thus have chosen to frame these constructs as "mind-body flexibility/inflexibility" and/or "psychophysiological flexibility/inflexibility" (as opposed to just psychological). Our intent here is to reflect that these dynamics are represented by/embedded in physiology and the lived experience of the body.

Additionally, the six components of ACT are often presented in a linear order, which is best avoided as a reminder that human processes are non-linear. Working with the six components of the hexaflex model may be learned and woven into our lives in various patterns and endless combinations based on changing BME conditions. Introduced above, ACT aims to identify and address the many ways in which these ingredients of "inflexibility" show up. ACT teaches pivots (enactive solutions) to these dynamics. These pivots are trained through a variety of metaphors and experiential learning strategies. With practice and support, it becomes more natural and intuitive to recognize which of the pivots serve the experience the best.

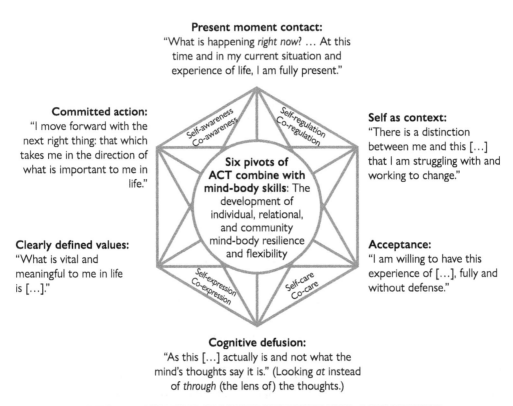

Present moment contact:
"What is happening *right now*? … At this time and in my current situation and experience of life, I am fully present."

Committed action:
"I move forward with the next right thing: that which takes me in the direction of what is important to me in life."

Self as context:
"There is a distinction between me and this […] that I am struggling with and working to change."

Clearly defined values:
"What is vital and meaningful to me in life is […]."

Acceptance:
"I am willing to have this experience of […], fully and without defense."

Cognitive defusion:
"As this […] actually is and not what the mind's thoughts say it is." (Looking *at* instead of *through* (the lens of) the thoughts.)

Self-awareness Co-awareness

Self-regulation Co-regulation

Self-expression Co-expression

Self-care Co-care

Six pivots of ACT combine with mind-body skills: The development of individual, relational, and community mind-body resilience and flexibility

FIGURE 17.2: ACT MODEL IN COMBINATION WITH MIND-BODY MEDICINE

Figure 17.2 goes further into detailing the components of ACT in relation to mind-body medicine (MBM). How might we transform these tendencies? For each one, an example statement that reflects a "pivot" that can be learned/enacted is included. As you read it, you can insert "pain" or "anxiety" or any other topic that reflects a challenge in your life. We have embedded foundational concepts from within MBM and IRP to underscore additional context. For example, learning to self-regulate one's psychophysiological state can enhance one's ability to learn and apply the ACT model (more on this later). Notice how each "self-" construct is presented as a "co-" construct to convey individual relationship as well as community-based, collectivist perspective.

ACT AND EMBODIED ACCEPTANCE

In the ACT model, acceptance is presented as a willingness to have one's experience *as it is*, *right now*, and *without defense*. Consistent with wisdom teachings (Chapter 2), added suffering occurs when aversion/avoidance to an internal (e.g., bodily sensation, thought) or an external (e.g., environmental, circumstantial, conditional) situation or experience is present and negatively impacting the workability of one's life. Aversion/avoidance may occur on a spectrum from subtle/minor to strongly influential in one's behavior and their relationship to any part of their experience. In ACT, a metaphor of "driving the bus" is sometimes used to convey core ACT concepts.

> **Experiential pause:** Using faculties of thought, imagery, and body awareness, imagine you are a bus driver. You have many passengers getting on and off your bus. Some get on for short rides, others for long rides. Some are pleasant, perhaps even superstars, while others are rowdy, distracting, and upsetting. You might even have a threatening passenger get on. Bring to mind a "passenger" in your life who is sometimes loud and unruly. This passenger is causing you discomfort. Sometimes you are frequently distracted, looking back, and losing sight of the road and the controls of the bus. Other times you are trying to pretend that the passenger isn't there but the tension persists. At the same time, you have forgotten about the nice passengers on your bus. What is this like? What happens? Now, can you envision a different way of driving the bus and relating to the passengers? If possible, describe a new approach to driving the bus to another person and, if not, write it down.

The tendency to find ourselves living out the six challenges of ACT is normal; given the choice, most would prefer to not be present to pain, sadness, or other types of distress. Enacting acceptance is certainly not an easy feat. Further, "acceptance" can paradoxically become a cognitive defense itself—something we give lip service to but we don't actually reach a lived experience of acceptance. Using the ACT pivots, individuals can work towards a deeper, somatic, and more genuine version of acceptance, reframing their relationship to their (pain/health/other) experience in an empowered way.

The old adage "What you resist is more apt to persist" gives context to the potential benefit of learning and applying skills that promote embodied acceptance. For example, Mikel may avoid getting together with old friends because he feels ashamed of his current circumstances. Some cognitive-behavioral approaches suggest the need to change one's thoughts and feelings. However, ACT focuses on accepting thoughts and feelings and relating/responding differently to them. ACT aims to help Mikel to accept and be present to his discomfort, evaluate and change his relationship to the thoughts, feelings, and sensations that he is experiencing, and connect with his values to engage in increased social activity. Such a process is benefitted when it is connected to bodily sensations and awareness of how it is reflected in one's mind-brain-*body* patterning.

When we engage in avoidance/aversion behaviors, it creates and adds tension—psychophysiological tension—including physical patterns of holding, constricting, guarding, posturing, and/or restrictions of movement. Posturing, body language, and movement patterns will also reflect these dynamics. Connecting the cognitive-behavioral pattern to what is happening in the body through awareness training reflects a somatic approach to ACT. It is theorized that such a combined (ACT and mind-body regulation) approach affords a less forced and more natural way to bring about changes in biobehavioral patterning.

Conceptually, embodied acceptance has potential to support restorative biological processes such as reducing allostatic load, improving circulation, and/or reducing protective/defensive physiology. One way of framing this is found in the concept of cultivating "comfort with discomfort." By helping a patient to identify their value system, the formulation of realistic committed actions that support well-being is enhanced.

Experiential pauses: ACT has a variety of concepts and techniques that you can practice yourself. Here are several examples.

- Allow feelings, sensations, thoughts, and external stimuli to happen without acting on the impulse to fix or avoid them (except when the impulse is proportional to real threat!). Start small...for example, try not scratching the sensation of an itch; or see what it is like to look *at* a problematic thought instead of experiencing yourself *through* the lens of that thought. For the latter, you might visualize yourself placing the thought on a leaf that is floating by on a stream. Stay as "soft" in the body as you can as you practice relating to thoughts and sensations in this way.

- Depersonalizing our challenging experiences and seeing that we are more than challenged parts can be useful. In ACT, this is known as "self as context." For example, shifting one's language from "my anxiety" (reflects "self as content") to "I am experiencing something called anxiety" demonstrates this pivot. While this language may be cumbersome to start with, it opens the door to experiencing oneself in a larger context. Give this a try for a part of your experience that you may be overly identified with, such as "my back pain" or "my depression." The earlier bus metaphor can be developed further to work with and convey the "self as context" pivot: "back pain and anxiety are passengers on my bus, and there are other passengers coming and going too." Consider developing your own meditative presentation of the bus metaphor now and then present it to others for feedback.

- For a guided experience that introduces all of the ACT pivots, on a device with an internet connection, search for "Healthflix Embodied Acceptance and Commitment" on YouTube. You will find a 45-minute video presentation that includes an introduction to the ACT pivots, presented in a somatic-focused and meditative way.

There is decidedly more to ACT. While we can't cover everything here, to get a sense of ACT at work, consider Mikel's story again. In working with the ACT skills, Mikel initially identified value in re-establishing relationships in his life as the motivating factor for seeking support and taking actions towards his own well-being. With guidance, Mikel determined that, despite his pain, scheduling a social event once a week was feasible: "I'm 85% certain I can do this, starting this week, for a three-week trial, to see how this goes." Mikel also identified two other important values: returning to his career and staying physically active. As such, he also made a commitment to work on movement retraining. When given the choice between structured and unstructured exercise, Mikel chose to trial a structured approach with ten minutes of graded exercise lessons three days per week. As the relationship between Mikel and his therapist advanced, and Mikel's relationship with the pain shifted, doors were opened to explore even larger contextual questions in relationship to his pain experience. Examples of questions built upon RFT and ACT are found in Appendix C.

ADDITIONAL TOPICS RELEVANT TO COGNITIVE-BEHAVIORAL INTEGRATION

There are several subtopics that offer additional insight into mind-body processes as they relate to building capacity for cognitive-behavioral integration. These include:

- self-control and physiological regulation
- mindfulness
- affect labeling
- appraisal/reappraisal
- affirmations and intentions
- placebo/nocebo and Hawthorne Effect
- stigmatization.

Let's review each one before further connecting dots and wrapping up.

Self-control and physiological regulation

Our ability to manage psychophysiological tension (as mentioned above) is an important consideration within cognitive integration. Doing so can be seen as involving both the ability to regulate one's physiological stress response in relation to demand/perceived demand and a correlated cognitive dynamic (perceived self-control capacity). "Self-control refers to a person's capacity to override and inhibit socially unacceptable and undesirable impulses and to alter and regulate one's behavior, thoughts, and emotions."[19] Additionally, motivation derived from a sense of truly valuing and enjoying one's pursuits ("want to") as opposed to motivation tied to external demands or others' expectations ("have to") is associated with an increased sense of success and overall well-being.[20] The degree to which one demonstrates a sense of self-control (autonomy, will, empowerment) in part predicts the relationship between well-being and "want-to" motivation.[21] Recalling the relevance of social determinants to health (Chapter 4) is vital to approaching this discussion.

Researchers have examined how self-regulatory strategies correlate with perceived success in one's life, despite the presence of avoidance of unpleasant aspects of our lives.[22] When research participants imagined tackling aversive challenges (e.g., an intense mental exam, a rigorous physical activity, or an existing unpleasant activity in their lives), the strategies that correlated with the best test outcomes were:

- thinking about the positive consequences of getting to the end of the difficult task (the most popular strategy)
- thinking that the end of the task is near (the second most popular strategy)
- cognitively monitoring one's goal progress
- regulating one's emotions.[23]

In contrast, distracting oneself from the aversive challenge was associated with less perceived success in completing the task. Understanding each person's unique cognitive structure is important in exploring how they view the challenges they face.

Introduced as part of the embodied ACT construct, mind-body skills play an important role in self-regulatory strategies. Mind-body skills can assist us in "softening into" our experience when appropriate and useful. This softening includes regulating the physiological basis of somatoemotional tension, such as breathing habits or patterns of protection. For example, with guidance, Mikel may notice that he begins to clench his jaw every time he thinks about his financial situation. With awareness, Mikel can now learn to practice releasing this habit of tension. Although this approach can be beneficial for patients to gain awareness and empowerment in relation to their health experience, the addition of regulation skills must not inadvertently reinforce aversion (as discussed in the section on ACT), where relaxation training (for example) then becomes another avoidance pattern. It is equally important to not set up a belief or expectation that staying relaxed 24/7 is necessary or desirable. Using mind-body skills in this way is not merely another "pill" used to "fix" the problem.

Mindfulness

As noted, key facets of mindfulness are embedded into ACT and other CBT-related therapies. Unto themselves, however, mindfulness practices have equally been shown to carry neurocognitive ("top-down," mind-brain-body) effects in the scientific literature.[24] Mindfulness-Based Stress Reduction is one such model that is commonly in use in health-care settings, including within rehabilitation professions.[25] Mindfulness (see Chapter 12 for more) supports exploring cognitive-behavioral dynamics; cultivating our ability to come into the present moment supports the ability to appraise and reappraise challenging BME content (i.e., thoughts, emotions), enhancing our relationship with ourselves, our bodies, others, and the world around us.

Meta-analytic research demonstrated that CBT and mindfulness are effective in pain management, with minimal side effects compared to pharmaceutical approaches.[26] The authors also suggest that mindfulness is just as effective as CBT when it comes to improving physical functioning. Mindfulness and CBT were equally beneficial in reducing pain and synergistic conditions such as depression (recall Mikel). These findings underscore that there are many avenues for rehabilitation professionals to positively address and support the influence of cognitive processes.

Affect labeling

Studies have shown that labeling feelings influences the way such emotions get expressed through the brain, body, and behavior.[27] This relatively simple skill of identifying and naming an emotion appears to work as well as more complex approaches, such as reframing (or changing) thoughts about a situation. Affect labeling is considered an implicit way of self-regulating. Evidence suggests that the areas of the brain associated with self-referential processes (e.g., "What feeling do I have right now?") are capable of generating inhibitory pathway activity that effectively regulates emotional (limbic), stress (autonomic), and pain (nociceptive) physiology in diverse distributions through the nervous system and body.[28] This labeling and self-referential process can impact our experience of, and subsequent response to (behavior around), our emotions and the bodily sensations that accompany them.

Cultivating the skill of labeling our emotional experience supports the higher cognitive capacity to appraise and reappraise our experience. In Mikel's case, he benefitted from simple assistance around understanding what emotions he was feeling in order to identify the thoughts and behaviors associated with that emotion. He identified feeling anxiety (fear, though this was a harder word for him to identify with) around attempting to go back to work, given his current challenges. His therapist asked: "Do you have any sense of what that anxiety is about?" Mikel quickly identified: "That I won't measure up. It is overwhelming to consider that."

Appraisal/reappraisal

We have used the general concept of "appraisal and reappraisal" to denote psychological flexibility in relating differently to perceptions and thoughts. More specifically, appraisal theory posits that how we evaluate events is inseparably linked to our emotional dynamics. For example, we appraise experiences based on past events, our personal history, and/or our belief systems. Our capacity to reappraise an event lies in the space between a stimulus and our subsequent reaction or response to that stimulus. In Mikel's case (speculative), seeing his children (the stimulus) evoked a sadness and emptiness (a negative appraisal) based on his comparison to his past ability to see them more frequently. If being asked "Is there another way of relating to seeing your children?" brought about a positive reappraisal, he may experience joy, gratitude, or hope for their presence in his life.

The appraisal concept is often studied separately from affect labeling, but is best approached as being inter-related within the whole of mind-body regulation. Using mindfulness or ACT skills builds awareness in which Mikel can identify how he is appraising the situation with his children and allows him the opportunity to pay attention to that awareness without judgement. If our patterned responses to certain stimuli, which many people call "triggers," are regularly reinforced, it not only affects our emotional reactions, but also strengthens the underlying neural circuitry. This is consistent with the saying: "Nerves that fire together tend to wire together." Or, in a more ancient form borrowed from Chinese medicine: "Where the mind goes, chi flows." If we are given the opportunity to reappraise our evaluation of a relationship to any type of event, we can relate differently to and/or even alter these neural pathways by way of neuroplasticity. Regardless, amelioration of distressing and unhelpful patterns promotes well-being.

Affirmations and intentions

For some, but not all, people,[29] affirmations and intentions may reflect a simple way of utilizing cognitive skills. Affirmations are best seen as resonant and supportive phrases that carry individualized meaning. As with pain neuroscience education, phrases like "Hurt does not equal harm" can assist in the transformation of cognitive-behavioral patterns. It is vital that any use of affirmation be self-selected, as there is a dynamic known as *toxic positivity*. Toxic positivity occurs when individuals use seemingly positive statements and frameworks disingenuously, or in a way that reinforces experiential avoidance as taught within the ACT model.

Looking back at Mikel's experience, we see a good example of affirmations. In observing how tense Mikel's system was, his clinician included experiential mind-body skills learning in the form of guided meditation combined with body awareness training (Chapter 13) and simple therapeutic education (Chapter 16). Mikel's learning also included touch-based therapies (Chapter 23) designed to demonstrate that decreased neuromuscular tension was a possibility. In one such session, the phrase "Now is not an emergency, soften…release…and let go" was included. A positive shift in somatic tension was immediately noticed by both Mikel and the clinician. At the end of the session, Mikel expressed that the words deeply resonated with him. The clinician suggested: "When you notice you're getting tense, activated, or the pain is increasing, you might consider reminding yourself: 'It's not me [depersonalizes the pattern], it's those protective circuits kicking in again; now is not an emergency…'" Mikel later reported that setting up a repetitive practice assisted him in responding differently to his triggers.

Placebo, nocebo, and Hawthorne Effect

We'll now connect a few dots from earlier discussions about placebo/nocebo and the Hawthorne Effect to what we have now learned about cognitive-behavioral integration. Think back to Chapter 7 where placebo was explored. The study of the placebo effect is, at its core, the study of how psychological processes shape brain-body processes and how body-mind thoughts, emotions, and values have physiological bases.[30] Supporting the professional's ability to navigate the reality of placebo, and its opposite, nocebo, is vital. Identifying belief systems, reappraising, and/or relating differently to thoughts, beliefs, and expectations serves to positively influence placebo/nocebo patterns.

"Be sure to use a new treatment while it still works" is a frequently heard joke about the placebo effect. Expectations carry significant physiological weight. If the color of a pill,[31] its shape and size,[32] and one's beliefs about how much it costs[33] impact its effectiveness, we must be willing to acknowledge how our underlying cognitive processes affect our physical health outcomes. We must also explore how the placebo effect influences our own (as professionals) beliefs as to the care approach and techniques that we deliver to our patients (e.g., how our expectations of their wellness or illness may influence their healing).

Additionally, the Hawthorne Effect, which is either a reduction or over-expression of symptoms due to being observed, reflects a similar dynamic. For example, if we know we are being observed, we may be more likely to report symptoms. Our experience of symptoms can arise out of the mind's conscious or unconscious factors.[34] Practical examples of the Hawthorne Effect include the desire to: be taken more seriously; receive greater consideration of priority management status; or conform to related cultural factors. There may also be secondary benefits to staying "ill" that can influence one's health status.[35]

The development of self-awareness around these dynamics is best achieved in unforced ways. In gently investigating and identifying cognitive patterns, we can subsequently influence them using various facets of cognitive-behavioral approaches. Thinking back to Mikel, when the clinician had an observational sense (through heightened symptom behavior) that the dynamic to be taken more seriously *might be* at work, a simple question—"What do you notice in yourself right now?"—brought an invitation into present-moment awareness without assuming, naming, or blaming.

Stigmatization

In Mikel's case, his own upfront pre-emptive statement "It's not all in my head" appeared to the therapist to reflect an attempt to control the potential for shame or blame. As introduced in Chapter 6, such statements may carry a history of: minimization, marginalization, a failure of prior health-care providers to adequately explain normal psychophysiological processes,[36] and/or more simply a common sociocultural dynamic at work. Through cognitive-behavioral integration, Mikel was able to determine "triggers" to his response, as well as new insight into his beliefs and subsequent emotional-behavioral responses. For Mikel, cognitive-behavioral integration also reflected an opportunity to become aware of physiological correlates to these patterns, increasing his ability to gain mastery in relation to his mental, emotional, and physical-state interactions. In essence, Mikel developed greater resilience and a more effective skill set for coping with his life challenges.

MOVING FORWARD

We have covered a lot of territory in our efforts to introduce you to cognitive-behavioral constructs and models. This may appear daunting if you are new to this. The good news is that you can start small by being curious about how your patients' thoughts are linked to their emotions and behaviors. You might also draw from the preceding chapter and include the provision of simple education around the research that demonstrates that the inclusion of cognitive-behavioral skills is a useful and evidence-based approach—and gauge a patient's interest and readiness. Simple opportunities for affect labeling, emotional expression, and mindfulness practices reflect additional entry points.

How one weaves these concepts together within a supportive and non-fixing therapeutic experience has no precise recipe. Seeing cognitive-behavioral integration as both an approach and a dot in the context of a larger whole reflects the IRP approach. When connected to other dots, fuller pictures may emerge, assisting in our capacity to understand and support the whole of a person's experience of health, injury, illness, or disease. Patient self-selection remains paramount. In closing, to support moving forward, regularly ask yourself these questions.

- What level of comfort do I currently have in exploring and engaging the realm of thoughts, feelings, and behaviors in those who come to me for help?
- If there is discomfort, what part of *me* does that arise from? Is it from a lack of adequate training? Is it discomfort in exploring these facets of my own self and experience?
- What do I need to move forward into a deeper exploration?

Experiential pause: Having read this chapter, identify and write down at least one actionable item of interest to you. In doing so, consider ways in which applying the material first to yourself, and then to patients, might serve those who come to you for care.

RESOURCES

- These are good resources for ACT training: www.actmindfully.com.au, https://psychwire.com, https://catalog.pesi.com/category/actacceptance-commitment-therapy, www.integrativepainscienceinstitute.com/act-for-chronic-pain-waitlist, www.laurarathbone.com.

- There are many models/strategies to consider beyond the ones introduced in this chapter. Many learning resources exist. You may wish to explore/search online for training resources in CFT, MBCBT, EAET, and others.

- For a patient-focused and ACT-based guide to working with persistent pain, see *Radical Relief* by Joe Tatta, PT, DPT, CNS.

CHAPTER 18

Exploring Spirituality

Marlysa Sullivan, PT, C-IAYT

A story: "Yoshi" has suffered with persistent pain for over ten years. She has disk herniations in both her lumbar and thoracic spine and she has seen numerous doctors and physical therapists for her pain. She experiences "knife-like" sensations in her back and legs, numbness in her arms, and has difficulty sitting for extended periods of time. Her pain limits her function at work, including her ability to concentrate and think clearly. She also finds she has a diminished ability to participate in social activity in the way she would like to. She is a research scientist whose job requires extensive international travel. While she does find satisfaction and joy in both her job and travel, the pain has diminished this enjoyment. She has been referred to me by her physical therapist to explore a mind-body approach through yoga therapy. Over the time we work together, she finds that she can manage her pain so that it both lessens in intensity and creates less interference in work and social activities. She learns practices to relax her body and mind, increase her concentration, and increase her function. She also comes to understand her pain and her own self differently. Her experience of yoga therapy is captured in her statement: "I no longer see myself as someone with chronic pain with a few good days. Instead, I see myself as someone who enjoys a meaningful life while sometimes experiencing pain."

A PHYSICAL THERAPIST/YOGA THERAPIST'S EXPERIENCE

Yoshi's story and insight into no longer being defined by her pain is one I have heard in various ways since I integrated spiritual concepts into therapeutic care. Yoshi was able to work with values that were important to her, such as patience, acceptance, and compassion for self and other. This work empowered a redefinition of identity such that the experience of pain no longer created a disconnect from herself, her relationships, and her sense of a meaningful life.

These realizations of the importance of working with spiritual concepts such as meaning, purpose, values, inner resourcing, and interpersonal connection reinforce the importance of moving beyond the biopsychosocial approach to the biopsychosocial*spiritual* model of care,[1] as embedded in integrative rehabilitation practice (IRP). It is crucial to find accessible and appropriate ways to bring spiritual well-being into patient care in order to address the complex, whole-person experience of pain or illness.

Figure 18.1 demonstrates the various interacting domains that exist in relationship to each other in cultivating well-being. In examining the graphic, you are encouraged to consider that each sub-circle is part of the whole, as well as the reminder that the psychosocial and spiritual facets of individuals' lives are also represented by biological/ physiological substrates.

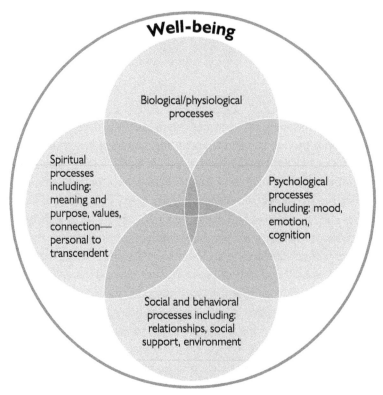

FIGURE 18.1: INTERACTING DOMAINS OF WELL-BEING

In my personal search to find ways to understand and bring the spiritual into the therapeutic space, I discovered the practice of yoga therapy. Yoga therapy integrates the wisdom teachings and practices of yoga with current scientific and biomedical thought. This perspective provided a portal through which I could shift from a more structurally based paradigm to the integrative lens of well-being. The capacity to incorporate aspects of spiritual well-being has been of immense benefit to patients as part of an integrated care model.

SPIRITUALITY IN HEALTH CARE

Spirituality can be a difficult subject to introduce into health-care settings. However, these discussions provide an important and essential foundation for change, for transformation, and to support whole-person well-being. Rather than separating and labeling spirituality as a distinct "thing," it may be helpful to weave the physical and mental health benefits as well as the themes attributed to spirituality into conversations with clients. These themes are discussed in detail in the next section and can include the patient's experience of their pain or illness and its impact on their identity, social relationships, work, life enjoyment, meaning, and purpose. Discussions of how the person can align with their personal values, meaning, and purpose through the healing process are part of these spiritually based conversations. For example, someone may want to bring qualities such as compassion, contentment, peace, or ease into their body and life. The session can then include an exploration of movements, meditations, and other practices that will help support this purpose and intention.

Ultimately, the intention within IRP is to provide an accessible, supportive environment to explore spiritual concepts in alignment with the person's perspectives, beliefs, and values. The patient is encouraged to find their own language and ways of expressing these concepts, which are then brought into the session. In order to create this accessible and patient-centered approach, it is necessary to understand the definition of spirituality and its significance for inclusion in rehabilitative therapies. This chapter begins by defining spirituality for health-care contexts. Subsequently, we will introduce the growing body of research supporting the inclusion of spirituality for improved health and well-being. Lastly, generalized ideas for the practical application of spirituality based practices in patient care will be offered.

DEFINING SPIRITUALITY

Defining spirituality, and its distinction from and/or overlap with religion, is of vital importance to its inclusion in health-care contexts. Puchalski *et al.* provide a look at both the process involved and the resultant consensus definition of spirituality from an international conference. The intention of the conference was to improve the inclusion and accessibility of the topic of spirituality in health care. The definition that came from this consensus was:

> *Spirituality* is a dynamic and intrinsic aspect of humanity through which persons seek ultimate meaning, purpose, and transcendence, and experience relationship to self, family, others, community, society, nature, and the significant or sacred. Spirituality is expressed through beliefs, values, traditions, and practices.[2]

Both this definition and other seminal research on this topic highlight common themes that are part of spiritual rather than religious teachings. Shared themes help us operationalize spirituality for health-care contexts. Themes of spirituality include the following.[3]

- **Seeking ultimate meaning and purpose**: Spiritual philosophies often support a process of inquiry into the meaning of life events and situations. This insight into meaning making from adverse life events such as pain, injury, or illness can support positive and adaptive physical, mental, and behavioral states. A sense of personal empowerment can be discovered as the individual explores meaning and purpose in response to life events. Significantly, purpose and meaning are linked to many positive health benefits, including decreased risk of all-cause mortality, improved inflammatory and immune processes, and improved function.[4] These benefits are also detailed later in the chapter.

- **Seeking relationship with the transcendent, nature, the sacred**: Certain positive psychological and behavioral attributes, such as acceptance, trust, and contentment, can be fostered through the relationship with a transcendent quality. Trust in something bigger than oneself—be it nature, energy, or an entity—can help the person find a greater sense of ease, equanimity, or contentment through hardship or adversity.

- **Relationship to self, family, others, community, society, nature, the sacred**: Spiritual teachings often emphasize and provide teachings of connectedness extending from an internal resourcing and inner wisdom—to other people, a transcendent entity, energy, or nature. Greater connectedness can support the emergence of many positive psychological and prosocial behavioral traits. There is a reciprocity between the experience of connection with oneself, others, and something greater. As one finds compassion, empathy, acceptance, and understanding for oneself, one often finds a natural expression of these positive qualities towards others, and something greater. Likewise, finding these qualities of compassion or acceptance in relationship with others, or something greater, supports these qualities in relationship to oneself.

- **Expressed through beliefs, values, traditions, and practices**: Values are often significant to spiritual teachings and include attributes such as forgiveness, patience, love, gratitude, kindness, optimism, and hope. As mentioned above, these values benefit relationships to oneself, others, and life situations by helping cultivate positive psychological and behavioral attributes and responses. Additionally, beliefs that the patient holds about oneself and their relationship to healing are important influences in the therapeutic process. We can help the person develop insight into their beliefs and values that hinder or foster greater physical, mental, or social well-being. As this discovery unfolds, the patient can find personal alignment with their beliefs and values to foster positive meaning making and a purpose-filled life for whole-person well-being.

SPIRITUALITY VERSUS RELIGION

It is important to differentiate between religion and spirituality in this therapeutic context. The research literature points to *spirituality* being defined through broader concepts such as the above ideas of meaning, purpose, and relationship with oneself, others, and the transcendent. On the other hand, *religion* is often described as a more organized system of beliefs, rituals, and symbols.[5] Religion, as distinguished from spirituality, has been examined in relationship to health with mixed results. Underscored in the research on religion is the need to focus on person-centered care where the patient self-selects the concepts that are relevant to them and directs how religious concepts are best articulated and integrated into care.[6] On the other hand, there are many benefits of spiritual well-being, which are detailed below, after a discussion on what can be termed "secular spirituality."

SECULAR SPIRITUALITY: EUDAIMONIA AND EUDAIMONIC WELL-BEING

In exploring concepts that dovetail into the broad concept of spirituality and to continue to differentiate spirituality from a discussion of religion, it may be useful to work with a secular terminology. "Eudaimonia" and "eudaimonic well-being" are terms that provide an accessible platform to discuss spiritual themes with both patients and other health-care professionals—and offer a more secular perspective.

Eudaimonia is a teaching from Aristotle that suggests everything has an ultimate, or final, purpose, aim, or goal. When the ultimate aim or goal of a "thing" is fulfilled then it is actualizing its purpose and the highest expression of itself. For example, the ultimate aim of a desk is to provide a stable surface for work including writing or reading. When a desk fulfills these needs, it has fulfilled its optimal expression and goal. Translating this to humans, a person who has achieved eudaimonia would be one who has fulfilled their greatest purpose—they are living "excellently," and flourishing. For each person this can be very different, but it is the fulfillment and actualizing of one's purpose that brings them to the realization of eudaimonia.

Aristotle differentiated two types of happiness—eudaimonic and hedonic. *Eudaimonic happiness* is a steadfast expression of contentment and joy. This non-fluctuating form of happiness is not always related to short-term pleasure and comfort, but provides a more lasting expression akin to contentment. *Hedonic happiness*, on the other hand, is transitory and linked to short-term comforts that may not always relate to long-term flourishing or well-being. In the research literature, the definition of eudaimonic well-being parallels many of the above-mentioned themes of spirituality, including:[7]

- meaning and purpose
- personal connectedness through concepts of authenticity and personal expressiveness
- promotion of ethical principles and values
- meaningful social relationships
- existential connections through concepts such as self-realization or self-actualization.

In a moment, we will look at the health benefits of both spiritual and eudaimonic well-being and explore their significance for inclusion in health-care contexts. However, it is helpful to first emphasize the importance of eudaimonic well-being as a way to increase the accessibility for introducing spiritual themes in discussions with patients, students, and rehabilitation and medical professionals.

The capacity to introduce any aspect of eudaimonic and spiritual well-being through the lens of secular spirituality has been beneficial in introducing these ideas to patients, as well as in professional presentations and exchanges with colleagues. Introducing spirituality through Aristotle's ideas and terminology decreases the potential stigma or resistance to discussing spirituality. The person is then able to both relate to and become engaged in finding their own expression of these concepts of spirituality and eudaimonic well-being. Because eudaimonia allows these topics to be discussed without words like "spirituality," there is no added pressure or potential barrier around individual religious expression. Some patients will bring up religious practices to help connect to these ideas, while others find more secular practices to work with these themes of spirituality or eudaimonic well-being.

RATIONALE FOR THE INCLUSION OF SPIRITUALITY AND EUDAIMONIA IN HEALTH CARE

A growing body of research supports the importance of spiritual well-being (as defined by the above themes of purpose and meaning; values; and connectedness from personal, interpersonal, transcendent) for improved physical and mental health including:[8]

- improved experience of pain in terms of decreased severity and sensitivity, as well as improved tolerance
- improved coping and adjustment to persistent pain and illness
- improved quality of life
- improved symptoms of anxiety and depression
- improved systemic physical health including cardiovascular, endocrine, and immune
- decreased mortality
- improved quality of social relationships and social support.[9]

Eudaimonic well-being, including the component measure of *meaning and purpose*, has also been linked to many positive health benefits including:[10]

- decreased all-cause mortality, independent of factors such as age, race, gender, physical inactivity, and chronic conditions, including cardiovascular disease, cancer, or stroke
- improved inflammatory and immune processes, including mitigating the negative physiological effect of perceived social isolation on these processes
- improved overall well-being and function with pain conditions
- lower levels of fatigue, disability, pain intensity, and pain medication use; improved well-being, function, adjustment to chronic pain, and depressive symptoms
- less amygdala activation and more engagement of higher cortical structures, which may demonstrate an improved capacity for greater discernment to transform habitual reactions to more constructive behaviors.

These significant systemic physical, psychological, and social health outcomes of spiritual and eudaimonic well-being demonstrate their importance for inclusion in health-care contexts. Moreover, as many of the component measures and benefits are shared between spiritual and eudaimonic well-being, the latter may provide an accessible language to help people understand spiritual concepts outside of a religious context. This ability to use secular language enables and empowers the patient to choose the direction and application of these concepts. Understanding these concepts and their health benefits has been immensely helpful in articulating these ideas to many different patient populations and health-care/medical professionals.

SPIRITUAL AND EUDAIMONIC WELL-BEING IN REHABILITATIVE CARE

There are many ways to introduce spiritual and eudaimonic themes that are independent of religious traditions or practices. Noted earlier, as these themes are introduced, some clients will offer religious practices which have helped them to integrate these ideas into the intervention. There are many other useful forms of contemplation, inquiry, and meditation to address these themes in a more secular manner. For some, their choice may be either/or—sticking with existing practices or learning more generic ones as part of care; for others, there is a both/and experience. As such, flexibility to be present to, learn about, understand, and support all experiences and choices remains the backdrop.

Significant to this discussion is research demonstrating a difference in effect between meditations that include a spiritual foundation and those that do not. Spiritually based meditations have greater effectiveness for decreasing frequency of migraine headaches, anxiety, and negative affect, and increasing pain tolerance, positive mood, self-efficacy in coping with headaches, and existential well-being when compared with non-spiritual meditation or relaxation.[11]

Many contemplative and spirituality based wisdom traditions have emerged throughout history and offer paths and practices to help foster such qualities as healthier relationships to oneself, including: greater authenticity and personal connection to body, mind, and identity; improved social relationships; sense of existential or transcendent connection; a meaningful and purpose-filled life; development of positive psychological and prosocial qualities through ethical principles. Mind-body contemplative practices, such as yoga, offer a valuable resource as a spiritual intervention, as they integrate spiritual care with physical activity, mental-based practices, and meaningful social connection. Next, we will look at some practices that can help prime the person for these qualities of spiritual and eudaimonic well-being.

As we explore these practices, it is important to emphasize an open and process-driven approach to weaving spirituality into the therapeutic space. As a foundation, we will look at the promotion of positive psychological and prosocial behavioral attributes through virtue ethics and ethical inquiry. Then we will explore the development of personal connectedness to one's body, mind, and identity for greater authenticity and inner resourcing. This will be followed by discussions of integrating meaning and purpose, existential and transcendent connection, and improved social relationships.

As we go through these we will integrate examples of how to work with these ideas in the above case study. My vehicle for these learnings has been yoga therapy and that is the lens I offer for these practices.

YOGA THERAPY

Yoga therapy is a spiritually based mind-body practice that is innately built upon an integrative perspective.[12] Yoga's philosophical foundation and its relationship to eudaimonic well-being were explored in a recent paper.[13] This explanatory framework for yoga therapy describes how the development of discriminative wisdom, and work with ethical principles such as kindness or contentment, enables the person to find a renewed sense of meaning and purpose—positive connection to themselves, others, and life situations. The result is the realization of eudaimonic well-being and lessening or alleviation of suffering. Spiritual well-being is attained as individuals discover healthy and adaptive connections with themselves—such as greater authenticity and an improved relationship to their body-mind-environment (BME) and their sense of identity within that experience. In addition, relationships with others are strengthened, resulting in more meaningful social connections. Finally, greater existential/transcendental connections are formed as the person finds a renewed sense of a meaningful and purpose-filled life.

The inclusion of yoga as a practice to foster spiritual well-being may be advantageous for many reasons. First, it is a popular practice that is both perceived and used as a complementary health practice by the general population.[14] Second, research on yoga demonstrates the importance of including the spiritual, philosophical, and ethical components for health benefits.[15] When compared with yoga as solely physical exercise, the inclusion of its spiritual foundations has demonstrated increased positive health effects, including: greater psychological well-being such as meaning in life; fewer depressive symptoms; greater mindfulness; heightened positive effect on anxiety levels.[16] Lastly, researchers reveal that the public recognizes yoga as a spiritual practice and, while people may often start the practice for physical reasons, these spiritual aspects are reported as motivators for continued practice and adherence.[17] The potential for the spiritual components to help promote continued participation in physical activity for populations experiencing persistent pain conditions is an interesting potential added benefit to the practice of yoga.

Inherent to the definition of yoga therapy by the International Association of Yoga Therapists is that it is a process of empowering individuals. It is therefore imperative for these intentions to be offered in a manner that honors, respects, and builds upon the patient's values, needs, and perspectives. In other words, this process of incorporating spiritual themes and intentions is not therapist driven, rather it is a patient-led exploration. For those interested in further exploring the landscape of the growing yoga therapy profession, we have committed a full chapter to the topic in Section Three of our journey (Chapter 24).

PRACTICAL APPLICATION: ETHICAL INQUIRY

Both spiritual teachings and contemplative traditions include an emphasis on the development of certain values, ethical attributes, or positive psychological qualities, such as: love, hope, awe, joy, optimism, forgiveness, honesty, gratefulness, patience, humility, and compassion.[18] A starting place for working with spirituality is through inquiry and contemplation on values and ethical principles, as they are foundational to many of the other aspects of spiritual and eudaimonic well-being. For example, asking clients about intentions for their sessions and providing examples such as contentment, patience, acceptance, and compassion is useful. The intentions become points of focus for practices such as meditation, contemplation, and journaling. This allows the client to have an opportunity to consider a value that would be important for them to foster through their healing journey. This patient-led ethical inquiry provides practical steps and a foundation from which to move into other topics of spiritual and eudaimonic well-being such as: meaning, purpose, and personal, interpersonal, existential (or transcendent) connection.

Reflection, inquiry, and contemplation on any ethical principle or value can provide insight into the roots of suffering and facilitate change and transformation towards the alleviation of suffering. The person may find a shift in their perspective and relationship to oneself, others, and life circumstances. This process can result in:

- an improved personal connectedness for greater authenticity and self-understanding
- greater patience, compassion, and tolerance of others in promotion of more meaningful social relationships
- the facilitation of meaning making such as the positive reappraisal of life circumstance for a more purpose-filled life.

An example practice that underscores this work is Aristotle's golden mean. In this practice the person reflects on any ethical virtue, such as forgiveness. The person contemplates any excess or deficiency of this virtue in their life. In the case of forgiveness, a deficiency might be the inability to understand, have compassion for, or absolve any wrong-doing. An excess might be seen in a premature forgiveness where the person does not adequately stand up for their needs or does not create healthy boundaries of safety for the relationship or situation. It could also be seen in the tendency to instantly forgive everything—a form of maladaptive coping that may unconsciously be reinforcing avoidance of certain emotions, challenges, or experiences. Each person decides where the middle ground of the virtue of forgiveness is found in their life. Once that is discerned, the person needs to consider their own nature and where they fall on the continuum to see what needs to happen to find the middle.

Looking at Yoshi from our opening story, we worked with the ethical virtues of contentment and acceptance in relationship to her experience of pain and resultant inability to participate in activity as she would have liked. An excess of contentment or acceptance might be seen in her not taking any action to help her pain or to help her function in the activities in which she wanted to participate. The deficiency might be seen in excessive worry or anxiety with an inability to find ease in the situation. Yoshi reported a tendency towards the deficiency, as she became worried and anxious when pain arose about what might happen, how bad it might become, what she needed to do, and the potential loss of work or enjoyable activity. She noticed how these anxious and worried thoughts and emotions created even more tension in her body and resultant loss of function. Over time, she developed the ability to inquire into the felt sensations of her body and mind to discern what was needed in that moment. She developed insight into her body-mind sensations as she learned to listen to her body and mind and honor what was needed. As a result, she found her body and mind carried less stress, her anxiety lessened, and her pain did not last as long and did not interfere in her life activities. She was soon able to rejoin and participate in activities with less loss of function. You may recognize that this process, entered into through the lens of ethical inquiry, is similar to the processes of Acceptance and Commitment Therapy as described in the last chapter. Shared and overlapping themes become more apparent as we explore integrative care constructs and models. These kinds of parallels and similarities between integrative models speak to shared truths and substrates of human experience that we can support consciously when we are informed, as well as practice in the application of these principles with our own journeys.

> **Experiential pause:** Ethical inquiry
>
> 1. Take a virtue or ethical principle such as compassion, forgiveness, patience, kindness, gratefulness, gratitude, hope, or another that comes to mind that brings meaning for you.
> 2. Consider the excess and deficiency of this virtue. Create clarity for the continuum of excess → middle → deficiency for this ethical principle.
> 3. Reflect on your own nature along this continuum. Write down your insights followed by your responses to the following questions.
>   - How does this quality, and your nature on the continuum, show up in the relationship you have to your body, your mind, your state of health and wellness—or its opposite?
>   - How does this show up in your relationship with others?
>   - How does this show up in relationship to your life circumstance?
>   - If you were to develop the mean of this virtue in each of these relationships (to yourself, others, life), what practices might you create?

PRACTICAL APPLICATION: PERSONAL CONNECTEDNESS, INNER WISDOM, AND AUTHENTICITY

Developing greater personal connectedness, inner wisdom, and authenticity is a natural next step from working with ethical inquiry. Through reflection on ethical qualities, the person gains insight into the values that are important and meaningful to them. This enables a greater self-understanding and personal connectedness, facilitating greater self-confidence, self-surety, and authenticity as the person learns to live and express themselves in alignment with these values and attributes. For example, a person may choose to explore the attribute of kindness. Through this process they learn what kindness means in their relationship with their body, thoughts, emotions, beliefs, relationships, and life situations. Over time, the person finds an authenticity in how they express themselves in the world through this value of kindness.

Both movement (see Chapter 15 for review) and body-based meditations (see Chapter 12 for review) can combine with ethical inquiry to foster this personal connectedness, self-confidence, and self-understanding. Meditations such as body scans are helpful in facilitating positive and non-reactive connections and relationships to bodily sensations. Bringing ethical qualities and attributes into these practices supports one's relationship to one's body for positive personal connection. Movement also reflects a particularly powerful methodology to cultivate positive attributes such as self-confidence and inner trust, and to challenge negative beliefs. For example, using movement to find a sense of strength to challenge the mind's belief of being weak, or finding a bodily sense of peace or calm to help the person see that this is a possible experience for them. The portal of bodily experience offers a potent experience to actualize this positive personal connection and greater self-confidence and self-understanding, and supports the larger backdrop of IRP—exploring our experience of mind as fully embodied.[19]

In reflecting back once again on Yoshi, we worked with finding ways to connect to bodily sensation in a safe and positive manner. She was interested in the qualities of kindness and acceptance. We found restorative, comfortable, supportive postures where she could spend time experiencing these qualities in her body. She explored what kindness meant to her and what the physical sensations of kindness would be in her body. Over time, she found that when she was actualizing this quality her body felt light, spacious, and open. She was able to then find ways to be in alignment with this value within life situations. Sometimes this meant creating boundaries, saying "no" to certain activities, or finding times to rest. Ultimately, she became proficient at assessing her bodily sensations in any moment and experienced greater self-confidence and self-understanding in expressing her needs.

Experiential pause: Body inquiry for personal expressivity, connectedness, and authenticity

1. Find a comfortable position—this could be laying down, sitting, or standing.
2. Notice the outline of the body and then go through each body part—head, face, jaw and mouth, throat, neck, shoulders and arms…left and right…, the chest and middle back, the abdomen and lower back, the pelvis, hips and legs…left and right—simply noticing the quality of sensation—heavy/light; fluid/rigid; light/dark; warm/cool; constricted/open, and so on… You may want to start at the crown of your head and work down to your feet or at your feet and work up to the top of your head.
3. Bring an intention that you are working with—this may be the ethical principle

you worked with in the above activity, or a new one. Notice how the quality of this principle (such as kindness, openness, acceptance) is located, is felt… in your body—is it light/heavy; spacious/compact; bright/dark? Come back to the body scan and bring this quality into each part of your body—offering the sensation from the crown of your head to your feet. Where is this easier or harder to do?

4. Imagine what it would be like to go through your day, talk to others, and relate to yourself from this quality in your body. As you go through your day, notice when you are in alignment with this quality, when you veer away, and how you can come back to this quality.

PRACTICAL APPLICATION: MEANING, PURPOSE, AND SELF-ACTUALIZATION

Two teachings on meaning and purpose may be helpful in developing strategies to bring these concepts forward to clients. *Dharma*, a foundational concept in yogic teachings, has a complex meaning that includes the notion of a *harmonious expression of right action*. Rather than a static concept, dharma is a process whereby one's actions may be in various degrees of alignment with one's inner authentic nature and with the outer world. This includes in relationship with others and with nature and the physical environment, such that all are supported in their optimal flourishing. Dharma is very much aligned with Aristotle's concept of eudaimonia, where a path of right action guided by the virtue ethics leads towards the actualization of one's full potential. Viktor Frankl in *Man's Search for Meaning* adds that meaning is important to the alleviation of suffering, it must be found in the world rather than isolation, and be a tangible, non-abstract concept in order for it to be constructive.[20]

These teachings offer us ways to discuss and describe topics of meaning and purpose and consider how to apply these in relation to ourselves and our particular life circumstances. Discussions on meaning and purpose are natural outgrowths of working with ethical attributes and personal connectedness.

Yoshi reflected on how she felt when she experienced the resonance of connection to herself, to her relationships, and in her life activities. She experienced this connection as an expansion and lightness in her body, a brightness and calm in her mind, and a fluidity in her relationship with her environment and actions in the world. We found physical postures, movements, and mind-body experiences that helped to strengthen the feelings of expansion, lightness, brightness, calm, and fluidity. We also worked with affirmations and visualizations to strengthen these experiences. She learned to notice when she was veering away from these feelings through her choices, thoughts, emotions, and activities and became able to use this to reinforce and move back towards what brought her mind and body to these states of expansion, calm, and fluidity.

PRACTICAL APPLICATION: EXISTENTIAL OR TRANSCENDENT CONNECTION

Topics such as transcendent/existential connection can seem like rather esoteric concepts to bring up in therapeutic settings. In working with ethical inquiry, personal connectedness, or meaning and purpose, the topic of existential/transcendent connection will often naturally arise. For example, working with intentions of trust, allowing, or acceptance will often lead into an idea of transcendent/existential connection—or can be an entry point for exploration. Possibility exists for using established practices or co-creating new ones that help cultivate connection to something greater and/or to foster attributes such as trust or acceptance.

One client might use a passage from the *New Testament* that brought her an experience of greater ease, as well as a sense of meaning, purpose, and transcendent connection. Another client might use the cycles of the natural world and nature visualizations to help realize a sense of trust, allowing, and connection to something greater. These practices are supported in scientific research as potentially contributing to processes of health and well-being.[21] Whether the connection is a transcendent energy or entity, or an existential connectedness to life, it serves to provide an experience of trust, allowing, and acceptance to benefit the person in their current situation. This can create a positive reappraisal of the situation, and can provide positive meaning making to help foster a sense of purpose within any facet of one's circumstances and experience in general.

> **Experiential pause:** Meditation for transcendental/existential connection
>
> Find a comfortable position sitting or lying down. Your eyes can be softly open or closed. Briefly scan the body to notice if you might adjust to become more comfortable. Allow the breath to be easeful and soft.
>
> What might it mean to you to connect to something greater—nature, the universe, something transcendent? Do you already have an image, feeling, word, or sensation that encapsulates that connection? If it helps, you can use the concepts of trusting, allowing, or accepting to notice what images or feelings arise that might help to experience this kind of connection. Take a moment to allow the felt sensations of this to become stronger and notice if an image or affirmation arises. Examples that you might try: "I am connected to all that surrounds me," "The world holds me in safety," "I trust and allow the cycles of life to move through me," "I am part of the cycles of life." Stay in this experience for a few moments, noticing when your attention wanders, and simply bringing it back. Consider journaling about this experience.

PRACTICAL APPLICATION: MEANINGFUL SOCIAL CONNECTION AND SOCIAL SUPPORT

Meaningful social relationships have been found to have significant positive physical and mental health effects. One of the most extensive studies on this topic, the Harvard Grant and Glueck study, found that good relationships keep us healthier and happier, and are a predictor of successful aging, independent of variables such as smoking, alcohol use, exercise, BMI, and education.[22] This study, in addition to others, demonstrates the many significant adverse health effects of perceived social isolation. This includes a negative effect on both inflammatory and immune processes contributing to cardiovascular, autoimmune, neurological disease states, and cancers.[23] Researchers demonstrate the importance of meaningful relationships, social support, and connection of any kind (e.g., pets) for longer, happier, and healthier lives.

Social and spiritual well-being are intertwined, as meaningful social relationships are part of the themes and constructs embedded within spiritual well-being scales. Additionally, the positive psychological and prosocial attributes emphasized by spiritual traditions, such as compassion, forgiveness, and patience, help to strengthen positive relationships.

For clients, including Yoshi, compassion or loving-kindness meditations have been beneficial for moving through an exploration of ethical inquiry, into personal connectedness, meaning/purpose, existential connection, and finally to that of fostering meaningful social connection. These meditations are often taught by saying the intention to oneself and then others. However, for some it may be difficult to offer these intentions to oneself as it can feel forced or fake. For this reason, it can help to start by sending the intention to a loved one or animal first and later move it towards oneself.

Experiential pause: Compassion meditation

There are many ways to do compassion meditation. This one is adapted from different teachers. With practice, you may create your own unique variations.

1. Find a comfortable position either lying down or sitting. The eyes can be softly open or closed. Scan the body, noticing if there are any parts that might find a little more comfort. Allow the breath to be easeful and soft.
2. Picture a person or animal with whom you feel a positive connection. Notice the feeling of that positive connection in your body. Offer the following intention to this person or animal: "May you be happy. May you be healthy. May you be free of suffering. May you find peace."
3. Picture all of the people you know and feel close to and again feel the positive connection in your body. Repeat the same intention to all of these positive connections.
4. Picture anyone you may have difficulty with or a difficult situation and extend this intention to this person or situation.
5. Finally, picture yourself, noticing what it is like to feel that positive connection in your body, and offer this same intention to yourself. Consider journaling about this experience.

CONCLUSION

The importance of the biopsychosocialspiritual approach, person-centered care, and shared decision making is becoming more apparent in current perspectives on health care. The spiritual domain of health is of interest, as it is supportive of physical, mental, and social health and well-being. Working with spiritual concepts necessitates a person-centered and shared decision-making approach, as it requires recognition and emphasis of each person's unique needs and values for integration into intervention approaches. The concept of eudaimonic well-being is beneficial for this conversation, as it opens the discussion into a secular spirituality. This enables the practitioner to meet the patient where they are and to allow the concepts to become intrinsic to the patient's own experience. Working with spiritual and eudaimonic well-being includes: practices of ethical inquiry to explore the client's needs, beliefs, and values; the cultivation of personal connectedness for greater authenticity, personal resourcing, self-understanding, and self-expression; meaning making and purpose; existential and/or transcendent connection; promotion of quality, meaningful social relationships.

Experiential pause: Having read this chapter, identify and write down at least one actionable item of interest to you. In doing so, consider ways in which applying the material first to yourself, and then to patients, might serve those who come to you for care.

RESOURCES

- The University of Minnesota Center for Spirituality and Healing: www.csh.umn.edu.

- Institute for Spirituality and Health at the Texas Medical Center: www.spiritualityandhealth.org.

- The Greater Good Science Center at the University of California, Berkeley: https://greatergood.berkeley.edu.

- Mind and Life Institute: www.mindandlife.org.

- To explore a forgiveness meditation: https://jackkornfield.com/forgiveness-meditation.

- To explore gratitude practices, the Yale Center for Emotional Intelligence: https://ei.yale.edu/what-is-gratitude.

- Kristin Neff's self-compassion exercises: https://self-compassion.org/category/exercises.

CHAPTER 19

Avenues of Expression

Dena Rain Adler, BEd, MA, ATR

A story: I was teaching a graduate art therapy class and discovered that one of my students, "Luna," had a lifelong natural practice of using the arts as a form of self-expression and reflection. She entered the program with a background in art and graphic design. Luna deeply connected to using the process of art as therapy. She spoke of her life history and the effects of trauma from being a survivor of child sexual abuse and growing up in a home with a step-parent who was a veteran who suffered from PTSD and alcoholism. Luna described her saving graces throughout her childhood as coming from writing, drawing, and reading. Later in life, she endured grief and loss from a tragic death of a beloved friend. Luna described periods in her life where she eased her pain with substance use. During the course of the art therapy graduate program, Luna was also diagnosed with bipolar disorder. She tried numerous medications; however, due to severe side effects, she and her psychiatrist worked together to implement an integrative care plan that included a multifaceted approach. This approach embraced a process-oriented lens, as well as reinforced innate wholeness and capacity. Luna described her creative process, visuals, and narrative as essential elements for her overall health and well-being. One of her nightly rituals was to write in her journal with a quick sketch as a way of: "clearing her mind before sleeping." She shared that her starting point began by following either a word, a line, or a shape. From there, she expressed and explored with curiosity and intention, giving shape to her inner voice.

Since the beginning of time, expressive-creative arts have been used universally to give voice and visual images to life's beauty and chaos. Ceremonies and rituals involving healing arts were used globally by shamans and communities in indigenous cultures. In the field of expressive therapies, imagination is viewed as a fundamental phenomenon of human existence and as having the innate ability to transform human suffering.[1] In the transformative process, creative expression leads individuals to opportunities for ways to find wellness.[2] The gift we all share, from our first breath and first scribble, is our innate ability to express ourselves. This chapter invites all to walk the path of an artist; the artist, unofficially and simply defined as one who expresses oneself through a medium.

There are times, however, when we may struggle to express what we feel. Stress, pain, trauma, or sociocultural conditioning are examples of dynamics that can lead to the suppression of self-expression. There are various avenues that carry potential to open up or deepen our capacity for expression.

Drawing, as means of creative self-expression, is one such avenue that provides us with a form and space to become more aware of what we know and do not yet know. Similarly, writing uses words as form and space, providing us with a contemplative strategy to enhance our processes of becoming and knowing. From simple drawings to writing, a portrait takes shape by painting a personal story of an individual's thoughts, feelings, and physical experiences. This process invites opportunities to find alternative ways to look and listen to what is experienced and felt within—on emotional, physical, cognitive, and spiritual levels. Within the message or image lies the capacity for integrating life's experiences and challenges into our lives. It is at this place where pain, fear, loss, and angst meet acceptance, self-efficacy, and hope. The essence of creative modalities is that they may enlighten the search for understanding the vastness of our human condition.

The visual and narrative methods are avenues for self-expression and self-awareness that play an important role within the scope of integrative rehabilitative practice (IRP). The expressive process supports compassion and understanding from the voices of the patient, providers, family members, caregivers, and the community as a whole. The arts have been described as a natural resource, often underutilized, that reflect clarity of the patient's narrative of the pain experience and the suffering felt within the soul.[3] With continued research into the mind-body connection and developments in the field of neuroscience,[4] the healing journey becomes grounded in our understanding of how expressive-creative processes can support overall psychosocial and functional health and well-being.[5]

LUNA'S PROCESS

Luna's life experience offers insight into the ways in which various *avenues of expression* can be woven into rehabilitation practice. The excerpt below is from Luna's journal, created at a transitional time upon entering graduate school. This excerpt includes a drawing (Figure 19.1) that Luna made to accompany her words, reflecting the use of creative self-expression for supporting the learning process in becoming a health-care practitioner. The excerpt also reflects the personal search for hope, healing, and well-being. In her journal entry, Luna humbly describes the learning and healing process needed for one's professional role. Emotional development and self-compassion for both the patient and the provider connect us on the same path of the meaningful search for self-awareness.

> **Experiential pause:** Take a few moments to be in the role of "bearing witness" to the created picture and words. Let your eyes look slowly over the two figures; move your eyes from left to right and bottom to top. Note the feelings and words that arise and resonate within you as you look at the sketch and read the journal entry. Then, consider using your own journal to sketch or write about your own process.

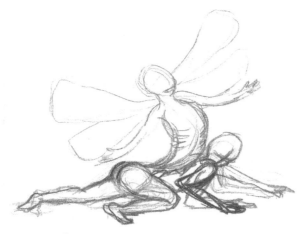

FIGURE 19.1: LUNA'S SPONTANEOUS FREE SKETCH AND JOURNAL ENTRY

I look forward to this time not only to learn, but to heal the wounded healer. I choose to immerse myself into this program—its teachings & experiences—to break myself apart, to slough off all the deadweight I've accumulated these past 36 years, and emerge anew, raw wounds & all, not necessarily healed, but healing. I know my own failures, mistakes and shortcomings will be of assistance to me, and them, for I have traveled many dark roads thus far, and will be able to recognize many journeys. Will it be enough? I know as I search to heal my own soul, I will cross the paths of other wounded seekers, regardless [of] the forum of our intersections, and we will both learn, and travel onward...

On the day that Luna received word of the bipolar diagnosis, she walked into the art therapy studio and gravitated toward the first objects she saw—a large coffee can and a mound of clay. Rooted in her felt sense, she took her time, kneading and working the clay. It became a vehicle to shape and form the rising images of her thoughts and feelings. She created a drum out of her clay sculpture (Figure 19.2) and described this as her symbol of "connection to the earth." Since that day, Luna speaks openly of the challenges of living with mood swings and the physical difficulties she experienced with medication. The drum is displayed in a sacred spot in Luna's art studio and symbolizes acceptance and resiliency of nature's rhythms.

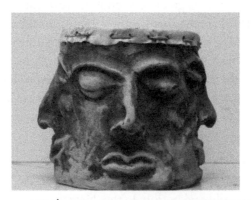

FIGURE 19.2: LUNA'S CREATION OF A DRUM AND JOURNAL ENTRY

One thing I can appreciate about myself is my ability to be fully joyful and fully depressed & and that I do not have to apologize for either. I am a person who swings to the extremes, it is who I am. The last two weeks the pendulum is swinging high, the last 6 months it was very low. I just hang on & go for the ride, wherever I go...

Contemporary history of therapeutic self-expression

Pioneers, pain, and passion

Brazilian psychiatrist Nise da Silveira (1905–1999) was a pioneer in the development of creative, expressive therapies. As reflected in the docudrama *Nise: The Heart of Madness*, Dr. da Silveira devoted her life to helping others heal from stress, adversity, and trauma. Silveira had an innate sense of compassion and integrity as she joined patients who were isolated and lost in their inner worlds. Her creative methods pioneered a path for integrative mental health treatment and policies. Vitor Pordeus, MD, described Silveira's work as advancing a: "deeply humanistic approach to understanding and working with patients."[6]

After becoming a psychiatrist in 1926, Silveira became a political prisoner for having books on communism and spent eight years in exile. In those years of exclusion, she delved into the work of Baruch Spinoza and developed an integrative philosophical perspective that changed her views on psychiatry and her own sense of self.[7] Upon her return to work in a psychiatric institution, Silveira resisted the trial procedures of electroconvulsive therapy (ECT) and lobotomies. As a result, she was sent to work in an old, unused area of the hospital that had been used for occupational therapy and was full of art materials. Silveira adapted the art activities by inviting patients to engage freely in self-directed creative expression and began to witness the healing and unconscious process of art and creativity. In 1946, Silveira created the Museum of Images of the Unconscious, honoring the patients' illustrations of their deepest feelings, traumas, and visions. The museum, located in Rio de Janeiro, continues to thrive as a research center for integrative mind-body health and has an archive of over 360,000 artworks.

Pordeus shared Silveira's words and perception of holistic treatment and the potentiality of the arts to bridge meaning and understanding:

> I can't conceive how it would be possible to make contact with a man or woman, and treat them, by whatever method, without having at least an idea of how this person is living in time and space, without hearing about the strange thoughts that come to him and the images that overwhelm his mind. One of the less difficult pathways to access the internal world…is to give him the opportunity to draw, paint or sculpt with all freedom.[8]

From a similar but different lens, the renowned artist Frida Kahlo (1907–1954) also serves as a source of inspiration to others to persevere with life's adversities and health challenges. The world has an intimate look into her life story, as she poured her emotional and physical pain and trauma into her artwork. Kahlo suffered throughout her life, first after contracting poliomyelitis in childhood, and then as a survivor of a devastating streetcar accident that resulted in significant damage to her spinal column and pelvic organs. Kahlo's paintings, "Broken Column" (1944) and "Henry Ford Hospital" (1932), illustrate the depth of her vulnerability, authenticity, and resiliency.

In the health-care community, Kahlo's life and artwork has been used to encourage patients to express their lived experience of pain and helped providers to find authentic ways to better understand the experience of pain from the patient's perspective.[9] A group of physical therapists created an exploratory inquiry into Kahlo's pain history and artwork.

They noted how looking inquisitively at the imagery and symbols increased their awareness of how pain is experienced. Their investigation highlighted how this may impact their role as health-care providers who are searching for alternative ways to prevent or reduce patient suffering and the need to integrate care in a holistic and skilled manner.[10]

Luna's practice of art and writing exhibits the use of the expressive-creative process for healing and self-care and illustrates how it may be used to support personal and professional growth. It is significant that Luna saves all her artwork, poetry, and journals, as this shows how they can become a visual narrative of a life journey, deepening self-awareness by seeing and noting change over time.

In Luna's painting and words below (Figure 19.3), the affirming life message expressed is how we can find ways to live in greater balance in times of darkness and calm. Luna shares her art pieces and life story with the restorative hope that others are inspired to dabble or delve with these forms of expression, especially as a way of searching for meaning with and through shadows, pain, and life hardships.

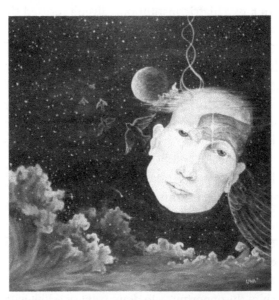

FIGURE 19.3: LUNA'S ACRYLIC PAINTING AND PERSONAL REFLECTION OF SYMBOLS
The moon watches beside me in the dark, my constant witness and protector. Birds are flying away into the night, as if they were able to break free and escape, and the DNA strand has me connected to the Universe, which for me indicates a very spiritual sense of connection. This painting to me has more elements of the battle I most often feel of my depression vs the healing presence of my higher spiritual self. The painting has a dark feeling to it, but also a sense of calmness to me.

THE ARTS IN HEALTH CARE

Over the past 50 years, the therapeutic use of creative modalities has developed into professional organizations and associations with certification and credentialing programs for each course of study. These include: art therapy, expressive arts therapy, creative arts therapies, music therapy (see Chapter 21), drama therapy, and poetry therapy. A shared perspective in these associations is that they embrace the arts as an aspect of integrative health care. As the fields are recognized for their contributions, the emphasis on evidence-based research and trauma-informed care has increased.

The use of arts in health care and in medicine programs is included in many hospitals and community-based wellness centers. In 2015, the National Organization for Arts in Health was established. In a 2017 paper, NOAH highlighted all of the creative arts therapies as significant therapeutic interventions as well as art-based programs facilitated by artists and art educators that support:

- prevention and management of illness and chronic disease
- improving patient experience
- humanizing the health-care environment
- developing empathy and compassion for the overall well-being of the patients, the caregivers, and the professional community.[11]

From a public health perspective, the growing concern around prevalence and burden of chronic disease and associated psychosocial difficulties (see Chapters 3 and 4) links to the growing investigation of relationships between the arts and health. This line of inquiry underscores the need for the expressive arts to be part of whole-person approaches to sustain health and wellness.[12]

PROCESSES OF SELF-EXPRESSION AND SELF-AWARENESS

Consider the following: "Artistic expression leads to mindfulness, mindfulness leads to creative anxiety, creative anxiety leads to change and action, change and action foster expression, and expression deepens mindfulness."[13] What does this imply?

> **Experiential pause:** Reread the preceding quote several times. How do you respond to this quote? What, if any, meaning does it carry for you? How does this quote tie in to preceding chapters and topics, such as creative wisdom (Chapter 2) or mindfulness (Chapter 12)? Jot down your response, even if it is one of judgment or confusion. Consider drawing or sketching a picture of the feelings and sensations that arise in response to this quote. Consider any relevance this quote might have in relationship to approaching rehabilitation as part of larger individual and collective processes.

Much like taking a photograph, creative expressions capture the present moment in a mindful way. An example of this is reflected in "Joe" who, in the midst of high stress, doubt, and self-criticism during graduate school, chose to use poetry for the first time as an expressive outlet. As a science major, Joe was encouraged to explore "uncertainty." Within a few short lines, he was able to view a self-created alternative way of looking at things—moving from "uncertainty" to "curiosity." Joe shared that the poetry supported a shift from the constant inner critic monologue of his worried mind and anxiety. Joe later shared that the poems he had written had brought about change and action in his family as well, deepening connections and healing from shared life stories.

The creative process engages the individual in the act of creating, destructing, reshaping, exploring, and searching for personal meaning making. The path may be seen as spiraling rather than linear. Making space to hold "creative anxiety" may be metaphorically envisioned with the paper or canvas acting as the framework to provide a safety measure in the process of healing. It is here, in this creative space, where the capacity to hold space for tension, fear, or anxiety of the unknown is generated. For most, experiencing a health challenge of any kind weighs heavily on one's sense of spirit or being. Self-expression is a way of externalizing the unconscious. It may open up new ways to vision life situations, as well as healthier means to manage the pain, distress, or suffering that one is experiencing. Pain, be it physical, mental, or emotional, has potential to become a teacher, guide, or messenger in navigating both our inner and outer worlds. The creation of words, images, or objects is not a destination. Rather, in process we can work and rework expressed images and symbols over time.

The self-inquiry process uses elements of creative expression as healing agents to cultivate awareness, acceptance, and the potential for change. As inner thoughts and feelings move towards expression, they may be processed internally and/or may move outward into some form, such as emoting, verbalizing, moving, and more. In relation to our exploration at hand, the avenues of drawing, art creation, or writing reflect mediums that support expression. However, for many, beginning with a blank slate (piece of paper, writing instruments, crayons, or other supplies) can be intimidating. Often, the first response when encouraged to write or draw is feeling not creative enough or not good enough. It is important to acknowledge that this dynamic may arise and emphasize that there is no prerequisite to use the arts as an avenue of self-expression. Shaun McNiff, one of the founding "grandfathers" in the field of creative arts therapies, explains that the skill required for creative expression is the ability to respond with spontaneity, self-compassion, and sensitivity to inner judgments. His guiding premise is to trust the process.[14]

The process of trusting and letting go opens up space for authentic self-expression. If in a stressed or tense state, meaningful engagement with oneself or others may be restricted.[15] Building on this understanding, authentic self-expression may be supported by regulation and relaxation response training, such as those that come through many of the mind-body techniques found elsewhere in this book.

Learning how to respond to what is created develops self-awareness. It is a gradual process that gives time for the emergence of self-discovery where feelings and thoughts are identified and named. From a phenomenological framework of therapeutic expression, this process has been described as: "looking in order to see"—seeing intentionally.[16]

As artwork and writings are shared, with one person or collectively in wider communities, the meaning-making process has reciprocal benefits. The dialogue spoken about the artistic expression lies within a triangular relationship made up of the creator, the art form, and the viewer or witness. In a health-care relationship, the need arises for patients to find their voice and for providers to learn how to listen. Similar to the phenomenology of seeing intentionally is the hermeneutic approach to understanding the human experience, which guides that the: "listener is listening openly for the truth."[17]

AN ART THERAPIST'S EXPERIENCE

As an art therapist who has been practicing for many years, it continues to be an honor to be in another's presence in front of a blank piece of paper and bear witness to the unfolding process of the inner spirit. Images, symbols, colors, forms, metaphors, and words become the groundwork that invites exploration for personal meaning making. Working collaboratively with other professionals increases the scope and depth of understanding and the potential of what holistic care can be. Integrating the arts into other health-care realms can be done very simply and with minimal supplies. Essential elements to support art expressions include the principles of creating a safe relational space (Chapter 8). Safety is also met by observing how the art materials are being experienced and used and assessing whether modifications are needed.

In my practice, incorporating mind-body skills, such as breathing, physical movement, and mindfulness meditations, supports the process of awareness and working with and through arising strong emotions and challenges. After the art making, reflection comes from being in silence and sitting with the created piece. Verbal or written reflections are encouraged—to describe associations to the color and created form, and note what symbols and images showed up and how the process felt. In a simple yet meaningful way, giving the piece a title is an act of mindfulness and clarifies the self-awareness process.

One client, "Peg," began therapy due to the grief and loss she was experiencing since the recent death of her mother from cancer. At this time, her brother-in-law was also nearing the last stages of brain cancer. Peg was very involved in her career and described herself as being very organized and a taskmaster. She had taken on the caregiver role in her family and was the one trying to keep things in order. At the same time, she was feeling overwhelmed and hoping to gain insights so she could make change. She had stated that she struggled in past therapies, when it was "all talk." Peg was willing to try painting, even though she felt that she was "not creative." In her first spontaneous painting (Figure 19.4), her process began with colors and symbolic shapes that reflected the directions and relationships in her life. She then moved to a free-form manner of working, blending and covering what she began with more kinetic lines and swirls. She titled the piece, "Mess." Through the art medium and process, Peg was able to externalize what she embodied at an emotional level and began to gain greater clarity of how she was truly feeling. In ongoing sessions, she remarked that she continued to struggle with the appearance of this art piece, but saw it as an honest reflection of her need to "let go" and shift from "fixing and doing."

As I painted alongside Peg, sharing the same palette of colors, I intuitively felt both a tightness of energy and inner strength. I deeply resonated with the emotional pulls between compassionate caregiving and the heart breaking open with loss and sadness. My painting movements led to a swirling circle shifting inward. At the same time, I had a sense of growth forming and let the lines rise and move. I noticed that at this time, Peg was adding her top layer of brush strokes and "S" shapes. Within the core of my circle, I saw the image of the "third eye" and brought that to the surface (Figure 19.5). As Peg continued in therapy, she was still meeting the needs of her family and supporting their emotional stress and physical ailments; however, she was also opening up to designating self-care time for herself for yoga, meditation, and visiting friends. She spoke of her hope to begin to "let go" and was reflective of the ways she was beginning to integrate change into her life.

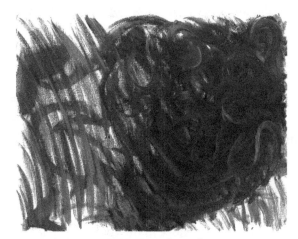

FIGURE 19.4: "MESS"

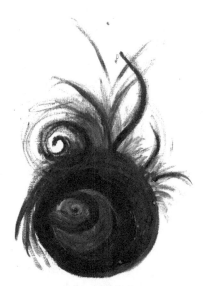

FIGURE 19.5: "THIRD EYE"

Experiential pause: Obtain a piece of blank paper (or use your journal if preferred) and some materials to draw with (preferably crayons or colored pencils, but anything will do). Find a quiet spot to be in. If you prefer to have some sound, you may play some relaxing music in the background. Close your eyes if you feel comfortable, or gently gaze downward with the eyes open. Soften into the present moment, relaxing the body and breath. Open your eyes. With the drawing materials, use colors, shapes, and lines freely. If an image arises, you can let yourself follow what you see to let it emerge. Draw for about seven to ten minutes. At the end of the drawing time, lay the art piece a little bit away from you. You might turn the paper around to see if other angles offer varying viewpoints. Explore the result. As you look, allow some descriptive words, metaphors, or feelings to surface to reflect what you see and feel. You may want to journal these or write about what the drawing process felt like. Explore whether you sense a connection between what you spontaneously created and how that relates to, or gives new insight into, yourself and your present state and experience(s). Give your sketch a title and date your piece. You may want to try this several times during the week and observe how your drawings may change.

RESEARCH AND USES FOR VARIOUS AVENUES FOR CREATIVE SELF-EXPRESSION

Drawing and art making

Over the past several decades, there has been a wealth of research using art and expressive drawing with various medical conditions and populations. Researchers have looked at the creative process for individuals and within group settings. The use of creative modalities ranges from open expression in an unconscious spontaneous manner to more guided approaches, with directive themes targeting awareness, perceptions, and solution-focused techniques. The following examples reflect a small sampling that demonstrates how these avenues for expression can alleviate the burden of chronic diseases and how they may improve quality of life.

A great benefit from drawing is that it helps people to externalize their experiences and feelings that are difficult to express verbally. Traditional health-care questionnaires often rely on emoji ideograms and numerical rating scales to assess levels of pain. Researchers had patients draw the part of their body affected by illness and how they perceived their condition. Drawing aided the provider's sense of understanding the patient's illness experience, served as a source of information for clinical interventions, and helped to determine how well patients were to cope with their condition.[18] Seeing and listening to what is expressed in patient drawings and writings helps to improve overall health interventions and support empathic care.[19] Beyond drawing a body part, one might consider creating a drawing of their pain, their diagnosis, or virtually any other topic they would like to explore.

Researchers illustrate the improvement of health factors, decrease in stress response, and significance of personal affirmations from art making. In one study, it was shown that a brief art experience lowered cortisol levels, regardless of level of art experience.[20] Perhaps more importantly, this study reflected that participants found the process to be: calming, promotional for understanding oneself, enjoyable, freeing from constraints, and capable of supporting movement through struggle to resolution. Changing and reformatting creative expressions may lead to greater well-being as the process utilizes the brain's executive functions to shift from negative views towards empowering relationships.[21]

Forms of creative self-expression have been examined in pilot studies to support individuals with a variety of presenting illnesses and conditions. Findings from art making and focusing techniques for women with breast cancer suggested that the multimodal process could have a positive impact on the functional level of the immune system.[22] The emotional expression through the arts also provided a safe and creative place for the women to illustrate the depth of feelings of anxiety, loss, and uncertainty.[23] Tarr studied engagement in an arts workshop for individuals suffering from autoimmune disorders, such as rheumatoid arthritis and kidney conditions, Crohn's disease, brain and spinal injury, and low back pain.[24] Participants used art making to externalize their relation to pain to find more bearable versions of the pain experience. As mentioned earlier, a public health lens on these findings reinforces a call to utilize a range of holistic practices to reduce the stress, emotional, and psychological challenges embedded in the chronic disease epidemic.[25]

Coming together in groups is healing in itself and supports connectedness and reduces social isolation.[26] Group-based care and support, covered in Chapter 25, reflects an important forum for exploring self-expression. In a study for people living with HIV, an expressive arts group was formed to support those dealing with illness, a poor sense of psychological well-being, social isolation, and existential conflict. Results indicated that existential meaning was made and participants experienced an increase in quality of life.[27] In the study, the art activities and themes focused on overcoming aversions to the participants' challenges by highlighting their lived experiences and striving towards their potential.[28]

Resiliency is another indicator of the capacity to cope with adversity. One study focused on how the arts support resiliency and one's ability to adapt to the experience and depth of suffering of persistent pain. Using a qualitative method to gain insight from participants, several responses included:

- using art served as a positive distraction and escape from an attentional focus on pain
- creative endeavors can change how life is viewed and help one to feel less isolated
- integrating the pain experience into artwork expands art expression
- "even in the gray times to still create even when you don't feel like it because sometimes that is what you really need to be doing at that time in your life."[29]

These studies suggest that further research is worth doing to support the promising practices. Limits identified in the research include: variation in drawing instruction; lack of methodological consistency; small group sample size; control group needed; and lack of assessment of long-term effect of the intervention. In a study on using art for those suffering from chronic migraines, many participants recognized that art was not always a healthy outlet. The authors stress that while we say "art heals," we need to be mindful that there are certain conditions where the art-making process and products can trigger pain.[30] Consistent with the foundations of IRP, using approaches and techniques from a non-fixing stance, in context, and via person-centered self-selection remains true here as well.

Experiential pause: Gather together some crayons and your journal or blank paper. Start by sitting or standing for a few minutes, sensing the body, and inviting the relaxation response. Then, open your eyes and choose to create one of the following options (or one with a similar theme that speaks to you today).

- Draw your relationship with your body.
- Draw a health challenge such as anxiety, neck or back pain, or indigestion.
- Draw any issue or challenge that you are navigating in your life.
- Draw your relationship with food and eating.
- Draw your relationship with exercise.

You might start with colors, lines, or shapes to express yourself; no art talent is needed. If an image arises, you may want to let it take shape. After you are done, reflect on your drawing. What do you notice? What feelings come up for you? Where are your eyes drawn to? Is there a message within it that speaks to you? Perhaps give your drawing a title. Consider sharing with it a trusted person.

Expressive writing

As in creative arts research, writing has been demonstrated by investigators to have impact as an avenue for mind-body expression. Writing forms include expressive writing, journaling, and poetry. Pennebaker and Smyth, pioneers in the field, have reviewed the utility of expressive writing in support of mind-body health, noting that both physiological and qualitative measures of well-being exist.[31] The benefits may be more significant when the writer expresses in an open and honest voice, reflecting who they truly are.[32] Being honest with oneself takes practice and helps one to recognize patterns and the roots of any critical or judgmental thoughts.

A sampling of findings from research presents us with a picture of both complexity and individuality when it comes to the usefulness of writing as an avenue for expression. Consider the following points.

- A 2012 study examining women with metastatic breast cancer and significant psychological distress found no statistically significant differences between participants who wrote about their deepest thoughts versus those who wrote neutrally about daily activities. However, the more expressive/emotional writing was positively correlated with use of mental health services.[33]
- A 2006 meta-analysis of 146 studies examined the effect of disclosing information, thoughts, and feelings through writing and sharing using various strategies. Results revealed a beneficial effect for one's psychological and physical health and overall functioning with a modest average effect size of 0.075.[34] Perhaps of more importance was the characteristics of participants that most strongly correlated to effect size. Persons with an existing health problem and/or history of trauma, persons who were overtly supported in their comfort with/during disclosure, paid participants, a larger dose (at least three successive experiences that included

disclosure of writing content), disclosure of more recent events that had not yet been adequately processed, and/or clear directions as to purpose and approach for disclosure all mediated the benefit.[35]

- Writing about stressful experiences reduces health-care utilization in healthy samples, but not in samples defined by medical diagnoses or exposure to trauma, stress, or other psychological factors.[36]

- Persons with innately high emotional expressiveness showed greater reduction in anxiety from therapeutic writing, whereas participants with low expressiveness experienced an increase in anxiety.[37]

- Cultural differences are found across populations in terms of who benefits from expressive writing.[38] However, successful writing studies have been reported across multiple countries, languages, and ethnicities and: "people dealing with strong emotional and cognitive reactions to important events, likely to be a universal condition, can benefit from translating the experience into narrative language."[39]

- In a generally healthy population of college students, participants utilizing expressive writing demonstrated lower depression symptoms at two months, but not at subsequent follow-up after they had ceased participation. Participants did not demonstrate significant changes in physical health complaints, anxiety, stress symptoms, or academic performance.[40]

The preceding sampling of interesting findings from research suggests that matching a person's naturally elected coping approach with interventions is important and beneficial.[41] The translation of inner experience to more outward forms may occur through many avenues that may or may not include disclosure in the presence of others. Smyth and Pennebaker, in their work on expressive writing, presented some important questions around assumptions that must be examined.[42] What follows is a list of their questions and their short answers, with input from IRP principles. In reading them, keep in mind that these were presented in the context of writing, but are applicable to drawing and other forms of creative self-expression as explored in this chapter.

- Do people need to write about traumatic/negative experiences? "Probably not."[43] Instead, it may be more important to write about what is important to you and to include positive experiences as well. Expressive writing may be encouraged by letting individuals decide what approach they would like to take. This perspective on trauma as it relates to expressive writing research does not forego the potential value of working with a trauma narrative as part of healing processes such as may occur in various forms of Cognitive Behavioral Therapy.[44]

- Is expressive writing a process that requires multiple days to accomplish? "Probably not."[45] Research has shown that both short- and longer-term/spaced writing strategies can be useful.

- Is there a single theoretical process that explains the research findings on therapeutic writing? "Probably not."[46] Scientific inquiry has tended to seek/favor simple explanation over multiple or complex explanations. Recall the values for IRP and other foundations of integral thinking as covered in Chapter 1.

- Is expressive writing only effective for some? "It is hard to tell"[47] from the research. It is best to explore and experiment in mindful, considerate ways, with each person. Simple education about treatment options that support our larger process, followed by self-selection, remains the rule. For those with limited writing ability, modifications may be tried by recording the voice following the expressive writing formats.

Experiential pause: Adapted from a technique taught by The Center for Mind-Body Medicine, the following technique reflects the establishment of a conversation with an issue, symptom, problem, or challenge. Bring to mind a topic that you would like to explore. It could be: a physical symptom, illness, or diagnosis; a topic such as anxiety or an emotional tendency towards anger; a problem, such as at work, with a relationship, etc. The topic should reflect a challenge that you would like to explore from a new lens. The first step will be to write a letter to the issue, symptom, problem, or challenge. What do you want it to hear? As you write the letter, stay aware of your bodily sensations and emotions that accompany the words. Once you're done, set it aside. Take a second piece of paper, and write a letter that comes from the voice of the issue, symptom, problem, or challenge. Let it share with you its experience, and its lens. As before, stay rooted in your bodily sensation and emotions. Once done, reread both letters. How do the voices interact? Do any new insights arise into your relationship with the issues, symptom, problem, or challenge? Moving forward, these letters can serve as a foundation for an ongoing dialogue that reflects the cultivation of a relationship over time.

CONCLUSION

Art therapy as a formal profession is a wonderful resource. When art therapy is not accessible, and even when it is, IRP advocates that all professionals deepen their understanding of the importance of supporting processes of and avenues for self-expression.

Paint flows on paper,
Colors mingle together creating new forms,
Suggestive of dreams which accompany me
Through open and closed eyes.
Clay smells of earth,
It receives the caress of my fingers
And the strength of my fist.
Wood splinters rough
Like my bristling emotions
Until it is sanded smooth,
The beauty of its grain revealed.
Metal burns white hot,
Explosive and angry

Needing the force of the hammer to shape it,
Cooling to a dull gray,
Only to be heated and reworked again.
My voice speaks and sings
With words of pain, love
Abandonment and isolation
Can you hear what I'm saying?
My creativity is expressed in these ways,
Exposing me, cleansing me.
I destroy in order to create
And inside the paint,
The clay,
The wood,
The metal,
The word, I look in
And I see me.

Luna

Self-expression is an important part of human experience. From spoken word, to emotional release, to movement…to our current emphasis on creative self-expression in the form of art making, drawing, and expressive writing, there are many avenues via which we express ourselves. In this chapter, we have only touched the surface when it comes to these topics. The hopeful intention is to inspire and tap into the source within. In Luna's poem, look in and see you.

> **Experiential pause:** Having read this chapter, identify and write down at least one actionable item of interest to you. In doing so, consider ways in which applying the material first to yourself, and then to patients, might serve those who come to you for care.

RESOURCES

– For an insightful ten-minute film that portrays Frida Kahlo's story from the lens of potential for transformation of disabilities by honoring creative self-expression, see *Frida Kahlo's Corset* (2000) at www.roaring-girl.com/work/frida-kahlos-corset. You may also enjoy the films *Frida* (2002) and *Nise: The Heart of Madness* (2015).

– American Art Therapy Association (AATA): https://arttherapy.org.

– National Association of Poetry Therapy: https://poetrytherapy.org.

– American Dance Therapy Association: https://adta.org.

– Focusing and Expressive Arts Institute: www.focusingarts.com/about-us.

– International Expressive Arts Therapy Association: www.ieata.org.

– Trauma-Informed Expressive Arts Therapy® and Trauma-Informed Art Therapy®: www.trauma-informedpractice.com.

CHAPTER 20

Finding Your Voice

Sherril Howard, MS, CCC-SLP

A story: "Jaylen," a 38-year-old female, was diagnosed with muscle tension dysphonia as well as unilateral vocal fold polyp. She was a professor with a PhD in the sciences and worked with an all-male staff in her university department. Jaylen explained that in addition to the amount of talking her job requires, she purposely lowered the pitch of her voice to sound more authoritative and "believable" around her male colleagues. Through her integrative speech therapy approach, she realized parts of her story were limiting. It was not a lower pitch that made her more "believable." She recognized that this false belief was not serving her well and was actually contributing to her internalized stress. With this insight, she was able to let go of false beliefs and work on finding her natural pitch and resonance in her voice, her life, and the world. This work brought beauty and power to everything she had to say. While healing her external voice, she was also supported in exploring how mind-body dynamics were a component of the overall condition of her voice. Jaylen reached inward to assist the healing of her voice.

As we see in Jaylen's story, the voice is a complex representation of each individual's larger being. It is not "just a voice" nor "just a polyp." The structure and meaning of voice are deeply intertwined with much more. The understanding that voice can reflect more than just the physical voice reinforces integrative rehabilitation practice's (IRP's) emphasis on considering a multitude of factors within each person's experience of their health condition. A dispositional theory of causation (Chapter 3) reminds us that causation arises out of the intersection of many ingredients, and similarly we are reminded of complexity in case formulation and clinical reasoning processes (Chapter 5).

The physiology of voice is shared with breathing, swallowing, and hearing, and is linked to our movement, posture, thinking, feeling, and patterns of self-expression. All these components are strongly linked to survival and safety, as well as shared with the physiological processes underlying intimacy, sustenance, and digestion.[1] Voice reflects stress,[2] emotion,[3] personality,[4] and voice behavior.[5] Speech and verbal expression are intimately wrapped up in cultural, social, gender, and racial contexts.[6] Voice, for example with song or prayer, links to one's spirituality.[7] Consistent with reminders across this book, sorting out causality, such as whether personality factors play causal, concomitant, or consequential roles in voice disorders, is less important than offering a person-centered, whole-person model of support. Going further, attempts at the assignment of causality is outright discouraged.

This chapter will take us on a journey into voice as a vital component of the larger whole. We will examine the ways in which physical voice and sound, as well as the abstract, symbolic, and metaphorical uses of "voice," interact as part of the body-mind-environment (BME) construct that we've become so familiar with throughout this journey into IRP. We will continue to explore our theme of connecting dots in support of rehabilitation professionals' capacity to understand and support the larger picture of each person's "voice." We will close the chapter by exploring practical ways for using the inter-related topics of voice, sound, and music within IRP, regardless of your primary discipline.

A SPEECH-LANGUAGE PATHOLOGIST'S EXPERIENCE

The field of speech-language pathology is quite broad, ranging from pediatrics to geriatrics and spanning areas from communication to swallowing. I have been a practicing speech-language pathologist (SLP) since the early 1980s, with a specialty in voice disorders. The prevalence of voice disorders is quite small, estimated to be only approximately 1% of speech disorders.[8] However, in a large study looking at self-reported rates of voice problems in individuals who are heavy voice users (e.g., teachers) versus the general population, ~57% and ~29% respectively reported challenges that interfered with their experience of communicating.[9] These findings are similar to my clinical experience practicing in an ear, nose, and throat department at a major university hospital, where I estimated more than 50% of my clients presented with voice disorders.

While voice disorders are undoubtedly physical, what I'm writing about is deeper associations within voice disorders. Far too often, professionals look at the physical domain only. Yet underneath, within emotional and/or personal psychospiritual levels, there may be other dynamics in the person's life that are linked to the whole of the voice disorder. Certain voice disorders (such as muscle tension dysphonia) are more strongly linked to stress, personality traits, emotion, anxiety, and/or depression.[10]

I had a voice disorder. Perhaps this is why I studied speech-language pathology. I was the youngest of three children in a very outgoing and boisterous family. In order to be heard, I felt I needed to be loud. I was a "type A" personality, never one to say no to a challenge, and very energetic. I enjoyed singing and dancing in school choir and theater. I was that "wannabe cheerleader" at school sporting events, yelling my lungs out while cheering on the team. At around age 14, I became quite hoarse, to the point where people mistook me for a male on the phone or told me I had a "sexy frog-like voice"! Upon seeing an ear, nose, and throat physician, I was formally diagnosed as having a voice disorder: bilateral vocal fold nodules. Vocal fold nodules are benign tissue masses that form on the vocal fold, thought to be the result of vocal fold tissue stress, including repeated or chronic vocal overuse, abuse, or misuse.

In short, I was told that I yelled too much and too hard. It was recommended that I see a speech-language pathologist. My parents were so relieved that nothing serious was wrong that we never pursued treatment when I was a youngster. I only received treatment nine years later when I entered graduate school and received voice therapy from a fellow student. Graduate school taught me the physical "cause" and treatment of my voice. However, in 30+ years of practice, I discovered that voice is so much more than just sound…

My deeper education started with a big jolt. In 1981, while I was working on my Master of Science degree in speech-language pathology at the University of Arizona, I attended a lecture by a well-known and highly recognized visiting professor, the late Dr. Arnold Aronson. A comment he made completely challenged my belief system and started my journey toward a deeper understanding of the mind-body connection. This comment actually changed my life trajectory. Dr. Aronson declared his estimate that 90–95% of voice disorders have a psychological element. As a young graduate student with vocal nodules, I was irate! I thought to myself: "I have an organic medical problem and my psychological state has nothing to do with this!" Was I ever wrong!

Such thinking remains pervasive—the splitting of mind and body as explored in the earliest chapters of this book. We must remember the call to repeatedly consider the benefit and flexibility that comes when considering the possibility of "both/and." This early reaction that I had was rooted in the black-and-white dichotomy of "either/or." As covered across earlier chapters, there is a growing science supporting the understanding that our psychology is both embedded within and influential upon biological processes.[11] In particular, the science of emotion and self-expression lays a backdrop to understanding the voice in the mind-body and integrative context.

As my career and experience progressed, working with hundreds of voice clients, I began to recognize the profound truth in Dr. Aronson's comment. What he meant, and what I now understand, is that many of our vocal pathologies need to be addressed using the integrative lens. For example, we must look deeper into our emotional and mental state in relation to what is manifest physically. Our voices are an expression of our inner life. Let me repeat that: our voices are an expression of our inner life! This deeper understanding took many years of learning from my clients, who many times were my best teachers; it also took years of self-exploration, meditation, and spiritual retreats to explore and understand my own mind-body reality as well. This does not mean that correlation implies causation. We simply cannot grasp all the variables that go into emergence, but the possibility of addressing parallel processes in support of the potential for healing processes is foundational in IRP.

It is interesting how a childhood issue or a single comment from one lecture can change the trajectory of both personal and professional life. As a 14-year-old, I would have never thought I would be working with clients with similar voice issues. As a graduate student, I never thought I would spend a great deal of my therapy efforts helping clients get in touch with the emotional aspects of their disorders. Having a voice disorder has led me and many clients on a journey of self-discovery. This journey is consistent with an integrative care construct: to consider that whatever is found in our embodied experience, regardless of the question of causality, can be seen as an opportunity for looking at and addressing the interactions between levels within the whole of our being.

THE SCIENCE OF VOICE AND SOUND

Communication involves both the expressive and receptive domains. Voice is one of many avenues for the expressive domain and sits alongside body language, movement, writing, art, and more. The receptive domain is most commonly associated with listening and hearing (auditory). However, we receive and comprehend communication in many other ways, as individuals who experience any spectrum of hearing challenge will emphasize. The receptive domain also includes visual input, reading and interpreting language, sensation (including touch), symbols, and more. Understanding, being aware of, and supporting the importance and relevance of voice, sound, and the many other avenues of communication that occur on a spectrum is critical in mind-body and integrative medicine constructs. Doing so supports the biological underpinnings of stress, safety, autonomy/empowerment, and nurturance/intimacy/relationship.

In graduate school, SLPs, the specialized leaders in caring for the voice, are taught the normal and abnormal anatomy and physiology of speech, language, voice, and swallowing. SLPs learn how to evaluate these areas and then how to treat the various diagnoses. They learn that the diagnosis and treatment of communication and swallowing disorders includes a multidisciplinary approach, working with other clinicians, including but not limited to: neurologists, otolaryngologists, internists, nutritionists, occupational therapists (OTs), physical therapists (PTs), and social workers. Now, as with other professions, the field has progressed into the transdisciplinary arenas of psychology and psychiatry, presenting valuable influence in helping us understand the entire spectrum of disorders. For example, Dietrich states: "From a clinical perspective, there is consensus that if psychological and emotional factors that *initiated*, *exacerbated*, or *maintained* a voice disorder are not addressed…the chance of long-term treatment efficacy decreases even if short-term success is achieved for the patient."[12] This call for attention to mind-body factors, as discussed elsewhere in the book, often falls on a spectrum; any exploration of such dynamics must occur with education and through invitation. In the case of voice disorders, muscle tension dysphonia has been given the greatest emphasis in this regard.[13]

Identifying when to refer to another discipline is part of the skill set we must learn. *And*, consistent with the integrative medicine movement, transdisciplinary education and capacity is important, regardless of the extent of other-discipline involvement. Broadening from traditional treatment to integrative options is relevant to speech therapists. Equally, other professionals benefit from learning foundations of speech, hearing, and more. For example, evidence-based ways to incorporate mindfulness and meditation practices into speech-language and voice therapy for the adult population are emerging.[14]

Persons experiencing voice issues, such as hoarseness, may have a number of contributing factors. This reminds us of the need to explore complexity without making assumptions, especially around assignment of causality to any one factor. From the physical level, there could be vocal nodules or polyps, vocal fold edema or erythema, and perhaps even neuromotor paralysis. Simple functional education around the three main physical structures needed for voice production can be a starting point for moving deeper into integrative constructs. This is done following the principles of therapeutic education as found in Chapter 16.

First, there is the respiratory system. In order to produce voice, we need a steady flow of air coming from the lungs. The respiratory system is the power source of airflow for voice production. This bridges us back to Chapter 11 on the breath. Second, there is the larynx or voice box. The larynx is comprised of many muscles and ligaments and is largely innervated by the vagus nerve. Within the larynx are the vocal folds. The pharyngeal and laryngeal muscles work to control the mechanisms of respiration, swallowing, and vibrating to create voice or sound. Lastly, there are the resonators and articulators. These structures form and shape our sounds and tones: our pharynx, nasal sinuses, and oral cavity amplify the vibrating energy, creating a fuller, more resonant quality; our tongue, lips, and cheeks adjust our vibratory sound into speech. We need all three of these components, respiration, vibration, and resonance, to have a normal voice, as well as normal inter-related function of breathing, oral motor function, swallowing, and hearing.

We know that excessive muscular effort leads to altered vibratory patterns of the vocal folds, which impacts our voice production or vocal quality. When there is an imbalance of tension between the intrinsic and extrinsic muscles surrounding the larynx, the imbalance may cause challenges with voicing, swallowing, and breathing. A well-researched mind-body phenomenon lies in understanding that the infrahyoid muscles activate during stress and that there are differences in these patterns between more introverted and extroverted personality types.[15] In general, our intrinsic and extrinsic laryngeal and pharyngeal muscles react to emotional triggers such as stress and anxiety. This reaction occurs in integration to the other facets of an integrated BME, whole-organism stress response. One common result is tightness or other restrictions in our voice, such as changes in prosody (rhythm, pitch, intonation, stress, and volume of speech).

More on the neuroscience of this in a bit, but first a broad reminder: becoming aware of, feeling, expressing, and regulating our emotions in flexible ways that are uniquely suited to individual disposition can improve health and well-being.[16] In metaphorical essence, healthy emotional dynamics support bringing forth each person's beautiful resonant voice—"finding one's voice." Consistent with other examples throughout this book, it is important to contemplate a shift away from the tendency to want to analyze or fix problems. This is especially true if we are only addressing the issue from a physical/structural lens. In doing so, we are only addressing one portion of a much larger equation. As the concepts and skills have shown us thus far, we need to delve further—to not just inquire about, but also support the client's psychosocial history, their emotional state, and various levels of stress (social, economic, relational, environmental). Yes, with tight musculature, the voice is constrained and we can assist in decreasing muscle tension through various exercises; we cannot forget to explore why the muscle tension might be there in the first place.

> **Another story:** "Claire" was a 54-year-old female presenting with little to no voice for over 30 days. A medical exam revealed normal-appearing and functioning vocal folds. After delving deeper, we discovered that she was going to receive a national award in two weeks and would be seeing someone from her past for whom she had some very troubling feelings. She had last seen this person 25 years ago when they had a business fallout that left Claire devastated. Once we uncovered her emotions around this situation, I asked if she had cried or released any of her emotions around this troubling situation. She said she hadn't, as at the time she simply had to get on with business. As I attuned and created space, she began sharing, and tears welled up. I encouraged her to cry, really cry, and let it out as a "necessary rinsing." As she released her emotions, her voice began to reveal itself. We worked together for several sessions and helped her recognize the connection of her emotions to the constriction of her voice. With her inner work, her voice returned and she was able to express her inner strength through her true voice.

POLYVAGAL THEORY, VOICE, AND SOUND

As covered in various contexts across earlier chapters, polyvagal theory (PVT) provides an integrated biological view of human behavior and mind-body processes. PVT offers significant relevance to an integrative view of voice and hearing. PVT is worth a deeper look in relation to voice, as it is rooted in core science that informs processes of healthy attachment, communication, emotion, social engagement, and self-/co-regulation.

PVT emphasizes that one's physiological state dictates the range of behavior accessible to an individual.[17] In essence, if defensive, survival-oriented physiology is dominant, it may restrict the effectiveness of higher cognitive processes, prosocial engagement, and/or communication.

Going further, the neuroscience underlying PVT links voice (vocal communication, sharing) and hearing (active listening) to:

- the neurological regulation of the heart and viscera
- affect and emotion
- facial expressivity and body language
- breathing
- motor control of the face, head, ear, throat, and neck for BME orienting
- social behavior that is responsive to the behavior of others.[18]

Phew! PVT, while far more complex than a single transmission line, is named for the vagus nerve. The vagus nerve ("wandering" in Latin) is a cranial nerve (CN), the 10th of 12 such nerves arising out of the brainstem. It carries autonomic/visceral efferent (motor) and afferent (sensory) input/control to nearly all organs, as well as skeletal muscle control of speech (recurrent laryngeal nerve—muscles of the larynx such as the cricothyroid). The vagus nerve interfaces with two source nuclei—the dorsal motor nucleus (DMN) and the nucleus ambiguus (NA). Divisions of the vagus contribute to sound modulation in the middle ear via the levator veli palatine muscle, and breathing control via the posterior cricoarytenoid muscle, the only abductor of the vocal folds. In sum, the vagus nerve is responsible for such varied tasks as heart rate, gastrointestinal peristalsis, sweating, auditory/sound filtering, and quite a few muscle movements in the mouth, including speech and keeping the larynx open for breath control. Of interest, the vagus nerve is strongly lateralized. Specifically, the right-side division, which is controlled by the right hemisphere of the brain (greater dominance over emotional regulation), also has predominant neurological control for vocal intonation.[19] Considering just how reflective tone of voice is of emotional states, this reminds us of a biological basis to something rather obvious—emotion is embodied and reflected in numerous ways within the mind-body connection.

Looking even deeper, the "ventral vagal complex" (VVC) reflects a cluster of brainstem nerves that derive from the same embryological division.[20] In addition to the previously described motor (outgoing) pathways of the vagus nerve (CN X) (controls the larynx, pharynx, and middle ear for mechanisms of speech, swallowing, and hearing), the NA is also the source of outgoing pathways for the glossopharyngeal nerve (CN IX) (controls swallowing) and the spinal accessory nerve (CN XI) (controls head/neck rotation). The VVC also includes the trigeminal nerve (CN V) (controls mastication/chewing, as well as contributes to hearing) and the facial nerve (CN VII) (controls facial expressivity, as well as contributes to hearing). These pathways also regulate the physiological processes of salivation, tearing, respiration, and heart rate. Collectively, this "complex" provides us with the biological foundations of emotional expression.[21] Thus, the neurological regulation of speech/vocalization and hearing/sound are inseparable from emotional physiology, visceral function, and our ability to self-regulate stress physiology. This science underscores an integrative lens for this chapter.

WHAT AM I NOT HEARING?

An integrative view of communication includes the receptive domain, which may or may not involve the auditory system. Certainly, if the hearing mechanism is intact, hearing is a key component of listening. And, we are capable of "hearing," "listening," receiving communication, and understanding (receptive language) in many other ways. Further, listening, whether it is auditory or via other means of reception, does not imply comprehension. As discussed in Chapter 6, we must check for gaps in communication and understanding in any relational interaction.

With that said, the basic mechanism of hearing is physiologically linked to the voice. Hearing involves the collection and concentration of sound waves by the earlobes. In an amazing demonstration of engineering, the sound waves are converted to neurological signals. This begins with vibration of the tympanic membranes, followed by movement of three "ossicle" bones as a lever system, and then the in/out movement of the footplate of the stapes at the oval window of the cochlea. In the final step, displacement of fluid in the cochlea allows conversion of the sound wave into nerve transduction via movement of specialized "hair cells," which float in the water like seaweed that moves with a current.

The impact of the muscles controlled by the vagus nerve complex, and their influence on hearing and the perceived acoustic environment, has to do with the ability to extract higher frequency sounds (human voice) from the lower frequencies (background "noise") of the environment. This extraction of voice is achieved by tensing of the eardrum and the modulation of middle ear (Eustachian tube) pressure. This feat is largely carried out by the earlier mentioned tensor veli palatine muscle, part of the VVC.[22]

Human voices may range from 60 Hz to 1100 Hz ($\sim F_2$ to C_6 on a musical note scale).[23] For females, an average speaking pitch range is 110–255; for males, it is 85–180.[24] The related frequency band is similar to the frequency band that composers have historically selected to express melodies, but also the frequency band that mothers have unconsciously used to calm their infants by singing lullabies![25]

PVT posits that the modulation of the acoustic energy within human voice will recruit and modulate the neural regulation of the ear muscles. What does this mean? Features of human voice and hearing are able to functionally calm one's behavioral and physiological state. The simplified take-away: sharing, listening, and engaging with others in consciously attuned ways directly contributes to the physiological regulation of self and other in relationship. This regulation reflects a critical backdrop of IRP—focusing as much on the attuned relationship as therapeutic, as any technique.

To support these therapeutic effects, modulation of voice is critical. The characteristics of one's voice reflect physiological state, and stress is detectable at both subconscious and conscious levels. There is both an upside and downside here:

> **Experiential pause:** Bring to mind someone you know who has a tendency for a harsh tone of voice. Imagine this person now. As you do this, notice how you feel. What happens in your body? Now imagine someone whose voice is naturally soothing. "Listen" to this person now. How does your body respond?

We feel and respond to others' tone of voice! This can be seen as an *exchange of affect*. Voice can either diminish or support the regulation of the listener. Think co-regulation. We saw this in our exploration of guided imagery (Chapter 14). It is imperative that professionals not just be aware of, but also consciously work with, their voice, including in relation to their body awareness/language.

In some cases, these physiological underpinnings of the integrated voice/listening system may be compromised.[26] Examples include:

- anxiety and depressive disorders
- post-traumatic stress disorder
- autism spectrum disorders
- personality disorders.[27]

These conditions often coexist with other diagnoses commonly presenting in rehabilitation practice as described in Chapter 3. For example, states of persistent pain may reflect as difficulty in reading and attending appropriately to social cues, communication difficulties, poor emotion/affect recognition and/or regulation, and overall poor regulation of the autonomic nervous system/physiological state.[28]

THE INTEGRATIVE LENS: PUTTING THINGS BACK TOGETHER

Our overall state of being not only affects the quality of our voice, but it can also potentially contribute an *ingredient* to somatic tissue changes, such as our earlier example of vocal nodules. This is "mind-body 101"! Just as we often need to understand drug interactions and their impact on communication and swallowing, we also need to understand non-motor influences. The BME picture points to an overall state of being that affects things such as sleep patterns, motivation, diet, relationships, and willingness to interact with others. As such, it is important to have a solid understanding of these many other relevant symptoms and patterns that may exist. These patterns and lifestyle factors may *influence* the person's chief presenting physical concern/symptom. Other such influences include the presence of fatigue, indigestion, depression, stress, anxiety, apathy, or maladaptive coping patterns. When working with our clients, we want to help them to explore all symptoms to maximize the greatest potential for well-being to emerge. In this process, we must know when to make an appropriate referral to another discipline.

SYMBOLISM, METAPHOR, AND MEANING: CONNECTING DOTS

We often hear things like: "Has the cat got your tongue?", "What are you not swallowing?", "Lost your voice, huh?", and "I'm all choked up." We have used these here purposely, as they point towards mind-body union. These metaphors can lead us into a deeper understanding of voice.

The voice is not our only "voice." For example, we may find "voice" in movement (Chapter 15) or the avenues of expression explored in Chapter 19. We can also represent voice as *inner voice*: the internal, more hidden, quiet, or silent aspects of our voice and thus our being.

And, as referenced earlier, the actual physical voice reflects a great deal of these subtle or more hidden notions of voice. Our external voice, what it is today, right now, expresses a lot about us. In a sense, we are our voices: the physical, real-time quality of our voice is part of our identity.

We can learn to more fully connect inner voice to our actual voice—giving voice to our interior outward into the world. When we teach about the components of voice production—that we have the respirator, vibrator, and resonator—we can concurrently contemplate the notion of a "soul-erator," the internal place of authenticity where we access our inner voice and give outward expression to our inner world. Recognizing this, we realize that our voices are so much more than just the physical mechanism. Our voices are an indicator of our larger physiological and mind-body (cognitive, emotional, etc.) states.[29] This brings us right back to what Dr. Aronson said in that graduate school lecture: that 90–95% of voice disorders have a psychophysiological connection. Going further, we might consider voice as reflective of each person's unique and continuously changing and evolving psychospiritual experience.

WORKING WITH "VOICE"

There are numerous entry points and avenues for exploring and transforming health challenges from the mind-body lens. We are not foregoing foundations of the rehabilitation professions, such as speech-language pathology. Instead, mind-body integration adds depth and potential. Explorations of physical challenges, such as a voice issue, benefit from looking at the larger context of the client's life experience. Past trauma, patterns of stress, embedded beliefs, emotions, and personality traits may exist as influential in the overall ingredients that inform the health manifestation.

In exploring these dynamics as opportunities for transformation, individuals are more able to reveal their most resonant, healthy-sounding voice—and their highest self in the process. In modeling the "both/and" construct, a goal is to simultaneously educate and address how the physical voice works alongside skills that support accessing and expressing one's inner voice—to integrate the two as a guide toward their own insight and to create healing dynamics.

Experiential pause: These experiences can be used to help others to find their "inner voice." However, to use them with others, we must first use them for ourselves. Consider documenting your experiences and responses in your journal.

1. **Get quiet**: Getting quiet is a great place to begin. Coming into stillness helps us to hear our inner voice. The world can be a very loud and overwhelming place. Sitting in silence allows us to hear *our* voice and not the hubbub around us. Getting quiet doesn't require sitting in a cross-legged position; it can be an active practice. Being aware or mindful in the moment with curiosity, without judgment, and with kindness. Once we become quiet, we can investigate the stories and beliefs that lay hidden. Once we become quiet, we can get in touch with our true, authentic self. Once we become quiet and discover our true self, we can be freed up to express the beauty that lies within. Leon Brown, a former Major League Baseball player, said it well: "Listen to your own voice, your own soul. Too many people listen to the noise of the world, instead of themselves." Take a moment, come quiet, and listen…

2. **Self-reflection**: As we begin the journey of self-reflection through quieting our mind, we get closer to knowing our inner selves. We begin to recognize

that we are more than the roles we play. We are more than a mom or dad, more than a therapist, doctor, or teacher. These roles are just an outer aspect of who we are and are often based on what others expect us to be or to look like. We need not be limited by the labels we are given. We can help others to recognize that they are not here to imitate others but to create their own authentic selves. Zen Master Dogen said it well: "Do not follow the ideas of others but learn to listen to the voice within yourself." Take a moment and reflect on the places where you suppress your voice…

3. **Work with your own voice**: Through self-awareness, self-listening, and self-regulation, you can learn to modulate your voice in ways that convey physiological calm. Combine this with body awareness of facial expressivity, postural and movement habits, and breathing practices. The next time you are in dialogue with another, pay attention in the lens of this chapter…

4. **Breathing exercises**: Breath is more than staying alive. As we learned in Chapter 11, across languages the word breath carries deeper meaning. For example, in Latin the word for breath is "spiritus" or spirit. Building on the Latin definition, we might contemplate how exploring breath and voice works with the spirit that animates it. Additionally, as we breathe, we're working with exercising the vagal pathways of the larynx and pharynx—pathways that are shared between vocalization, swallowing, and breath control. This carries implications for larger effects on systemic self-regulation processes. Becoming curious about one's breathing is a first step. Our breath, like our body, is our oldest, steadiest friend.

   - Take in a breath with full awareness…inhale…exhale…and as you continue, consider the idea of taking the breath from your "soul-erator," from your heart space. In other words, take in a *loving breath*—the intention of love, in the breath. Can you feel, sense, a difference? Consider using this loving breath meditation regularly.

   - There are many breathing practices, some of which were covered in Chapter 11. The potentially positive physiological impact continues to be documented.[30] In the context of this chapter, notice how these breathing practices impact your voice, as well as your ability to listen to and connect with others.

5. **Full expression of self**: Encourage those you work with to express themselves, to fully release their voices. This does not necessarily mean to let it all out fast and hard—to lambast or blame others. Rather, we work on creating inner awareness and voicing our truth lovingly and with clarity. You may feel that you are right and justified in anger or blame of another. In fact, you may be right. But it doesn't help you to express it with negativity. If expressed with negativity, our voice can become tight, constricted, or strained. Instead, voice your thoughts with compassion and love. This process also requires deep listening—to ourselves and to others. Take a moment of meditation and

consider a place that may be ripe to express yourself in this way. Imagine what this would look and feel like…

6. **Vocal toning, humming, chanting, and singing**: Exercises for the vocal mechanism may improve the physiological foundations of regulation. The mechanisms involved are complex and in part are due to regulating effects via vagal nerve modulation, which innervates vocal prosody and breath control.[31] As with breathing, many forms exist, ranging from yogic practices, to religious chanting, to group singing.[32]

   – Borrowed from the mind-body based therapy known as Somatic Experiencing (SE) (covered in Chapter 13), a simple practice known as the "voo" exercise represents a good example of a generic approach to vocalizing. Other similar sounds that are easy to vibrate, like "ooohmmm," "hummm," or "zzzzz," are OK too! If desired, adjust your posture to feel supported, stable, and relaxed. Take notice of your current sense of the mix of mental, emotional, and physical energies. Now, call to mind the sound of a ship's foghorn, or a similar sound, and imagine the depth and vibration that it conveys. Then slowly inhale and, on the out breath, gently vocalize the sound you've chosen, sustaining it throughout the entire exhalation. Vibrate the sound as though that vibration is arising from your belly and into your vocal cords as the sound is expressed into the space all around you. At the end of the breath, let the next breath arise naturally. You can repeat the sound every breath or every few breaths if desired. When it feels like enough, check back in with your sense of self and notice any impact on your mental, emotional, and physical state. This exercise can be used as needed to contribute to self-regulation and to get "unstuck" from any unhelpful pattern/state that you are working on transforming.

CONCLUSION

Many may have heard the statement: "Your eyes are the window to your soul." In an embodied view of mind and spirit, every part of our physical being can carry such a reflection. This includes our voice, and the window can be opened wide to allow the sound of our soul, our expression, to come forth. This sometimes also comes in silence— knowing when to exercise the voice and when to withhold it. Either way, the voice can be the expression of our deepest sense of self. In relationships, this also involves the connection to attunement and deep listening…listening beneath the words for the depth, the feelings, and the meaning. The phenomenological heuristic of IRP, in general, supports these constructs, and, in this chapter, we have looked at an integrative view of finding our voices—individually and together in heart-centered spaces of care and mutual support.

While current evidence related to IRP and voice is limited, science is revealing fuller, though sometimes-hidden meanings and relevance to our voices.[33] These meanings can be explored from both the intra- and interpersonal lens. It is possible to use our voices in directed ways. Voice and sound can help us to reduce stress, create a deeper sense of presence, and promote healing and well-being in ourselves and others.

We live in a complex world. What we can do to balance that complexity is to offer our healing voice to others. Finding depth within ourselves can translate into letting our hearts and voices, minds and bodies, "sing" together. The loving vibration of our voice can be heard and felt by others, and as we grow, we can increasingly let others hear our clear, strong, yet relaxed voices—giving a subtle but profound gift to others. We all carry a light within, and when we sense it, we create greater harmony within ourselves and our lives that is passed on to others. This process of self-discovery does not happen overnight; it is a lifelong journey, and we are reminded of the wisdom of patience, kindness, and gentleness with our own and others' voices in the process.

Experiential pause: Having read this chapter, identify and write down at least one actionable item of interest to you. In doing so, consider ways in which applying the material first to yourself, and then to patients, might serve those who come to you for care.

CHAPTER 21

Music as Medicine

Alicia L. Barksdale, MS, MT-BC, NMT

A story: "Alejandro" is an 18-year-old male who experienced a traumatic brain injury (TBI). Five months post-injury, Alejandro presented with acute aphasia, hemiparesis on his right side, and acute depression with pseudo-seizures. Alejandro's speech-language pathologist observed Alejandro's consistent participation in music and his natural rhythm and movement skills and referred him to music therapy. The hope was that engagement in musical activity would facilitate Alejandro's engagement in physiotherapy, occupational therapy, and speech-language therapy, which he had begun resisting as his awareness of his injury increased. Alejandro also reported increased depression symptoms. Alejandro did in fact engage in learning to play the drum set, which helped him to retrain gross motor control and strengthen muscles. He also engaged in singing, first vocalizing freely, then shaping vowel sounds, and then adding consonants and short syllables, which motivated him to engage wholeheartedly in speech-language therapy. The musical endeavors Alejandro seemed to value most though were the piano pieces he was able to improvise along with his music therapist. These became a primary expressive outlet for him when he was unable to verbalize. Early on, Alejandro selected from a menu of choices (with words and pictures) for the parameters of the piece to match the emotion he was currently experiencing. Alejandro would point to select the volume, tempo, and feeling of the piece. The therapist would begin playing on black keys only (a naturally harmonic pentatonic scale), to match Alejandro's choices, and asked Alejandro to play along on any black keys. The therapist offered feedback and reassurance as Alejandro played using his left hand. Eventually, with encouragement, Alejandro began using his right hand as well when playing piano. Soon Alejandro was beginning the pieces, and the therapist would join in and match Alejandro's music making. Through these musical interactions, Alejandro expressed his emotional state without needing to say anything. As Alejandro increased his ability to express himself musically, his expressive language increased and he was able to verbally express emotions, needs, and ideas. He began to engage in counseling to help him plan for independent life as a young adult. Three years after his injury and work with music therapy (MT), Alejandro had regained 95% of his expressive language, completed culinary training, and been offered a job as a cook in a hospital cafeteria. He was considering forming a band with friends. He was excited to be alive.

Alejandro's story is inspiring and reflective of a best-case scenario. However, consider that Alejandro's progress through musical intervention is reflective of a valuable contribution towards the possibility of health and well-being, irrespective of outcome. Connecting with the many dimensions of each person's unique health journey, including the emotional inner life of the experience, is vital to that person's recovery and wellness. Music, like other avenues presented within the pages of this book, can speak volumes to those in rehabilitation care.

This chapter will describe select aspects of the MT profession relevant to integrative rehabilitation practice (IRP), explore MT interventions in integrative health care, and offer a sampling of strategies for the non-MT reader to explore and integrate into practice. Towards the latter, there are many ways in which music is used as part of the general environment and/or specific to a component of a treatment session. Especially when self-selected by the patient and chosen from options, music is an important part of an integrative care approach. Subtle attention to musical style, volume, tempo, and context is needed. Music therapists may offer guidance for the types, uses, and applications of these musical interventions by other practitioners; however, many uses of music such as music listening are available to all practitioners to enhance their clinical work, with clients' input. Here is an example:

> **Experiential pause:** Bring to mind a favorite piece of recorded music that you have access to. Prepare to play the music. Before starting the piece, take a minute or two to settle into a favored, comfortable posture/position. Deepen awareness into and through the sensations of the body. Notice your breathing. Now, play your chosen piece of music, staying attuned to the felt senses of body and being. How does the music act on, in, and through your being? What thoughts arise? What emotions do you notice are evoked? Do images arise? Do any memories or associations in relation to this music get evoked? When the piece is finished, inquire into any overall changes in your mind-body state.

A MUSIC THERAPIST'S EXPERIENCE

MT is attaining growing prominence as a treatment within integrative health care. The American Music Therapy Association defines MT as: "the clinical and evidence-based use of music interventions to accomplish individualized goals within a therapeutic relationship, by a credentialed professional who has completed an approved MT program."[1] As a practitioner of MT for 35 years, with clients of all ages, I feel that while this definition provides an accurate description of MT, it does little to capture the spirit of the practice and profession as I know it and as clients experience it.

If I were to highlight the most important words of the aforesaid definition, "relationship" and "music" have equal importance. Musical engagement facilitates the formation of the therapeutic relationship, which facilitates further exploration on the part of the client and their willingness to take part in a new experience that yields self-discovery and self-awareness. One of the most powerful applications of music can be seen in a client's use of music to transform physical and emotional pain into an experience that is profoundly beautiful and healing.

My journey as a music therapist has taken me across many settings and allowed me the privilege of witnessing many miracles. Alejandro's story is just one of many that I carry with me. Working with elderly residents of a nursing care facility to create a musical art show opening, engaging teens with neurological difficulties in playing instruments and songwriting, using music to help a client illustrate their life story and work through grief, singing to my own father when he was in a coma and watching him wake up—these events have shown me the true power of music. When music is harnessed as a vehicle for positive change, great things are possible.

What I have learned through these experiences is that I am a facilitator. More than implementing an intervention, I am offering an opportunity and creating an environment where the client can participate in a musical experience on their terms, in ways that work for them, and as part of the larger process of their life experience. This engagement may include only me and the client, or it may include other clients or professionals. My job is to provide a structure through their journey toward wellness where the client feels safe to express, to relax, to engage, and to be who they are without judgment. Consistent with the principles of mutual learning inherent to IRP, there is reciprocity within MT practices, which is that the therapist is both a facilitator and a recipient of the musical experience. In this way, the therapeutic relationship deepens.

SOME BACKGROUND ABOUT THE MT PROFESSION

Music can be viewed as a system of time, energy, and space that is defined by form and perception. From in utero to the final moments of our lives, music provides a way to create order, to make sense of one's experiences, and support meaning and comfort. It is likely that every culture in history has identified music as a possible connection to the Divine and has used music in rituals for enhancing spirituality.

Although the MT profession is built on the heels of the ancient history of music, MT has developed since its inception in the 1940s as an evidence-based practice. Music therapists play an integral role in health, healing, and social connections for their clients.

As integrative practitioners, music therapists create individualized treatment plans for each client, with specific therapeutic goals and objectives designed in an appropriate way for the client and setting. MT interventions may be designed for the individual, or for a group when appropriate, and may be delivered collaboratively, co-led, or one on one. Example interventions used by music therapists include: music improvisation, music listening, song writing, lyric discussion, music and imagery, singing, music performance, learning through music, music combined with other arts, music-assisted relaxation, music-based patient education, electronic music technology, adapted music intervention, and movement to music. MT interventions may be receptive in nature, such as music listening or music-assisted relaxation, or they may be designed to facilitate active engagement and interaction through music making or movement. The use of live music interventions demands that the professional possesses not only the knowledge and skills of a trained music therapist, but also the unique skill set of a trained musician in order to manipulate the MT intervention to fit clients' needs. This understanding is reflected in Alejandro's story, where formal MT was accessible within the health-care setting. MT clinical practice may be found in developmental, rehabilitative, habilitative, medical, mental health, preventive, wellness care, or educational areas.

Music therapists in integrative health settings function as independent clinicians within the context of the interdisciplinary team, supporting the treatment goals of the client and/or co-treating with physicians, nurses, neurologists, psychologists, psychiatrists, social workers, counselors, behavioral health specialists, physiotherapists, occupational therapists, speech-language pathologists, audiologists, educators, clinical case managers, caregivers, and more. Specific MT assessment, treatment planning, and implementation are undertaken with consideration for the client's diagnosis and history, are performed in a manner congruent with the client's level of functioning, and address client needs across multiple domains including communication and speech/language, social, emotional, cognitive, behavioral, physical/sensorimotor, occupational, and spiritual.

MT METHODS IN INTEGRATIVE HEALTH CARE

Music therapists are highly qualified through their extensive training to use a variety of methodologies. Many music therapists become specialized in advanced methods which are designed for specific client outcomes. MT has established itself as an evidence-based field;[2] three evidence-based MT methodologies that are frequently utilized by trained music therapists are as follows.

- **Neurologic MT (NMT):**[3] NMT is a series of prescriptive, standardized musical interventions to address specific diagnosed neurologic dysfunctions through music and rhythm. NMT is the application of music for rehabilitation of brain and behavior functions and development and maintenance of mental and physical health. Researchers have found that music and rhythm affect multiple areas of the brain at once;[4] thus, music and rhythm can be used by IRP practitioners to help build new neural connections and more organized processing in the brain/body, and improve a client's overall functioning and quality of life.
- **Nordoff-Robbins MT (NRMT):**[5] The NRMT approach is based on the belief that everyone possesses a sensitivity to music that can be utilized for personal growth and development. In NRMT, clients take an active role in creating music together with their therapists. Through this approach, therapists enhance and support clients' expressive skills and ability to relate to others. Improvisations are created in the moment that relate to the client's presentation at that time, supporting and recognizing the client's musical expression, and entering into the client's world with them through musical interaction.

- **Guided Imagery and Music (GIM):**[6] The Bonny Method of GIM is a music-assisted therapy which uses guided imagery scripts to help clients to work on significant life issues, such as disturbing memories, grief, trauma, interfering health conditions, and relationship issues. While being guided to find helpful resolutions, strong emotions are sometimes processed with this method. The approach was founded on the theory that disturbing imagery left in the unconscious can lead to emotional and physical difficulties, and that the more one is able to bring images to consciousness, the more healing occurs.

AN INTEGRATED MT APPROACH

A "one-size-fits-all" approach to MT does not meet the needs of all clients. For example, while the NMT, NRMT, and GIM specific methods may fit well for some, they do not offer an optimal approach for every need/situation. This understanding is important in relationship to IRP's advocacy for recognizing the uniqueness of each individual's body-mind-environment (BME) experience, thus promoting individualized strategies for whole-person wellness.

One MT theory that aligns well with IRP is known as Music-Centered Music Therapy, developed by Kenneth Aigen (2005).[7] NRMT is a methodology that falls under the category of Music-Centered Music Therapy. Aigen asserts that clients have the right to engage in "musicking," or music making for its own sake, just as anyone who wants to make music would, and that music therapists may facilitate this music making for their clients. He writes:

> The music therapist's art consists of creating opportunities for musicking in which the dynamic forces of music can be encountered by the client in an I-Thou relationship. And the music-centered therapist embodies this relationship to music in two ways: first…with a consciousness of the dynamic forces inherent in music; and second, in the way that the therapist's own life represents an I-Thou encounter with music…because as music therapists, "we are also bound to the laws of music, tying our own destinies…to the dynamic play of forces which lie at its heart."[8]

In MT practice, although individuals typically experience the nonmusical benefits of engaging musically (e.g., lower blood pressure, increased strength and control over gross/fine motor skills, increased expressive language), clients are engaged in the music because they are naturally drawn to it. Feelings of relaxation, exhilaration, or joining with others are often reported. In Alejandro's story from earlier, his connection with the musical part of his formal rehabilitation care was evident to his entire care team; however, his personal recovery in nonmusical areas was not apparent to Alejandro until much later in the treatment process.

The musical experience takes on a life of its own that carries deep individual meaning and value, especially when it occurs in relationship with others. Trust becomes established, within which musical engagement occurs and grows.

The following factors reflect integrative-minded care in relation to MT:

- The therapist creates, adjusts, and adapts the musical experiences to fit the skills, interests, structural requirements, needs, and preferences of each specific client, such as providing adapted or labeled instruments, or choosing instruments that are accessible to the client.

- The therapist reflects the experience back to the client, nonverbally through music and/or verbally through discussion of the process, affirming and reaffirming the client's experiences and helping guide the client forward toward insight, health, and growth.

- The therapist facilitates the client's own stated wishes, values, and needs within the musical experiences, creating musical endeavors in which the client feels empowered, moved, successful, and/or relief from physical or emotional discomfort.

THE SCIENCE OF MUSIC

Neurologic research affords us a greater understanding of why music making is beneficial for its own sake. The overall neurophysiological effects of music and MT continue to be delineated and explored.[9] In a literature review, Chanda and Levitin[10] suggest four interacting domains via which music may act on whole-person biology:

- positive influence upon survival-oriented motivations, mechanisms of reward, and/or pleasure seeking
- enhanced regulation of stress and arousal states towards homeostatic processes
- enhanced immune function
- mechanisms related to positive social engagement.[11]

Consistent with the integral view of science presented in Chapter 7, similar research into MT demonstrates integrated impacts on inflammation and immune function. MT research has shown potential benefits across a wide range of conditions,[12] including: serious mental illness,[13] dementia,[14] emotion regulation,[15] general rehabilitation,[16] pain,[17] autism spectrum disorders,[18] brain injury,[19] and critical care.[20]

MUSIC AND THE POLYVAGAL THEORY

Writings by Stephen Porges regarding MT as it relates to the polyvagal theory (PVT) shed further light on the idea that making music within a therapeutic relationship supports growth, wellness, and healing. See the preceding chapter on the voice for the core PVT science that equally supports MT.

Porges asserts that the PVT is particularly important in understanding the mechanisms underlying MT, which requires both the processing of acoustic stimuli and face-to-face social interactions.[21] He states that the PVT offers insight into the beneficial effects of MT, since the PVT provides an understanding of the neural control of structures involved in the two features of MT: social interactions between the client and the therapist; listening to and expressing music.[22]

Porges explains that, through the lens of PVT, MT can be viewed as two concomitant and integrated processes. First, the therapeutic environment involves the face-to-face interaction between the therapist and the client. This face-to-face interaction, if effective, will trigger the client's perception of safety. Next, the auditory frequency band associated with sung melodies duplicates the frequency band conveying information in the human voice, to which the human nervous system is sensitive and selective. Music, particularly when sung, produces melodies by modulating these same auditory frequencies. This process stimulates the neurobiological correlates of social engagement in a way that carries potential to enhance social interaction skills and emotional regulation.

Interestingly, the phrasing of music is also an important component of the process of emotional regulation in PVT, since singing or playing a wind instrument results in short inhalations and extended durations of exhalations.[23] Such changes in breathing (see Chapter 11) increase a sense of calm and safety. In this way, singing and playing wind instruments may promote positive outcomes, improving several features related to quality of life.

Finally, and as explored in Chapter 20, research about the therapeutic effects of music overlaps with research regarding health benefits of solo singing, chanting, and choral/group singing.[24] PVT provides a science-informed lens for multiple levels of interactions within and between individuals' BME conditions and experiences. PVT provides additional insight into how and why music may yield therapeutic impact when explored in rehabilitation.

MUSICAL INTERVENTIONS FOR HEALTH AND WELL-BEING

How does this information about MT relate to one's everyday life? Can a person engage in music therapeutically without a music therapist to guide them? Are there ways in which other health practitioners may use music within their practice with clients? The answer is, of course, a resounding "yes." The therapeutic benefits of music are available to all of us. We know this intuitively. The following is a list of suggested activities for ways in which we may use music to improve our own lives and the lives of our clients, even if a music therapist is not present or available.

- **Create your own wellness playlists**: Many of us have a large listening library contained in our cell phones or other electronic devices. However, there is a way in which we may curate our own specific playlists to effect and support positive changes in mood, energy, and concentration, by paying attention to our own responses to music and making note of them:
  - **Keep a listening journal**: When listening to a song or a musical piece that has a *strong, positive effect* on you, write down the name of the song and artist, and the effect that it had (released sadness, increased energy, increased relaxation, etc.). Do not include songs that make you feel worse after listening.
  - **Add songs that remind you of specific joyful times that you feel happy to think of**: Such songs might include milestones, childhood, teen years, celebrations.

- **Categorize your songs by function and create different lists**: Here is one example list that was created that included labels for music to use at different times as needed: songs for sleeping; woman empowerment; early morning wake-up; enhancing concentration; cry it out/let it go; relieve anxiety.
- **Burn CDs or create playlists on your devices**: You may want to suggest this playlist activity for your clients or use it yourself as part of much-needed self-care. Music listening is free and requires no medication. The act of attentive and mindful listening is a stabilizing intervention in itself, even if you don't have much time. In a recent study, The British Academy of Sound Therapy sought to identify whether specific types of music would help people feel better in specific ways.[25] Among 7,581 participants, 89% reported feeling happy and uplifted after only nine minutes of listening to songs with a fast tempo, a driving rhythm, and positive lyrical content. The majority of participants who experienced improved concentration, relaxation, or sleep needed only 13 minutes on average of their preferred focusing, calming, or sedating music to feel the desired effect. Participants reported that classical music of Mozart and Bach was best for improving their concentration, while participants with improved mood reported that songs with lyrics that they could personally relate to were the most effective type of music for releasing sadness. Ultimately, self-selection of music combined with the cultivation of awareness around one's response to that selection is what matters most.

- **Use of calming instruments/sounds**: There are many musical instruments that require minimal skill to produce ambient, calming tones. As a health practitioner, you may want to have some instruments available or suggest some to your clients to use to induce mindful relaxation. Rain sticks, Remo Lullaby Ocean Discs, Remo Ocean Drums, soft-sounding shakers, wind chimes, ocarinas, or flutes have quiet sounds and offer kinesthetic feedback and visual input which clients may find calming. The use of such instruments can enhance breathing patterns and overall psychophysiological state (see Chapter 11).

- **Use a steady beat to enhance physical movement**: Using music that matches the speed of the movement you are targeting—whether it is your own workout at the gym, or a client's physiotherapy, occupational therapy, or speech-language skills—can support neuromotor function. You can use recorded music, beat a drum, use a metronome, or strum a guitar. Moving to a steady beat results in improved regulation, muscle output, endurance, and motivation.[26] Drawing[27] (also see Chapter 19) and/or moving/dancing[28] (also see Chapter 15) may be combined with music to support and facilitate fine and gross motor movement, not to mention processes of self-expression and other impacts as explored in earlier chapters.

MUSIC IN THE CLINIC

Sounds including environmental "noise" can impact us deeply. Attention to your work environment is important in this regard. Further, and depending upon your setting and the nature of your individual work, the use of music in the clinic presents another opportunity to yield positive effects from music outside of direct access to a music therapist in your setting/community.

Whether in individual sessions or group experiences, well-chosen music enhances the overall experience and may yield positive combined physiological influence for both the clinician and client(s) during: meditation or biofeedback experiences; manual therapy; guided imagery. Patient preference is important. Having two or three options for soothing music that your client can choose from (if music is desired in the first place—check this too) is encouraged. Music designed for meditation or relaxation, and/or ambient sound (like rain or ocean waves), reflect good choices. Volume is important, so check regularly to make sure it is "just right." Sensitivity to music in shared spaces is also important.

MUSIC IS MEDICINE

Music is vital to human experience, an intrinsic human need. All people naturally respond to rhythm or melody in some way. The value of music in IRP is in the overall positive quality of the musical experiences, within a therapeutic relationship, that can move clients forward toward health and wellness. Such musical experiences may be provided by a music therapist, as was the case for Alejandro. Formal MT experiences may include evidence-based uses of rhythm, melody, and phrasing through listening, singing, playing instruments, analyzing, or creating music.

One need not be a music therapist, however, to harness the benefits of music in the clinic. There are many ways to support therapeutic effects from music within IRP through client-chosen music listening and music-making endeavors that enhance or improve the overall well-being of the client(s). Through a shared musical-listening or creative experience, the practitioner can meet clients where they are emotionally and spiritually, and together progress forward toward the attainment of therapeutic goals and improved quality of life.

Experiential pause: Having read this chapter, identify and write down at least one actionable item of interest to you. In doing so, consider ways in which applying the material first to yourself, and then to patients, might serve those who come to you for care.

CHAPTER 22

Exploring Nutrition and Food

Brigid Titgemeier, MS, RDN, LD, IFNCP and Matt Erb, PT

A story: "Cherise" is a nurse in her mid 50s. She is thin and seemingly "healthy" but had been struggling with constant pain as a result of multi-joint arthritis. As a health-care practitioner herself, she had access to some of the best rheumatologists, all of whom prescribed nonsteroidal anti-inflammatory drugs (NSAIDs) and corticosteroids. As a conventionally trained nurse of 25 years, Cherise was skeptical of integrative approaches, but her husband encouraged her to seek answers. After a thorough nutritional assessment and presentation of potentially beneficial approaches, Cherise chose to follow an anti-inflammatory diet and nutraceuticals, such as turmeric and omega-3 fish oil. In addition, she committed to five minutes of daily morning meditation and breathing to assist in deepening connection with her body. She had some hesitancy around the effort required, but with guidance she was able to link her commitment to her life values. At her 12-week follow-up, Cherise smiled with tears in her eyes and said that she felt a sense of renewal, had started golfing again once a week, and had notably increased her engagement with household activities.

In this chapter, we will take a look at food, eating, and nutrition, and explore each person's unique relationship with food in support of each person's mind, body, and spiritual health. Food represents a powerful, cost-effective, underappreciated, accessible form of medicine, yet a majority of the population does not take advantage of its potential medicinal properties. Eating a diet rich in micronutrients, polyphenols, and phytonutrients can synergistically alter multiple pathways and prevent inflammatory cascades.

While food carries vital healing benefits, it may be a source of shame for some. The question of why the topic of food and eating carries challenges such as shame represents another area for engaging complex thinking; the reader is invited to review the discussion on shame and stigma in Chapter 6. Additionally, factors related to the sociocultural determinants of health, such as food production, access, and security, must be considered. The choices that people make around food may be subject to their food environment, government food subsidies, and food advertising, as well as a host of complex individual dynamics.

Cherise's experience reflects the possible upside of lifestyle change. Even when there are no sociocultural or economic barriers, change around food and eating does not necessarily come easily. As with the whole of this book, start with yourself first. If your relationship with food is already optimal, stay alert for the possibility of self-inflation that negatively influences how you support others' relationships with food.

FOOD INFLUENCES CHRONIC CONDITIONS

While diet and nutrition play a clear role in chronic health conditions, most people's experience with food stems from restriction and weight loss.[1] This includes frequent challenges with body image and/or weight. Historically, nutrition was simplified into a calories-in/calories-out weight-loss equation. While calorie deficit and energy balance play a role in weight loss to various degrees, there are potential flaws with oversimplifying this equation.

- Calories are not created equal.
- Inadequate caloric intake can decrease energy expenditure and lead to weight gain.
- Food provides information for cells, having the ability to regulate genetic expression and modulate risk of disease (epigenetics, from Chapter 7).
- Food quality and soil quality can significantly influence the body's response to foods.
- There are other factors to consider for weight loss such as imbalances in hormones and the gut microbiome.

Nutrition plays an important role in helping people achieve and maintain optimal body weight. But the role of food goes much deeper than weight. What you feed your body changes its physiological state by modulating risk of disease, feeding diverse strains in the gut microbiome, influencing genetics, supporting immunological resilience, lowering inflammation, helping with pain management, and more.[2]

In recent years the literature has become clear: in order to decrease inflammation, enhance immunity, and decrease the risk and prevalence of chronic disease, the medical system and the larger society are in dire need of learning effective ways to leverage the power of food, without creating more shame. This is an important part of integrative solutions to health promotion that can produce more effective outcomes at lower cost.

Experiential pause: Take a moment and become aware of your body. Connect with the many sensations of your body—the whole body. Take a minute or two to contemplate the experience of your body, and your sense of relationship with/to your body. How would you define your "body image"? Take time to write down your insights. Now, contemplate how your relationship with yourself and your body might be interacting with food, nutrition, and eating… Continue writing down what comes to you around these questions.

THE NUMBERS

Approximately six out of ten adults in the US have a chronic disease and four out of ten adults have two or more.[3] It is estimated that seven out of ten of the top causes of death in the US are associated with poor nutrition.[4]

Optimal nutrition can combine with three other modifiable risk factors (never smoking, having a body mass index below 30, and performing 3.5 hours per week of physical activity) to support an estimated 78% lower risk of developing chronic disease (diabetes, myocardial infarction, stroke, and cancer).[5] As covered in Chapters 3 and 4, chronic stress is also implicated in chronic disease. It follows that support for mitigating any presence of toxic stress is of equal importance.[6] Together, these topics reflect a recipe for health promotion with nutrition as an essential ingredient. What conventional medicine fails to actively embrace is that being thin does not make you healthy. In Cherise's case, she was not overweight but nutrition and stress management were still vitally important for modulating inflammatory mediators and improving her quality of life.

PAIN AND NUTRITION

Of importance to the topic of chronic health challenges is the prevalence of persistent pain. In the integrative framework, "pain" can be experienced in a variety of forms: physical/sensory, emotional, cognitive, social, or spiritual. While persistent pain does not influence mortality rates as obviously as chronic disease does, it is a large contributor to suffering, disability, dependence on NSAIDs and opioids, and low quality of life.[7]

As we've seen in prior chapters, pain is complex and the contributing factors to pain are vast and highly individualized. When exposed to various stress inputs, the body is designed to adapt. When adaptation capacity is exceeded, a person's risk of developing health issues, including persistent pain, increases.[8] The integrative lens reminds us of interdependence within body-mind-environment (BME) interactions, as well as the importance of taking committed actions in support of general health and well-being. At a minimum, addressing nutrition and mindful eating reflect this rationale.

PAIN, WEIGHT, AND OVERLAPPING CHALLENGES

We don't have to look far to see the general challenge of obesity in our society, nor its relevance to the topic at hand. Looking further in examining relationships of comorbidity, one of many risk factors for developing persistent pain is obesity. Carrying excess weight has been associated with an increased risk of persistent pain conditions including: fibromyalgia, osteoarthritis, rheumatoid arthritis, and low back pain.[9]

As discussed in Chapter 3, multimorbidity and syndemics are topics that reflect the complicated and often "stacking" interactions of multiple chronic diseases. Such dynamics set up negative interactions that demand contextual capacity in the health-care provider, if meaningful change might be realized.

While persistent pain frequently occurs independently from obesity and/or other chronic disease, the presence of chronic disease(s) increases the risk of persistent pain onset, and chronic disease and pain interact in complex ways.[10] In the cases of cancer-related pain, neuropathic pain (such as diabetic neuropathy), and visceral pain, pain is thought to emerge secondary to chronic disease.[11] This is common in individuals with single chronic conditions (such as cancer, diabetes, and hypertension) and multiple chronic conditions.[12] Regardless of whether pain is the primary health challenge or not, when the topic is of interest to the patient, exploring nutrition has potential to impact BME relationships.

INFLAMMATION, IMMUNITY, AND FOOD: ALLIES OR ENEMIES?

One component of physiology that is increasingly seen as a shared factor in disease is inflammation.[13] Chronic inflammation can ensue in the presence of non-degradable pathogens, persistent viral infections, and autoimmune reactions as examples. It can occur when acute inflammatory mechanisms fail to eliminate tissue injury, and this increases the risk of chronic diseases and persistent pain.

In today's environment, we are frequently exposed to a large number of inflammatory mediators such as processed foods, heavy metals, air pollution, and unfiltered water. When there is excess adipose tissue, which is an active endocrine organ involved in the regulation of inflammation, the impact may be increased.[14] As noted earlier, toxic stress can also enter the equation via various entry points, such as individual or collective psychological, historical, social, physical, environmental, and/or *nutritional* stress, impacting regulation of the hypothalamic-pituitary-adrenal axis.[15]

In regard to the pressing topic of pain, when inflammation is present, it can increase neurophysiological sensitivity in both the body and the brain in relation to pain processes.[16] This sensitivity is mediated by chemicals, peptides, and other cellular substances such as cytokines and prostaglandins.

The immune system is also involved in health and disease processes.[17] Inflammation and immune function interact with the many other factors listed, influencing overall health state and underscoring complexity. Ultimately, exploring nutrition can help within a comprehensive plan to mitigate the interrelationships between inflammation, immune function, and other conditions.[18]

THE WONDROUS GUT: ECOSYSTEMS WITHIN ECOSYSTEMS

The gut microbiota composition affects a person's biology and overall health in profound and, perhaps, previously unexpected ways. As first explored in Chapter 7, the *microbiome* influences all aspects of health (physical, mental, emotional) via systems-wide influence. This direct influence includes immune system function as well as brain health via the gut-brain axis.[19] The digestive tract hosts trillions of bacteria, fungi, and other organisms. It has the largest collection of immune cells—approximately 70% of all lymphoid tissues in the body.[20] The gut is where the majority of neurotransmitter production occurs.[21] The gut/microbiome environment is also where electrolytes are reabsorbed, water is extracted, and nutrients are produced by bacteria, such as vitamin K and B vitamins such as biotin (B7), folate (B9), and cobalamin (B12).[22]

Liang *et al.* demonstrate that gut microbiota also help to regulate visceral and peripheral pain responses.[23] Research among individuals with an altered gut microbiome indicated that supplementing with probiotics may be associated with a decline in the level of pain.[24]

Diet and probiotics are two factors that play an important role in altering the gut composition, carrying potential impact on risk of chronic disease, pain processes, and numerous mental and neurological diseases.[25] Therapeutic nutrition interventions can play a critical role in improving psychiatric symptoms and cognitive impairment that are associated with the changes in the gut-brain axis.[26] Foods act as a direct source of fuel for the bacteria living in the gut microbiome. Dietary interventions change the distribution of bacteria, gut microbial activities, stress-related differences in energy metabolism, and the excretion of cortisol and catecholamines.[27] In essence, food is a key component of the microbiome's environment. Think *interacting levels of* BME: interdependence of an ecosystem within a larger ecosystem.

Recall Cherise, who struggled with widespread joint pain attributed to arthritis. There is growing inquiry into associations between diet, the microbiome, and arthritic conditions.[28] The possibility of such associations had never been mentioned or explored in Cherise's conventional medical care. After several months of dietary and lifestyle changes, Cherise began to experience improvements in her symptoms. While we can't say for sure to what extent the dietary changes impacted her microbiome and thus systemic inflammation, evidence is pointing us towards potential links.

RECIPES

There are many factors to consider when identifying ingredients that impact the "recipe" of any given state of health or illness. While there's growing evidence that chronic disease and pain are associated with inflammation, the gut microbiome, the immune system, and stress, there are still uncertainties around the ways in which they mix. When we approach our efforts towards health promotion from the lens that shifting ingredients in the recipe alters the "taste," we see nutrition and one's relationship to food as influential ingredients. There is ample opportunity to incorporate the principles and strategies found in this chapter into self-selected care approaches as you discover the recipe that is unique to your own needs.

A NEED FOR PERSONALIZED NUTRITION

When it comes to exploring the role of food and eating in the promotion of health and well-being, a personalized approach is necessary. When Cherise was first seen, her dietitian understood complexity and considered many variables that might have been impacting Cherise's health. In regard to nutrition, public health recommendations tend to be generalized and do not sufficiently address complexity. As adapted from Minich and Bland,[29] Table 22.1 demonstrates numerous complex interacting factors that may impact a personalized nutrition approach.

Table 22.1: Factors Influencing Personalized Nutrition

Age	Life cycle	Gender	Past medical history
Family history	Ethnic background	Stress history and levels	Genetics/epigenetics
Lifestyle habits	Nutritional status	Medication use	Supplement use
Physical location	Travel/transportation	Home environment	Individual values/goals
Microbiome state	Food sensitivities	Nutrient deficiency	Nutrition knowledge
Cooking experience	Taste preferences	Food accessibility	Socioeconomic status

Adapted from Minich and Bland[30]

> **Experiential pause:** Table 22.1 is thorough but not exhaustive. As you review each item, contemplate how each topic informs your current nutrition/food experience. Are there areas that carry more or less perceived impact on your current nutritional status? Or areas you've never considered? Jot down your ideas. Ask yourself what factors you would add. What about the ways in which you might use food and eating as a form of coping? How might this apply to you?

FOOD AS MEDICINE
Overview

Food provides both a source of energy and nourishment for the body and vital information for cells and genes. The food choices made each day can become one of the best ways for a person to care for themselves and their family members. The easy choices in the short term are ultra-processed, calorie-dense, and/or fast foods. However, when considering choices that pay off in the long term, shifts towards increased whole/unprocessed, plant-based, and nutrient-dense foods reflect starting principles. While nutrition is best personalized, additional foundations to consider include incorporating dietary fiber, omega-3 fatty acids, and anti-inflammatory herbs and spices. Let's look at a few of these subtopics, noting that there are many more to explore as you deepen your understanding of individualized nutrition.

Can you recognize the original form of the food you eat?

The increased consumption of processed foods hijacks the body's normal physiology. At one point in time, people viewed 100 calories of spinach and 100 calories of soda as comparable, when in fact they carry very different messages and influences. Foods and beverages that are processed and/or high in simple sugars have adverse biochemical effects, especially in the context of high caloric intake and a sedentary lifestyle.[31] A diet high in refined carbohydrates, like soda, can lead to the impaired production of hormones like leptin, ghrelin, neuropeptide Y, and insulin, which can drive more food consumption.[32] When it comes to eating 100 calories of spinach, the opposite is true.

Eating a diet that is high in ultra-processed foods puts a person at risk of being undernourished in terms of fiber, antioxidants, and other beneficial components. These foods, known as empty calories, lack the fiber, protein, phytochemicals, and other nutrients that help to slow down digestion, balance blood sugar levels, decrease production of reactive oxygen species (aka free radicals, part of inflammation), and signal feelings of fullness to the brain.[33] On the other hand, eating *whole foods* that arrive in their original unprocessed state leads to a very different gut environment. Whole foods provide the body with the natural forms of micronutrients, phytonutrients, and dietary fiber that feed the bacteria and beneficial metabolites within the gut microbiome—and in turn, the body's cells.

Fiber—a fabric for the gut

Eating a diet that is high in fiber can be beneficial for weight loss, the gut microbiome, heart health, and more. The best sources of fiber come from legumes, nuts and seeds, vegetables, and fruits. Additional fiber sources may be warranted, such as psyllium husk fiber, unmodified potato starch, or acacia. Fiber intake should include both soluble (dissolves in water to form a gel-like consistency and slows passage of food from the stomach to the small intestine) and insoluble (does not dissolve in water and is bristlier, providing roughage and adding bulk and softness to stool) sources.[34]

Reduction in pain may be another benefit of eating foods that are higher in fiber.[35] Fiber intake should also be considered when patients are prescribed opioids for pain management. Opioid-induced constipation (OIC) is the most common adverse effect of opioids, and it is increasingly unresponsive to laxatives.[36] This makes it imperative for patients who are taking opioid medication to increase consumption of fiber-rich foods. Fluid intake should also increase unless contraindicated.

Omega-3 fatty acids—lotion for cells and tissues

Omega-3s take a few different forms. The short-chain version of alpha linolenic acid (ALA) is found in plant foods such as chia seeds, flax seeds, and walnuts. The long-chain versions include eicosapentaenoic acid (EPA) and docosahexaenoic acid (DHA) and are found in fatty fish and fish oil supplements. These fatty acids have been shown to impact pain because of their ability to increase anti-inflammatory eicosanoids, resolvins, and protectins while lowering pro-inflammatory eicosanoid production. They do so through various mechanisms, all of which are primarily associated with changes in the fatty-acid composition of cell membranes.[37]

When using a food-first approach, a person will benefit most from incorporating two to three weekly servings of fish that are high in omega-3 fats and low in mercury. Examples of foods rich in EPA and DHA include wild salmon, sardines, herring, oysters, anchovies, and cod. Regular consumption of plant-based sources of ALA, such as chia seeds, ground flaxseeds, hemp seeds, and walnuts, is also beneficial.[38] Many people may require fish oil supplementation to obtain an adequate intake and the beneficial impact that can come from omega-3s.[39]

The average Western diet tends to fall short on omega-3 intake while also including an abundance of omega 6-polyunsaturated fats.[40] A higher omega-6 to omega-3 ratio is pro-inflammatory.[41] As such, many individuals may need to consume more omega-3s while concurrently eating fewer omega-6 polyunsaturated fats to lower the omega-6 to omega-3 ratio. The most common sources of omega-6 fats include soybean oil, corn oil, safflower oil, sunflower oil, peanut oil, and other vegetable oils, in addition to grains.[42]

Turmeric, ginger, and spices, oh my…

Spices and herbs have anti-inflammatory properties that can help to lower inflammation.[43] Two examples that stand out are turmeric and ginger. Turmeric is a spice made up of the active component curcumin. Curcumin has been found to decrease pain and inflammation related to osteoarthritis, in a similar way to medications like ibuprofen and COX-2 inhibitors.[44] Typical doses are 1500mg Curcuma domestica or 1000mg of a combination of Curcuma longa with Boswellia serrata.[45] Curcuma longa is produced in supplement form, called Meriva®.[46] While supplementing is the best route for increasing the absorption of turmeric, there may be some benefits to including turmeric root in foods with black pepper and a source of fat such as extra virgin olive oil.[47]

Ginger has long been used in traditional medicine as an anti-inflammatory agent. Along with being a rich source of vitamins and minerals, ginger contains anti-inflammatory compounds such as gingerol, shogaol, paradol, and zingerone, which inhibit the synthesis of pro-inflammatory compounds, cytokines, and can down-regulate the expression of genes that cause inflammation.[48] Ginger has been shown to reduce many different types of pain, such as menstrual cramp pain and exercise-induced muscle injury.[49] Fresh ginger root can be incorporated into an anti-inflammatory diet as a flavoring agent for a variety of dishes.

The world of spices and the larger landscape of herbal and plant-based medicines reminds us of the healing properties found in the plant world. Biochemical plant compounds are powerful; while carrying potential health benefits, they can also be toxicogenic.[50] It is important, if exploring the addition of herbal/plant-based supplements delivered in concentrated forms, to work with a registered dietitian or other health-care practitioner who understands their properties, as well as potential interactions with medications and other supplements.

WHAT IS YOUR RELATIONSHIP WITH FOOD?
Overview

All of the preceding information is of limited use unless it is explored through an approach that defines one's relationship to food and eating first. While food has high potential to serve as powerful medicine in our lives, many people experience shame, disconnect, or other associations when it comes to food choices and eating. This is partially why overly prescriptive diets often fail, setting up cycles of negative feelings and behavioral patterns.[51] In order to improve one's long-term relationship to food, formulating a baseline picture of one's unique relationship to food is necessary. Clarity in this picture might be followed by applying principles of motivational interviewing,[52] mindfulness, and personalized nutrition recommendations that stem from an intention to create positive connection to food and eating.

> **Experiential pause:** Take a moment and indulge in a few slower, fuller breaths to invite the relaxation response. Now close your eyes and contemplate: What does my past and current relationship with food look like? Is it positive, neutral, or negative? Are there areas where judgment is at work? See if any images come, not just words and thoughts. Consider writing down, sketching, or drawing what you come up with. Repeat these steps to conceptualize what your relationship to food might look like in the future.

Creating a positive relationship with food

Nutrition knowledge alone does not explain or dictate one's eating behaviors, for example in relationship to body weight.[53] Establishing a nourishing, non-judgmental, and loving relationship with food is just as important as what you eat when it comes to harnessing potential benefits and promoting well-being. When a person's relationship with food is judgmental and controlling, it leads to an increase in stress around food. Chronic stress can arise from pervasive negative thoughts and feelings around food, eating, body weight, and/or negative body image. Such stress can contribute to high/prolonged hypothalamic-pituitary-adrenal axis activation. This increase in stress can negatively impact the gut microbiome.[54] As noted earlier, there are correlations between pain and the gut microbiome. There are also correlations between eating disorders and the gut microbiome.[55] In these associations, and others, dots can sometimes be connected; however, correlation does not imply causation. Allowing patients to determine relevance is always a best practice.

Disordered eating versus eating disorders?

When the prevalence of individuals who suffer with an eating disorder and functional gastrointestinal disorders (FGIDs) was examined, rates of overlap were high but it wasn't initially understood which occurred first.[56] Perkins and colleagues found that 83% of participants had developed an eating disorder prior to irritable bowel syndrome (IBS).[57] Eating disorders often occur before the development of gastrointestinal symptoms, suggesting that the stress from controlling one's foods, in addition to poor food consumption, may alter gut microbiome and health (e.g., inflammation), contributing to the manifestation of FGIDs.[58] Stress history, such as that found in adverse childhood experiences or trauma exposure (Chapter 4), impacts autonomic physiology, reflecting another glimpse into possible relationships that impact FGIDs.[59]

Diagnosable eating disorders, such as anorexia nervosa or bulimia, are not extremely prevalent in the general population, but *disordered eating patterns* are more common than uncommon. While food can serve as medicine, people experience complex relationships around food and eating, including possible patterns of shame, as discussed earlier. Overly restrictive eating plans can further perpetuate disordered or judgmental eating patterns. Contributors to obesity and poor eating choices are unrealistic nutrition goals, negative feelings around food, body image, stress/emotional eating as a form of maladaptive coping, and lack of ability to listen to one's body.

The way that a person approaches their diet can have a large impact on their lived experience. Rather than approaching wellness and nutrition from a place of lack, it's important to approach it from a place of abundance, respect, and love. When a person comes from a place of lack, they would be more likely to focus on caloric restriction, force, and more willpower. Unfortunately, this is more likely to create a negative experience that adds tension, creating a downward food spiral. When a person embraces wellness and nutrition from a place of care and concern, the focus shifts to nourishment, intention, and increased acceptance of body and self.

The starting place for approaching food without judgment is to defuse thoughts such as: "I had a bad food day," "I was bad," "I cheated on my diet," "This food is bad," and "I have no willpower or control." Food has no moral value and such thoughts only have influence if we fuse these thoughts as belief or truth. The choices made around food (and the thoughts that accompany them) do not reflect a person's innate value. These things do not go hand in hand. There is no such thing as "bad" food, and eating a certain food does not create a "bad" person.

Approaching food from a non-judgmental place should not be confused with giving permission to eat endless amounts of processed foods. There are many foods that lack nourishing properties, like ultra-processed, nutrient-deficient foods that can perpetuate FGIDs. However, instead of viewing these foods as "bad," which fuses self-value to consumption, try to approach them as "less optimal" or "nutritionally empty." Create space to ask: Is this an optimal choice for my body? This also helps with reframing thoughts such as: "Should I eat this?", "Is this right/wrong?", and "Is this food good/bad?"

Food cravings and addiction—a personal or societal problem?

Intellectually, most people know that processed foods are not an optimal choice. The issue is that processed foods are designed to be addictive and cause people to consume more of the same.[60] When Cherise returned for her recheck visit, she expressed that the hardest thing for her in shifting her food patterns was realizing just how much she craved snacks such as packaged pastries, cookies, and crackers through the day. Previously, she saw this as a personal weakness. The addictive nature of processed foods has been strategically created by the food industry using a 5-A equation.

1. **Availability**: Making the substance available everywhere 24/7.
2. **Affordability**: Making it as cheap as possible.
3. **Addictive** properties in the product ingredients.
4. **Advertising**: Spending millions of dollars on marketing to create a norm in society.
5. **Age of onset**: Targeting young consumers.[61]

When Cherise learned of this, it made it easier to assess and more effectively respond to urges through the adjustment phase of not relying solely on these foods to boost her mood and energy.

Additional factors that interact in processed food addiction and that reflect a greater degree of individuality than the preceding systemic issues include being disconnected from oneself and/or the present moment, and the tendency to use food as a stress and emotion coping strategy, which was true in Cherise's case. Comforting or otherwise pleasant effects may arise from food choices and the eating experience; direct effects may also come from the impact of the food's properties on our neurophysiological state, impacting mood.[62]

Additional insight into these associations may come from the understanding that oral motor activity (the physical use of the mouth) carries remnants of infant regulation strategies due to shared developmental and neuroanatomical processes.[63] Simplified: when our mouth is in motion, it may be delivering self-soothing neurophysiological effects for stress/emotion coping. Even simpler: the Japanese language has a word *kuchisabishii*, which infers a dynamic where one is not necessarily hungry but would like to eat because the "mouth is lonely."[64] The preceding systemic dynamics combine with such individual tendencies to point us towards the importance of mindfulness in relationship to food and eating.

> **Experiential pause:** View the sample food images in Figure 22.1. Do any associations arise? Are there feelings, memories, thoughts, beliefs, or judgments? Notice any bodily response as you look at each food item (remember the lemon imagery in Chapter 14?).

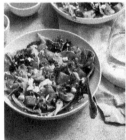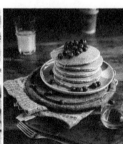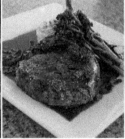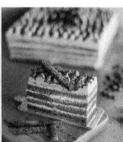

FIGURE 22.1: FOOD IMAGES

MINDFUL EATING

Overview

The idea of mindful eating is often applied to the act of consuming food. Digestion, however, starts with a *cephalic phase*—awareness of the mental/emotional processes that inform the when, where, why, what, and how of eating. "What sounds good? What's in the fridge? Shoot, I need eggs for that dish. I'm tired, maybe we'll get takeout tonight. Ooh, yeah, pizza sounds good." Similar to whether we are stressed/tense, or relaxed, such mental processes can inform digestive processes.

Mindful eating allows a person to be more present with food choice and food preparation. Mindful eating then extends to the consumption phase, affording increased awareness of textures, flavors, and colors of the food, and increased intentionality with how one feels before, during, and after eating various foods or portions. Slowing down and paying attention also help to optimize digestion and absorption of nutrients, prevent gluttony or overeating, and allow for checking in on one's mind-body state regularly.

> **Experiential pause:** Write down your own insights around the following questions, which are modified and shortened from a yogic presentation on mindful eating.[65] The questions aim to support the gradual development of individualized values that inform your relationship to nutrition, food, and eating. Identify any other values and qualities that you have that can inform the taking of committed actions that serve an improved relationship with food and eating. Starting small is recommended. You may only work with one or a few of these at any given time.
>
> - Am I honest about my relationship with food? Am I willing to compassionately examine the patterns of emotions, thoughts, and beliefs that influence my relationship with food and with my body?
> - Do I eat more or less than what is needed for my body's energetic needs? If so, why?
> - Where and how do I invest the fuel from what I eat? Is this energetic equation in balance?
> - How does past and/or current stress interact with the when, where, what, and why behind my eating?
> - Do I experience gratitude for the nourishment that I receive? Am I aware of the people, land, and other resources that went into the production of the food I eat? Am I aware of the fact that many individuals may not have the same access to food that I do?
> - Can I pay enough attention to notice how certain foods that I eat impact how I feel and/or any symptoms that I have like bloating, joint pain, or headaches?
> - Do I choose to eat foods that support me in serving others and myself in the highest way?

Principles of mindful eating

There are a number of mindful principles that can be applied to food and nutrition. These principles assist in revealing hidden patterns in one's relationship with food. Incorporating mindfulness principles can also help in the larger process of learning about and proactively meeting one's unique and changing needs. A few examples to get you started are given below.

- **Sit down**: Whenever possible, sit down to eat. Become mindful of your posture while eating. Ask yourself, am I upright yet fully relaxed? Does my posture support healthy attention, chewing, and digestion?
- **Partake in breathing, meditation, and/or prayer**: Before you begin eating, bring awareness to the breath. Check in with your mood and overall mind-body state. Is your energy fast? Inhale and exhale more slowly. Doing this helps to activate the "rest and digest" state, allowing you to better digest and absorb your food. Consider integrating meditation, intention, or prayer practices into the start of your meal.
- **Bring fuller attention to the meal**: Try not to view mealtimes as opportunities for multitasking. This is a time to be present as much as possible. Are you multitasking or focused on the food choice and the act of eating? Can you put away other objects of attention?
- **Listen to your body**: The more attuned one is to the subtle sensations, cues, and messages of the body, the more able one is to detect the influence of foods, dietary patterns, and habits on health.
- *Hara hachi bu:* *Hara hachi bu* is a Japanese phrase and practice that encourages you to chew your food thoroughly and eat until you are ~80% full. This requires pausing while eating to support attunement to interoception (see Chapter 13).
- **Relate**: When possible, link your meals and eating to relationship and connection.

Awareness experiments

Awareness experiments assist in learning more about one's individuality in relation to food, including food sensitivities that are linked to neuroinflammatory and immune responses. Temporary selective elimination of certain foods, followed by reintroduction of that food, may allow a person to see more clearly how their body responds. In an elimination program, foods are typically removed for a minimum of three weeks and then reintroduced one at a time. During this time, noticing overall symptom patterns, emotional dynamics, and/or thoughts/beliefs is useful. It is recommended to keep a daily diary of this process, including food consumption, timing, and anything else you notice.

You can also devise your own awareness experiments and discover what your body is telling you. Remember that health is complex and these experiments do not occur in isolation. Also remember that nocebo, the opposite of placebo, can sometimes be at work, and can lead to the formation of faulty, negative beliefs and associations about food(s). Thus, the point here is to explore and contemplate and not create negative associations that may not exist. Here are a few example experiments.

- **For people who eat on the run, while reading or watching TV, or multitasking**: Try slowly eating a meditative meal in a quiet environment: breathe, relax, and appreciate.
- **For people who love processed and fast foods**: Try eating only whole foods for one week and see what it brings up for you.
- **For people who eat high sugar/carbohydrate meals**: Try eating a high-protein meal such as eggs, salmon, or unsweetened yogurt.
- **For people who tend to be irritable between meals**: Try to stretch, shift, and use movement first, and if the irritability persists, try snacking on smaller amounts of whole foods such as vegetables, nuts, and fruit.

Considerations

To best support your patient's needs, we encourage you to refer to or collaborate with skilled and licensed integrative and functional dietitians and certified nutritionist specialists whenever possible. This helps in creating a multidisciplinary team-based approach to health that leverages the expertise of specialists. At the same time, with appropriate training, exploring the foundations of general nutrition and mindful eating can be within the scope of many rehabilitation professionals. Creating a strong therapeutic relationship, in addition to sharing some basic information, can go a long way.

Clinicians must assess if/when the extent to which they are addressing nutrition falls outside of their level of training or expertise level. For example, in working with individuals using nutrition interventions for diseases, such as type 2 diabetes or rheumatoid arthritis, it is vital that the professional has the necessary training to understand the individual needs of the patient. Similarly, if an individual has an eating disorder, specialized training is needed to ensure safety.

DIGESTING THIS CHAPTER

While the information we have presented is a lot to digest, this chapter offers only a taste of a massive topic. Nutrition impacts a person's basic physiology on a day-to-day, meal-to-meal basis and each of us is given daily opportunities to consume a natural form of medicine through the power of our fork. Rather than getting overwhelmed, when exploring a food as medicine approach, it's important to start small; to do so in a way that is non-judgmental, compassionate, and informed by patient, persistent practice. We must bridge the gap (or for some of us, the chasm) between idealism and realism. The true goal is to participate in an ongoing experiment of coming to know oneself—and one's relationship to nutrition, food, and eating—better. At the end of the day, nutrition is always personal and dependent on supporting well-being based on each person's unique needs.

Experiential pause: Having read this chapter, identify and write down at least one actionable item of interest to you. In doing so, consider ways in which applying the material first to yourself, and then to patients, might serve those who come to you for care.

CHAPTER 23

Reframing Manual Therapy

Cheryl Van Demark, PT, C-IAYT

A story: The therapist walks towards the waiting room to greet the next patient, holding an intention to notice the many factors that have the potential to influence each therapeutic encounter. To refresh and focus attention, the therapist's breath is released in a long slow exhale. Footsteps are deliberate. The ground is sensed. This feels good.

The patient is greeted with a smile that softens the therapist's eyes. As the patient is escorted to the treatment room, the therapist focuses their five senses as if experiencing the clinic for the first time, like the patient. The therapist recognizes that the state of the patient's nervous systems will influence if, when, and how to use manual therapy.

The patient story is allowed to unfold through a biopsychosocialspiritual interview process. The therapist has learned the art of listening with their whole body. How the patient uses their body and breath to emote their story also becomes an invaluable observation for the attuned manual therapist. This feels good.

The physical examination begins with permission for the therapist to lay hands on the patient's body. This signals an important aspect of safety and patient control in introducing therapeutic touch. The patient's experience of posture and movement is assessed with open-ended questions. Their answers reveal a level of body awareness that will profoundly guide the use of any manual therapy in the overall treatment plan. Is weight held evenly on both feet? How does it feel to move into that direction? What sensation stops the motion at that point? Is this sensation concerning? An environment of curiosity about perception of body position in space, movement quantity, quality, and perceived power is established. As the body part is moved or palpated, the patient is prompted to share emotions, images, and beliefs about what is happening in response to movement.

The process of simple and well-placed pain neuroscience education is initiated; the patient's responses are sensed and checked along the way. The profound impact of the various interacting facets of our neurophysiology upon healing is introduced. The role of manual therapy to influence movement among other factors is explained. The patient's concerns, aspirations, and expectations for participating in therapy are discussed. The foundation for shared decision making is established. The patient is asked if they believe that this plan might be helpful. They are willing to participate and do all they can to help themselves. The therapeutic alliance is established. Conducting the initial therapeutic encounter in this way reflects the integrative rehabilitation practice (IRP) paradigm and opens our minds to how we might rethink manual therapy in this chapter. This feels really good!

As mentioned in the first chapter, the etymology of the word "rehabilitation" evolved from the medieval Latin "re," again, and "habitare," to make fit. Such a description can invite the association of a need to fix or remodel the body of the patient. Historically, the biomechanical perspective of manual therapy (MT) as a tool to address pathomechanical models for understanding pain in rehabilitation medicine has indeed implied this association. For example, the *Guide to Physical Therapist Practice* defines MT in this way:

> Manual therapy techniques are skilled hand movements and skilled passive movements of joints and soft tissue and are intended to improve tissue extensibility; increase range of motion; induce relaxation; mobilize or manipulate soft tissue and joints; modulate pain; and reduce soft tissue swelling, inflammation, or restriction. Techniques may include manual lymphatic drainage, manual traction, massage, mobilization/manipulation, and passive range of motion.
>
> Physical therapists select, prescribe, and implement manual therapy techniques when the examination findings, diagnosis, and prognosis indicate use of these techniques to decrease edema, pain, spasm, or swelling; enhance health, wellness, and fitness; enhance or maintain physical performance; increase the ability to move; or prevent or remediate impairment in body functions and structures, activity limitations, or participation restrictions to improve physical function.[1]

Many rehabilitation professionals beyond physical therapists utilize MT, including massage therapists, osteopaths, chiropractors, and occupational therapists. The current controversy in the literature around MT challenges its efficacy as it is described above. The evidence suggests that some of these claims are theoretical,[2] which reinforces the need for rethinking MT through the integrative lens.

The overlap of the chronic pain and opioid crises has revealed the many challenges of effectively treating populations that are experiencing persistent pain. MT, a key component of rehabilitation, and other non-pharmaceutical interventions are being critically evaluated as alternatives to opioids for musculoskeletal pain.

REASONS TO UTILIZE MT

There are a number of reasons to use MT; however, there are a number of reasons that using MT within a biomechanical paradigm is considered an outdated mode of clinical reasoning. For example, determining biomechanical dysfunction using clinical examination of the lumbar spine is unreliable, does not positively influence outcomes, and has a poor association with imaging.[3] Even the methodology of using clinical prediction rules to establish groupings of patients with musculoskeletal complaints that may benefit from receiving MT has been deemed questionable.[4] Clinicians choosing to apply MT based on these biomechanical premises should consider rethinking their rationale.

Mechanistic models for MT may be useful if clinicians take a broader neuroscientific view of the influence of tissue movement imparted with MT techniques. MT is typically utilized by clinicians to influence movement, and movement-evoked pain does generally lessen with MT. Movement-evoked pain, more so than spontaneous pain at rest, is associated with decreased physical function and quality of life.[5] It has long been accepted that targeted movement in the spine cannot be isolated with spinal manipulative therapy (SMT), known to produce movement in the spine above and below a spinal level targeted for particular techniques. Additionally, during the posterior-to-anterior mechanical force produced by MT, activation is observed in medial parts of the postcentral gyrus (S1) bilaterally, the secondary somatosensory cortex (S2), posterior parts of the insular cortex, different parts of the cingulate cortex, and the cerebellum.[6] Taking the constraints of the biomechanical model for MT into account, clinicians wanting to continue to use MT might choose to look upon its influences using a broader lens.

Another reason to utilize MT might be to modulate pain via a so-called bottom-up approach of sensory input to the nervous system. In a systematic review of MT's analgesic effects for musculoskeletal pain, the authors concluded that MT applied to spinal joints can produce short-term positive effects on "local" pressure pain thresholds (PPT).[7] Such local effects should be understood by the clinician to likely be short term and therefore capitalized upon within the treatment session. With pain temporarily diminished from application of the MT techniques, the patient could possibly be taught to pay attention to and learn something useful about the experience of more comfortable or greater motion.

A more integrative understanding of the effects of MT is found when we consider its influence upon the brain from a so-called top-down perspective, involving the processing or perception of pain. As covered in Chapter 7, placebo and nocebo effects reflect embodied psychophysiological responses that are influenced by contextual factors such as: expectations; patient history, conditioning, beliefs; the clinician's behavior and rapport; and more.[8]

Placebo effects reflect a powerful influence within the MT experience. Manual therapists are therefore encouraged to embrace placebo as a potential active mechanism that can influence MT treatment effects.[9] Placebo is known to have the capacity for hypoalgesia, but the strength of this effect varies based on the context of how it is introduced, patient expectations and conditioning, personality traits, mood, and genetic factors that influence reward and opioid systems.[10] To take these factors that influence MT into account, Jacobs and Silvernail suggest taking a perspective of manual therapist in an interactor model with the patient and the contextual environment of the therapeutic encounter, rather than a historic model of manual therapist as an operator applying a technique to a patient who is playing a passive role.[11] A prudent manual therapist will see opportunity in setting the stage for manual interventions to improve the likelihood of a positive effect from any manual technique. Within ethical bounds, the patient's expectations about manual technique could be enhanced and potential obstacles related to prior conditioning about MT identified and mitigated.

Other top-down neural modulation occurs via the brain's pain-processing network. This includes the thalamus, and cortices of the primary and secondary somatosensory, cingulate, and insular regions.[12] This network is responsible for encoding cognitive, sensory, and emotional processing of the pain experience and for communicating with descending modulatory pathways, including the periaqueductal gray (PAG). MT is postulated to have cortical descending modulatory effects and changes the communication between cortical regions involved in conditioned pain modulation. Such communication between brain regions is described as functional connectivity.

Bialosky *et al.*[13] describe the relevance of a study[14] using fMRI to explore resting-state connectivity before and after MT given to participants with exercise-induced low back pain:

> Common to all MT interventions (spinal thrust, non-thrust, and therapeutic touch), the coupling of cortical activity decreased between sensory discriminant and affective regions (primary somatosensory cortex and posterior insular cortex), while increases were observed between affective regions (posterior cingulate and anterior insular cortices) and affective and descending pain modulatory regions (insular cortex and periaqueductal gray). The results of this study suggest that MT alters cortical interactions within nociceptive processing networks at rest, such that subsequent stimuli are received within the cortex in an altered state. Future studies should attempt to further clarify how MT disrupts maladaptive cortical patterns and functional connectivity associated with chronic pain.[15]

Studies of individuals with chronic pain suggest the need for further investigation into how pain is processed. Patients with chronic pain shift away from nociceptive processing regions towards emotion regulation centers.[16] Study results show shifts in attention to the mind wandering and self-evaluative brain regions collectively referred to as the default mode network, as well as to the emotional regulatory centers of the limbic system.[17] Curious clinicians might wonder about the effect that MT has upon the patient's ability to bring attention to physical and emotional habits associated with problematic movement. Perhaps it would be useful to investigate if MT influences the level of mindfulness of movement and how the movement experience is altered by "maladaptive cortical patterns," generating catastrophic thinking patterns, misbeliefs, and fear of movement.

Another potential reason for the use of MT is reflected in biochemical effects. MT may exert influence upon the circulatory biomarkers known to influence pain and inflammation.[18] Patients with chronic low back pain, fibromyalgia, and temporomandibular disorder are known to have altered neuro-immune-endocrine system function that includes dysregulation of cortisol.[19] Questions remain regarding whether this dysfunction is responsible for deterioration of vertebral end plates versus aging processes. Altered chemical biomarkers influenced by MT include substance-p, neurotensin, oxytocin, and interleukin levels. MT may also increase cortisol levels post-intervention; however, the collection methods for sampling cortisol are being re-examined across studies to determine consistency of methodology in future methods. There is a need for researchers to examine these MT effects on patients with pain, in addition to healthy subjects.[20] Astute clinicians will recognize the role that MT can play in restoring freedom and comfort to movement so that the patient is empowered to return to greater activity. There is strong evidence that regular physical activity helps to reduce inflammation and improve endogenous opiate production, and acts as an effective antidepressant.[21]

Returning to the story at the outset of this chapter, recall how the therapist was interacting with the patient during the physical examination. Consider the reasons to utilize MT that are presented in this section. The therapist repeatedly cued the patient to sense various qualities of their static and dynamic movement during the examination. When the therapist used touch, it was not only applied for the therapist to discern information about the tissues, but also for the patient to pay attention to the body areas receiving touch in new ways. The therapist's examination gathered information in the usual domains of range of motion and provoking factors but did so in a way that also illuminated the patient's psychoemotional experience of the movement and their beliefs about the nature of their complaints. This type of top-down and bottom-up involvement of the patient in the examination process provides the therapist with opportunities to consider the use of MT in the more novel ways described in this chapter.

MT AND "SENSITIZATION"

The experience of persistent pain is sometimes described as a sustained physiological state of vigilance of portions of the individual's nervous system. The concept of nociplastic pain was introduced in Chapter 16. *Nociplastic pain* is defined as: "pain that arises from altered nociception despite no clear evidence of actual or threatened tissue damage causing the activation of peripheral nociceptors or evidence for disease or lesion of the somatosensory system causing the pain."[22]

Similarly the concept of *central sensitization* (CS) has been defined as: "an increased responsiveness of nociceptive neurons in the central nervous system to normal and subthreshold afferent input."[23] The meaning and utility of these terms continues to evolve as researchers and clinicians seek to understand the complexity and mysteries of pain.

The concept of sensitization is implied in both nociplastic pain and CS. Both terms have been characterized by altered or heightened neurophysiological activity associated with painful sensations. While questions have been raised around the theoretical and scientific basis of CS as an isolatable construct in the nervous system,[24] a persistent pain experience is understood to carry underlying neurophysiological changes for which these terms are often used to attempt to describe mechanistic changes in the nervous system.[25] The general notions of hypervigilance, learned overprotection, or sensitization all point towards the same understanding. Current models of pain care encourage the inclusion of treatment objectives to recognize and reduce neurophysiological sensitization via various means including contextually framed and well-thought-out MT approaches. The embedded concepts of IRP are well suited to support these efforts.

SENSITIZATION, THE AUTONOMIC NERVOUS SYSTEM, AND MT

Manual techniques influence the integrated central-autonomic-peripheral nervous system. For example, when manual techniques are applied in a comforting manner, there is potential to facilitate optimal parasympathetic nervous system responses.[26] A systematic review examining the effect of osteopathic manual therapies and myofascial techniques suggests that there are impacts upon the autonomic nervous system as reflected in changes in heart rate variability.[27]

Some MT techniques may increase sympathetic arousal. For example, neural mobilization techniques (using the slump position) have been tested in a small group of healthy subjects and found to have a sympathetic effect on the ANS as demonstrated by increases in blood pressure.[28] Researchers have questioned whether sympathetic stimulation might account for the reported analgesic effect of such techniques.[29] However, specific to joint mobilization techniques such as high-velocity thrust manipulations, currently there is low evidence for significant or lasting effects on ANS activity.[30]

While these questions continue to be researched, most clinicians agree that hands-on techniques carry potential to inform the patient's overall nervous system about the state of sensitivity and accuracy of their sensory perception. Consider how manual inputs cue the position in space of body parts and connection to the whole of the body and movement, as well as the ability to direct attention, including the breath, to where hands are laid upon the body. In a small study of 30 "normal" subjects, 15 experimental subjects received manipulation and massage, and 15 subjects (controls) received massage alone, and were examined for changes in joint-position sense. Joint-position was measured using a digital clinometer. Results suggested that joint-position sense could be improved with manipulation and massage, but not massage alone, in both the cervical and lumbar spine.[31]

Consider the story at the beginning of this chapter in light of this discussion on the influence of MT upon the nervous system. If we understand nervous system sensitivity on a spectrum and in context, we understand the potential for the effect of inner, outer, and other environmental conditions to be influential upon the patient's physiological state and how this will in turn influence the movement experience for the patient. In the story, the therapist was not only observing the patient's movement, but also the patient's interaction with the clinical environment to look for signs of hypervigilance. The therapist was also taking a fresh look at how the clinic environment might influence physiological state in favorable or unfavorable ways. Such influences might guide the choice of manual techniques for the given session, as well as the therapeutic outcome of the MT over the episode of care. Additionally, the therapist checked in with the state of their own nervous system and took steps to refresh themselves/balance their own ANS to receive the patient. Such considerations might prompt the health professional to adapt their clinical environment and perhaps even adopt personal practices that can bring states of calm presence.

THERAPEUTIC ALLIANCE AND CONTEXTUAL FACTORS INFLUENCE MT

Thus far, this chapter has focused on primarily intrinsic or internal mechanisms that influence MT. There are also significant external factors, including therapeutic alliance and other contextual factors that are often described as "non-specific."

Therapeutic alliance considers the working rapport between the therapist and patient. It describes the relational processes at play in treatment which can act in combination or independently to influence interventions, including MT. Therapeutic alliance is characterized by collaboration, communication, therapist empathy, and mutual respect. It has three components which include agreement upon goals of treatment, tasks, and the development of connection (reciprocal positive feelings) between the client and therapist.[32] As covered in Chapter 8, therapeutic alliance also plays a role in treatment adherence and has an impact on treatment outcomes in rehabilitation.

Experiential pause: Consider how components like MT and exercise can be viewed and linked when the focus is on the therapeutic relationship, as well as other contextual factors, and not as much on the technique and the perceived rationale for it being delivered. The next time that you are in the clinic, resolve to identify one contextual factor and observe its influence upon how you utilize MT to inform the patient's movement experience. Take a moment to make some notes about how this awareness contributed to your ability to integrate MT with patient movement quality. Include any observations of how this integration possibly enhanced therapeutic alliance.

Introduced earlier, contextual factors include:

complex sets of internal, external, or relational elements, encompassing: patient's expectation, history, baseline characteristics; clinician's behavior, belief, verbal suggestions, and therapeutic touch; positive therapeutic encounter, patient-centered approach, and social learning; overt therapy, posology of intervention, modality of treatment administration; marketing features of treatment, and health care setting.[33]

These factors can be appreciated as establishing a treatment atmosphere that supports the context of environment in healing processes. For example, by eliciting expectations and memories, patients' nervous systems consciously and unconsciously interpret these factors in ways that can produce either placebo or nocebo effects. These effects have significant capacity to influence therapeutic outcome.[34]

Providers can influence contextual factors through the nature and quality of the therapeutic relationship. Relevant concepts and skills include: the use of empathy; enactive compassion; language, quality of therapeutic touch, active listening; extra time spent with the patient; more face-to-face therapeutic contact, warmth, attention, care, encouragement, and support. The environment in which care is given is also an influential contextual factor, reminding us of the inseparability of body-mind-environment (BME) interactions. Such considerations include architecture, interior design, furnishings, sound, and outside views.[35]

> **Experiential pause:** Consider again the opening story and the reference made to the intention of the therapist to notice how therapeutic alliance and the contextual factors might influence how MT might be utilized in the treatment session: a warm smile and the degree of self-awareness, empathy, and active listening that the therapist embodied (listening with the whole body). Review the story and then jot down any other ingredients that you see that support the themes of IRP. To conclude, consider the idea that the result of all therapeutic interactions comes from a combination of what we do, how we do it, and the intention we bring to modulate our own nervous system to adapt to the needs of the patient's nervous system.

THE IMPACT OF TOUCH AND IMAGERY
Touch

As explored in Chapter 13, the human being has an amazingly sensate design. Human beings are deeply tactile creatures and need touch to thrive.[36] As we age, tactile needs can be neglected. MT is obviously a form a therapeutic touch. Endorphins are released and substance-p is inhibited. Touch also elicits emotion. Anthropologist Ashley Montagu asserts: "it is through the emotional involvement of touch that one can reach through the isolation and communicate love, trust, affection, and warmth."[37] Many a good manual therapist has heard patients request to take the therapist home with them!

Inter-individual touch can range from highly desirable to profoundly aversive. Touch combines with many other sensory, contextual, and motivational cues. External and internal states, both of which are impacted by history/conditioning, influence the experience of touch. Like pain, the neurophysiological basis of touch implies bidirectional communication between brain and body. The neurochemistry of touch involves the μ-opioids and oxytocin systems, implying potentially profound relevance to the sensory, affective, and social components of pain and other health experiences.[38]

Results from a meta-ethnographic study across several health professions indicate that the therapeutic impact from touch is enhanced when touch is caring, sensitive to power differentials, and delivered in a safe space.[39] As a hands-on form of care, MT imparts caring by humanizing the health-care experience using compassion. Power is demonstrated via technical competence, and safe space is created by upholding personal and professional boundaries.[40]

Tommaso makes a memorable claim that clinicians should begin to utilize MT less as a "tool" to fix the patient's body and more as means to communicate with the patient's brain, in a similar way to words.[41] The touch component of MT is described by Tommaso as having three dimensions: *analgesic*, *affective*, and *somato-perceptual*. *Analgesic* touch is regarded as being instinctive throughout human history. The laying on of hands as part of healing processes is part of many cultures. At a neurophysiological level, touch is considered to be an expression of tactile pain modulatory capacity of A-delta, beta, and C fibers; it also acts via down-regulation of emotional processing regions within the central nervous system.[42]

For this latter component, we see that touch is fundamentally relational. *Affective* touch is understood to carry information from sender to receiver. This is conceptualized to include the physiological state and the intention of the sender. This is capable of conveying a sense of support, safety, concern, and care. Such touch, provided with appropriate parameters and feedback from the recipient, has high potential to induce:

- neurophysiological changes rooted in the parasympathetic relaxation response
- a reduction in stress biomarkers as measured through salivary amylase, heart rate, and salivary cortisol
- a reduction in negative affect.[43]

It is well known that the *somato-perceptual* component of regions commonly associated with persistent pain (e.g., the lower back) is generally poor. Humans perceive pain to be more intense when they cannot see the body part or origin of the pain. Additionally, any region that has already developed a persistent pain state is known to have decreased or altered somato-perceptual representation in the brain.[44]

As mentioned when discussing MT and processes of sensitization, touch can be used from the lens of helping to reorganize the mental representation of the body and to teach the patient to discriminate between safe and threatening sensation. Hands-on techniques can help to improve the patient's sense of body ownership (this is my body) and body agency (I control my body). This relevance is underscored in Tommaso's paper: "There is the need to state firmly that touching a person is a therapeutic act per se, delivered according to precise theoretical constructs (e.g., neurophysiological, biomechanical, psychological) to insure its results."[45]

Imagery

Given that humans are also highly visual, it should not be surprising that the visual component of mental imagery can function as a valuable skill that could be used to enhance MT. Imagery enhances athletes' performance[46] and treatment and immune responses in cancer patients,[47] and reduces anxiety that plays a significant role in the pain experience in surgical patients.[48]

As covered in Chapter 14, guided imagery describes the use of techniques that can involve visualization, other senses, the suggested use of images and symbols, metaphor, and even storytelling. Imagery is a language embedded in every facet of our experience—how we think, experience our environment, and move. Imagery affects the physiology of multiple body systems through its influence on and through the central and autonomic nervous systems. One study examined the effects of imagery compared with a structured touch protocol for post-operative joint replacement pain and anxiety. The study found that both the imagery and touch protocols carried significant benefit, with touch performing slightly better.[49] While not the preceding study's design, consider how combining techniques such as touch-based therapies *with* guided imagery may improve both patient experience and potentially clinical outcomes.

WEAVING EDUCATION AND OTHER INGREDIENTS INTO MT

Pain neuroscience education and its larger framework of therapeutic education (Chapter 16) has been demonstrated to have beneficial effects in pain management. Similar to the suggestion of combining MT with guided imagery, applying MT alongside pain neuroscience education carries potential to influence sensitization and perhaps refresh the patient's body awareness.[50] Moving further, this chapter advocates for clinicians to employ MT alongside *multiple* ingredients and contextual considerations.

Just as we are being asked to re-examine pain, rehabilitation professionals must examine historical presumptions about MT. Even more so, we must co-explore with the patient to uncover systemic factors that may be informing the state of the tissues, increase self-efficacy, and support lasting changes in BME patterning.

Using the IRP perspective, clinicians become more able to reframe the rationale for the involvement of MT in the plan of care. Rather than framing MT as something we *do to* the patient, we can present our hands-on therapy as one component of a "make-fit-to-live-in-again" rehabilitation interactive process. Such an approach carries potential to refresh and reintegrate BME relationships in multiple ways.

MOVING FORWARD AFTER LOOKING BACK

Using physical therapy as an example, in earlier days MT courses were a major focus. Aspiring rehabilitation therapists (especially physical therapists) often entered post-professional MT education tracks, some of which culminated in a certification in that particular MT guru's vein of instruction. Currently, recognition is growing of the limitations of following MT guru lineages or delivering predominantly MT approaches. Other manual-based professions (massage therapy, chiropractic, osteopathy) have also begun to recognize these limitations, moving towards more balanced and contextual perspectives on the relevance and role of MT.

Continuing to use physical therapy as a useful example, in the first decade of this century, it appeared necessary for those who considered themselves manual therapists to become adept at specific thrust manipulation techniques that followed clinical practice rules. This movement was intended to improve clinical decision making as to which patients might benefit the most from spinal manipulative therapies. Academic physical therapy programs took a closer look at how curriculums were preparing students to perform manipulation. Inter-professional debates ensued. For a time, cavitation or no cavitation with manipulation became a point of pride or frustration.

In more recent years, physical therapy academic programs have emphasized exercise and patient education to an extent that may have overshadowed the simple therapeutic effect of human touch. Hands-on care is even being discussed in contrast to hands-off care.[51]

In the IRP lens, which advocates for complexity, non-dual thinking, and the "middle ground," we can consider the value of human touch via hands-on care in light of our early presentation of human needs: safety, empowerment, and nurturance. MT, used in the context of relationship, intention, and mind-body effects, can be seen as providing experiences of safety and nurturance. When MT is combined with other empowering skills such as movement retraining, breath regulation, and neurocognitive skills (Acceptance and Commitment Therapy, mindfulness), we see a recipe for the integrated use of MT that fits well into the overall IRP constructs.

FUTURE EXPLORATIONS OF MT WITHIN AN IRP PARADIGM

A look forward to future research would explore how MT impacts healing via additional neglected or poorly understood mechanisms. The "National Institutes of Health, Healing Experience of All Life Stressors" (NIH HEALS) model is the first of its kind to examine factors related to psychospiritual healing. It identified these factors as relevant:

> 1. Connection—belief in and connection to a higher power, religion, religious community, and family; 2. Reflection & Introspection—finding meaning, purpose, gratitude and joy in nature, activities including those that connect mind and body, interconnectedness, present moment orientation, and an increased sense of awareness about the fragility of life; and 3. Trust & Acceptance—accepting what is, feeling resolved, feeling at peace, and trusting that caregivers, friends, and family will respond to needs as they arise.[52]

In view of the NIH HEALS research, curiosity arises as to how MT might be examined for its role in promoting psychospiritual healing. How might manual techniques influence the *connection* we have to our body as a possible creation of a higher power? How might manual techniques be delivered to facilitate an inner, outer, and other environment that encourages *reflection and introspection* upon movement as a type of sacred gift? Can manual therapies, as a form of healing touch, be used more intentionally and taught more broadly to care extenders?

In light of the importance of the psychospiritual dimension of healing, future integrative perspectives of MT should investigate its impact upon the entire dimension of the human experience. There is actually precedence for this when we examine the yoga tradition. Its model of the human being, known as the Pancha Maya Kosha model, articulates five dimensions of the human being. From this perspective, a witnessing faculty of consciousness is present that includes not only the body, but also the energies that animate and operate the body, mind, and emotions. These *koshas* are described as "treasures" or "sheaths" that obscure their catalyst—the fifth treasure of spirit. In this model, all gross form is derived from the subtle, which thereby attributes the source of all health, healing, and relief of suffering to the spirit.[53] A MT model that embraces such understandings of the psychospiritual nature of the human would have an entirely different intention beyond mechanistic, central, or contextual factors as discussed in this chapter. Future models of MT might integrate this perspective of the human as five treasures to raise awareness of MT's potential scope of influence. Such an approach also stands in support of the NIH HEALS key factors of connection, reflection, introspection, trust, and acceptance as that which supports human healing.

For example, the human as the sensate organism could be educated to receive MT as a stimulus to be explored on the basis of the phenomenological effects upon each of these five treasures. Instead of limiting our MT reassessment to the effect of a technique upon physiological and accessory joint motion or pain experience, the effect of the manual technique could be expanded to more of an interoceptive assessment. Does the manual technique enhance the patient's mindful connection to the state of the five senses? Is there a different emotional appreciation of, and connectedness to, the treated body area or body as a whole? As a gateway into reflection and introspection, did the manual technique influence parasympathetic responses, including vagal tone?[54] Does the tactile mode of the manual technique build the healing factors of trust and acceptance? Do our handling skills also influence the body's kosha/treasure of metabolic energies? For example, stretch-gated ion channel PIEZO2 has been shown to be essential for aspects of mechanosensation in model organisms.[55] Unexplored aspects of MT related to healing abound. While the metaphysical roles of touch are presently non-putative, new technologies will likely reveal a whole new realm of considerations for the influence of therapeutic touch.

MOVING FORWARD

Choosing how to move forward naturally depends on your perspective of which direction constitutes forward! MT reframed in the ways discussed in this chapter has an important role in expanding our understanding of rehabilitation (to make fit to live in). Looking back to the opening story in this chapter, it concludes by asking if the patient believes that the therapy will be helpful and affirms their commitment to participate in their rehabilitation. As we engage in all of these potential ways to rethink MT, we would be wise to embrace an understanding that the patient's story is always being written by them. The patient is the source of their healing. End of story, or is it the beginning?

Experiential pause: Having read this chapter, identify and write down at least one actionable item of interest to you. In doing so, consider ways in which applying the material first to yourself, and then to patients, might serve those who come to you for care.

ADDITIONAL DELIVERY MODELS FOR A CHANGING PRACTICE

A note for Section Three: The content of this section seeks to offer several examples of looking larger—of progress and expansion of thought and application of integrative rehabilitation practice (IRP). This section aims to present models that can hold the whole. Reinforcement of earlier principles and approaches, alongside new and expanded examples and ideas for expanding the reach of IRP, will be presented. Section Three will end with a short chapter aimed to support readers in taking the next steps.

CHAPTER 24

Yoga Therapy in Rehabilitation

Matthew J. Taylor, PT, PhD, C-IAYT

OVERVIEW

For many readers, either personal or clinical experience may have generated curiosity about the therapeutic potential of yoga therapy (YT), and consequently how best to bridge that experience with traditional paradigms or as an integrative rehabilitation practitioner? How can this long-established wisdom tradition for navigating life inform our development today as an integrative rehabilitation practitioner? This chapter brings together many facets of integrative rehabilitation practice (IRP) and summarizes the arc of my journey in utilizing YT in rehabilitation, essentially describing what I wish I had known when my interest was first piqued in 1996.

We will follow this sequence of material.

- Define YT and discuss its increasing popularity.
- Review how IRP and the rehabilitation professions are abuzz with the finding of whole-person or biopsychosocialspiritual approach to care.
- Describe the relationships between YT, mind-body science, and modern physical rehabilitation.
- Explore how such an approach is the heart of YT in a brief history and description of the paradigms shaping yoga therapeutic principles.
- Share the most common personal self-care practices, and examination and intervention principles, and offer some functional detail.
- The chapter concludes with a vision for the future of YT and IRP.

THE DEFINITION OF YT

What is YT? Who can provide YT? How is YT like traditional rehabilitation? The short answer is that while YT is rooted in ancient principles, it is quite embryonic in its emergence into Western culture and medicine. Right now (at the time of publication), anyone may claim to be a yoga therapist because there are no regulatory restrictions. This is true even though the International Association of Yoga Therapists (IAYT) initiated standards for schools' accreditation, a definitive scope of practice, and the credentialing of individual therapists. There has also been a natural, and often unconscious, enculturation/ appropriation of yoga into the Western health-care model through various means and in numerous representations. Unfortunately, this scattered process has constrained YT's full therapeutic potential. More on that later.

In December 2007, the IAYT offered its first definition of YT following 18 years of discussion and discernment.[1] Each word was carefully chosen to provide an in-depth understanding of YT relative to rehabilitation:

> Yoga therapy is the process of empowering individuals to progress toward improved health and wellbeing through the application of the teachings and practices of Yoga.

To be clear, YT is a subset of the larger body of yoga, not separate or distinct from yoga. Conceptually, it is important to know that yoga refers to an enormous body of precepts, attitudes, techniques, and spiritual values developed in India for over 5000 years.[2] Yoga describes a method of discipline or means of discovering the integral nature of the body and mind (i.e., modern mind-body science). Yoga is one of the oldest and largest bodies of work from the wisdom traditions.

The paradigm within which yoga is held maintains that it must be both known conceptually and enacted in order to truly be practiced. That perspective reflects Walsh's wisdom definition that states that wisdom is the deep and accurate understanding of oneself and the central existential question of life, and skillful, benevolent responsiveness.[3] Just knowing the teachings isn't sufficient. Enacting or engaging the practices in one's life fulfills the practice. Reminiscent of the early chapters on IRP, isn't it? And, of course, it is only our parochial perspective that then makes YT appear "new" or foreign as a therapy in the West.

Presently, reflect on how the definition of YT in 2007 and our description of IRP relate to one another.

- **Process/progress toward**: YT is an ongoing process versus an event or focal "fix" of a complaint. The primary complaint is understood to be merely a singular manifestation of imbalance in health of which there are many other related facets. Hence, an extended YT inquiry is the adaptation of unfolding health behaviors that can provide relief and prevention beyond the resolution of the original complaint. In general, YT is better suited for persistent lifestyle-related complaints, rather than acute maladies or traumas. This principle is expanded in the "yogopathy" discussion that follows.
- **Empowering**: A YT practice rejects the disempowering "expert fixes the broken" model of sick care and rightfully restores the responsibility and power of healing to the individual through a person-centered orientation in both assessment and planning care.
- **Toward health and well-being**: YT is health care, not sick care. It is a wellness model for optimizing the health of not only the individual, but also the individual's relationships, community, and planet. YT is not a pathology-based model fixated on alleviating diagnosis-related symptoms…that is "yogopathy."[4] *Yogopathy* is

the use of yoga practices based on a medical diagnosis to affect amelioration of symptoms, without including the teachings of yoga or identifying the root cause(s) of the complaint. Yogopathy isn't "bad" or wrong, but it isn't YT either. The isolated use of techniques, void of context for etiology and ethical incorporation, sells short the broader and deeper value of YT. Additionally, YT focuses on what is working, versus what is lost, symptomatic or dysfunctional, and optimizes what can be optimized. YT even offers a person in late-stage terminal disease various processes and practices to move toward healing and wholeness.[5]

- **Application**: YT is a practice that requires action and discipline. Passivity, dependence, and detachment by the client is not YT.
- **Teachings (philosophy) and practice**: YT is more than practices, as noted above regarding yogopathy. YT is a holistic life science. It is a biopsychosocialspiritual model of wellness that covers every aspect of the human experience from pre-gestation to death. Practice of the methods and technologies of yoga, without the study and integration of the philosophy, reduces YT to yogopathy…just another mechanistic model of pathology-based care. Of note, all philosophy and no practice, or all practice and no teaching integrated into the lifestyle, is not YT.

So, how do YT and modern rehabilitation interface? First a broad overview proposal, then specifics described in the YT assessments and applications.

YT AND CONVENTIONAL REHABILITATION MODELS

The previous definition of YT is neither exhaustive nor complete, and there is now a much more detailed definition with the IAYT standards. Having discussed how the definition contrasts with yogopathy, let's now look more specifically at rehabilitative paradigms. In my experience as an orthopedic physical therapist, as recently as the 1980s, any suggestion that the hip may actually influence function in the shoulder would have been heretical. Slowly, through my career, the discussion of what else might influence the client's presentation began to broaden. In a guest editorial in the November 2007 *Journal of Orthopedic and Sports Physical Therapy*, the editors proudly proclaimed: "Regional interdependence: A musculoskeletal examination model whose time has come."[6] Most importantly, the editorial concludes: "Further investigation of the regional-interdependence concept in a systematic fashion may add clarity to the nature of many musculoskeletal problems and guide subsequent decision making in clinical care. Regional interdependence is a model whose time has come."[7]

That was just over 13 years ago. And they were only heralding the biomechanistic component of influence on musculoskeletal challenges. No mention of the psychosocial or spiritual influences. In that proclamation, which does have merit, albeit limited, a biomechanistic interdependence model can be helpful in managing rehabilitation cases. However, the historical context has been lost. Over 3000 years ago, the *Taittiriya-Upanishad* of the Indian Vedanta describes the model of human integration, or the five yogic sheaths, or koshas.[8]

The kosha model of human integration extolls the value of understanding that not only is physical regional interdependence important in optimizing health, so too are all of the other aspects of the human experience, including social, emotional, psychological, and spiritual influences. The kosha model bears many similarities to both the regional interdependence model and the biopsychosocialspiritual model used in IRP. Historically, though, it is more accurate to say that the new models in rehabilitation resemble the earlier kosha model from India! One more example of our need for humility around "discovering" and "new" principles to inform IRP.

A more recent example of "rediscovering" what is very old is that the present pain crisis in the US has led to the formation of a collective of over 65 stakeholders in pain care. This congress (now undergoing reorganization after one of the host organizations went bankrupt from lack of funding from, ironically, the pharmaceutical industry) has established a consensus definition of comprehensive, integrative pain management (CIPM). The "new" definition again contains the kosha aspects of being human:

> Comprehensive, integrative pain management includes *biomedical, psychosocial, complementary health,* and *spiritual care.* It is *person-centered* and *focuses on maximizing function and wellness.* Care plans are developed through a *shared decision-making model* that reflects the *available evidence* regarding optimal clinical practice and the *person's goals and values.* [*Emphasis* added][9]

The CIPM definition overlays with how we've described IRP and defined YT. All of these brilliant minds came together and essentially said: "This CIPM is how to relieve suffering/pain." In this context, not exactly news, right? Or said another old way: "Nihil novi sub sole" ("There is nothing new under the sun"), as written in Ecclesiastes 1:9. Truly, nothing is new under the sun. Given that dose of humility making, how then does this ancient YT model and its paradigm and technologies fit in with traditional rehabilitation and mind-body medicine in the West?

YT IN A WESTERN MEDICINE CONTEXT

In the US, the National Center for Complementary and Integrative Health (NCCIH) classifies yoga (and therefore YT) as a complementary health approach. Complementary approaches reflect a group of diverse medical and health-care systems, practices, services, and products that aren't currently a part of conventional medicine. One survey revealed that of those who used yoga specifically for therapeutic purposes, 21% did so because it was recommended by a conventional medical professional, 31% did so because conventional therapies were ineffective, and 59% thought it would be an interesting therapy to explore.[10] Through such means, YT has gained popularity in Western culture and is now the most commonly used mind-body therapy in Western complementary medicine. It has been suggested that YT's unique ability to facilitate spiritual, physical, and psychological benefits is appealing as a cost-effective alternative to conventional interventions, though to date there is no good cost-comparison research.

YT is an emerging field with a professional association of over 6000 members, 40+%

of whom have dual training, including physical therapists, occupational therapists, and speech-language pathologists. The organization has sponsored annual research and clinical application symposiums since 2007 with researchers from around the world to build its evidence base and solidify its rightful place in the Western conversation of health and medicine. IAYT's annual *International Journal of Yoga Therapy* has been indexed on PubMed since 2011. IAYT is also actively participating in several national task forces to include pain and oncology, as well as numerous international yoga organizations.

Experiential pause: Pause to consider that a yoga therapist utilizes posture, movement, breathing, and education principles as methods for supporting their clients. That reads quite a bit like the scope of a physical or occupational therapist, doesn't it? So, with such a close-knit overlap of techniques, what is it about the teachings (philosophies) that differentiate what might look to be very similar professions on a silent video observation of a clinical interaction? Does the reflection create confusion for you as to what's the difference or to whom you should make a referral for those services? If those are your professions, is there any sense of fear or "turf" infringement? Can you identify with the post-normal time (PNT) experiences of uncertainty, contradictions, etc. from Chapter 2?

GUIDING YOGA PHILOSOPHY CONCEPTS WITH REHABILITATION IMPLICATIONS

One major barrier for the acceptance of yoga is concerns regarding it being a religion or conflicting with the faith practice of clients. This is but one common misunderstanding of yoga, but a crucial one when examining the foundational principles. Yoga originally developed with origins from the Hindu, Jain, and Buddhist traditions. However, yoga is not a religion itself, but a psychospiritual practice.[11] Yoga is a philosophical life science with practical applications that invites discovery, evaluation, and updating of one's spiritual beliefs. Yoga may help to answer "Who am I? What am I?" and, given those answers, "How shall I move/act in the world?" Thus, the practice of yoga is congruent with all religious traditions and demands no belief in deities or practices that would conflict with an individual's spiritual tradition. Yoga is practiced by people of all faith traditions when properly understood as such.

Moving from the subtle spiritual pole to the other grosser pole of attraction to Western sensibilities would be the physical postures (asanas) and motor-performance outcomes which characterize so much of yoga. These asana and motor-performance factors are a byproduct of what is more accurately described as a technology for the evolution of the mind and consciousness. Therefore, YT provides an experience of the emerging mind-body science of current pain and motor theories. Said another way, the felt sense or awareness of the individual of the mind-body connection is actually the rediscovery of what has been the basis of the practice of yoga for thousands of years. The basic tenet of all branches of yoga focuses not just on conceptualization of this connection, but also on literally experiencing the unity of the mind and body, as well as developing spiritual, psychological, and physical health. This process is indeed transformational for clients, producing a transcendent experience of the connection between and across their full living experience.

While there are many yoga philosophies (six others) that won't be described here, the most popular one in the West is that of the eight-limbed path of yoga outlined by Patanjali. In Chapter 2, Sutra 29 of his *Yoga Sutras*, he lists a practical science for the relationships between thoughts, emotions, memories, intentions, and actions.[12] As seen in Table 24.1, each limb emphasizes moral and ethical conduct, as well as self-discipline.[13] Traditionally, the client began with the yamas and niyamas. When well grounded in the practice of the first two limbs, the client would then embark on the other six limbs in a recursive and inclusive application, not unlike the processes often employed in life coaching. In modern postural yoga sold in yoga studios, however, typically the entry has been through asana, with maybe a small bit of pranayama and dhyana thrown in.

Table 24.1: Patanjali's Eight-Limbed Path of Yoga[14]

Limb	Description
Yamas	Moral precepts with others: Non-harming, truthfulness, non-stealing, chastity, greedlessness.
Niyamas	Qualities to nourish oneself: Purity, contentment, austerity (exercise), self-study, devotion to a higher power.
Asana	Postures/movements: A calm, firm steady stance in relation to life.
Pranayama	Breathing exercises: The ability to channel and direct breath and life energy (prana).
Pratyahara	Decreased reactivity to sensation: Focusing senses inward; non-reactivity to stimuli both internal and external.
Dharana	Concentration; unwavering attention, commitment.
Dhyana	Meditation; mindfulness, being attuned to the present moment.
Samadhi	Ecstatic union; flow; "in the zone"; spiritual support/connection.

Yoga includes techniques for participants to question and verify the nature of reality through their direct experience. Table 24.1 demonstrates how practices and techniques are intended to go beyond the Western stereotype of yoga as complex poses and meditation. Since its introduction into Western culture in the late 1880s, there has been a significant shift in emphasis from spiritual outcomes of practice to more physically based outcomes. This shift toward more physical outcomes is the result of the adoption of the West's mechanistic reductionistic world view. This is, of course, analogous to what we see in medicine via yogopathy, as already discussed. An authentic practice of yoga combines a rigorous practice discipline with a wide array of physical and mental exercises rooted in moral and ethical principles that address every aspect of modern life, including consumer patterns, nutritional decisions, and vocational choices. Therefore, when discussing the utilization of YT in rehabilitation, one can see how it allows the patient and therapist to embody a holistic approach to life and health. YT is a wellness and prevention practice designed to generate a lifelong series of healthy lifestyle choices. Curiously, as science advances, it is now coming to reveal that this yoga model offers a balance of both a Western linear perspective and a more Eastern non-linear perspective of holism as it relates to human health. The specifics of this broad statement are supported in the following section.

THE PRACTICE AND TECHNOLOGIES OF YT

What you know of as yoga is probably tainted by what is sold as yoga. YT is being used as a treatment in Western culture from major university hospitals to boutique yoga studios. What is commonly referred to as "yoga" in the West is usually Hatha yoga, which is comprised of various styles including, but not limited to: Vinyasa, Ashtanga, Bikram, Power, Iyengar, etc. Hatha focuses on physical postures, deep breathing, and meditation. These practices are what is popular in the media and is sold in the gyms. Hatha's popularity is attributed to its physical familiarity with a typical Western athletic workout. It should be understood not to be the equivalent of YT, as YT includes other forms of yoga which focus on ethics, mudras (hand movements/postures), bhavana (guided imagery and meditation), jnana (self-study), and/or diet. All styles of yoga are said to lead to the same path of personal fulfillment through self-transformation, yet as described below in the context of health challenges, these techniques of YT are far richer and broader than mere yoga-like postures adapted as therapeutic exercises.[15]

A central feature of YT is that each practice can be modified, depending on the participant's abilities, needs, and state of health. These characteristics make YT ideal, accessible, and easy to utilize for all age groups. The only prerequisite for participating in YT is that the participant be breathing. YT stresses the importance of the client's developing awareness of how what they think, believe, perceive, and have been told influences their physical posture and mobility, the quantity and quality of breathing, and the level of central nervous system vigilance. All of these behavioral skills trainings ultimately affect their flexibility, health, and vitality.[16] How to arrive at these outcomes requires first assessing with the client where they are, then, as follows in the next section, the shared decision of what to do and how to get there.

YT PRINCIPLES OF EXAMINATION AND ASSESSMENT IN REHABILITATION

This section examines the key principles of YT for both examination and assessment in language familiar to the rehabilitation professions. The following principles suggest entry points where one may begin a seamless integration into even the most conservative rehabilitation practices in order to practice as an integrative rehabilitation practitioner. The adoption of any of these practices will, of course, be dependent on your profession and scope of practice. Obviously, this is a small sampling, but it should offer insight into the value of the perspective and approaches of YT in relation to the concepts of IRP that preceded this chapter.

Examination principles

Global postural assessment is foundational and begins from the base(s) of support (BOS) in all standard postures (sitting, standing, gait, supine, and prone). Key is that imbalances in the BOS are identified first by the client and then, if not recognized or sensed, illuminated by the therapist both through proprioceptive cues and visual feedback. A fundamental principle of YT is that alignment of structure dictates the flow or communication of prana (one's life force) or what in present-day language would be described as ground reaction forces and Newton's third law of motion. Hence, postural assessment is done as an embodied lived experience for the client, versus a passive declaration by the therapist.

Postural holding habits are where the individual discovers postural holding patterns within the assessment with open-ended questions such as: "Where do you feel the most tension in your body in this position?" and "Which leg is tighter and denser feeling than the other?" The therapist's questions empower the individual to become aware of themselves. The therapist is facilitating the identification of not only postural but also breathing, emotional, and spiritual patterns that reflect the hypervigilance and old postural setting patterns. These patterns become the touchstone for the home-care programs because, once discovered, the client has a felt baseline.

Postural awareness and accuracy is where the individual learns to accurately describe asymmetries in their various postures without having to first visually look or merely repeating what they have been told, but by what they can sense in the moment. This includes regional areas such as: which foot is turned in or out; the higher shoulder; the shorter rib cage; greater seat pressure on right or left; which shoulder is higher off the table; which palm faces more backward, etc. Active participation by the individual during assessment introduces topics such as neuroplasticity and the discovery that the individual's own awareness may even correct itself on the spot. Through an introspective attention, they sense, then confirm visually, and then re-sense if the corrective postural choices were accurate or inaccurate, which assists in refreshing cortical sensory and motor maps.

Breath assessment includes standard parameters of rate, volume, and quality, while together they study closely the regional movements associated with the act of respiration. The therapist may ask: "Is there movement in the abdomen? How much and in which directions?" And there are similar questions for the upper quarter: "Is there movement of the rib cage that creates arm movement? What about the sternum, scapula, head, or clavicles? What is the tension level of the tongue, eyes, facial musculature? Is there thoracic or diaphragmatic recruitment?" Again, questions invite the individual to sense and assess for themselves the dysfunctions. This recursive pattern of observation, sensing, and discovery exists throughout all of the assessments. The introduction of the importance of respiration patterns with its over 19,000 movements a day is essential to providing an efficient and stable BOS that will make all other attempts to alter function more effective.

Self-assessment of the organs of sensing (eyes, ears, nose, tongue, and skin) is fundamental for YT as "stabilization of the mind stuff." A preponderance of focus on the thoughts (one of the senses in yogic theory) generates a lack of awareness of the other sensing fields or an "instability" of the senses/lack of embodiment. Awareness of these fields moves attention off a fixation of thinking. When tension is noted, further questions refine perception and stimulate insights into patterns. This process is then applied in the practices that follow as well.

These are only a small percentage of the available assessments for the yoga therapist. Other assessments include observation of movement patterns, strength, and flexibility, which are redundant to traditional physical rehabilitation assessments. Other YT assessments, however, require extensive training and study beyond the scope of this chapter. In YT, there are blurred boundaries between evaluation, assessment, and interventions. Additionally, the roles where the individual becomes a partner with the therapist in assessment, and the therapist takes on the role of learner in addition to the role of expert, mirror our IRP discussions.

YOGA TECHNOLOGIES OF INTERVENTION

As promised, below are descriptions of some of the most frequently used yoga technologies available to the rehabilitation professional to use with the client following their discussion about the findings. The pronunciation of the practices is included for reader confidence in approaching local yoga referral sources.

Asanas (Ah·sah·nas), or physical postures, are the third limb of Patanjali's classical eight-limbed system mentioned in Table 24.1. Asanas have been demonstrated to generate greater cardiovascular fitness, strength, mood modifications, and flexibility.[17] Asanas are used to increase body awareness and discover one's unique optimal biomechanical positioning of the body in space both in static and dynamic movement. Beyond alignment, each asana enhances awareness and the skill to identify the effect of thoughts, emotions, memories, and breathing on comfort and stability. Therefore, selection of an asana is far more complex than just addressing stability and inflexibility of the musculoskeletal system. Asanas for deep relaxation are initially chosen to facilitate perception, reflection, and quieting of the central nervous system. Sustained expression of some selected postures allows for the relaxation of muscles safely and naturally with gravity assistance, as well as further discovery of previously unknown patterns of holding. The sequencing of asana includes not only principles that correlate to therapeutic exercise progression, but also those that affect breathing patterns, thoughts, emotions, and spiritual insights.[18]

To differentiate YT asana from the standard rehabilitation use of exercise, note that asana:

- includes mindful procedures for entering into, holding, and emerging from each asana
- coordinates and slows down movements while breathing to sustain ease and comfort
- explores related breath and other bodily sensations to decrease the agitation

and increase focus, as well as top-down discovery of the deeper patterns of fear, attraction, and revulsion that exist as mind-body connection

- has a counter-asana where if, say, a back bend is performed, a form of a forward bend is included. Attention is brought to the experience to explore the polarities of each. These ancient processes are now in modern rehabilitation terminology and are being implemented as pacing, scaling, graded exposure, and desensitization to address fear avoidance, hyperesthesia (increased sensitivity to stimuli), and kinesiophobia (fear of movement)

- shares similar therapeutic progression in terms of load and imposed challenges/perturbations, but then seeks to also identify the emotional, intellectual, and spiritual responses. Asana selection varies widely by respective yoga lineages to add further complexity

- can be adapted with props such as belts (gait or yoga), blocks, and blankets for the individual to approximate a more complex posture like the way orthotics, assistive devices, and prostheses are employed in conventional rehabilitation.

Pranayama (Prah·nah·yah·ma) are breathing practices and the fourth limb of yoga. There are over 100 different practices of yoga breathing patterns. Each is designed to enhance awareness of the lived experience of breathing, related not only to respiration, but also consciousness and action. Breathing techniques in YT are energy management tools to note and manage the effects of increased stress, mood imbalance, threats, and pain. Patterns of inhalation and exhalation can bridge the connection between breathing, the mind, and the emotions but in conventional rehabilitation tend to not be utilized beyond instruction in diaphragmatic breathing.[19]

In YT, modifying breathing patterns through pranayama can decrease related postural loads and facilitate self-reflection to discover the source of the threat (real or perceived) that is eliciting the sympathetic response. The individual can then address the source of the response, rather than just "plow through" the rehabilitation or biomechanical limitations of the moment. The development of such introspection creates new insights for both the individual and therapist, from which new strategies for action emerge (i.e., movement with intention and diminished fear).

> **Experiential pause:** Stay just as you are, don't move a bone. Sense the distance from your sitting bones (ischial tuberosities) to the crown of your head. Then sense the distance between the front of your right shoulder and the front of your left shoulder. Those are your baselines: height and width. Now, gradually begin to increase the length of your exhale and then wait and allow a natural inhale to occur. Repeat this ten times. Recheck your baselines of height and width. Anything change in that regard? Notice anything else that changed (breathing rate, volume, ideation, energy level, etc.). Do note that you weren't instructed to "Take a deep breath"… that's the Western approach to dominating the breath rather than surrendering to the emergence of breathing.

Pratyahara (Prut-yah-hah-ruh) (withdrawing of the senses) and dharana (dhah-ruh-nah) (concentration) are important behavioral health skills. They are the fifth and sixth limbs of yoga. They are important skills during both rehabilitation and activities of daily living. They offer top-down and bottom-up integration of the limbic system with the prefrontal cortex and the resultant interplay afforded by awareness. These practices decrease reactivity to stimuli, increase one's concentration and focus, and create adaptive motor strategies beyond habituated patterns of response. These technologies are more volitional and therefore differ from meditation.

Dhyana (Dhy·ah·na) (meditation) is a collection of conscious mental processes that results in uninterrupted concentration aimed at quieting both the mind and body. Siegel states that this intra- and interpersonal attunement increases awareness, promotes muscle relaxation, encourages the adoption of more efficient postures and patterns of movement, and results in the prevention and reduction of misalignment, cumulative stress, and pain.[20]

Meditation is not, as is often mistakenly thought, the elimination of all thoughts. Siegel suggests that meditation practice impacts the therapeutic relationship. He cites the deleterious effects on the patient's ability to breathe well and attain mindfulness if the therapist is stressed, distracted, and lacking in personal integration.[21] The literature indicates that when teaching not only meditation, but all YT technologies, the therapist has a tendency to assume similar introspective, self-reflective qualities that mirror the desired outcomes to the client. Consequently, the state of the mind of the therapist influences the patient's ability to integrate the intervention. Kind of sounds like IRP, right?

Mudras (Moo·drahs) are precise ways of holding the hands, fingers, tongue, and/or body to produce specific effects and embodied experiences. YT views hands as a delicate interface between the individual and the rest of reality. The fingers and hands are far more than just a robotic tool or claw, and of course there's a large amount of brain dedicated to the fingers and hands in the cortices too. The practice of mudras offers a gateway to discovering the subtle realities of experience through interoceptive practice. Their gentle nature, non-threatening experiences that often arise at a distance from areas of threat, and constant availability for practice are ideally suited to rehabilitation. Mudras offer a natural segue to visual and motor imagery below as the perception of these internal experiences is often most easily described by images and metaphor rather than words.

Experiential pause: Sit up tall but relaxed. Note the location of related movement and volume of breath. That's your baseline. Now, gently fist both hands with your thumbs extended. Place each hand, palm down, on the respective thigh, thumbs pointing at one another. Recheck your baseline experience of breath movement location and volume of breath. Now, turn both hands palm up, thumbs pointing away from one another. Recheck baseline again. What is different? Be skeptical and repeat and sequence as you like. How's that work? Fun, no?

Bhavana (Bah·vah·na) (imagery) and yoga nidra (deep rest) are YT technologies that provide conscious and subconscious integration of memories, emotions, and conceptual limitations of the individual. Closely related to motor imagery in current rehabilitation, these are approaches of mental representation of sensation and movement without any body movement and/or in conjunction with movement. YT utilizes image, metaphor, imagination, visualization, and sensation to invite whole-brain participation and discovery. The therapist's language requires creativity in the experience for the individual, while the sharing of the experience by the individual deepens their embodied experience and communicates potential clinical information for decision making with the therapist.

Chanting (vocalization) requires attention, top-down focus and direction, and bottom-up sensory awareness of the head and neck, as well as auditory integration. As explored in Chapter 20, auditory integration enhances both sensory and motor function of the glottis and thoracic outlet, which impacts autonomic regulation and has other effects. The chants should be in culturally appropriate language and have meaning for the individual. Like mudra, they are portable, always available (silent chanting is part of the skill), and non-threatening when matched to client preferences.

In conclusion, these technologies of YT may seem far removed from traditional rehabilitation, but closer study and practice yields many commonalities. An integrative, biopsychosocialspiritual approach to care such as IRP indeed revisits the very old and also becomes the new evolution of rehabilitation. That said, what do "treatments" look like? The following summary description of intervention principles addresses that important element.

Intervention principles

Interventions and treatment plans in YT intervention strategies include, but are not limited to, the following, as described in conventional rehabilitation.

Manual therapy in YT is not considered a unidirectional fixing intervention from the therapist to client. Manual contact in YT is seen as, in the language of Siegel, intrapersonal attunement.[22] The state of the therapist's mind and body is an equal concern in determining the effectiveness of the intervention. The therapist self-monitors their state, their intention, and that of the patient throughout hands-on care for sensory awareness or physical support. Touch is not intended to move or alter tissue position or quality. A sense of reverence of touch, intention, and gentleness creates a state of therapeutic presence allowing for greater sensitivity and reduced sensory overload, as well as unintentional violence of what might be described as impersonal manipulation.

Therapeutic exercises as asana focus on movement precision as facilitated through concentration and specificity of movement. Traditional therapeutic exercises become asana when they are synchronized with the breath and studied for the relationship between the distal and proximal segments of the extremities and the relationship between the extremities and the spine. The intention of the action in an asana is held clearly, as the mind scans for sensations, emotions, and thoughts that arise during and after the posture. Thus, asana is a very detailed process in comparison to merely counting and completing repetitions. Asana also doesn't strive to reach some increased motion goal.

Directed therapeutic activities are "off-the-mat" yoga. The client's entire experience beyond just gross movement is attended to around the BOS, thoughts, emotions, and other sensations. If the activity reveals gaps in awareness or new insights, those are explored in real time. For instance, difficulties in reaching for a seatbelt may reveal a lack of side bend and rotation to the opposite side. In response, an asana that incorporates those components could be explored to enhance weight shifting and side bend. The activity is then revisited and explored. If the process fails to transfer, they might look for any perceived fear, hesitancy, or additional insights. In YT, limitations are teaching points with successive layers of inquiry going beyond mechanical barriers. Tying one's shoes, reaching for the milk, and grooming one's dog take on a playful sense of discovery and many levels of exploration, experimentation, and discovery about one's self rather than failure or a sense of setback. Intention, attention, and action weave together, creating fun and cycles of inquiry for both patient and therapist.

Home exercise programs are composed of the various YT technologies to reinforce new learning or invite new awarenesses that both therapist and client believe will foster additional understanding. For example, an individual with a persistent right shoulder joint disorder has a habit of clenching the left hip at rest. An asana that opens and stretches the left hip may enhance the mind-body connection to a level that the clenching becomes an activity that raises the patient's awareness, allowing for change of the previously unconscious habit. This iterative process informs the next step of interventions. Besides the formal home program, the individual is encouraged to regularly return to awareness throughout their day, especially when frustrated or during an exacerbation of symptoms. The potential benefit of this is that individuals actually begin to ask for additional home practices. This is a sharp contrast to the usual frustration of non-adherence to conventional home exercise programs. Again, this off-the-mat yoga generates for the client a full list of experiences to explore and introduce into the next YT session, versus waiting for the therapist to create the agenda. Like the patient interaction of an integrative rehabilitation practitioner, isn't it?

Internal "passive" exercises include bhavana and yoga nidra that augment the qualities of non-reactivity and equanimity to stimuli and environments. These modalities require participation by the patient and should match their lexicon and life experiences. They can also be incorporated during otherwise passive modalities such as ice, electrical stimulation, and/or ultrasound. These "passive" practices can broaden their vocabulary of description for sensation, movement, and activities and are congruent with the guidelines of guided and/or motor imagery to use precise, detailed visioning and other senses. This "exercise" of attention engages connectivity between the frontal cortex, memory centers, limbic regions, sensorimotor pathways, and self-regulation (e.g., breath) processes. Here, "passive" reflects the cultivation of active resiliency by demanding a fully engaged patient. These "exercises" can be reinforced with current technology by recording guides on the client's phone or tablet.

The assessments, technologies, and intervention strategies of YT are, of course, far more varied and nuanced than this cursory introduction. Hopefully, though, a new context is available to explore both yoga and IRP within a richer weave of relationship and possibilities. Such possibilities prime for the surprises of the creative process that each of us finds ourselves engaged and embedded in today.

VISION FOR YT IN MEDICAL REHABILITATION

Now you have been introduced to YT on top of all of this IRP material. So what? The what is that the way to change systems is through the personal practices of those that make up the systems.[23] Might we consider that how we become integrative practitioners could be augmented through a personal practice of yoga? Start small (five to ten minutes a day), and then explore through classes, self-study, and creating space for a contemplative/meditative practice. Repeat—over and over! These domain practices prime for your and our collective creativity.[24] So, practice.

Beyond inspiring a regular practice, the intention of this chapter is to bridge the worlds of YT and IRP, and to stimulate creative discovery of the possibilities of YT. In 2015, I wrote: "Please understand that this summary of YT and traditional rehabilitation is only a rearview mirror look at what has already been…and what stretches out ahead is even more exciting!"[25]

Today, more than five years since that quote, I see the interface of YT and IRP as a laboratory for the emergence of genuine health reform. The study of both YT and IRP holds the potential for making our individual and collective lives in this world "more fit to live in" in expressions and depths that we can't imagine. The time has arrived and we are all needed to step forward to allow our best future to emerge.

> **Experiential pause:** Having read this chapter, identify and write down at least one actionable item of interest to you. In doing so, consider ways in which applying the material first to yourself, and then to patients, might serve those who come to you for care.

RESOURCES

– Free 15-week course on integrating yoga therapy into rehabilitation for graduate students and practicing therapists: http://courses.smartsafeyoga.com. Use "practicingiytir" coupon code for complimentary registration.

– Khalsa, S. B. S., Cohen, L., McCall, T., & Telles, S. (2016). *The Principles and Practice of Yoga in Health Care*. Edinburgh: Handspring Publishing.

– How to find a certified yoga therapist: www.iayt.org/search/custom.asp?id=1156.

CHAPTER 25

The Power of Groups

Matt Erb, PT and James S. Gordon, MD

We are a social species. Social engagement is not just a philosophy; it is embedded within our biology and being.[1] Despite individual variability in relational needs, we are hardwired for connection, and how well we are connected with others has implications for our health. The impact of social and community relationships on health is delineated in numerous scientific and theoretical publications.[2] In fact, the likelihood of survival (decreased mortality risk) can be up to 50% higher for individuals with stronger social relationships, a finding consistent across age, sex, initial health status, cause of death, and differences in follow-up periods.[3]

In the body-mind-environment (BME) construct, *environment* includes not just the physical environment but also other levels (Figure 25.1). In this ecosystem, interdependence, as well as interaction, is the rule. In this chapter, the relational/social environment is emphasized.

Typically, *prosocial* denotes qualities seen as positive, helpful, or intended to promote social acceptance. Prosocial applied to others (one's social environment and experience) reflects intent and/or capacity to relate and respond to others in friendly, caring, and supportive ways. Prosocial applied to self can be seen as reflecting self-compassion. Prosocial applied to one's physical environment and/or other various parts of one's experience reflects an intrapersonal value, ethic, or general stance as to how to conduct BME relationships and interactions as a whole.

Prosocial behavior reflects enacting the preceding components of prosocial: "helping, sharing, and other seemingly intentional and voluntary positive behaviors…"[4] Prosocial behavior reflects general or social behavior that benefits others and/or society as a whole. Helping, caring, supporting, serving, cooperating with, and/or intending and seeking to understand others and their experiences are examples that reflect prosocial behavior.

One way that integrative rehabilitation practice (IRP) can contribute to the evolution of health care is through offering greater support for prosocial engagement and experiences in the form of group- and community-minded care options. These options are informed by a collectivist view of human life and health. The pioneering work of The Center for Mind-Body Medicine (CMBM) provides a solid example of group-based support. CMBM's approach combines many core integrative constructs: evidence-based mind-body medicine; self-care and self-regulation principles rooted in an understanding of interdependence and co-regulation; and the power of group connection and mutual support. The CMBM small-group approach can be delivered in many settings. Increasingly, these mind-body skills groups are being delivered in a community-based way in which they are deployed as part of organized, community-wide health, well-being, and resilience initiatives. With adequate training and support, this approach can be delivered effectively by a wide range of individuals: licensed health-care professionals, educators, clergy, and more. We will come back to the structure of this small-group model shortly, but first, a bit more on the science of social support and prosocial behavior.

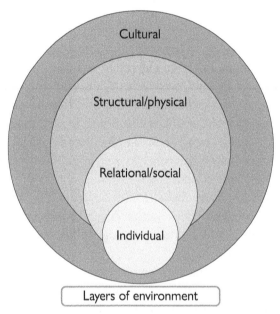

FIGURE 25.1: INDIVIDUALS EMBEDDED WITHIN LAYERS OF ENVIRONMENT
Adapted from Ranjbar *et al.*[5]

THE POWER OF SOCIAL SUPPORT

Research into the health effects associated with general social support[6] frames the scientific background that supports collectivist-minded health care. Findings include the following.

- Potential health-related *behaviors* do not appear to be primarily responsible for the positive health associations derived from increased social support, suggesting a primary effect from social interaction.
- Positive, familial sources of social support may be particularly important for beneficial health effects.
- Emotional support is an important dimension of social support.

- Down-regulation of the stress response and mitigation of allostatic load occurs from positive social interactions.
- Positive social experiences improve coping with negative social experiences.

Looking further into the physiological interactions linked with social support, considerable evidence shows that inflammatory processes and social dynamics are powerful regulators of one another.[7] In particular, consider the following points.

- Inflammation may specifically enhance sensitivity to potentially threatening dangers in one's social environment and/or may promote social withdrawal from unfriendly others during times of sickness.
- Inflammation and sickness do not exclusively induce social withdrawal (prior bullet) but in some cases may encourage the approaching of close/safe others in order to elicit care (tend and befriend). This is consistent with attachment theory (see Chapter 4).
- Exposure to social stress increases pro-inflammatory activity.
- Individuals who are more socially isolated or lonely show increased inflammation.[8]

As presented in Chapter 7 and across this book, using an integral lens on scientific inquiry assists in connecting dots and reinforcing principles of interdependence within each individual's overall biological functioning. Expanding principles of interdependence in BME interactions, including in the sociocultural context, moves us even further into understanding the complexity of each person's health experience.

> **Experiential pause:** Before moving on, consider the following questions, and jot down your ideas.
>
> 1. How can we have a positive effect on the physiological correlates of social engagement beyond that derived from cultivating positive relational experiences in the individualized model of health care?
> 2. What parts of the larger picture of social engagement in your patients' lives can be addressed, and can or should they be addressed directly or indirectly?
> 3. Are there elements of these dynamics that are outside the realm of our influence?

DEEPENING THE NEUROBIOLOGY OF SOCIAL ENGAGEMENT

The core science underlying polyvagal theory (PVT), a subject that we have explored in several chapters, brings general understandings of social support together to form a more cohesive picture of social behavior. PVT links the evolution of the autonomic nervous system (ANS) to the emergence of social behavior in mammalian species. The theory posits that emotional and affective states require specific physiological shifts to facilitate their expression in individual behavior, including prosocial behavior. In examining PVT, we see connections between the evolution of the neurophysiological regulation of the heart and viscera with affect regulation, interoception, emotional expression (facial gestures, body language), breathing, expressive and receptive communication, and responsive social behavior.

Early-life development affects how we relate to others and the world around us. As we develop and grow, all the following processes become intimately integrated and support our ability to function in groups and with each other:

- sensorimotor development
- oral motor behavior
- eye contact/visual feedback
- head turning
- facial expression
- vocalization and tone of voice
- hearing and modulation of sound in the environment (including human voice)
- movement
- touch.[9]

In optimal conditions, these processes combine to support the development of healthy, autonomous self-regulation. As development progresses, higher brain pathways develop and begin to contribute to regulation of the brainstem nuclei and their integration into the larger framework of the ANS. These pathways help to shape personality, psychophysiology, higher cognitive processes, the infant's relationship to its environment (including social/relational), and, ultimately, the development of a larger sense of self.

At the biological level, how does this all happen? In individual relationships? In the presence of group experiences? Current neuroscience presents us with simplified "transmission-line" conceptualizations. Noting this reduction, a more complex, nuanced view is useful. All available sources of afferent information are relayed from the internal/external environment to central processing/interpretive regions. Here, processes of active filtering determine the answer to "questions": friend or foe?, pleasant or unpleasant?, novel or normal?, respond or disregard?, and so on. It is important to note that incoming information includes cues arising from social interactions such as others' behaviors, movement patterns, facial expressions, tone of voice, and body language. All information is compared unconsciously through memory filters that are, ultimately, survival oriented. See Figure 25.2 for a sample simplified schema of relevant neuroscience presented from the integral lens of BME.

It is important to emphasize that the underlying neurophysiology of social engagement is happening outside of conscious awareness. Understanding what contributes to safety in any relational experience, including the whole of medical care and the environments in which it is provided, is crucial. Any approach or intervention that has potential for increasing the experience of safety has equal potential for recruiting the evolutionarily more advanced neural circuits that support the prosocial behaviors of the social engagement system. This means that it is crucial for clinicians to understand and proactively work to support the emergence of safety.[10]

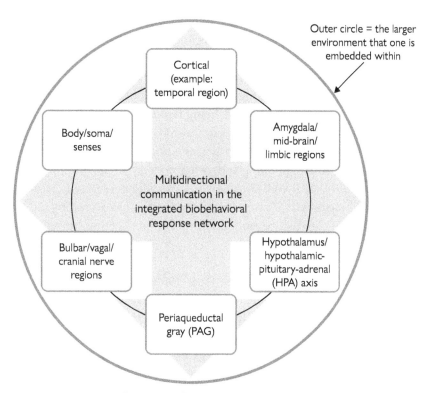

FIGURE 25.2: "PATHWAYS" OF SOCIAL ENGAGEMENT

Because the professional is embedded within the patient's environment, it is necessary to develop the professional's *presence*, as well as the safety of the environment in which care is given. Together, these will support the biological underpinnings of safety, nurturance, and empowerment. What does all this look like when it moves beyond the typical one-to-one provision of health care into a model that supports our collectivist nature?

LEVELS OF AGENCY: SOCIAL COGNITIVE THEORY AND INDIVIDUALITY

Social cognitive theory examines various forms of "agency" and the ways in which individuals are both producers and products of social systems. Agency can include: individual responsibility; proxy agency, in which people secure needs and outcomes by influencing others to act on their behalf; and a collectivist engagement, in which people act in interdependence. It can be tempting, when looking at self-care constructs, to miss the relevance of relational interdependence. We encourage a non-dual (both/and) lens, an understanding that these constructs work well together.

There is notable intercultural and inter-individual variability in one's psychosocial experience. Thus, it is important to define our own experience and support others' experiences in ways that address uniqueness. This uniqueness includes one's agential relationship to the culture to which one belongs. Valuing a person's culture and their distinctive place within it is a feature of *cultural humility*,[11] an approach to understanding the ineffable nature of culture as embedded in individual BME. We don't look at "culture" as something that determines behavior or attitudes, or that is neatly categorized or learned, as may be implied in constructs of cultural *competency*. Cultural humility, by contrast, entails supporting and serving others' complex life processes and how they find agency within them, rather than claiming to fully understand them. Feeling a sense of cultural belonging can contribute to the well-being that comes with social support, but not all people find comfort in their cultural community.

Ultimately, building and strengthening social support, including through group medical visits, group support, and other forms of community, is an important consideration within IRP. Well-designed group experiences recognize individuality, while also meeting shared needs. As we proceed, we encourage co-creating individualized ways to offer a blend of care that accommodates these intersecting concepts.

GROUPS AS POSITIVE SOCIAL ENGAGEMENT

Group-based support broadens the scope of social engagement in health care from provider and patient to larger levels of interaction. Groups come in many forms, including psychotherapeutic groups, self-help groups, support groups, rehabilitation therapy-based groups, educational groups, exercise classes, yoga classes, group medical visits, and more.

The concept of *coherence*, or harmonious relationship(s), can be applied to explorations of individual physiology, as well as socially.[12] Social coherence reflects harmony between pairs or groups of individuals, and even larger units, such as communities, organizations, or societies.

Group-based approaches are increasingly regarded as an important part of integrative health care and there is growing evidence to support this valuation.[13] In particular, researchers are examining the "group inclusion effect," the biological impact of the group environment over and above the effects of the skills or techniques delivered.[14]

In addition to the potential mechanisms that can be derived from the general positive social supports discussed above, being in a supportive group environment can improve health outcomes, partially through physiological mechanisms that underlie belonging and feeling supported.[15] When loneliness is "treated," positive health effects such as analgesia are seen.[16] Published studies on group approaches in health care include benefits for pain management,[17] increased resilience in health-care workers,[18] lessening of anxiety,[19] and reduced insomnia.[20]

These variables have collective relevance *and* are highly individual. Models of care that consider social environments must be able to address the uniqueness of each person's BME experience. In identifying and meeting needs, consider how personality, prior experience, conditioning, and individual beliefs interact.

MIND-BODY SKILLS GROUPS

Peacemaking, talking, or healing circles reflect an important component of social life within indigenous populations around the globe.[21] Such circles recall us to our human roots and establish a different style of relating and communicating than the more individualistic European traditions and the hierarchical model of conventional Western medicine. These circles are designed to create a safe, non-hierarchical place in which all present have the opportunity to voice and express themselves (recall Chapters 19 and 20). Circles are not just a space in which to express oneself, but rather they aim to support the prosocial capacity to understand, learn from, and serve one another. Circles that are led from a non-analyzing, non-pathologizing, and non-fixing stance remind us to consider the limitations of the modern biomedical tendency to "fix the broken." We are encouraged to adopt a wisdom-rooted perspective and practice that assists others in their capacity to learn and discover things for themselves.

In the authors' experience, the example of mind-body skills groups (MBSGs) as taught by CMBM reflects a contemporary version of healing circles. MBSGs reflect a reparative and transformative opportunity for healthy attachment and safe communication that teaches, encourages, and facilitates regulation *within ourselves and between us and others.*

The CMBM approach is taught internationally and combines small-group structure with principles of meditation, facilitated sharing, simple education, and experiential learning—all rooted in the evidence-based, self-care skills that are the heart of mind-body medicine. Though self-care may appear individualistic, self-care in context supports "co-care." CMBM describes this concept succinctly: "a supportive group is the medium in which self-care flourishes."[22]

The CMBM group model was first used in the early 1990s with individuals navigating cancer and other life-threatening illnesses. Since then, the work has expanded into numerous populations and settings and reflects a wellness-oriented group approach that is applicable and accessible to a wide range of settings, conditions, cultures, and experiences. Through CMBM training, MBSGs have been delivered throughout the world to support individuals and communities impacted by war, natural disaster, other forms of trauma, or persistent high levels of stress.

Numerous studies have been published on the efficacy of MBSGs in addressing a number of challenges, conditions, populations, and settings.[23] These studies demonstrate the benefits of MBSGs in post-traumatic stress disorder, depression, and anxiety, as well as in burnout prevention in health-care professionals.

Groups ordinarily have one or two leaders and up to ten participants and include a variety of evidence-based mind-body skills, among them: meditation and relaxation techniques, biofeedback, autogenic training, drawings, written exercises, movement practices, and guided imagery. These skills are tailored to support the person-centered approach as defined and explored throughout this book—enabling people to become more aware of themselves and giving them the techniques and strategies for acting on what they're learning. These "skills" are presented as experiments, opportunities for learning about oneself, and simple ways of using one's imagination and intuition to identify solutions to challenges or problems that one is experiencing.

The model focuses on each individual's capacity to know themselves better—through individual awareness, expression, and regulation. This occurs in the context of mutual support and reflects the understanding of humans as interdependent social beings. Self-regulation becomes co-regulation, and healing is embedded in the intersubjective space that connects us to each other.[24] In essence, the MBSG invites the emergence of each person's presence, recognizing that it arises organically in the amplifying presence of others.

MBSGs can be tailored to virtually any population, setting, or culture. MBSGs are generally held for two hours, once or twice a week, for eight to ten weeks. Shorter and longer durations can be offered, as well as various workshop formats. Group leaders set ground rules that contribute to safe exploration and discussion. In examining the CMBM model, consider the relevance of the following ground rules:

- confidentiality
- mutual respect (refraining from interrupting others or interpreting or analyzing what they say or do, and focusing on what arises in oneself)
- the role of the leader as both teacher and participant (leaders do exercises along with participants and take their turn in the check-in process)
- the option of "passing" if one does not wish to speak and the opportunity to share at a later time if desired
- the importance of attending all groups and arriving on time or informing the instructor of extenuating circumstances
- an emphasis on being with present-moment experience, developing the capacity to observe one's own real-time thoughts, feelings, and sensations and bring the same attentive presence to the shared words and experiences of other group members.

Each MBSG carries the same basic structure.

1. Opening meditation.
2. "Check-in," in which participants, including the facilitator(s), share what they are experiencing or processing, with a focus on present-moment attention.
3. Provision of simple, practical, and interactive education on a specific evidence-based mind-body medicine topic.
4. Experiential learning of a mind-body skill or approach.
5. Sharing of the experience with the understanding that all experiences are welcome and encouraged, including challenges, and without any attempt to convince, change, or fix each person's experience.
6. Closing meditation.

While the preceding structure is specific to the CMBM model, the principles carry direct relevance to the general principles described for IRP and may carry benefit to other group offerings. In the MBSGs, learning a variety of mind-body techniques enables participants to see that there are many ways in which they can interact with their experience to improve well-being. Individuals can choose which skills are most appealing and/or effective for their current experience and lay a foundation for accessing other skills as needed in the future.

Facilitators of MBSGs report that individuals often start out in a group experience with hesitancy about, aversion toward, and/or discomfort with sitting in a circle and sharing their lives with strangers. Gradually, however, participants begin to feel connection, support, and meaning. For some, this is a first experience of physiological self-regulation, self-awareness, and self-expression in a safe, accepting, non-judgmental space of connection and community.

The term "community withdrawal syndrome" was coined by one of CMBM's faculty members to denote a feeling that sometimes arises as a MBSG ends. Individuals are faced with transitioning back to their regular life patterns that may lack a similar forum of relational support that the MBSG experience offered. It is speculated that processes of early-life attachment patterns and needs (see Chapter 4) may inform this dynamic.[25] The MBSG design recognizes and addresses the possibility that, for some, the end of the group experience may come with a sense of loss around a nurturing sense of secure/safe attachment and expression. For this reason, group experiences "end" with a closing ceremony designed by the facilitator to assist in transitions out of the group and enhanced integration back into the "next right thing" in one's life.

Experiential pause: Using your faculties of imagination, consider the relevance of PVT in relation to mind-body skills training, interpersonal support, and the dynamic of a supportive group setting as described below.

Imagine you are sitting in a circle with a group of ten other individuals who have come together to explore the cultivation of well-being. The group begins with a short meditation rooted in basic present-moment awareness of the body, combined with a simple breathing practice: silently think the word "soft" as you breathe in, and the word "belly" as you breathe out. Take a moment now and practice this for a minute or two as you imagine being in the group…and then proceed through the rest of this script.

Following the meditation, each person has the opportunity to share what is happening in their life: what they are experiencing (thinking, feeling, processing, etc.). This is prefaced by an instruction: each person is asked to share with present-moment awareness, as well as to not respond, interject, give advice, or fix others' emotions and experiences when others are sharing. You are listening, considering what you will say, and noticing how it feels to be in the presence of others and what is happening in your body.

When it is your turn, you begin to share with the others…

Based on your current life experience, what might you be sharing? How might it feel to express your experience in a group of people? Have you had other experiences with groups that would make this feel easy or hard, comfortable or uncomfortable?

CHALLENGES AND CONSIDERATIONS

Including group-based options as part of the integrative care model has many potential advantages, such as cooperation and mutual support. But doing so is not without challenges and important considerations.

Individual dynamics and differences (e.g., personality, sociocultural environment, perceived importance, and durability of social support) may impact a person's interest in experiencing and receiving group-based care options and their motivation. In addition, persons experiencing high-stress conditions and/or other mind-body health states, including post-traumatic stress disorder (PTSD), personality disorders, and autism spectrum disorders, may have psychophysiological patterns that affect their interest in and/or capacity for social engagement in both individual and group settings. Still, it is appropriate to encourage hesitant individuals to consider a group setting, as the experience may later turn out to be highly rewarding. We approach the exploration of group membership in accordance with the same principles laid out throughout this book: education, encouragement, nurturing support, empowered decision making, and stepping back.

CONCLUSION

The cost of health care as currently delivered is economically unsustainable and at crisis levels. Access to service is limited, and the need for lifestyle and whole-person approaches that support and expand the biomedical model is increasingly urgent. Further, our individualistic health-care model, while necessary, misses the collectivist nature of human beings. Social engagement can expand beyond the cultivation of the patient-professional relational space as presented in Chapter 8.

We offer this chapter on group-based options as a creative, bold, and necessary response. Group-based health care reflects a cost-effective way to deliver evidence-based care to multiple people.[26] One-to-one care will always be with us, but the group model is poised to become a necessary and vital companion and enhancement of it.

MBSGs present us with a case study in group-based care. MBSGs offer an evidence-based blend of mind-body medicine in a small-group format. Consistent with the broad intentions that inform IRP, the MBSG model approaches individuals as being capable of discovering their own solutions and answers. Exploring our experience in relationship to others' experiences also helps us to see that we are not alone in our challenges. While not optimally suited for all individuals, group-based options can expand the reach of IRP while simultaneously supporting the innate needs of connection and belonging.

Experiential pause: Having read this chapter, identify and write down at least one actionable item of interest to you. In doing so, consider ways in which applying the material first to yourself, and then to patients, might serve those who come to you for care.

RESOURCES

For more information about The Center for Mind-Body Medicine, the availability of in-person and online MBSGs, and training to lead them, you can consult the CMBM website (www.cmbm.org) and read Dr. Gordon's book *The Transformation: Discovering Wholeness and Healing After Trauma.*[27]

CHAPTER 26

Integrative Rehabilitation Practice and Mental Health

Matt Erb, PT and Noshene Ranjbar, MD

OVERVIEW

Integrative rehabilitation practice (IRP) is well suited to contributing to improved mental health. In this chapter, the term *mental health* applies to the whole of mental, emotional, social/relational, behavioral, and other psychological facets of human experience. Individual spirituality, encompassed in the term *psychospiritual*, is also included within our encompassing definition of the purview of mental health.

Practicing IRP means developing a skill set capable of supporting foundational psychospiritual needs by empowering others through challenging times, utilizing a non-pathologizing lens, and acting in service to overall well-being. The psychological facets of our lives do not exist in isolation from each other, nor from our bodies and the environments that we are embedded within. Think ecosystems within ecosystems. Therefore, we must apply an approach informed by a dispositional theory of causation (Chapter 3). A dispositional theory of causation reminds us that it is short-sighted to think that any one effort aimed towards fixing a perceived ingredient in causality will adequately or wholly address a health challenge. In looking at mind-body connection in general, there is great risk of over-reducing causality solely to a personality trait, an emotional tendency, or a past trauma…to give a few examples.

Alongside the growth of integrative health care models, the provision of *integrated* care (physical and mental health care together) is developing. Across this book, we have discussed issues such as the benefits and limitations of transdisciplinary education/ practice, scopes of practice, the rise of multimorbidity and syndemics, public health topics, and more. This chapter explores the following topics to support the use of IRP both as part of general mental health promotion and within systems of mental health care:

- rejoining mind and body in support of mental health
- body-mind-environment (BME): an ecosystem view of mental health

- the role of the body in mental health
- the role of IRP in mental health
- a collaborative model of integrative and integrated mental health care.

REJOINING MIND AND BODY IN SUPPORT OF MENTAL HEALTH
Transforming a long history

As covered in Chapter 3, the philosophy of mind-body has a long and complex history. Here we wish to curiously notice and then walk past this rabbit hole, in favor of engaging in practical discussion about the benefits and challenges of greater mind-body integration in ourselves, in our collective culture, and as applies to clinical rehabilitation practice in support of mental health.

With an entrenched tendency to compartmentalize psychological and social facets away from physical health, we can see how professionalization (e.g., *physical* therapist versus *psycho*therapist, or internal medicine versus psychiatry) has inadvertently reinforced the mind-body divide to the potential detriment (shame, stigmatization, as covered in Chapter 6) of patients. The stark dichotomy of common biomedical pain interventions versus psychosocial practices for pain reflects this dynamic. Often, people unconsciously believe pain is either/or—either a physical issue that can be fixed by manual medicine, surgery, or drugs…*or* a purely psychological problem, existing "all in one's head." Recall the story of Massoud in Chapter 6 as a good example. This dynamic represents a common blind spot within our current health care system, which left unaddressed can contribute to a cascade of additional stress, cost, and challenges for the patient, professionals, and the system as a whole.[1]

While each professional discipline contributes key insights and approaches to overall well-being, splitting mind and body in practice comes with a price when professionals fail to adequately acknowledge and support the whole of each person. In IRP, disciplines can establish a core scope of practice and solid starting points for professional development. Subsequently, transdisciplinary education and skill development improves whole-person care within and across professions. Transdisciplinary education as translated into clinical care supports the capacity of all professionals and aims to improve patient experience, safety, and quality of care. Knowing how to practice in a transdisciplinary way that minimizes inadvertent harm necessitates continual self-appraisal.

The upside to the dis-integration of mind and body is that it precedes the creation of something new in the process of re-integration—hence the ongoing development of integrative care constructs in general. Across this book, we have explored many avenues for whole-person support. From functional education, to integrative-minded interviewing, to mind-body medicine skills, we have presented a foundation for "human care" that stands equally in support of "mental" and "physical" health. We have reached a point where the historical dis-integration of mind and body is giving way to the process of their re-integration. Another way of saying this is reflected in the notion that destruction is part of ongoing creation. And…what is old is new again too—as none of this is entirely new, just reinvented for contemporary conditions.

Clarifying potential problems

Whether care is *primarily* directed towards mental or physical health, properties assigned to each category are inseparable. The idea of bottom-up (body impacts mind) and top-down (processes in the psyche impact the body) can be useful. This language is commonly used in the research and academic world.[2] However, without clarification, we see here that "top" is either being equated to brain, or not defined at all. This equating comes with the aforementioned rabbit hole around the nature of mind and the reduction of mind solely to brain, stirring up philosophies, opinions, emotions, and thus heated debates—a rabbit hole indeed.

While the brain is "top" in regard to an upright orientation of the body in space, and indeed is considered vital and necessary to our experience of mind, we must be flexible in not reifying that the brain is necessarily the sole origin of mind. Integral thinking encourages the view that, wherever our experience of consciousness and psyche originates, the mind is distributed within the whole of one's bodily experience, as well as inseparably connected to, and influenced by, the environments in which it is embedded.[3]

From a neuroscientific standpoint, in addition to the intricate neuronal connections within the brain and spinal cord, there are powerful and extensive neural networks found throughout the body, for example in the heart, gut, and other viscera.[4] The embodied view of mind encourages us to understand the brain as being extended throughout the body. The expanding neuroscientific literature on interdependent body-brain connectivity supports an understanding that there are layers and levels of "intelligence" housed within the human body. Theories and strategies supporting individualized, narrative-based explorations of distributed somatic intelligence exist to assist in navigating the psychological/material divide that the mind-body problem reflects.[5]

BME: an ecosystem view of mental health

Self-organization and the influence of environment

Self-organization refers to an innate or spontaneous drive towards overall patterning, pattern change, and order in living systems. Self-organization arises from the interactions of components into the formation of greater overall order or coherence. In human studies, self-organization can be used to define how one makes sense of self and the experience of living.[6]

An integral understanding of self-organization demands the linking together of not just body and mind but also *environment* (BME) as we have done across the book. In relation to mental health, and building on Dr. Dan Siegel's recent exploration of mind, integration—whether within a view of the brain itself, an individual, an organization, or within the larger society—is fundamental to any notion of healthy BME states.[7]

The mind as distributed and extended

What does it mean to say that the mind is distributed and extended? To say that the mind is *distributed* first refers to the idea that it is not just in the head/brain, but also integrated into the whole of the body. To say that the mind is *extended* suggests that it is interacting with and dependent upon the physical and social environments being experienced.[8] Take, for example, cognition as one component of our experience of mind. The distributed and extended view suggests that cognitive function:

- involves coordination between the whole of internal (somatic/bodily) and external (environmental) structures
- is not just intra-individual, but is also linked to relationships and social interactions across various levels, as illustrated in Figure 25.1 in Chapter 25.

Without getting lost in philosophy here, what is the simplified relevance to mental health? What we say (our words) extends our mind to others and can carry significant impact on mind-body interactions at both intra-individual and inter-individual levels.[9] Supporting changes in one's physical and/or socioeconomic environment can influence health in the absence of personal effort.[10] Towards the latter, and recalling Chapter 4 (social determinants of health), individualistic cultures see mental illness as a *personal* challenge or worse: as a weakness or failing. Often, scientific inquiry reduces mental states such as fear, focus, affection, or memory to specific psychological faculties presumed to be found solely in the individual brain. However, growing evidence suggests that mental states emerge from large-scale mind-brain-body-environment networks. That is, the state of the body and both its relationship to and movement within its environment are necessary for cognition.[11]

Clinical relevance
When treating patients, we must take into account the ecosystem that the person is a part of. When supporting parts, we understand that the parts are comprised by a larger whole, and there is uncertainty in what may emerge in the picture of the whole. Mental health care, similar to physical health care, often *dis*-integrates a person's experience into parts and overly reduces the cause of illness to a part, such as disturbed chemistry. Further, it fails to acknowledge the collectivist lens on health, including sociocultural and ecological models of mental health.[12] This understanding is vital to counteract self-blame tendencies around mental health, which are shaped by multiple factors within an ecological system.[13]

Simplifications, though at times useful, typically miss this larger interplay of contributing factors. Mentioned earlier, the clinical application of the dispositional theory of causation assists clinicians in addressing the larger scope of influences. To paraphrase a quote found elsewhere in this book, for every problem there are simple, neat, and tidy solutions—that are at best faulty, and at worst plain wrong.[14] With simplified solutions, we often miss both the reality and the fullness/wholeness of the person sitting in front of us.

Experiential pause: Invite a contemplative state by settling into the support beneath you, softening bodily tension as you are able, and taking a few slower, fuller breaths. Now, reading slowly and mindfully, contemplate the following examples, looking deeper into the mind-body connection of mental health. You might even place yourself into each imagined scenario.

- If I touch your painful knee, am I touching other parts of you within the whole of your experience? What part(s) of your mind has been touched? What beliefs, feelings, associations, expectations, and/or memories might be held or evoked in/with/from this part of the body? What is the relevance and meaning of your knee to the larger landscape of your life?

- If you have a chronic migraine/headache condition, how does that interact with your individual psychology? How does it interact in relationship to others such as an intimate partner or family unit? How does it interact with your work or sense of purpose?

- Imagine that wildfires have suddenly become frequent in your geographic region. How does this affect your state of mind? How do these environmental conditions and each person's experience of them "land" in the body?

- If depression is found to have somatic correlates in posture and movement, can changing the posture and movement habits of the body in turn change the state of the mind?[15] Try the following: collapse your whole body and imagine feeling defeated or down. Then move your posture in a more upward, outward, and opening way and see how that feels.

- Recall the phrase: "I'm shouldering a lot." Now, tense your shoulders upward and/or forward—just a slight amount—enough to feel that you are purposely holding your shoulders in a tense way. What happens? How is your breathing? What else do you notice? What happens when you release that tension? How often do you link physical patterns to mental, emotional, social, or environmental stressors in your life? And in the lives of your patients? How might the development of contemplative attention on the body help a person navigate their experiences of stress?

The role of the body in mental health

Mental illness can be viewed as a chemical imbalance of the brain. While this lens (the biological model of psychiatry) has clearly brought advances that improve workability and quality of life for some, it also has challenges and limitations[16] that an integral lens can help to overcome. Indeed, efforts to enhance psychiatric and psychological care, such as the power threat meaning (PTM) framework,[17] carry direct parallels to the efforts of this book with regard to rehabilitation practice. The approach of the PTM framework is summarized in six questions that can apply to individuals, families, or social groups.

1. What has happened to you? (How is power operating in your life?)
2. How did it affect you? (What kind of threats does this pose?)
3. What sense did you make of it? (What is the meaning of these situations and experiences to you?)

4. What did you have to do to survive? (What kinds of threat response are you using?)
5. What are your strengths? (What access to power and resources do you have?)
6. What is your story? (How does all this fit together?)

This is another way of presenting many of the same principles found throughout this book. However, one vital point relevant to the mind-body split is missing here. Where is the body? What is the role of the body? The aforementioned "all in the head" phrase reflects a high societal stigma that exists around psychiatric and psychological experiences and states, implying weakness, begetting shame, and in some cases reflecting "mind" as an arbitrary, loosely defined construct with no somatic origin or correlate.

Experiential pause: Reread items one to six from the PTM framework above and then add the following questions to the original questions.

1. And, how has it/is it impacting your bodily experience?
2. And, how might it be influencing the stress and tension patterns in your brain and body now?
3. And, what do you notice in the felt sense of your body as you contact these past experiences?
4. And, how did the innate intelligence and built-in survival physiology of your body assist you in managing and coping with these challenges? How has your body helped and supported you? What burden has it absorbed?
5. And, how are these strengths found in your body, and your relationship to your body, in the present?
6. And, as you share your experience, how does it feel in the sensations of your body? Be sure to not forget the holding of strengths along with any challenges.

With the growth of numerous disciplines exploring the mind-body connection, a variety of mental health approaches are shifting to include the role of the body.[18] Numerous experts from across the fields of physical medicine and rehabilitation, nutrition, and mental health have written on the topic, largely focusing on trauma and neuroplasticity.[19] There is also ample research into the role of exercise in mental health conditions, such as anxiety and depression.[20] Further, as explained in Chapter 3, depression often coexists with somatic conditions (comorbidity, multimorbidity, and syndemics) in a bidirectional way; a wide range of physical activity approaches demonstrate benefit.[21]

For many rehabilitation professionals, structured physical activity is easily understood to confer a wide range of protective health benefits. However, mind-body dynamics function at a deeper level than just the physical and psychological benefits of exercise. Consider the following examples of research into the way that the body is implicated in mental health.

- Movement patterns reflect and influence emotions.[22]

- Personality characteristics are associated with back pain, muscle-firing patterns, muscle pain, and fatigue.[23]
- Poor nutritional status, either from poor intake or problems with nutrient absorption related to gut problems, can impact mental and physical health and recovery.[24]
- Yoga and other movement-based contemplative practices that integrate combinations of exercise, physical postures, breathing, body awareness, and/or meditation principles have been shown in a growing body of research to have direct impact on psychological health.[25]

As touched on across this book, a growing number of evidence-supported theories and/or models of mind-body union are being used in both mental and physical health care arenas. These theories and models include polyvagal theory, neurovisceral integration theory, preparatory-set, sensorimotor psychotherapy, Somatic Experiencing, yoga therapy, contemplative movement practices, body awareness training, and eye movement desensitization and reprocessing (EMDR), among others. Taken together, these examples only scratch the surface of both a body of evidence and a movement towards embodied approaches to mental health.

The role of IRP in mental health

The current landscape of mental health care in rehabilitation

The field of occupational therapy (OT) is rooted in whole-person theory and mental health practices.[26] In the US, due to a variety of factors (primarily changes in payor dynamics), OT is unfortunately less frequently included in the provision (referral and coverage) of mental health care services. That being said, clinical and OT researchers tend to strive for whole-person models, assessments, interventions, and outcomes.

As mentioned earlier, the dichotomy between *physical* therapy (PT) and *psycho*therapy reflects perhaps the starkest professional split of body and mind. We will therefore use the example of these two professions to paint the picture of a landscape shifting towards transdisciplinary education, rooted in mind-body integration, while maintaining professional identity and scope of practice.

The World Confederation of Physical Therapy recognizes the role of physical therapists in mental health through the International Organization of Physical Therapists in Mental Health (IOPTMH) subgroup. A biennial conference, The International Conference of Physical Therapy in Psychiatry and Mental Health, highlights emerging research and forums for work on mental health within PT. Valuable overviews of this field have been published.[27] A majority of this work arose out of European efforts and in many ways overlaps with existing and developing OT models and approaches. While the content is largely shared with similar work that is developing in the US, there are some variations rooted in systemic and cultural differences. In particular, the model proposed in IRP draws strongly on the contemporary fields of evidence-based integrative medicine, mind-body medicine (MBM), and yoga therapy, which have a solid and growing foundation in the US. As a result, depending on your locale, facets of these practices may be more or less accessible for training and implementation.

Recognition of the need for psychologically integrated practice (PIP) in PT has grown slowly over time, with an increase in attention in the last few years.[28] And paradigms shift slowly. Data suggest that it takes an average of 17 years for some evidence to be integrated into clinical practice.[29] Further, the dissemination of clinical practices through passive methods, such as journal articles, is generally ineffective, resulting in minimal changes in the uptake of new practices.[30] Many agree on the need for a more holistic approach to care, but, with some exceptions (especially within OT), the average rehabilitation professional is challenged to successfully address the complex psychosocial dynamics and social determinants of health (Chapter 4) that inform patients' experiences.

"I'm not a psychologist"

Acknowledgement of challenges in the current landscape presents an opportunity to creatively solve the question of how to best integrate psychosocial support in rehabilitation professions. This is especially true if the clinician is not able or interested in enacting a PIP and/or mind-body approach to care. Comfort with psychology is variable within the general population. For rehabilitation professionals, interest might range from engaged to absent. In social media groups for non-mental-health rehabilitation professionals, aversion to PIP can present as extreme, exemplified by the not uncommon comment: "I'm not a psychologist." True, you are not. But this type of response misses the point.

With this dynamic in mind, the possibility of deepening the use of IRP as part of mental health care models might be seen as an even bigger hurdle. Wait! Let's start smaller, with basic competencies in understanding and supporting, in normalizing ways, the whole of each person. This book is designed to help to build this type of capacity, but it must come with an important reminder.

As noted in Chapter 2, the learning that is needed to assist in the development of whole-person support is best done from an understanding of oneself first, the other later. This approach supports co-regulation: concurrent self-awareness and self-regulation practices in the clinician that influence the experience and psychophysiological state of the patient. Think *presence*. Self-awareness in this regard includes examining the presence of attachments to outcomes and/or the implicit drive to fix the other, which implies that the other is broken—a paradigmatic blindness that may contribute to burnout.[31] In essence, if we do not know what we feel, we are less able to know or relate to what others feel, a concept inherent to models of affective neuroscience, relational attunement, and embodied, enactive compassion.[32] Even if we are not psychologists, developing self-awareness is a critical first step to being able to support our patients as whole people in IRP.

Strategies matter

As stressed throughout this book, it is vital that rehabilitation professionals develop the understanding and capacity to deliver safe interventions in collaboration with those who come to them for support. This capacity must fit a *phenomenological heuristic*: an approach and set of strategies and interventions that enable individuals to come to know, relate to, and respond to their own experience. Said another way: a person-centered approach that supports individuals in discovering, learning, and deciding things for themselves. An important part of this approach is understanding how to support unconditional acceptance and validation of the patient's experience (recall the relational space from Chapter 8). It is equally important to uncover ways of speaking about the mind in relation to the body that are safe, supportive, and useful *to the patient*. We must learn to allow each person to define this in a way that serves their needs.

In the development of IRP, we have also asked (and must continue to ask) if the way in which we are serving patients is considerate of individual cultural, religious, philosophical, and spiritual beliefs. The whole of this book has been aimed towards such consideration. It may not be perfect (nothing is) and, as noted in the opening chapter, it will change, evolve, and transform too, as all things do. You are actively contributing simply by reading this book and participating in the exercises.

There are many evidence-supported strategies and interventions that are directly beneficial for psychological and behavioral well-being (see the next section). These approaches are available to and useful for both professionals and patients and may be especially important for working with persons experiencing chronicity and/or states of physical/mental health comorbidity (see Chapter 3). Also, consider that by its very nature, deploying care that operates from the IRP perspective *is* supporting mental health.

Bridge-building skills

Here is a sampling of concepts selected to underscore how IRP supports mental health care. Stay mindful that our advocacy is not intended to reinforce the splitting of mental health care away from physical medicine. These topics are presented in review through a lens of mental health care.

- **Exploring values, motivation, and commitment**: In Chapter 17, we introduced Acceptance and Commitment Therapy (ACT) as an example of a skill set that can enhance IRP. ACT encourages the identification of one's values, motivations, and plans for committed action. In doing so, we need to pay attention to bridging the gap between idealism and realism; setting realistic expectations becomes important. We also need discernment around the delicate balance of inaction and action. For example, embodied acceptance in essence is an act of empowerment as opposed to passivity or "giving in." ACT and other cognitive-behavioral integrated skills offer us the capacity to relate to the unpleasant aspects of our lives as passengers on a bus. There are also other passengers, including some neutral ones and some pleasant ones. Ultimately, a fuller sense of self can be developed as the larger context of the whole bus, its controls, a navigation system, and a valued destination.
- **Supporting purpose and meaning**: In Chapter 18, we explored a number of strategies to support individuals in the development of purpose and meaning.

These topics and approaches overlap and weave together with the preceding section on values and committed action.

- **Needs assessment and needs fulfillment strategies**: We all have basic needs, which are usually thought to consist of food, shelter, and water. Add to this safety, connection, nurturance, and autonomy, among others. Assisting individuals to contemplate their needs, advocate for them, and proactively contribute to meeting them is vital. One simple strategy is to show individuals a list of common needs (such as connection, honesty, enjoyment/play/fun, physical well-being, and a sense of purpose and meaning as reflected above) and invite them to discuss which are being met or not being met on a spectrum. This assessment then links to common affective patterns—where emotions/feelings and behavior intersect. When basic human needs are fulfilled, the door to positive, prosocial feelings and behaviors is opened. When needs are unfulfilled, the door gets heavy and might even lock. Finally, combining an exploration of needs with the embodied approach—such as discovering the impact of met/unmet needs on/in the body in the form of sensations, postural tendencies, and movement patterns—assists in formulating greater awareness of BME patterns. Such awareness can be the first step towards transforming patterns that are no longer serving the person's needs and experience.

- **Exercise and movement**: A growing body of literature in mental health focuses on structured movement, or exercise. Systematic reviews demonstrate the importance of exercise in depression, anxiety, schizophrenia, bipolar disorder, and eating disorders.[33] Exercise is a loaded topic for some, bringing up negative associations, such as excessive structure, time limitations, aversion, or even shame. For some individuals, it may be beneficial to use a less structured approach to exercise. For example, exploring the relevance of movement in our lives and developing inspired and creative relationships to moving our bodies in and through the world can be beneficial. Changing up patterns of bodily movement has great potential to influence the experience of mind. Dr. James S. Gordon, founder of The Center for Mind-Body Medicine, reminds us that often the challenging mental, emotional, or physical content of our lives is not the problem, but our relationship to that content is: we get stuck.[34] Movement as explored in Chapter 15 is one avenue that can assist us in learning the art of getting unstuck when a pattern has become habitual.

- **Breath awareness and other foundations of self- and co-regulation**: In Chapter 11, we explored the breath. Breathing is a vital entry point for influencing processes of physiological regulation. Applied regulation involves teaching individuals to shift maladaptive biobehavioral states that arise in response to inner and outer stimuli. When one can shift their physiological state, access to higher order self-referential processes such as the capacity to reappraise one's experience is enhanced. The self-regulation construct is considered foundational to current understandings in resiliency research. Autonomic nervous system dysregulation plays a part in compromised resilience,[35] and this has been linked to numerous mental and physical health problems.[36] Improving overall mind-body regulation is thus important for management of numerous conditions.[37] Finally, enhanced self-regulation supports comfort with discomfort—and thus the possibility of improved quality of life.

- **Body awareness**: In Chapter 13, we explored sensation. Sensing in all its forms can be seen as the primordial bedrock of our experience. We *feel* our way through this world. Tracking sensation in real time affords us:
  a. the ability to more skillfully navigate BME interactions
  b. the capacity to regulate unconscious neuromuscular tension patterns like guarding, holding, or clenching that are linked to mental patterns of tension
  c. improved emotional intelligence
  d. a sense of knowing what is happening, which facilitates optimal/informed decision making.

- **Affect labeling and emotional expression**: Because it is linked with sensory awareness and processing, we find the reality of *feeling* to be both physical and emotional. As covered in Chapter 17 and as linked to Chapter 13 and the preceding bullet, inquiring into a person's affective realm in a way that facilitates naming of the emotion(s) being experienced can release tension by inhibiting fear and stress centers in the brain.[38] Beyond the benefit to postural correction, balance training, coordination, and a host of movement challenges, exploring each person's unique relationship to body awareness is equally useful in both pain management[39] and mental health conditions.[40] Learning basic labeling strategies inherent to mindfulness practices has been shown to orchestrate similar effects.[41] Encouraging independent expressive writing (Chapter 19) about mental or physical health experiences may provide a more feasible alternative for modulating the stress response for individuals who may be less emotionally expressive, demonstrate variations of alexithymia, or simply prefer a less affectively oriented style of engagement.[42] These examples are provided to underscore the presence of simple ways to engage mind-body interactions in a supportive, person-centered approach.

Experiential pause: Consider the following simple ways in which to begin to add attention to the preceding subtopics within your practice (one from each section above). Often, the entry point is the use of simple, well-placed, and open-ended questions as invitations into awareness and exploration. If the patient bypasses the offer, move on to other avenues.

- Exploring values, motivation, and commitment: "What is most important to you in your life…in the big picture, what matters the most to you? What do you most value?" "Do you feel it is possible to work on 'X' (self-selected committed action(s)) with your motivation for doing so arising from these values? Can you work on X without an attachment to the idea that doing so will make the challenge go away?"
- Exercise and movement: "How would you describe your current relationship

to movement and/or exercise, which is really a label for a more structured approach to moving our bodies?"

- Breath awareness and other foundations of self- and co-regulation: "What do you notice when you become aware of your breathing?" "I'm wondering what strategies you utilize to regulate your body's stress response."
- Body awareness: "What do you notice is happening in your body right now as you share about these stressors in your life?" "You shared that this shoulder pain is very frustrating for you. Where do you feel that frustration in your body?"
- Affect labeling and emotional expression: "How are you feeling today? In general? How is this health challenge making you feel—in other words, what is the experience bringing up for you in terms of emotions?"
- Needs assessment and needs fulfillment strategies: "What needs do you feel are not getting met in relationship to your current health challenge?"

Scope of practice

Despite the potential benefits of increasing the number of rehabilitation professionals who can work with patients who have comorbid physical-mental health conditions, there are challenges to achieving this within the existing health care paradigm. These challenges are consistent with those discussed in Chapters 1–6, such as access to educational training, patient access issues, and third-party payor structures. In relation to scope of practice and psychological integration, earlier chapters (especially Chapter 6) present vital information in support of patient safety in whole-person care. In the development of whole-person care capacity, and especially if working more directly with mental health focused practice, ongoing clinical supervision and professional mentoring are strongly encouraged as well.

Several key points and clarifications are useful for discussing scope of practice and professional boundaries in the context of mental health. First, most rehabilitation professionals are not qualified to diagnose mental health conditions. However, with proper training, they can and often *are* treating patients referred with primary or secondary mental health diagnoses. Rehabilitation professionals' skill set is an especially important component of therapy for these patients as it can add a useful and often unaddressed layer of support for the embodied elements of comorbidity as described in Chapter 3.

Second, any attempt to psychoanalyze a person's life experience is unwarranted by anyone but a psychoanalyst. In contrast, seeking to understand human behavior through psychologically integrated practice, normalizing the stress response, and exploring emotions and cognitions within healthy boundaries enhances healing processes. The presence of psychological difficulties must never:

- be a reason to overlook a patient's complaint of pain or other symptoms
- cause the professional to forego medical screening and diagnostics

- lead to assumptions about a patient's life experience or their rehabilitation potential.

Instead, the awareness of the additional layers informing the patient's suffering should make the assessment and treatment of the pain or other symptom *more* comprehensive and efficacious. Hopefully, such awareness will reduce unnecessary tests and high-cost and unsustainable interventions.

Third, giving personal life advice, such as suggesting that someone quit a job or leave their spouse, is discouraged. In contrast, assisting patients to explore their needs and discover their own decisions, as well as supporting them with resources and strategies for getting such needs met, is appropriate.

Caring for the whole person

Given these foundational guidelines, it is important to note: in whole-person care, no profession has an exclusive license on active listening, being fully present, supporting feelings, demonstrating compassion, and delivering humanized treatment in general. An example is found in a person-centered approach to exploring adverse childhood experiences (ACEs).[43] In such a model, a starting point is the provision of simple education or questions.

Try questions such as: "Have you heard about the research that suggests that past stress, especially if it was early in life, may leave a lasting impact that we can positively address in the present? Would you like to learn more about that?"

Questions are followed by monitoring and responding to each person's response and interest level, while respecting choice. *Present-moment focus* is encouraged. When the past is impacting the present, we still address it through our current experience. In this flow, we are able to address the context (and the biological underpinnings) of such dynamics without necessarily needing to explore or address specific psychological content. The patient need not tell their story to address their current experience; however, the professional must not "shut it down" or react in discomfort if the patient self-selects to do so. The extent of interaction with each person and any content shared is on a case-by-case basis depending on each professional's core discipline, training level, experience, and comfort. If there is specific psychosocial content that is highly charged and/or needs a psychotherapy setting, referral to the appropriate mental health professional is warranted. This does not mean that if a patient chooses to share about a past traumatic experience, for example, the rehabilitation professional should shut it down out of fear that a professional boundary is being breached. Patients must always feel welcome to disclose their experiences.

Similarly, if strong emotions arise, which can happen in any setting regardless of whether one is taking a purposeful mind-body integrated approach, working with the orienting, regulating, and resourcing skills covered in Chapter 6 is appropriate. If the professional's response is to immediately suggest psychiatric/psychological intervention, we may have conveyed a message that the present therapeutic setting is not safe for expression; it can also give a destructive message by inadvertently suggesting that the nature of the content shared and/or the patient needs fixing.

An enacted compassionate response is to first implicitly accept the person and their experience as it is. At some point, ask a question such as: "Is there any support that you need or would like in relation to these experiences?" This is similar to the aforementioned importance of inviting, allowing, and supporting emotion in any health care setting— "How is that feeling for you right now?"—and/or simply allowing emotion to come if it comes, and not rushing, out of our own discomfort, to try to fix, avoid, or interpret the emotion. It is OK.

Experiential pause: As you read the following quotations, contemplate what the intended message is, followed by how it carries relevance to your own practice in relation to mind-body integration and general mental health.

- "More and more we ignore the clinical skills that detect, at all levels of awareness, what another person feels. The shift is clearly marked in our practice, research, teaching, literature, and ideal for professional identity. Brain replaces mind, miraculously erasing the great philosophic problem."[44]
- "Sensitivity to proper drug levels...has pushed aside sensitivity to emotional nuances."[45]
- "Many [professionals] can't decipher the subtle pervasive non-verbal communications that are the way humans express their interior." [46]

These statements speak to the often-unconscious oversimplification and failure to recognize the influence of the inner life in health care provision. Consider that we also miss these possibilities in our ourselves—and our relationship to our own experience.

A COLLABORATIVE MODEL OF INTEGRATIVE AND INTEGRATED MENTAL HEALTH CARE

Figure 26.1 demonstrates a collaborative and contextual model for increased utilization of IRP to enhance mental health. Bidirectional referrals that have no financial conflict of interest are established. Integrative evaluations on both sides lead to the co-creation of individualized support. A larger network for accessing care options that cut across traditional biomedical care and group-based complementary and integrative health options (e.g., yoga, Ayurveda, group support) may also be offered. Finally, models of mentoring and clinical supervision are recommended to ensure ongoing assessment of quality of care and observance of scopes of practice.

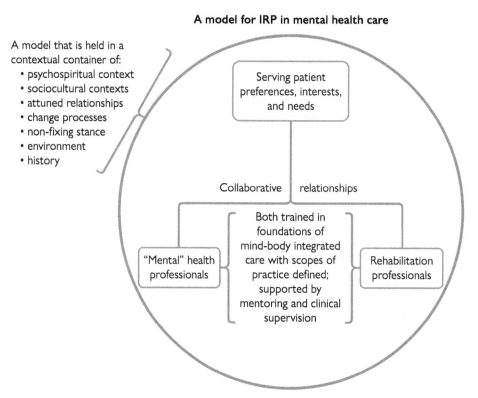

FIGURE 26.1: COLLABORATIVE CARE MODEL

CONCLUSION

Rehabilitation professions of all kinds are well positioned to play an increasing role in integrated and integrative care models that act in support of mental health and well-being. "Top-down" and "bottom-up" approaches are merging both within whole-person care models and across professions, optimizing the type and nature of support that is delivered. Adequate definitions, training, and boundaries are needed to maintain safety and quality in care provision for those experiencing mental health challenges.

The subtopics covered across this book combine with core principles of integrative care to create a person-centered approach that serves the mental health needs of both the patient and the professional. We must remember that "mental health" is fully embodied and that there are multiple avenues and entry points for support. When we are serving the body, we are serving mental health, and when we are serving the mind, we are serving the body.

Experiential pause: Having read this chapter, identify and write down at least one actionable item of interest to you. In doing so, consider ways in which applying the material first to yourself, and then to patients, might serve those who come to you for care.

CHAPTER 27

Wrapping Up and Opening Forward

Matt Erb, PT and Arlene Schmid, PhD, OTR, FAOTA

INSIGHTS

Integrative rehabilitation practice (IRP) aims to support *content in context*—to increase capacity for zooming out, even when zooming in is necessary and helpful. As Nora Bateson suggests in the main title of her book, individuals and the world that we exist in reflect: *small[er] arcs of larger circles*.[1] To navigate the relationships between smaller and larger circles, a grasp of the many levels and layers of context (complexity within a whole) is needed. Further, a skill set must be cultivated for successful navigation.

As such, IRP is devoted to safely increasing the range of professionals—a range informed by transdisciplinary capacity and aimed at enhanced service to the whole of each person. As Matthew J. Taylor suggested in Chapter 2, in a world of increasing information, complexity, and specialization, people who embrace diverse experiences and think both complexly and contextually are more primed for creativity and flexibility. Writer David Epstein, in his comprehensive exploration of what it takes to excel and thrive in this world, has come to similar conclusions.[2]

CHALLENGES OR OPPORTUNITIES?

Occasionally, cookbook techniques might (appear to) align well and meet a desired outcome. Complexity reminds us to examine if this might be a crapshoot, one that is also fraught with the dichotomy of "Yay me" (success) versus "I'm no good" (failure). Worse, we might unconsciously deflect the discomfort of the latter by blaming the patient. Looking into these dynamics further, we must look for hidden errors within the more linear biomedical paradigm where techniques = outcomes = predictability = control. Within this paradigm we must train ourselves to look for the ways in which the "fixer-of-the-broken" tendency may negatively influence the care we provide.

By definition, IRP is asking more of rehabilitation professionals. In particular, IRP asks us to consider the whole—aka holistic—in a grounded and realistic way. To borrow from the popular Star Trek series, the philosophy of the fictional Vulcan species reminds us that there is: "infinite diversity in infinite combinations." Any attempt to consider a whole must also embrace diversity. IRP seeks to improve our ability to navigate the vastness that informs diversity, brought down to the uniqueness of each individual provider or client.

Another challenge to be prepared to navigate was introduced in the opening chapter: labels, such as integrative or holistic, carry associations, beliefs, emotions, and thus challenges. For example, a history of exaggerated claims by "holistic healers," or a lack of scientific support for claims which can present as dogmatic or insipid, are frequently encountered. A lack of knowledge and/or a lack of epistemic humility may also present in individuals who are overly reified in their existing lenses on life, health, and science. This may be equally true of advocates of IRP as it is of critics of integrative care. Cultivating psychological flexibility as defined by Acceptance and Commitment Therapy (ACT) principles, along with the other principles and skills across the book, aim to support this capacity.

Finally, in looking at challenges, we add the presence of resistance within financial, organizational, or other power structures that are inextricably linked into health-care systems. IRP is not a newly opened fragrant rose, rather IRP reflects life and death cycles within ecosystems…processes within processes…and uncertainty. IRP does not align well with complacency or aversion to discomfort. Research, advocacy, commitment, and more will support the road ahead.

NATURAL DEVELOPMENT

Many health-care practitioners naturally move towards a more integral approach to their work over time. Perhaps this is the natural course of the development of wisdom within the larger life process. And, we should not assume that such wisdom will necessarily emerge. We must strive to train ourselves for greater capacity to honor and meet the reality of complexity. Ideally, this is done out of the gates in the academic programs of various disciplines. Some programs are moving in this direction now. Other programs have recoiled in the face of systems dynamics, where others recognize a need but aren't sure how to advance. Lags in the translation of research into clinical practice, let alone into the relationship between academic settings and board testing (programs are tasked with teaching to the test), also present challenges towards advancing whole-person care as described across this book.

In the opening chapter, we recognized barriers to IRP. Recently, Holopainen and colleagues[3] examined themes and categories of description for various phenomena that may arise in learning and integrating a cognitive-behavioral approach into physiotherapy. Examination of these dynamics provides a backdrop for approaching potential challenges as you launch from your review of this book into clinical translation. Table 27.1 provides a short summary as adapted through the lens of this book.

Table 27.1: Categories of Challenge in Developing Integrative Rehabilitation Practice

	Recognizing the differences of the new approach	Moving towards/ considering clinical integration	Actively exploring and experimenting	Commitment to practice transformation	Expanding applications of new approach
Examples of what can come up	Discomfort, aversion, loneliness, insecurity	Cultural, organizational, and/or systemic barriers Personal challenges Lack of support	Lack of a shared language The need for self-reflection and the need to more skillfully navigate turbulence and challenges	Support from colleagues, work setting(s), mentor(s) Strong patient relationships built on mutual learning Growing self-evident truths	Ongoing transdisciplinary education and interprofessional support Continuously reframing professional identity

Adapted from Holopainen et al.[4]

How do we address such dynamics in ourselves? In systems and structures? Process orientation (Chapter 1) and creative wisdom (Chapter 2) are needed across all categories. Softness, as a quality, can, well, soften that which is rigid. Softness is embedded in willingness, gentleness, flexibility, and patience. Aiming for the principles and engaging in the practices presented across the book encourage the development of greater balance between structure and flexibility in ourselves. Other foundations within IRP, such as non-dual and complex thinking, as well as principles of interdependence, further support navigating changed practice patterns towards integral/whole-person service. Self-application through ongoing experiential learning of the concepts reflected in the many pauses across this book must remain a backdrop to lifelong learning.

EMERGENCE, PATIENCE, AND MEETING NEEDS

We propose that the ingredients found across this book will prime the emergence of complex thinking, enhanced clinical reasoning, and greater flexibility in serving ourselves, our work, and our fellow human beings. Certainly, experience across time, and thus patience, are needed to navigate the challenges we face individually, in health care, and in the larger challenges of our shared world.

At the time of the writing of this concluding chapter, we find ourselves in unprecedented global dynamics with the Covid-19 pandemic. When viewed through the lens of living systems and complexity, we see several intersecting crises—of health, of climate, of truth. To meet these challenges, academic and healthcare systems are being asked to embody more open, diverse, and collaborative qualities,[5] as well as to operate in ways where identified values are congruent with actions. Think ACT (Chapter 17) applied at the systems level. "They will also need to go beyond producing knowledge about our world to generating wisdom about how to act within it."[6] Re-enter the need for Matthew J. Taylor's Chapter 2: Creative Wisdom as a vital orientation to the whole of the book. We are co-creating new realities and exploring and understanding ourselves from the constructs that we used to define IRP as an enhanced approach to care for post-normal times.

MALLEABILITY AND DUCTILITY

The development of an integrative approach to care is an ongoing process with no end. No two processes will look the same. Processes, when interacted with consciously, benefit from certain qualities or properties. We will use the examples of malleability and ductility to paint a picture for you to then personalize into your own framework for moving forward from the experience of this book.

Malleability reflects the property of a material or substance to deform under compression. We must be capable of adapting to discomfort as we examine, challenge, and transform existing patterns and beliefs. *Ductility* reflects the property of a material or substance to stretch without getting damaged. We must be capable of stretching and challenging ourselves (requiring the discomfort of malleability), without losing core structure and stability. What this core structure is…is unique to you.

IRP is not static and we must challenge the tendency to fall into complacency. We must challenge ourselves as an act of humility and service. As such, any core structure will be defined and redefined over time. Remember the Chapter 1 mention of research demonstrating that we carry a tendency towards avoiding stressful or uncomfortable information and/or experiences—even when they might benefit us or others.[7] IRP demands that we look closely at this dynamic in ourselves. Have we fallen into familiarity, comfort, or complacency? Are we ready to embody malleability and ductility in forging ahead in growing the way in which we support others?

Research suggests that: "the interplay between *how therapists treat themselves as a person* and *how they feel about a patient* during treatment affects patient outcome."[8] "Tentatively, the 'take home message' from this study could be formulated with the following words: 'Love yourself as a person, doubt yourself as a therapist.'"[9]

Consider how the information and ingredients found across this book might inform the development of this blend of loving yourself *as a person*, enacting compassion for self and other, and doing so with a healthy form of *self-doubt as a therapist*. Also consider what it might look like to receive ongoing feedback from your patients in comparison with your own experience.[10] Consider how staying active in the academic and scientific literature might afford for regular appraisal and reappraisal—and thus ongoing transformation and growth in the quality of the care offered to those who come to you for support.

THE EVIDENCE OF SERVING OTHERS

IRP aims to meet needs—both those needs that are obvious and those that are subtle. Attuning to the latter needs takes intent, hard work, and the development of a discerning "eye" (presence). Looking deeply into complexity and human behavior as an intentional stance supports our ability to meet others' needs that they may not (yet) have a conscious framework to describe.

Experiences of safety, nurturance, and empowerment reflect IRP's backdrop aim in serving others. Further, and as Cheryl Van Demark reminded us in Chapter 23, the "NIH HEALS" key factors of connection, reflection, introspection, trust, and acceptance are those that support human healing.[11] While teaching versus embodying these qualities presents a challenging gap, enacting the approaches across this book aims to support their emergence in a more widespread way in rehabilitation and the larger frameworks of health care.

Finally, regardless of the type, nature, and/or perceived quality of evidence that informs treatment options, the use of any intervention without full consideration of input from and respect for the person receiving the care falls short. In this process, kindness goes a long way.[12] The evidence that the patient presents is the most overlooked form of evidence, as we, as clinicians, often unconsciously presume to know what's wrong and what the best answer is. Naming and addressing this tendency both equalizes the power base and acts in support of clinician humility. As is sometimes said in yoga practices, when we are serving others, we are serving ourselves; when we are serving ourselves, we are serving all others. The latter reminds us that our commitment to self-application deepens and enhances the care that we offer and brings us into deeper understanding of interdependence.

NEXT STEPS

What qualities and characteristics do you have and/or wish to further cultivate in support of your ongoing personal and professional development? In Chapter 17, we introduced the ACT model which encourages individuals to define their core values—a framework for purpose and meaning. Doing this in relationship to your work and what you've learned across this book is a good next step in support of moving ahead in committed action.

Experiential pause: Following these instructions is a chapter-by-chapter list of what you have encountered across this book. This "summary" comes with one key word for each chapter to reflect a general theme. After reviewing, take a look back... thumbing through the pages of each chapter. Pause to read just a bit here and there for each chapter—randomly, wherever your attention lands—to jog your memory a bit. Then, create your own list of key word(s) that speak to your take-away meaning or relevance for each chapter.

Take the time now to complete your look back:

Chapter key word	My key words
Chapter 1 Frame	....

Chapter 2 Create   . . . .

Chapter 3 Deepen   . . . .

Chapter 4 Contextualize   . . . .

Chapter 5 Reason   . . . .

Chapter 6 Humanize   . . . .

Chapter 7 Analyze   . . . .

Chapter 8 Start   . . . .

Chapter 9 Relate   . . . .

Chapter 10 Regulate   . . . .

Chapter 11 Breathe   . . . .

Chapter 12 Meditate   . . . .

Chapter 13 Sense   . . . .

Chapter 14 Imagine   . . . .

Chapter 15 Move   . . . .

Chapter 16 Educate   . . . .

Chapter 17 Think   . . . .

Chapter 18 Expand   . . . .

Chapter 19 Speak   . . . .

Chapter 20 Express   . . . .

Chapter 21 Listen   . . . .

Chapter 22 Eat   . . . .

Chapter 23 Touch   . . . .

Chapter 24 Yoga   . . . .

Chapter 25 Connect   . . . .

Chapter 26 Support   . . . .

Chapter 27 Launch   . . . .

After completing your key word list, now consider what parts of the book stand out to you as being most applicable to your professional development at this point in time. To do this, apply the following steps.

1. Create a list of your values as applies to both your work and the larger scope of your life course and experience. What matters? Where do you derive purpose and meaning? Jot these down.

2. Where would you like to focus your next steps as you set this book down and move into deeper experiential applications? What committed action(s) do you now wish to take as the next right thing in follow-up to completing this book? Consider choosing actions that you are reasonably certain you can and will follow through on. Jot them down in your process journal.

3. Finally, ask yourself how the preceding two lists interact. Consider sitting in a meditative state, with a focus on the global body sense where all senses and sensations are perceived in a unified way. What insights arise as to how these interact? See if the wisdom needed can arise from this space that you create for yourself to *listen* as opposed to just "thinking." Bridge any gaps between idealism and realism. Avoid *should*. Once you have done this, jot down your insights.

A final note: How things actually proceed…how they will play out…may or may not look like this initial formulation. This is OK and expected. Things will in fact take their own course as the blend of unconscious and conscious dynamics interact to yield ongoing emergence. This does not forego regular efforts to frame your values, your intentions, and committed actions in the service of transformation, growth, and development. Your personal process in life parallels the professional; however, we often fail to see the relevance of parallel processes in this light.

To close, consider this famous quote, in light of completing your review of this book:

> We shall not cease from exploration
> And the end of all our exploring
> Will be to arrive where we started
> And know the place for the first time.[13]

A Note on Evidence

The topic of evidence is a complicated one. Exploring the topic of evidence in our health-care environment is as complex as exploring living systems! As philosopher Edgar Morin reminds us, science is built on controversy and always refutable. He reminds us that we have unsolved problems around the complexity of knowledge and: "scientific theories are not absolute, like religious dogma, but 'biodegradable.'"[1]

Said another way: the more we know (or think we know!), the less we understand. Cultivating epistemic humility is encouraged as an intellectual orientation. *Epistemic humility* is grounded in the understanding that our knowledge is *always* provisional and incomplete—and that it requires continuous revision in light of new evidence.[2]

EVIDENCE-BASED MEDICINE

The constructs and intentions behind evidence-based medicine (EBM) were first posited in 1978.[3] In the early 1990s, the concept was named EBM and rapidly expanded in use.[4] EBM carries many assets which do not need repeating here. EBM arose as a natural outgrowth of clinical epidemiology, and it can be generally defined as an integration of the currently available evidence with clinical experience, and guided by patient preferences/values.[5] This concept was designed to give equal emphasis to:

- the patient's situation
- the patient's goals, values, and wishes
- the best available research to draw from to assist in making clinical decisions
- the clinical expertise of the practitioner.[6]

This is consistent with integrative medicine (IM)/integrative rehabilitation practice (IRP) values, goals, and efforts. Given the diversity of sources from which the evidence on clinical decision making is derived, a useful reframing of the whole field with appropriate "epistemic humility" may be "evidence informed." The accent is immediately on the uncertainty and the ambiguity.

Over time, various dynamics and challenges in relation to EBM have arisen. For those who wish to take a closer look, a list of references covering a wide variety of topics are included.[7] These dynamics and challenges do not detract from the importance of evidence in our health-care system, rather they are seen as growing edges that we all are facing and that point us in the direction of problem-solving. We can all learn to take a critical eye on what we read.[8] An *open* eye is also invited.

IRP aims to interact with evidence through the lens of process and complexity; most importantly, from a person-centered approach that places support for enhancing well-being as the foundation. Evidence-informed practice necessarily interacts with patient preference and individuality, common sense, intuition, professional experience, wisdom, and creativity.

As is said in nearly every published paper, there are limitations to note, and more evidence is always needed. There are various layers, levels, and kinds of evidence that carry applicability to how health care is practiced. Some EBM practitioners tend to think: "There is no evidence to suggest…." We can replace such thinking with phrases that carry distinct inferences for decision making and improve clarity of communication:

- "scientific evidence is inconclusive, and we don't know what is best"
- "scientific evidence is inconclusive, but my experience or other knowledge suggests 'X'"
- "this has been proven to have no benefit"
- "this is a close call, with risks exceeding benefits for some patients but not for others."[9]

"EBM practitioners should abandon terms that may unintentionally mislead or inhibit [person]-centered care."[10] The preceding is consistent with the general tenets underlying IRP.

EVIDENCE IS A PROCESS

Evidence is continuously expanding and changing. Similar to the recent efforts of the functional medicine model,[11] the IM/IRP models need critical inquiry. Do not take what we have presented in this textbook freely. Challenge it. Look for bias, and, in doing so, observe how your own biases interact in that analysis. And, more importantly, help us advocate for funding and efforts to study integral care models and approaches.

In understanding the complexity of evidence, the benefits and limitations of any approach must be acknowledged and addressed on an ongoing basis so that it can be used effectively—and without doing harm. This latter task includes the challenging of beliefs about how and why we practice what we do. We run the risk of falling off either side of a knife's edge. On one side, we see the provision of ungrounded therapies, presented with unfounded pseudoscience. On the other side, we see a rigid, overly structured approach that is based on the current status of the evidence, but that misses the needs, beliefs, and preferences of the person in front of us. We encourage you to adopt a balanced perspective, demonstrate person-centered flexibility, and look for overly polarizing stances from either side. And, allow room for the possibility of mystery: there will always be unknowable factors influencing each person's health experience.

IRP embraces principles of: emergence in living systems; body-mind-environment

(BME) relational interdependence; and wisdom, creativity, and intuition as informants within the therapeutic process. Ultimately, what seems to help one person may prove useless for another. No matter what "evidence" we do or do not have to operate from, and even with the very best efforts, some individuals will "improve" and some will not. Moving forward with the grounding of current and emerging science, and the flexibility of beginner's mind, offers a mix for us all to strive for.

A Primer on Trauma-Informed Care

While estimates vary, trauma exposure is widespread in the population and carries potential impact on health.[1] Trauma-informed care (TIC) reflects a strength-based approach to addressing trauma. TIC aims to recognize the visible, as well as hidden, impact of past trauma on experiences for patients, families, and staff. Beyond clinical practice, embedding TIC principles into organizations (e.g., policies, procedures), systems (e.g., justice system, academic/education systems, political efforts), and public health (e.g., primary prevention efforts) is necessary. An enactive approach to TIC implies actively combating re-traumatization where environments and/or relational dynamics may reproduce facets of prior traumatic experiences, begetting further stress.

Certain principles underscore a TIC approach.[2] These include various facets to support the possibility of a greater experience of physical, social, and emotional safety. Cultural considerations are also vital to understand in relation to TIC.[3] In essence, these ingredients have been innately reflected in the integrative rehabilitation practice (IRP) model that serves foundational human needs, such as:

- cultivating empowerment:
  - using patients' strengths, skills, and preferences in the treatment process
  - provision of choice in all treatment options/approaches
  - graded experiential learning
  - regular opportunity for feedback, questions, comments, and concerns
- providing nurturance:
  - demonstration of a caring, attuned presence; enactive compassion
  - provision of treatment experiences that carry potential for feeling cared for
  - providing a physical care environment that reflects calming and caring qualities
  - identifying and/or supporting internalized care and concern
- communicating and collaborating:
  - using simple education to screen for trauma; following a person-centered strategy (self-determined relevance, including any desire for referrals or additional resources or services when applicable)
  - understanding and demonstrating the ingredients needed for effective, trustworthy communication
  - creating ample space and opportunity for self-expression

–   maximizing communication and collaboration between caregiver and patient, their family/social network, and other health-care professionals in support of patient well-being.

A FEW FINAL NOTES

Bring attention and pay attention—not too little, not too much. We are at risk of not recognizing the impact of past trauma and/or for making harmful assumptions about the relevance of past trauma that are not consistent with IRP's advocacy for patient self-determination.

Next, we are at risk of over-focusing on individuality in TIC and missing the systemic lens, as covered in Chapter 4. Without a systemic lens, trauma-informed practice may promote solutions that are individually targeted while missing the relevance of systems that cause or perpetuate trauma's effects.

Next, in TIC there is great benefit from staying in the present moment—what is happening *right now*? If the past has impacted us, it is found in the present-moment experience. Provision of TIC includes experiences that assist in regulation, resilience, and the recognition of strengths and possibilities.

Finally, trauma influence can be addressed by focusing on context over content, including offering the chance for mind-body skills learning that influences the underlying neurophysiological basis of trauma's influence on health without necessarily engaging specific psychological content.[4] For those who wish for the latter approach, referral to qualified mental health professionals is warranted.

Relational Frame Theory Interventions for Transforming Pain into Purpose

1. Conditional:
   a. *If* you could make room for this pain, *what would* that enable you to do that matters in your life?
   b. *If* you could use this pain to help others who are suffering, *how* might you go about doing so?
   Note: Conditional relations (cause/effect) are present in many of the following examples.

2. Coordination:
   a. What might this pain *be revealing* that you care about?
   b. If this pain *represented* a gap between the life you have and the life you want, what would the life you want look like?
   c. If you pull away from this pain, what *else* might you be turning away from that matters to you?

3. Comparison:
   a. Is the pain *more or less* present when you're doing something meaningful?

4. Distinction:
   a. How would your life be *different* if you were willingly open to having this pain?
   b. What would you have to *not* care about to *not* experience this pain?

5. Opposition:
   a. If this pain was on *one side* of a coin, what would be on the *opposite side* that's important to you?
   b. If this pain that you *don't* want was actually an indication of something you *do* want (in your life), what might it be pointing towards?

6. Spatial:
   a. *Where* (what important situations) in your life do you tend to experience this pain?
   b. If this pain was on the *outside* protecting something precious on the *inside*, what might that be?

7. Temporal:
    a. What have you learned from *past* experiences with pain like this that could be helpful *now*?
    b. How might experiencing this pain right *now* be of value to you in the *future*?
8. Deictic:
    a. *Ten years* from now, *you're looking back,* what do you want your life to have stood for in the presence of this pain?
    b. If *you* were *here* and *I* was *there* experiencing this pain, how would *you* respond to *me*?
    c. *Someone* you care about shares about *their own* experience of this pain, how do *you* respond?
    d. If your *dearest friend* or *family member* was *here*, how might *that person* respond to *your* pain?
9. Hierarchical:
    a. If this pain was *part of* something that really mattered to you, what would it be?
    b. How could you use this pain *in the service of* something greater, to enrich your life in some way?

Content developed by Lou Lasprugato and Phillip Cha, 2019, and reprinted with permission (inspired by and adapted from Villatte, Villatte, & Hayes, 2015[1]).

The Contributors

Matt Erb, PT, is a physiotherapist, Senior Faculty and Clinical Supervisor for The Center for Mind-Body Medicine, and instructor for the University of Arizona, Andrew Weil Center for Integrative Medicine, and also presents for the Departments of Psychiatry and Family Medicine. Matt has a clinical practice with Simons Physical Therapy and is Founder of Embody Your Mind, which is focused on writing, teaching, and consulting.

Arlene Schmid, PhD, OTR, FAOTA, has been an occupational therapist for over 20 years and is a Professor in the Department of Occupational Therapy at Colorado State University. Arlene develops and tests yoga interventions for people with disabilities and has nearly 100 publications, most of which disseminate yoga research.

Matthew J. Taylor, PT, PhD, C-IAYT, is a physical therapist and yoga therapist. He is the Director of MyRehab, LLC, Iowa City, IA (DBA SmartSafeYoga and consulting services). He's in a joint venture with a Fortune-100 health-insurance company to bring yoga therapy into rehabilitation. He serves on two national task forces for non-pharm pain management and is a board member of Accessible Yoga.

Daniel Winkle, MD, is a physician specializing in physical medicine and rehabilitation. He is certified in mind-body medicine by The Center for Mind-Body Medicine and working as Medical Director of acute inpatient rehabilitation. He is integrating mind-body skills into the practice of inpatient rehabilitation and professional development.

Andra DeVoght, PT, MPH, is a physical therapist, yoga instructor, educator, and the owner of Insight Physio, PLLC. Her clinical expertise is focused on women's health and trauma-informed care. Her teaching and consulting work aims to connect the dots between mind, body, and the social determinants of health.

Todd E. Davenport, PT, DPT, MPH, OCS, is Professor and Program Director of the Department of Physical Therapy, School of Health Sciences, University of the Pacific in

Stockton, California. Todd maintains a clinical practice focused on community-based outpatient orthopedic physical therapy with Kaiser Permanente in Stockton, California.

Bronwyn Lennox Thompson, MSc(Hons), PhD(Cant), DipOccTh(CIT), is an occupational therapist with an MSc in psychology and PhD in health sciences. She teaches postgraduate courses in pain and pain management at University of Otago, Christchurch, NZ.

Noshene Ranjbar, MD, is Assistant Professor at the University of Arizona, where she serves as Training Director of the Integrative Psychiatry Fellowship and Director of the Integrative Psychiatry Clinic. She is faculty at the Andrew Weil Center for Integrative Medicine as well as The Center for Mind-Body Medicine.

Shelly Prosko, PT, C-IAYT, is a physiotherapist, yoga therapist, author, and educator dedicated to enhancing health care by integrating yoga into rehabilitation. She is a pioneer of PhysioYoga, has a clinical practice in Canada, and teaches in various yoga and rehabilitation programs globally. Shelly is co-editor of *Yoga and Science in Pain Care.* www.physioyoga.ca

Geoff Sittler, OTR/L, BCN, is an occupational therapist and faculty member with The Center for Mind-Body Medicine. He specializes in mind-body modalities and has brought these approaches to inpatient behavioral health, various school settings, primary care, and community mental health with the Department of Veterans Affairs (US). He is certified in neurofeedback (BCIA) and mind-body medicine (CMBM).

Kellie Finn, MS, C-IAYT, ERYT-500, is a yoga therapist, Gateless Writing teacher, and Clinic Supervisor/Adjunct Faculty at Maryland University of Integrative Health. She serves on the board at Circle Yoga, where she teaches weekly classes, and has clinical practices in Easthampton, MA and Washington DC.

Betsy Shandalov, OTR/L, C-IAYT, is an occupational therapist, and a certified yoga therapist in private practice in the San Francisco Bay Area. Betsy lectures nationally to health-care and rehabilitation professionals on therapeutic yoga, mindfulness, and meditation. She has advanced training through The Center for Mind-Body Medicine and is currently training to be an Ayurvedic Wellness Counselor.

Peggy Ninow, OTR/L, SEP, CHTP, is an occupational therapist. She has additional certifications in Somatic Experiencing, Biofeedback, and Healing Touch. She brings to her practice a wealth of experience in the areas of trauma, sensory interventions, neuroscience, chronic pain, and autism. She currently works as The Sensory/Trauma Consultant at Regions Hospital in Minnesota.

Leslie Davenport, MA, MS, LMFT, is: a licensed marriage and family therapist; founding member of the Institute for Health and Healing at California Pacific Medical Center; author of *Healing and Transformation through Self-Guided Imagery* and editor of *Transformative Imagery: Cultivating the Imagination for Healing, Change and Growth*; and Professor at the California Institute of Integral Studies.

Rachelle Palnick Tsachor, MA, CMA, RSMT, is certified in Mind-Body Medicine, Movement Analysis (CMA), and Somatic Movement Therapy (RSMT-ISMETA). She is faculty at the University of Illinois at Chicago, Laban/Bartenieff Institute of Movement Studies, and Wingate College. She investigates body movement to bring a human, experiential understanding to how movement affects our lives.

Irena Paiuk, MscPT, BPT, CMA, is a physical therapist (MScPT), certified in Movement Analysis (CMA) and Rehabilitation Pilates (STOTT Pilates), certified DNS (Dynamic Neuromuscular Stabilization) practitioner, Integrated Contact Improvisation practitioner, and a performer ("Shlombal" ensemble). She is faculty at the Physical Therapy Department in Tel Aviv University and a clinician.

Molly J. Lahn, PT, DPT, PhD, is a pain clinical specialist and is the lead physical therapist with the Minneapolis VA Medical Center's Chronic Pain Rehabilitation Program. She has also served as associate faculty with The Center for Mind-Body Medicine and Saybrook University.

Margaret Gavian, PhD, received her PhD in Psychology from the University of Minnesota, specializing in trauma and resilience. She completed a fellowship in integrative behavioral health and held health-care leadership positions before starting her consulting business and private practice. She enjoys teaching psychology, directing wellness programming for the fire service, and is passionate about her work with CMBM.

Marlysa Sullivan, PT, C-IAYT, is a physical therapist, yoga therapist, Assistant Professor of Integrative Health Sciences and Yoga Therapy at Maryland University of Integrative Health, and adjunct faculty at Emory University. She is the author of *Understanding Yoga Therapy: Applied Philosophy and Science for Well-Being* and co-editor of *Yoga and Science in Pain Care.*

Dena Rain Adler, BEd, MA, ATR, is a registered art therapist and a special education teacher, and co-founder of a restorative practice, Spiral River. Dena provides in-home community-based supports, is a Behavioral Health Consultant for Head Start, and faculty and a Certified Practitioner of The Center for Mind-Body Medicine.

Sherril Howard, MS, CCC-SLP, has been a certified speech-language pathologist since 1984. She was Director of Speech Pathology at University Medical Center in Tucson and later a private practitioner specializing in head and neck cancer and voice disorders. Currently, Sherril is a clinical supervisor for Northern Arizona University's graduate speech pathology program. She also sees clients in her home office.

Alicia L. Barksdale, MS, MT-BC, NMT, is Lead Music Therapist at the Kennedy Krieger Institute in Baltimore. She is a Doctor of Musical Arts candidate at Boston University, guest lecturer on music therapy and musical strategies, and author of the textbook *Music Therapy and Leisure for Persons with Disabilities.*

Brigid Titgemeier, MS, RDN, LD, IFNCP, is a board-certified integrative and functional nutrition dietitian and adjunct instructor. In her virtual nutrition practice, Brigid delivers personalized food as medicine recommendations. She has helped nearly 4000 patients find health with nutrition. She was a founding dietitian at Cleveland Clinic Center for Functional Medicine. Learn more at: https://beingbrigid.com

Cheryl Van Demark, PT, C-IAYT, is health professional, teacher, and writer dedicated to integrating yoga therapy into health care and self-care. As a physical therapist, certified yoga therapist, yoga teacher, and Reiki practitioner with a Master's degree in physical education and exercise science, Cheryl is currently facilitating an inter-professional and integrative self-care program for chronic pain at Yavapai Regional Medical Center in Prescott, Arizona.

James S. Gordon, MD, author of *The Transformation: Discovering Wholeness and Healing After Trauma*, is an authority on post-traumatic stress and mind-body medicine. Dr. Gordon is a clinical professor at Georgetown Medical School and Founder/Executive Director of The Center for Mind-Body Medicine, where he created what may well be the world's largest and most effective program for healing population-wide psychological trauma.

Victoria Maizes, MD, is the Executive Director of the University of Arizona, Andrew Weil Center for Integrative Medicine, where she is a professor of medicine and public health. Internationally recognized as a leader in integrative medicine, Dr. Maizes is committed to helping individuals live healthier lives. She is editor of *Integrative Women's Health* and the author of *Be Fruitful: The Essential Guide to Maximizing Fertility and Giving Birth to a Healthy Child.*

Endnotes

CHAPTER 1

1   IOM Summit Provides Models for Health Reform. (2009, February 27). *Healthcare Finance*.
2   CDC (Centers for Disease Control and Prevention). (2018). *Chronic Diseases in America*. Retrieved October 7, 2020 from www.cdc.gov/chronicdisease/resources/infographic/chronic-diseases.htm.
3   Stussman, B. J., Nahin, R. R., Barnes, P. M., & Ward, B. W. (2019). U.S. physician recommendations to their patients about the use of complementary health approaches. *The Journal of Alternative and Complementary Medicine, 26*(1), 25–33.
4   NIH (National Institutes of Health). (2016, June 22). *Americans Spent $30.2 Billion Out-Of-Pocket On Complementary Health Approaches*. Retrieved July 22, 2018, from NIH News website: https://nccih.nih.gov/news/press/cost-spending-06222016.
5   Institute of Medicine (US) Committee on Quality of Health Care in America. (2001). *Crossing the Quality Chasm: A New Health System for the 21st Century*. Retrieved August 6, 2020 from www.ncbi.nlm.nih.gov/books/NBK222273.
6   McGlynn, E. A., Asch, S. M., Adams, J., Keesey, J., *et al.* (2003). The quality of health care delivered to adults in the United States. *New England Journal of Medicine, 348*(26), 2635–2645.
7   Anhang Price, R., Elliott, M. N., Zaslavsky, A. M., Hays, R. D., *et al.* (2014). Examining the role of patient experience surveys in measuring health care quality. *Medical Care Research and Review, 71*(5), 522–554.
8   Manary, M. P., Boulding, W., Staelin, R., & Glickman, S. W. (2012). The patient experience and health outcomes. *New England Journal of Medicine, 368*(3), 201–203.
    Kumar, S. & Nash, D. B. (2011). *Demand Better!: Revive Our Broken Healthcare System*. Bozeman, MT: Second River Healthcare Press.
9   *A Galveston Declaration*. (n.d.). Retrieved August 6, 2020 from http://galvestondeclaration.org.
10 Taylor, M. J. & Nova Science Publishers. (2016). *Fostering Creativity in Rehabilitation*. New York: Nova Science Publishers.
11 *What is Integrative Medicine?* (n.d.). Retrieved August 6, 2020 from https://integrativemedicine.arizona.edu/about/definition.html.
12 *Ibid.*
13 *What is Integrative Medicine?* (n.d.). Retrieved August 6, 2020 from https://dukeintegrativemedicine.org/about/what-is-integrative-medicine.
14 Integrative. (n.d.). In *Lexico*. Retrieved August 6, 2020 from www.lexico.com/en/definition/integrative.
15 *Constitution*. (n.d.). Retrieved August 6, 2020 from www.who.int/about/who-we-are/constitution.
16 Zhang, Q., Sharan, A., Espinosa, S. A., Gallego-Perez, D., & Weeks, J. (2019). The path toward integration of traditional and complementary medicine into health systems globally: The World Health Organization report on the implementation of the 2014–2023 strategy. *The Journal of Alternative and Complementary Medicine, 25*(9), 869–871.
17 Antonovsky, A. (1996). The Salutogenic model as a theory to guide health promotion. *Health Promotion International, 11*(1), 11–18.
18 Taylor, M. (2007). A fork in the road: "Doing to" or "being with"? *International Journal of Yoga Therapy, 17*(1), 5–6.
19 *A Galveston Declaration*. (n.d.).
20 Engel, G. L. (1977). The need for a new medical model: A challenge for biomedicine. *Science, 196*(4286), 129–136.
21 Waddell, G. (1987). 1987 Volvo award in clinical sciences. A New Clinical Model for the Treatment of Low-Back Pain. *Spine, 12*(7), 632–644.
    Fordyce, W. E. (1988). Pain and suffering. A reappraisal. *The American Psychologist, 43*(4), 276–283.
    Gatchel, R. J., Peng, Y. B., Peters, M. L., Fuchs, P. N., & Turk, D. C. (2007). The biopsychosocial approach to chronic pain: Scientific advances and future directions. *Psychological Bulletin, 133*(4), 581–624.

22 Engel, G. L. (1980). The clinical application of the biopsychosocial model. *The American Journal of Psychiatry*, *137*(5), 535–544.

23 Sulmasy, D. P. (2002). A biopsychosocial-spiritual model for the care of patients at the end of life. *The Gerontologist*, *42 Spec No 3*, 24–33.

24 Mescouto, K., Olson, R. E., Hodges, P. W., & Setchell, J. (2020). A critical review of the biopsychosocial model of low back pain care: Time for a new approach? *Disability and Rehabilitation*, 1–15.
    Gatchel, *et al.* (2007).
    Stilwell, P. & Harman, K. (2019). An enactive approach to pain: Beyond the biopsychosocial model. *Phenomenology and the Cognitive Sciences*, *18*(4), 667–668.

25 Deacon, B. J. (2013). The biomedical model of mental disorder: A critical analysis of its validity, utility, and effects on psychotherapy research. *The Future of Evidence-Based Practice in Psychotherapy*, *33*(7), 846–861. p.856.

26 *Ibid.* p.856.

27 Chalmers, K. J. & Madden, V. J. (2019). Shifting beliefs across society would lay the foundation for truly biopsychosocial care. *Journal of Physiotherapy*, *65*(3), 121–122.

28 Henriques, G. (n.d.). *Moving From the Biopsychosocial Model to the ToK System*. Retrieved April 1, 2019 from https://www.psychologytoday.com/us/blog/theory-knowledge/201510/moving-the-biopsychosocial-model-the-tok-system.

29 Sheldon, K. M. (2004). *Optimal Human Being: An Integrated Multi-Level Perspective*. Mahwah, NJ: Lawrence Erlbaum Associates.

30 Henriques (n.d.).

31 Sheldon (2004).

32 Kitwood, T. M. (1997). *Dementia Reconsidered: The Person Comes First*. In *Rethinking Ageing Series*. Buckingham; Philadelphia: Open University Press. p.8.

33 Morgan, S. & Yoder, L. H. (2011). A concept analysis of person-centered care. *Journal of Holistic Nursing*, *30*(1), 6–15. p.3.

34 Morgan & Yoder (2011).

35 Gusmini, C. (2019). Should you first cure your ignorance, healthcare professionals? *British Journal of Sports Medicine*, doi: 10.1136/bjsports-2019-101038.

36 Dewi, W. N., Evans, D., Bradley, H., & Ullrich, S. (2014). Person-centred care in the Indonesian health-care system. *International Journal of Nursing Practice*, *20*(6), 616–622.

37 Prochaska, J. O. & Velicer, W. F. (1997). The transtheoretical model of health behavior change. *American Journal of Health Promotion*, *12*(1), 38–48.
    Glanz, K., Rimer, B. K., & Viswanath, K. (Eds) (2015). *Health Behavior: Theory, Research, and Practice* (Fifth edition). San Francisco, CA: Jossey-Bass & Pfeiffer Imprints, Wiley.

38 Gosnell, F., McKergow, M., Moore, B., Mudry, T., & Tomm, K. (2017). A Galveston Declaration. *Journal of Systemic Therapies*, *36*(3), 20–26.

39 *Ibid.*

40 Bell, I. R., Caspi, O., Schwartz, G. E. R., Grant, K. L., *et al.* (2002). Integrative medicine and systemic outcomes research: Issues in the emergence of a new model for primary health care. *Archives of Internal Medicine*, *162*(2), 133–140.
    Institute of Medicine (US). (2009). *Integrative Medicine and the Health of the Public: A Summary of the February 2009 Summit*. Retrieved August 6, 2020 from www.ncbi.nlm.nih.gov/books/NBK219637.

41 Ho, E. H., Hagmann, D., & Loewenstein, G. (2020). Measuring information preferences. *Management Science*. Retrieved January 8, 2020 from https://doi.org/10.1287/mnsc.2019.3543.

42 Keefe, F. J., Main, C. J., & George, S. Z. (2018). Advancing psychologically informed practice for patients with persistent musculoskeletal pain: Promise, pitfalls, and solutions. *Physical Therapy*, *98*(5), 398–407.
    Holopainen, R., Simpson, P., Piirainen, A., Karppinen, J., *et al.* (2020). Physiotherapists' perceptions of learning and implementing a biopsychosocial intervention to treat musculoskeletal pain conditions: A systematic review and metasynthesis of qualitative studies. *Pain*, *161*(6), 1150–1168.

43 McGregor, S. L. T. (2004). *The Nature of Transdisciplinary Research and Practice*. Retrieved August 6, 2020 from www.kon.org/hswp/archive/transdiscipl.pdf.
    Montouri, A. (2012). Transdisciplinary reflections. *Integral Leadership Review*, 1–6.

44 Hartman, S. E. (2009). Why do ineffective treatments seem helpful? A brief review. *Chiropractic & Osteopathy*, *17*, 10–10.

45 Keefe, Main, & George (2018).

46 Institute of Medicine (US). (2009).

47 Miller, R. (2007). *Integrative Restoration* [6 CD Set]. iRest Institute.

CHAPTER 2

1   Taylor, M. J. (Ed.) (2015). *Fostering Creativity in Rehabilitation* (First edition). New York: Nova Publishing.
    Taylor, M. J. (2018). *Yoga Therapy as a Creative Response to Pain*. London: Singing Dragon.

2   Sardar, Z. (2010). Welcome to postnormal times. *Futures*, *42*(5), 435–444.

3   Cairns, G., Montuori, A., & Beech, N. (2001). Beyond and between nihilism and social hope: Stumbling on the edge of a positive postmodernity. In *EGOS Colloquium*, 5–7 July 2001, Lyon.

4   *Ibid.*

5   Walsh, R. (2015). What is wisdom? Cross-cultural and cross-disciplinary syntheses. *Review of General Psychology*, *19*, 278–293.

6   *Ibid.*

7   *Ibid.*

8   Sardar (2010).

9   Montuori, A. (2010). Transdisciplinarity and Creative Inquiry in Transformative Education: Researching the Research Degree. In M. Maldonao & R. Pietrobon (Eds) *Research on Scientific Research* (First edition). Portland, OR: Sussex Academic Press.

10   *Ibid.*

11   Barron, F. (1958). The psychology of imagination, *Scientific American*, September.

12   Barron, F. (1990). *No Rootless Flower: Towards an Ecology of Creativity*. Cresskill, NJ: Hampton Press.

13   Taylor (2015).

14   *Ibid.*

15   *Ibid.*

16   Halifax, J. (2012). A heuristic model of enactive compassion. *Current Opinion Supportive and Palliative Care*, *6*(2), 228–235.

17   Taylor (2018). p.155.
     Halifax (2012).

CHAPTER 3

1   Siegel, D. J. (2017). *Mind: A Journey to the Heart of Being Human* (First edition). New York: W. W. Norton.

2   Rejeski, W. J. & Gauvin, L. (2013). The embodied and relational nature of the mind: Implications for clinical interventions in aging individuals and populations. *Clinical Interventions in Aging*, *8*, 657–665.

3   Wade, D. (2006). Why physical medicine, physical disability and physical rehabilitation? We should abandon Cartesian dualism. *Clinical Rehabilitation*, *20*(3), 185–190.

4   Taylor, M. J. & Nova Science Publishers. (2016). *Fostering Creativity in Rehabilitation*. New York: Nova Science Publishers.

5   *Ibid.*

6   Vachon-Presseau, E., Berger, S. E., Abdullah, T. B., Griffith, J. W., Schnitzer, T. J., & Apkarian, A. V. (2019). Identification of traits and functional connectivity-based neurotraits of chronic pain. *PLOS Biology*, *17*(8), e3000349. p.2.

7   *Ibid.*

8   *Ibid.*

9   Finniss, D. G., Kaptchuk, T. J., Miller, F., & Benedetti, F. (2010). Biological, clinical, and ethical advances of placebo effects. *The Lancet*, *375*(9715), 686–695.
     Benedetti, F. (2014). *Placebo Effects*. Oxford: Oxford University Press.
     Price, D. D., Finniss, D. G., & Benedetti, F. (2008). A comprehensive review of the placebo effect: Recent advances and current thought. *Annual Review of Psychology*, *59*(1), 565–590.
     Benedetti, F. (2005). Neurobiological mechanisms of the placebo effect. *Journal of Neuroscience*, *25*(45), 10390–10402.

10   Kirmayer, L. J. & Gómez-Carrillo, A. (2019). Agency, embodiment and enactment in psychosomatic theory and practice. *Medical Humanities*, *45*(2), 169–182.

11   *Ibid.* p.169.

12   Tran, B. X., Harijanto, C., Vu, G. T., & Ho, R. C. M. (2020). Global mapping of interventions to improve quality of life using mind-body therapies during 1990–2018. *Complementary Therapies in Medicine*, *49*, 102350.
     Dossett, M. L., Fricchione, G. L., & Benson, H. (2020). A new era for mind-body medicine. *New England Journal of Medicine*, *382*(15), 1390–1391.

13   Taylor, A. G., Goehler, L. E., Galper, D. I., Innes, K. E., & Bourguignon, C. (2010). Top-down and bottom-up mechanisms in mind-body medicine: Development of an integrative framework for psychophysiological research. *Explore*, *6*(1), 29.

14   *Ibid.*
     Schore, A. N. (2019). The Development of the Unconscious Mind. In *A Norton Professional Book and the Norton Series on Interpersonal Neurobiology* (First Edition). New York: W. W. Norton.
     Castro, W. H., Meyer, S. J., Becke, M. E., Nentwig, C. G., *et al.* (2001). No stress—no whiplash? Prevalence of "whiplash" symptoms following exposure to a placebo rear-end collision. *International Journal of Legal Medicine*, *114*(6), 316–322.
     Muehsam, D., Lutgendorf, S., Mills, P. J., Rickhi, B., *et al.* (2017). The embodied mind: A review on functional genomic and neurological correlates of mind-body therapies. *Neuroscience and Biobehavioral Reviews*, *73*, 165–181.

Garland, E. L., Brintz, C. E., Hanley, A. W., Roseen, E. J., et al. (2019). Mind-body therapies for opioid-treated pain: A systematic review and meta-analysis. *JAMA Internal Medicine, 180*(1), 91–105.

Zhang, Y., Fu, R., Sun, L., Gong, Y., & Tang, D. (2019). How does exercise improve implicit emotion regulation ability? Preliminary evidence of mind-body exercise intervention combined with aerobic jogging and mindfulness-based yoga. *Frontiers in Psychology, 10*, 1888–1888.

15 O'Keeffe, M., George, S. Z., O'Sullivan, P. B., & O'Sullivan, K. (2018). Psychosocial factors in low back pain: Letting go of our misconceptions can help management. *British Journal of Sports Medicine, 53*, 793–794.

16 Bell, I. R., Caspi, O., Schwartz, G. E. R., Grant, K. L., et al. (2002). Integrative medicine and systemic outcomes research: Issues in the emergence of a new model for primary health care. *Archives of Internal Medicine, 162*(2), 133–140.

17 Martinez-Calderon, J., Zamora-Campos, C., Navarro-Ledesma, S., & Luque-Suarez, A. (2018). The role of self-efficacy on the prognosis of chronic musculoskeletal pain: A systematic review. *The Journal of Pain, 19*(1), 10–34.

18 Eisenberger, N. I. (2013). An empirical review of the neural underpinnings of receiving and giving social support: Implications for health. *Psychosomatic Medicine, 75*(6), 545–556.

19 Halifax, J. (2012). A heuristic model of enactive compassion. *Current Opinion in Supportive and Palliative Care, 6*(2), 228–235.

20 Fauchon, C., Faillenot, I., Quesada, C., Meunier, D., et al. (2019). Brain activity sustaining the modulation of pain by empathetic comments. *Scientific Reports, 9*(1), 8398.

21 Coleman, K., Austin, B. T., Brach, C., & Wagner, E. H. (2009). Evidence on the chronic care model in the new millennium. *Health Affairs, 28*(1), 75–85.

22 SAMHSA. (2006). *Morbidity and Mortality in People with Serious Mental Illness*. Retrieved August 7, 2020 from www.samhsa.gov/sites/default/files/grants/pdf/sm-17-008-revised.pdf.

23 Strosahl, K. (1998). Integrating Behavioral Health and Primary Care Services: The Primary Mental Health Care Model. In A. Blount (Ed.) *Integrated Primary Care: The Future of Medical and Mental Health Collaboration* (pp.139–166). New York: W. W. Norton & Company.

24 Arnow, B. A., Hunkeler, E. M., Blasey, C. M., Lee, J., et al. (2006). Comorbid depression, chronic pain, and disability in primary care. *Psychosomatic Medicine, 68*(2), 262–268.

25 Merikangas, K. R., Ames, M., Cui, L., Stang, P. E., et al. (2007). The impact of comorbidity of mental and physical conditions on role disability in the US adult household population. *Archives of General Psychiatry, 64*(10), 1180–1188.

26 *Ibid.*

Druss, B. G., Marcus, S. C., Olfson, M., Tanielian, T., Elinson, L., & Pincus, H. A. (2001). Comparing the national economic burden of five chronic conditions. *Health Affairs (Project Hope), 20*(6), 233–241.

27 Bair, M. J., Robinson, R. L., Katon, W., & Kroenke, K. (2003). Depression and pain comorbidity: A literature review. *Archives of Internal Medicine, 163*(20), 2433–2445.

Outcalt, S. D., Kroenke, K., Krebs, E. E., Chumbler, N. R., et al. (2015). Chronic pain and comorbid mental health condition. *Journal of Behavioral Medicine, 38*, 535–543.

Lerman, S. F., Rudich, Z., Brill, S., Shalev, H., & Shahar, G. (2015). Longitudinal associations between depression, anxiety, pain, and pain-related disability in chronic pain patients. *Psychosomatic Medicine, 77*(3), 333–341.

Asmundson, G. J., Coons, M. J., Taylor, S., & Katz, J. (2002). PTSD and the experience of pain: Research and clinical implications of shared vulnerability and mutual maintenance models. *The Canadian Journal of Psychiatry, 47*(10), 930–937.

Siqveland, J., Ruud, T., & Hauff, E. (2017). Post-traumatic stress disorder moderates the relationship between trauma exposure and chronic pain. *European Journal of Psychotraumatology, 8*(1), 1375337.

28 Asmundson, et al. (2002).

Siqveland, Ruud, & Hauff (2017).

Sharp, T. J., & Harvey, A. G. (2001). Chronic pain and posttraumatic stress disorder: Mutual maintenance? *Clinical Psychology Review, 21*(6), 857–877.

29 Asmundson, et al. (2002).

30 Bair, et al. (2003).

Boakye, P. A., Olechowski, C., Rashiq, S., Verrier, M. J., et al. (2016). A critical review of neurobiological factors involved in the interactions between chronic pain, depression, and sleep disruption. *The Clinical Journal of Pain, 32*(4), 327–336.

Kemp, A. H. & Quintana, D. S. (2013). The relationship between mental and physical health: Insights from the study of heart rate variability. *International Journal of Psychophysiology, 89*(3), 288–296.

31 Nemeroff, C. B. & Goldschmidt-Clermont, P. J. (2012). Heartache and heartbreak—The link between depression and cardiovascular disease. *Nature Reviews. Cardiology, 9*(9), 526–539.

Thayer, J. F., Yamamoto, S. S., & Brosschot, J. F. (2010). The relationship of autonomic imbalance, heart rate variability and cardiovascular disease risk factors. *International Journal of Cardiology, 141*(2), 122–131.

Porges, S. W. & Kolacz, J. (n.d.). Neurocardiology through the Lens of the Polyvagal Theory. In R. J. Gelpi & B. Buchholz (Eds) *Neurocardiology: Pathophysiological Aspects and Clinical Implications*. Amsterdam: Elsevier.

32 Holzman, J. B. & Bridgett, D. J. (2017). Heart rate variability indices as bio-markers of top-down self-regulatory mechanisms: A meta-analytic review. *Neuroscience and Biobehavioral Reviews, 74*(Pt A), 233–255.

33   Kemp & Quintana (2013).

34   Boakye, *et al.* (2016).

Halfon, N., Larson, K., & Slusser, W. (2013). Associations between obesity and comorbid mental health, developmental, and physical health conditions in a nationally representative sample of US children aged 10 to 17. *Academic Pediatrics, 13*(1), 6–13.

Halfon, N., Larson, K., Son, J., Lu, M., & Bethell, C. (2017). Income inequality and the differential effect of adverse childhood experiences in US children. *Academic Pediatrics, 17*(7S), S70–S78.

Halfon, N., Larson, K., Lu, M., Tullis, E., & Russ, S. (2013). *Lifecourse Health Development: Past, Present and Future* (Vol. 18).

35   Boakye, *et al.* (2016).

36   De Hert, M., Correll, C. U., Bobes, J., Cetkovich-Bakmas, M., *et al.* (2011). Physical illness in patients with severe mental disorders. I. Prevalence, impact of medications and disparities in health care. *World Psychiatry: Official Journal of the World Psychiatric Association (WPA), 10*(1), 52–77.

37   SAMHSA (2006).

De Hert, *et al.* (2011).

38   Whitty, C. J. M., MacEwen, C., Goddard, A., Alderson, D., *et al.* (2020). Rising to the challenge of multimorbidity. *BMJ, 368*, l6964.

39   Singer, M., Bulled, N., Ostrach, B., & Mendenhall, E. (2017). Syndemics and the biosocial conception of health. *The Lancet, 389*(10072), 941–950.

40   *Ibid.*

41   Davis, M. A., Lin, L. A., Liu, H., & Sites, B. D. (2017). Prescription opioid use among adults with mental health disorders in the United States. *Journal of the American Board of Family Medicine: JABFM, 30*(4), 407–417.

42   Institute of Medicine (US) Committee on Advancing Pain Research, Care, and Education. (2011). *Relieving Pain in America: A Blueprint for Transforming Prevention, Care, Education, and Research*. Retrieved August 7, 2020 from www.ncbi.nlm.nih.gov/books/NBK91497.

43   Chronic Pain Research Alliance. (2015). *Impact of Chronic Overlapping Pain Conditions on Public Health and the Urgent Need for Safe and Effective Treatment: 2015 Analysis and Policy Recommendations*. Retrieved August 7, 2020 from www.chronicpainresearch.org/public/CPRA_WhitePaper_2015-FINAL-Digital.pdf.

44   IASP. (n.d.). *IASP Terminology*. Retrieved August 7, 2020 from www.iasp-pain.org/Education/Content.aspx?ItemNumber=1698#Pain.

45   Cohen, M., Quintner, J., & van Rysewyk, S. (2018). Reconsidering the International Association for the Study of Pain definition of pain. *Pain Reports, 3*(2), e634–e634.

46   Karos, K., Williams, A. C. de C., Meulders, A., & Vlaeyen, J. W. S. (2018). Pain as a threat to the social self: A motivational account. *Pain, 159*(9), 1690–1695.

47   *Ibid.*

48   Vachon-Presseau, *et al.* (2019).

49   Tousignant-Laflamme, Y., Martel, M. O., Joshi, A. B., & Cook, C. E. (2017). Rehabilitation management of low back pain—It's time to pull it all together! *Journal of Pain Research, 10*, 2373–2385.

50   Karos, *et al.* (2018).

51   Nicholas, M. K., Linton, S. J., Watson, P. J., Main, C. J., & "Decade of the Flags" Working Group. (2011). Early identification and management of psychological risk factors ("yellow flags") in patients with low back pain: A reappraisal. *Physical Therapy, 91*(5), 737–753.

52   van Rysewyk, S. (2019). *Meanings of Pain Volume 2: Common Types of Pain and Language*. Cham: Springer Nature Switzerland.

53   Low, M. (2017). A novel clinical framework: The use of dispositions in clinical practice. A person centred approach. *Journal of Evaluation in Clinical Practice, 23*(5), 1062–1070.

54   Quintner, J. L., Cohen, M. L., Buchanan, D., Katz, J. D., & Williamson, O. D. (2008). Pain medicine and its models: Helping or hindering? *Pain Medicine, 9*(7), 824–834.

55   Low (2017).

56   *Ibid.*

57   Stilwell, P. & Harman, K. (2019). An enactive approach to pain: Beyond the biopsychosocial model. *Phenomenology and the Cognitive Sciences, 18*(4), 667–668.

58   Leknes, S. & Bastian, B. (2014). The benefits of pain. *Review of Philosophy and Psychology, 5*.

Bastian, B., Jetten, J., Hornsey, M. J., & Leknes, S. (2014). The positive consequences of pain: A biopsychosocial approach. *Personality and Social Psychology Review, 18*(3), 256–279.

59   Boersma, K., Södermark, M., Hesser, H., Flink, I. K., Gerdle, B., & Linton, S. J. (2019). Efficacy of a transdiagnostic emotion-focused exposure treatment for chronic pain patients with comorbid anxiety and depression: A randomized controlled trial. *Pain, 160*(8), 1708–1718.

60   Danese, A. & Lewis, S. (2017). Psychoneuroimmunology of early-life stress: The hidden wounds of childhood trauma? *Neuropsychopharmacology: Official Publication of the American College of Neuropsychopharmacology, 42*(1), 99–114.

Broyles, S. T., Staiano, A. E., Drazba, K. T., Gupta, A. K., Sothern, M., & Katzmarzyk, P. T. (2012). Elevated C-reactive protein in children from risky neighborhoods: Evidence for a stress pathway linking neighborhoods and inflammation in children. *PloS One, 7*(9), e45419.

Shonkoff, J. P., Garner, A. S., Siegel, B. S., Dobbins, M. I., *et al.* (2012). The lifelong effects of early childhood adversity and toxic stress. *Pediatrics, 129*(1), e232.

61   Schore (2019).

62   Miller, G. E., Chen, E., & Zhou, E. S. (2007). If it goes up, must it come down? Chronic stress and the hypothalamic-pituitary-adrenocortical axis in humans. *Psychological Bulletin, 133*(1), 25–45.
Cohen, S., Janicki-Deverts, D., & Miller, G. E. (2007). Psychological stress and disease. *JAMA, 298*(14), 1685–1687.
Aschbacher, K., Kornfeld, S., Picard, M., Puterman, E., *et al.* (2014). Chronic stress increases vulnerability to diet-related abdominal fat, oxidative stress, and metabolic risk. *Psychoneuroendocrinology, 46*, 14–22.
Song, H., Fang, F., Tomasson, G., Arnberg, F. K., *et al.* (2018). Association of stress-related disorders with subsequent autoimmune disease. *JAMA, 319*(23), 2388–2400.

63   Castro, *et al.* (2001).

64   Simotas, A. C. & Shen, T. (2005). Neck pain in demolition derby drivers. *Archives of Physical Medicine and Rehabilitation, 86*(4), 693–696.

65   Radley, J., Morilak, D., Viau, V., & Campeau, S. (2015). Chronic stress and brain plasticity: Mechanisms underlying adaptive and maladaptive changes and implications for stress-related CNS disorders. *Neuroscience and Biobehavioral Reviews, 58*, 79–91.

66   Danese, A. & McEwen, B. S. (2012). Adverse childhood experiences, allostasis, allostatic load, and age-related disease. *Physiology & Behavior, 106*(1), 29–39.

67   Shanafelt, T. D., Boone, S., Tan, L., Dyrbye, L. N., *et al.* (2012). Burnout and satisfaction with work-life balance among US physicians relative to the general US population burnout and satisfaction with work-life balance. *JAMA Internal Medicine, 172*(18), 1377–1385.
Stehman, C. R., Testo, Z., Gershaw, R. S., & Kellogg, A. R. (2019). Burnout, drop out, suicide: Physician loss in emergency medicine, part I. *The Western Journal of Emergency Medicine, 20*(3), 485–494.
Dyrbye, L. N., Thomas, M. R., Massie, F. S., Power, D. V., *et al.* (2008). Burnout and suicidal ideation among U.S. medical students: Medical student burnout and suicidal ideation. *Annals of Internal Medicine, 149*(5), 334–341.

68   Shanafelt, T. D. & Noseworthy, J. H. (2017). Executive leadership and physician well-being: Nine organizational strategies to promote engagement and reduce burnout. *Mayo Clinic Proceedings, 92*(1), 129–146.

CHAPTER 4

1   World Health Organization. (2019). *Social Determinants of Health: About Social Determinants of Health.* Retrieved August 10, 2020 from www.who.int/social_determinants/sdh_definition/en.

2   Schroeder, S. A. (2007). Shattuck Lecture. We can do better—Improving the health of the American people. *New England Journal of Medicine, 357*(12), 1221–1228.

3   World Health Organization (2019).

4   Artiga, S. & Hinton, E. (2018). *Beyond Health Care: The Role of Social Determinants in Promoting Health and Health Equity.* Retrieved August 10, 2020 from www.kff.org/disparities-policy/issue-brief/beyond-health-care-the-role-of-social-determinants-in-promoting-health-and-health-equity.

5   Braveman, P. & Gottlieb, L. (2014). The social determinants of health: It's time to consider the causes of the causes. *Public Health Reports 129*(Suppl 2), 19–31.

6   Davenport, T. E. (2020). Supporting our hike upstream: Special issue and recurring feature on social determinants of health in physical therapy. *Cardiopulmonary Physical Therapy Journal, 31*(1), 2–4.

7   McKinlay, J. B. (1986). A Case for Refocusing Upstream: The Political Economy of Illness. In P. Conrad (Ed.) *The Sociology of Health and Illness: Critical Perspectives* (Second edition, pp.484–498). New York City, NY: St. Martin's.
Jones, C. P., Jones, C. Y., Perry, G. S., Barclay, G., & Jones, C. A. (2009). Addressing the social determinants of children's health: A cliff analogy. *Journal of Health Care for the Poor and Underserved, 20*(4 Suppl), 1–12.

8   Stedman, T. L. (2008). *Stedman's Medical Dictionary for the Health Professions and Nursing* (Sixth edition). Philadelphia: Wolters Kluwer Health/Lippincott Williams & Wilkins.

9   Panza, G. A., Puhl, R. M., Taylor, B. A., Zaleski, A. L., Livingston, J., & Pescatello, L. S. (2019). Links between discrimination and cardiovascular health among socially stigmatized groups: A systematic review. *PLoS One, 14*(6), e0217623.

10   Diez Roux, A. V., Mujahid, M. S., Hirsch, J. A., Moore, K., & Moore, L. V. (2016). The impact of neighborhoods on cv risk. *Global Heart, 11*(3), 353–363.

11   Kim, H., Caulfield, L. E., Garcia-Larsen, V., Steffen, L. M., Coresh, J., & Rebholz, C. M. (2019). Plant-based diets are associated with a lower risk of incident cardiovascular disease, cardiovascular disease mortality, and all-cause mortality in a general population of middle-aged adults. *Journal of the American Heart Association, 8*(16), e012865.

12   Anda, R. F., Brown, D. W., Felitti, V. J., Dube, S. R., & Giles, W. H. (2008). Adverse childhood experiences and prescription drug use in a cohort study of adult HMO patients. *BMC Public Health, 8*, 198.
Anda, R. F., Felitti, V. J., Bremner, J. D., Walker, J. D., *et al.* (2006). The enduring effects of abuse and related adverse experiences in childhood: A convergence of evidence from neurobiology and epidemiology. *European Archives of Psychiatry and Clinical Neuroscience, 256*(3), 174–186.

13 Kaplan, R. M. & Milstein, A. (2019). Contributions of health care to longevity: A review of 4 estimation methods. *Annals of Family Medicine, 17*(3), 267–272.

14 *Ibid.*

15 Bronfenbrenner, U. (1979). *The Ecology of Human Development: Experiments by Nature and Design.* Cambridge, MA: Harvard University Press.

16 *Ibid.*

17 Ben-Shlomo, Y. & Kuh, D. (2002). A life course approach to chronic disease epidemiology: Conceptual models, empirical challenges and interdisciplinary perspectives. *International Journal of Epidemiology, 31*(2), 285–293.
    Biglan, A., Flay, B. R., Embry, D. D., & Sandler, I. N. (2012). The critical role of nurturing environments for promoting human well-being. *American Psychologist, 67*(4), 257–271.

18 Ben-Shlomo & Kuh (2002).

19 *Ibid.*
    Biglan, *et al.* (2012).
    Sullivan, K. J., Wallace, J. G., Jr., O'Neil, M. E., Musolino, G. M., *et al.* (2011). A vision for society: Physical therapy as partners in the national health agenda. *Physical Therapy, 91*(11), 1664–1672.

20 Felitti, V. J., Anda, R. F., Nordenberg, D., Williamson, D. F., *et al.* (1998). Relationship of childhood abuse and household dysfunction to many of the leading causes of death in adults. The Adverse Childhood Experiences (ACE) Study. *American Journal of Preventive Medicine, 14*(4), 245–258.

21 *Ibid.*

22 *Ibid.*

23 *Ibid.*
    Dube, S. R., Cook, M. L., & Edwards, V. J. (2010). Health-related outcomes of adverse childhood experiences in Texas, 2002. *Preventing Chronic Disease, 7*(3), A52.
    Dube, S. R., Felitti, V. J., Dong, M., Chapman, D. P., Giles, W. H., & Anda, R. F. (2003). Childhood abuse, neglect, and household dysfunction and the risk of illicit drug use: The adverse childhood experiences study. *Pediatrics, 111*(3), 564–572.
    Dube, S. R., Felitti, V. J., Dong, M., Giles, W. H., & Anda, R. F. (2003). The impact of adverse childhood experiences on health problems: Evidence from four birth cohorts dating back to 1900. *Preventive Medicine, 37*(3), 268–277 (12914833).
    Jones, G. T., Power, C., & Macfarlane, G. J. (2009). Adverse events in childhood and chronic widespread pain in adult life: Results from the 1958 British Birth Cohort Study. *Pain, 143*(1–2), 92–96.
    Kalmakis, K. A., Meyer, J. S., Chiodo, L., & Leung, K. (2015). Adverse childhood experiences and chronic hypothalamic-pituitary-adrenal activity. *Stress, 18*(4), 446–450.
    Danese, A. & McEwen, B. S. (2012). Adverse childhood experiences, allostasis, allostatic load, and age-related disease. *Physiology & Behavior, 106*(1), 29–39.

24 Afifi, T. O., Ford, D., Gershoff, E. T., Merrick, M., *et al.* (2017). Spanking and adult mental health impairment: The case for the designation of spanking as an adverse childhood experience. *Moving Beyond the Spanking Debate: A Call to Action, 71*, 24–31.
    Cronholm, P. F., Forke, C. M., Wade, R., Bair-Merritt, M. H., *et al.* (2015). Adverse childhood experiences: Expanding the concept of adversity. *American Journal of Preventive Medicine, 49*(3), 354–361.
    Finkelhor, D., Shattuck, A., Turner, H., & Hamby, S. (2013). Improving the adverse childhood experiences study scale. *JAMA Pediatrics, 167*(1), 70–75.
    Marsac, M. L., Kassam-Adams, N., Delahanty, D. L., Widaman, K., & Barakat, L. P. (2014). Posttraumatic stress following acute medical trauma in children: A proposed model of bio-psycho-social processes during the peri-trauma period. *Clinical Child and Family Psychology Review, 17*(4), 399–411.

25 Halfon, N., Larson, K., Son, J., Lu, M., & Bethell, C. (2017). Income inequality and the differential effect of adverse childhood experiences in US children. *Academic Pediatrics, 17*(7S), S70–S78.

26 Ranjbar, N., Erb, M., Mohammad, O., & Moreno, F. A. (2020). Trauma-informed care and cultural humility in the mental health care of people from minoritized communities. *FOCUS, 18*(1), 8–15.

27 Font, S. A. & Maguire-Jack, K. (2016). Pathways from childhood abuse and other adversities to adult health risks: The role of adult socioeconomic conditions. *Child Abuse & Neglect, 51*, 390–399.

28 *Ibid.*

29 Ellis, B. J. & Del Giudice, M. (2019). Developmental adaptation to stress: An evolutionary perspective. *Annual Review of Psychology, 70*(1), 111–139.

30 Bethell, C., Jones, J., Gombojav, N., Linkenbach, J., & Sege, R. (2019). Positive childhood experiences and adult mental and relational health in a statewide sample: Associations across adverse childhood experiences levels. *JAMA Pediatrics*, e193007–e193007.
    Bethell, C. D., Newacheck, P., Hawes, E., & Halfon, N. (2014). Adverse childhood experiences: Assessing the impact on health and school engagement and the mitigating role of resilience. *Health Affairs, 33*(12), 2106–2115.
    Bethell, C. D., Solloway, M. R., Guinosso, S., Hassink, S., *et al.* (2017). Prioritizing possibilities for child and family health: An agenda to address adverse childhood experiences and foster the social and emotional roots of well-being in pediatrics. *Academic Pediatrics, 17*(7S), S36–S50.

Lynch, B. A., Finney Rutten, L. J., Wilson, P. M., Kumar, S., *et al.* (2018). The impact of positive contextual factors on the association between adverse family experiences and obesity in a National Survey of Children. *Preventive Medicine, 116,* 81–86.

31   Bethell, *et al.* (2014).

32   Rees (2007) Childhood attachment. *Br J Gen Pract, 57*(544), 920–922..

33   Bowlby, J. (1969). *Attachment. Attachment and Loss: Vol. 1. Loss.* New York: Basic Books.

34   Kidd, T., Hamer, M., & Steptoe, A. (2011). Examining the association between adult attachment style and cortisol responses to acute stress. *Psychoneuroendocrinology, 36*(6), 771–779.
Bartholomew, K. & Horowitz, L. M. (1991). Attachment styles among young adults: A test of a four-category model. *Journal of Personality and Social Psychology, 61*(2), 226–244.

35   Grady, M. D., Levenson, J. S., & Bolder, T. (2016). Linking adverse childhood effects and attachment: A theory of etiology for sexual offending. *Trauma, Violence, & Abuse, 18*(4), 433–444.
Ehrenthal, J. C., Levy, K. N., Scott, L. N., & Granger, D. A. (2018). Attachment-related regulatory processes moderate the impact of adverse childhood experiences on stress reaction in borderline personality disorder. *Journal of Personality Disorders, 32*(Suppl), 93–114.
Dagan, O., Asok, A., Steele, H., Steele, M., & Bernard, K. (2018). Attachment security moderates the link between adverse childhood experiences and cellular aging. *Development and Psychopathology, 30*(4), 1211–1223.

36   Lin, H.-C., Yang, Y., Elliott, L., & Green, E. (2020). Individual differences in attachment anxiety shape the association between adverse childhood experiences and adult somatic symptoms. *Child Abuse & Neglect, 101,* 104325.

37   Pietromonaco, P. R. & Beck, L. A. (2019). Adult attachment and physical health. *Current Opinion in Psychology, 25,* 115–120.

38   Feeney, J. A. (2000). Implications of attachment style for patterns of health and illness. *Child Care Health and Development, 26*(4), 277–288.
Ahrens, K. R., Ciechanowski, P., & Katon, W. (2012). Associations between adult attachment style and health risk behaviors in an adult female primary care population. *Journal of Psychosomatic Research, 72*(5), 364–370.

39   Pietromonaco & Beck (2019).
Brenk-Franz, K., Strauss, B., Tiesler, F., Fleischhauer, C., *et al.* (2015). The influence of adult attachment on patient self-management in primary care—The need for a personalized approach and patient-centred care. *PLoS One, 10*(9), e0136723.

40   Dipietro, J. A. (2012). Maternal stress in pregnancy: Considerations for fetal development. *Journal of Adolescent Health, 51*(2 Suppl), S3-8.
Consiglio, C. R. & Brodin, P. (2020). Stressful beginnings with long-term consequences. *Cell, 180*(5), 820–821.

41   Field, T., Hernandez-Reif, M., Diego, M., Figueiredo, B., Schanberg, S., & Kuhn, C. (2006). Prenatal cortisol, prematurity and low birthweight. *Infant Behavior and Development, 29*(2), 268–275.
Bermudez-Millan, A., Damio, G., Cruz, J., D'Angelo, K., *et al.* (2011). Stress and the social determinants of maternal health among Puerto Rican women: A CBPR approach. *Journal of Health Care for the Poor and Underserved, 22*(4), 1315–1330.

42   Almond, D. & Currie, J. (2011). Killing me softly: The fetal origins hypothesis. *Journal of Economic Perspectives, 25*(3), 153–172.

43   Wadhwa, P. D., Buss, C., Entringer, S., & Swanson, J. M. (2009). Developmental origins of health and disease: Brief history of the approach and current focus on epigenetic mechanisms. *Seminars in Reproductive Medicine, 27*(5), 358–368.

44   Meaney, M. J. & Szyf, M. (2005). Maternal care as a model for experience-dependent chromatin plasticity? *Trends in Neurosciences, 28*(9), 456–463.

45   Yehuda, R. & Lehrner, A. (2018). Intergenerational transmission of trauma effects: Putative role of epigenetic mechanisms. *World Psychiatry, 17*(3), 243–257.

46   Combs-Orme, T. (2013). Epigenetics and the social work imperative. *Social Work, 58*(1), 23–30.

47   Marmot, M. G., Smith, G. D., Stansfeld, S., Patel, C., *et al.* (1991). Health inequalities among British civil servants: The Whitehall II study. *Lancet, 337*(8754), 1387–1393.
Ferrie, J. E., Shipley, M. J., Davey Smith, G., Stansfeld, S. A., & Marmot, M. G. (2002). Change in health inequalities among British civil servants: The Whitehall II study. *Journal of Epidemiology and Community Health, 56*(12), 922–926.

48   Braveman, P., Egerter, S., & Williams, D. R. (2011). The social determinants of health: Coming of age. *Annual Review of Public Health, 32,* 381–398.
Wilkinson, R. G. & Pickett, K. E. (2009). *The Spirit Level: Why More Equal Societies Almost Always Do Better.* London: Allen Lane.

49   Braveman, Egerter, & Williams (2011).

50   *Ibid.*

51   Wilkinson & Pickett (2009).
Pickett, K. E. & Wilkinson, R. G. (2015). Income inequality and health: A causal review. *Social Science & Medicine, 128,* 316–326.

52   Danese & McEwen (2012).

Castagne, R., Gares, V., Karimi, M., Chadeau-Hyam, M., *et al.* (2018). Allostatic load and subsequent all-cause mortality: Which biological markers drive the relationship? Findings from a UK birth cohort. *European Journal of Epidemiology, 33*(5), 441–458.

Epel, E. S., Crosswell, A. D., Mayer, S. E., Prather, A. A., *et al.* (2018). More than a feeling: A unified view of stress measurement for population science. *Frontiers in Neuroendocrinology, 49*, 146–169.

Geronimus, A. T., Hicken, M., Keene, D., & Bound, J. (2006). "Weathering" and age patterns of allostatic load scores among blacks and whites in the United States. *American Journal of Public Health, 96*(5), 826–833.

Kaestner, R., Pearson, J. A., Keene, D., & Geronimus, A. T. (2009). Stress, allostatic load and health of Mexican immigrants. *Social Science Quarterly, 90*(5), 1089–1111.

53   Epel, *et al.* (2018).

54   Geronimus, *et al.* (2006).
     Kaestner, *et al.* (2009).

55   Castagne, *et al.* (2018).
     Crimmins, E. M., Kim, J. K., & Seeman, T. E. (2009). Poverty and biological risk: The earlier "aging" of the poor. *Journals of Gerontology Series A: Biological Sciences and Medical Sciences, 64*(2), 286–292.

56   Taylor, S. E. (2010). Mechanisms linking early life stress to adult health outcomes. *Proceedings of the National Academy of Sciences of the United States of America, 107*(19), 8507–8512.

57   Hansen, H. & Metzl, J. (2019). *Structural Competency in Mental Health and Medicine: A Case-Based Approach to Treating the Social Determinants of Health.* Cham: Springer, p.vii.

58   Ebrahim, S. (2011). Surveillance and monitoring for chronic diseases: A vital investment. *National Medical Journal of India, 24*(3), 129–132 (21786838).

59   Rietveld, E. & Kiverstein, J. (2014). A rich landscape of affordances. *Ecological Psychology, 26*(4), 325–352.

60   Leventhal, T. & Brooks-Gunn, J. (2003). Moving to opportunity: An experimental study of neighborhood effects on mental health. *American Journal of Public Health, 93*(9), 1576–1582.
     Ludwig, J., Sanbonmatsu, L., Gennetian, L., Adam, E., *et al.* (2011). Neighborhoods, obesity, and diabetes—A randomized social experiment. *New England Journal of Medicine, 365*(16), 1509–1519.

61   Andermann, A. (2016). Taking action on the social determinants of health in clinical practice: A framework for health professionals. *CMAJ, 188*(17–18), E474–E483.
     Andermann, A. (2018). Screening for social determinants of health in clinical care: Moving from the margins to the mainstream. *Public Health Reviews, 39*, 19.

62   Kelly, M. P. & Barker, M. (2016). Why is changing health-related behaviour so difficult? *Public Health, 136*, 109–116.

63   López, N. & Gadsden, V. L. (2016). *Health Inequities, Social Determinants, and Intersectionality.* NAM Perspectives, Discussion Paper. Washington, DC: National Academy of Medicine.
     Hill Collins, P. & Bilge, S. (2016). *Intersectionality.* Malden, MA: Polity Press.

64   Pauly Morgan, K. (1996). Describing the Emperor's New Clothes: Three Myths of Education (In)Equality. In A. Diller (Ed.) *The Gender Question in Education: Theory, Pedagogy & Politics.* Retrieved August 10, 2020 from https://sites.google.com/site/natalyadell/home/intersectionality.

65   *Ibid.*

66   Ranjbar, N. & Erb, M. (2019). Adverse childhood experiences and trauma-informed care in rehabilitation clinical practice. *Archives of Rehabilitation Research and Clinical Translation,* 100003.

67   Foronda, C., Baptiste, D.-L., Reinholdt, M. M., & Ousman, K. (2015). Cultural humility: A concept analysis. *Journal of Transcultural Nursing, 27*(3), 210–217.

68   Ranjbar, *et al.* (2020).

69   Andermann & Collaboration (2016).
     Andermann (2018).

70   Andermann & Collaboration (2016).
     Andermann (2018).

71   Hansen & Metzl (2019).

72   Lopez, B. L. (2019). Unconscious Bias in Action. In M. Martin, S. Heron, L. Moreno-Walton, & M. Strickland (Eds) *Diversity and Inclusion in Quality Patient Care.* Cham: Springer.

73   Andermann & Collaboration (2016).
     Andermann (2018).

CHAPTER 5

1   Rogers, J. C. & Masagatani, G. (1982). Clinical reasoning of occupational therapists during the initial assessment of physically disabled patients. *The Occupational Therapy Journal of Research, 2*(4), 195–219.

2   Daly, P. (2018). A concise guide to clinical reasoning. *Journal of Evaluation in Clinical Practice, 24*(5), 966–972.

3   Norman, G. R., Monteiro, S. D., Sherbino, J., Ilgen, J. S., Schmidt, H. G., & Mamede, S. (2017). The causes of errors in clinical reasoning: Cognitive biases, knowledge deficits, and dual process thinking. *Academic Medicine, 92*(1), 23–30.

4   Sturmberg, J. P., O'Halloran, D. M., McDonnell, G., & Martin, C. M. (2018). General practice work and workforce: Interdependencies between demand, supply and quality. *Australian Journal of General Practice*, *47*(8), 507. p.508.

5   McKenzie, K., Pierce, D., & Gunn, J. (2018). Guiding patients through complexity. *Australian Journal for General Practitioners*, *47*, 8–13. p.8.

6   Bolton, D. & Gillett, G. (2019). *The Biopsychosocial Model of Health and Disease: New Philosophical and Scientific Developments*. Cham: Palgrave Pilot.
     Farre, A. & Rapley, T. (2017). The new old (and old new) medical model: Four decades navigating the biomedical and psychosocial understandings of health and illness. *Healthcare (Basel, Switzerland)*, *5*(4), 88.

7   Barry, E., Roberts, S., Finer, S., Vijayaraghavan, S., & Greenhalgh, T. (2015). Time to question the NHS diabetes prevention programme. *BMJ*, *351*, h4717.

8   Mitsikostas, D. D., Mantonakis, L. I., & Chalarakis, N. G. (2011). Nocebo is the enemy, not placebo. A meta-analysis of reported side effects after placebo treatment in headaches. *Cephalalgia*, *31*, 550–561.

9   Benedetti, F. & Piedimonte, A. (2019). The neurobiological underpinnings of placebo and nocebo effects. *Seminars in Arthritis and Rheumatism*, *49*(Suppl 3), S18–S21.

10   Tucker, C. B. & Hanley, B. (2017). Gait variability and symmetry in world-class senior and junior race walkers. *Journal of Sports Sciences*, *35*(17), 1739–1744.

11   Van der Velde, J., Laan, E., & Everaerd, W. (2001). Vaginismus, a component of a general defensive reaction. An investigation of pelvic floor muscle activity during exposure to emotion-inducing film excerpts in women with and without vaginismus. *International Urogynecology Journal*, *12*(5), 328–331.

12   Jain, N. B., Luz, J., Higgins, L. D., Dong, Y., *et al.* (2017). The diagnostic accuracy of special tests for rotator cuff tear: The ROW cohort study. *American Journal of Physical Medicine & Rehabilitation*, *96*(3), 176–183.

13   Jensen, R. K., Kent, P., Jensen, T. S., & Kjaer, P. (2018). The association between subgroups of MRI findings identified with latent class analysis and low back pain in 40-year-old Danes. *BMC Musculoskeletal Disorders*, *19*(1), 62.

14   Pan, F., Tian, J., Cicuttini, F., Jones, G., & Aitken, D. (2019). Differentiating knee pain phenotypes in older adults: A prospective cohort study. *Rheumatology*, *58*(2), 274–283.

15   Kirmayer, L. & Gomez-Carrillo, A. (2019). Agency, embodiment and enactment in psychosomatic theory and practice. *Medical Humanities*, *45*, 1–14.

16   Wade, D. (2006). Why physical medicine, physical disability and physical rehabilitation? We should abandon Cartesian dualism. *Clinical Rehabilitation*, *20*(3), 185–190.

17   *Ibid.* p.186.

18   Johnstone, L. & Boyle, M. (2018). The power threat meaning framework: An alternative nondiagnostic conceptual system. *Journal of Humanistic Psychology*, 0022167818793289.

19   Chockalingam, N., Thomas, N. B., Smith, A., & Dunning, D. (2011). By designing "blades" for Oscar Pistorius are prosthetists creating an unfair advantage for Pistorius and an uneven playing field? *Prosthetics and Orthotics International*, *35*(4), 482–483.

20   Benedetti, F. (2013). Placebo and the new physiology of the doctor-patient relationship. *Physiological Reviews*, *93*(3), 1207–1246.

21   Chockalingam, *et al.* (2011).

22   Ferreira, M. L., Machado, G., Latimer, J., Maher, C., Ferreira, P. H., & Smeets, R. J. (2010). Factors defining care-seeking in low back pain—A meta-analysis of population based surveys. *European Journal of Pain*, *14*(7), e1–e7.

23   Van den Bergh, O., Witthoeft, M., Petersen, S., & Brown, R. J. (2017). Symptoms and the body: Taking the inferential leap. *Neuroscience and Biobehavioral Reviews*, *74*, 185–203.

24   Keller, G. B. & Mrsic-Flogel, T. D. (2018). Predictive processing: A canonical cortical computation. *Neuron*, *100*(2), 424–435.

25   Orenius, T. I., Raij, T. T., Nuortimo, A., Naatanen, P., Lipsanen, J., & Karlsson, H. (2017). The interaction of emotion and pain in the insula and secondary somatosensory cortex. *Neuroscience*, *349*, 185–194.
     Ploner, M., Sorg, C., & Gross, J. (2017). Brain rhythms of pain. *Trends in Cognitive Science*, *21*(2), 100–110.

26   Higgins, K. S., Birnie, K. A., Chambers, C. T., Wilson, A. C., *et al.* (2015). Offspring of parents with chronic pain: A systematic review and meta-analysis of pain, health, psychological, and family outcomes. *Pain*, *156*(11), 2256.

27   Cagle, J. & Bunting, M. (2017). Patient reluctance to discuss pain: Understanding stoicism, stigma, and other contributing factors. *Journal of Social Work in End-of-Life & Palliative Care*, *13*(1), 27–43.
     Creighton, G., Oliffe, J., Ogrodniczuk, J., & Frank, B. (2017). "You've gotta be that tough crust exterior man": Depression and suicide in rural-based men. *Qualitative Health Research*, *27*(12), 1882–1891.

28   Atkins, D., Uskul, A. K., & Cooper, N. R. (2016). Culture shapes empathic responses to physical and social pain. *Emotion*, *16*(5), 587–601.

29   Benedetti (2013).

30   Winkelman, M. (2015). Shamanism as a biogenetic structural paradigm for humans' evolved social psychology. *Psychology of Religion and Spirituality*, *7*(4), 267–277.

31   Tsao, J. C., Evans, S., Seidman, L. C., & Zeltzer, L. K. (2011). Healthcare utilization for pain in children and adolescents: A prospective study of laboratory and non-laboratory predictors of care-seeking. *International Journal of Adolescent Medicine and Health*, *23*(3), 287–292.

32   Elnegaard, S., Andersen, R. S., Pedersen, A. F., Larsen, P. V., *et al.* (2015). Self-reported symptoms and healthcare seeking in the general population-exploring "The Symptom Iceberg." *BMC Public Health*, *15*(1), 685.

33 Cagle & Bunting (2017).
    Neuberg, S. L. & Kenrick, A. C. (2018). Discriminating Ecologies: A Life History Approach to Stigma and Health. In B. Major, J. F. Dovidio, & B. G. Link (Eds) *The Oxford Handbook of Stigma, Discrimination, and Health* (pp.125–145). New York: Oxford University Press.

34 Bostick, G. P., Dick, B. D., Wood, M., Luckhurst, B., Tschofen, J., & Wideman, T. W. (2017). Pain assessment recommendations for women, made by women: A mixed methods study. *Pain Medicine, 19*(6), 1147–1155.

35 Ahlzén, R. (2019). Narrativity and medicine: Some critical reflections. *Philosophy, Ethics, and Humanities in Medicine, 14*(1), 9.

36 Benedetti (2013). p.5.

37 Humphrey, N. (2018). Shamans as healers: When magical structure becomes practical function. *Behavioral and Brain Sciences, 41*, e77.

38 Hutchinson, P. & Moerman, D. E. (2018). The meaning response, "placebo," and methods. *Perspectives in Biology and Medicine, 61*(3), 361–378.
    Annoni, M. & Blease, C. (2018). A critical (and cautiously optimistic) appraisal of Moerman's "meaning response." *Perspectives in Biology and Medicine, 61*(3), 379–387.

39 Rimondini, M., Mazzi, M. A., Busch, I. M., & Bensing, J. (2019). You only have one chance for a first impression! Impact of patients' first impression on the global quality assessment of doctors' communication approach. *Health Communication, 34*(12), 1413–1422.

40 Schafer, G., Prkachin, K. M., Kaseweter, K. A., & Williams, A. C. de C. (2016). Health care providers' judgments in chronic pain: The influence of gender and trustworthiness. *Pain, 157*(8), 1618–1625.
    Sessa, P. & Meconi, F. (2015). Perceived trustworthiness shapes neural empathic responses toward others' pain. *Neuropsychologia, 79*, 97–105.

41 Moerman, D. E. & Jonas, W. B. (2002). Deconstructing the placebo effect and finding the meaning response. *Annals of Internal Medicine, 136*(6), 471–476.

42 Benedetti (2013).

43 Steinkopf, L. (2017). Disgust, empathy, and care of the sick: An evolutionary perspective. *Evolutionary Psychological Science, 3*(2), 149–158.

44 De Ruddere, L. & Craig, K. D. (2016). Understanding stigma and chronic pain: A-state-of-the-art review. *Pain, 157*(8), 1607–1610.

45 Olson, K. L. & Mensinger, J. L. (2019). Weight-related stigma mediates the relationship between weight status and bodily pain: A conceptual model and call for further research. *Body Image, 30*, 159–164.

46 De Ruddere & Craig (2016).
    Walton, J. A. & Lazzaro-Salazar, M. (2016). Othering the chronically ill: A discourse analysis of New Zealand health policy documents. *Health Communication, 31*(4), 460–467.

47 Nyblade, L., Stockton, M. A., Giger, K., Bond, V., *et al.* (2019). Stigma in health facilities: Why it matters and how we can change it. *BMC Medicine, 17*(1), 25.

48 Darlow, B., Dowell, A., Baxter, G. D., Mathieson, F., Perry, M., & Dean, S. (2013). The enduring impact of what clinicians say to people with low back pain. *Annals of Family Medicine, 11*(6), 527–534.

49 Caneiro, J., Smith, A., Rabey, M., Moseley, G. L., & O'Sullivan, P. (2017). Process of change in pain-related fear: Clinical insights from a single case report of persistent back pain managed with cognitive functional therapy. *Journal of Orthopaedic and Sports Physical Therapy, 47*(9), 637–651.

50 Jones, J. M. (2015). Refractory migraine in a "just world." *Headache, 55*(1), 183–185.

51 Low, M. (2017). A novel clinical framework: The use of dispositions in clinical practice. A person centred approach. *Journal of Evaluation in Clinical Practice, 23*(5), 1062–1070.

52 Pedler, A., Kamper, S. J., Maujean, A., & Sterling, M. (2018). Investigating the fear avoidance model in people with whiplash: The association between fear of movement and in vivo activity. *The Clinical Journal of Pain, 34*(2), 130–137.
    Buragadda, S., Aleisa, E. S., & Melam, G. R. (2018). Fear avoidance beliefs and disability among women with low back pain. *Neuropsychiatry, 8*(1), 80–86.

53 Vertue, F. M. & Haig, B. D. (2008). An abductive perspective on clinical reasoning and case formulation. *Journal of Clinical Psychology, 64*(9), 1046–1068. p.1047.

54 Maung, H. H. (2019). The Functions of Diagnoses in Medicine and Psychiatry. In S. Tekin & R. Bluhm (Eds) (2019). *The Bloomsbury Companion to Philosophy of Psychiatry* (pp.507–525). London: Bloomsbury Publishing.

55 Vertue & Haig (2008).

56 Jutel, A. (2011). Classification, disease, and diagnosis. *Perspectives in Biology & Medicine, 54*(2), 189–205.

57 Jutel, A. & Nettleton, S. (2011). Towards a sociology of diagnosis: Reflections and opportunities. *Social Science & Medicine, 73*(6), 793–800. p.793.

58 Undeland, M. & Malterud, K. (2007). The fibromyalgia diagnosis: Hardly helpful for the patients? A qualitative focus group study. *Scandinavian Journal of Primary Health Care, 25*(4), 250–255.

59 Pedler, *et al.* (2018).

60 Cano, A., Miller, L. R., & Loree, A. (2009). Spouse beliefs about partner chronic pain. *The Journal of Pain, 10*(5), 486–492.

61 Walton, D. M. & Elliott, J. M. (2018). A new clinical model for facilitating the development of pattern recognition skills in clinical pain assessment. *Musculoskeletal Science and Practice*, *36*, 17–24.

62 Nicholas, M. K. & George, S. Z. (2011). Psychologically informed interventions for low back pain: An update for physical therapists. *Physical Therapy*, *91*(5), 765–776.

63 Vertue & Haig (2008).

64 Peirce, C. S. (1867). On a new list of categories. *Proceedings of the American Academy of Arts and Sciences*, *7*, 287–298.

65 *Ibid.*

66 Stanley, D. E. & Campos, D. G. (2016). Selecting clinical diagnoses: Logical strategies informed by experience. *Journal of Evaluation in Clinical Practice*, *22*(4), 588–597.

67 Stanley, D. E. & Campos, D. G. (2013). The logic of medical diagnosis. *Perspectives in Biology and Medicine*, *56*(2), 300–315.

68 Nicholas & George (2011).
    Sharp, T. J. (2001). Chronic pain: A reformulation of the cognitive-behavioural model. *Behaviour Research and Therapy*, *39*(7), 787–800.

69 Low (2017).

70 Law, M. & Laver-Fawcett, A. (2013). Canadian model of occupational performance: 30 years of impact! *British Journal of Occupational Therapy*, *76*(12), 519–519.

71 Walton & Elliott (2018).

72 Baranowski, A. P., Lee, J., Price, C., & Hughes, J. (2014). Pelvic pain: A pathway for care developed for both men and women by the British Pain Society. *British Journal of Anaesthesia*, *112*(3), 452–459.

CHAPTER 6

1   Flink, I. K., Reme, S., Jacobsen, H., Glombiewski, J., *et al.* (2020). Pain psychology in the 21st century: Lessons learned and moving forward. *Scandinavian Journal of Pain*, *20*(2), 229–238.

2   Bem, D. J. & Funder, D. C. (1978). Predicting more of the people more of the time: Assessing the personality of situations. *Psychological Review*, *85*(6), 485–501.
    Sherman, R. A., Rauthmann, J. F., Brown, N. A., Serfass, D. G., & Jones, A. B. (2015). The independent effects of personality and situations on real-time expressions of behavior and emotion. *Journal of Personality and Social Psychology*, *109*(5), 872–888.

3   Deci, E. L. & Ryan, R. M. (2012). Self-Determination Theory. In *Handbook of Theories of Social Psychology, Vol. 1* (pp.416–436). London: SAGE Publications Ltd.

4   Russell, J. A. & Barrett, L. F. (1999). Core affect, prototypical emotional episodes, and other things called emotion: Dissecting the elephant. *Journal of Personality and Social Psychology*, *76*(5), 805–819.

5   Shouse, E. (2005). Feeling, emotion, affect. *M/C Journal*, *8*(6).

6   Porges, S. W. (2011). *The Polyvagal Theory: Neurophysiological Foundations of Emotions, Attachment, Communication, and Self-Regulation (The Norton Series on Interpersonal Neurobiology)* (First edition). New York: W. W. Norton.

7   Zolnierek, K. B. H. & Dimatteo, M. R. (2009). Physician communication and patient adherence to treatment: A meta-analysis. *Medical Care*, *47*(8), 826–834.

8   Dalgleish, T. (2004). The emotional brain. *Nature Reviews Neuroscience*, *5*(7), 583–589.
    George, M. S., Nahas, Z., Bohning, D. E., Kozel, F. A., *et al.* (2002). Vagus nerve stimulation therapy. *Neurology*, *59*(6 Suppl 4), S56.
    Zeng, X., Oei, T. P. S., & Liu, X. (2014). Monitoring emotion through body sensation: A review of awareness in Goenka's vipassana. *Journal of Religion and Health*, *53*(6), 1693–1705.

9   Kashdan, T. B., Barrios, V., Forsyth, J. P., & Steger, M. F. (2006). Experiential avoidance as a generalized psychological vulnerability: Comparisons with coping and emotion regulation strategies. *Behaviour Research and Therapy*, *44*(9), 1301–1320.

10 Gawande, A. (2018, June 2). Curiosity and what equality really means. *The New Yorker*. Retrieved August 12, 2020 from www.newyorker.com/news/news-desk/curiosity-and-the-prisoner.

11 Luminet, O., Bagby, R. M., & Taylor, G. J. (Eds) (2018). *Alexithymia: Advances in Research, Theory, and Clinical Practice*. Cambridge; New York: Cambridge University Press.
    Esin, R., Gorobets, E., Esin, O., Hayrullin, I., Gorobets, V., & Volskaya, Y. (2020). The comorbidity of back and cervical pain, anxiety, depression and alexithymia. *BioNanoScience*, *10*, 365–369.

12 Torrisi, S. J., Lieberman, M. D., Bookheimer, S. Y., & Altshuler, L. L. (2013). Advancing understanding of affect labeling with dynamic causal modeling. *NeuroImage*, *82*, 481–488.

13 Quintner, J. L., Cohen, M. L., Buchanan, D., Katz, J. D., & Williamson, O. D. (2008). Pain medicine and its models: Helping or hindering? *Pain Medicine*, *9*(7), 824–834.

14 Eisenberger, N. I. (2012). The neural bases of social pain: Evidence for shared representations with physical pain. *Psychosomatic Medicine*, *74*(2), 126–135.
    Kross, E., Berman, M. G., Mischel, W., Smith, E. E., & Wager, T. D. (2011). Social rejection shares somatosensory representations with physical pain. *Proceedings of the National Academy of Sciences*, *108*(15), 6270.

15 Rietveld, E. & Kiverstein, J. (2014). A rich landscape of affordances. *Ecological Psychology*, *26*(4), 325–352.

16 Castro, W. H., Meyer, S. J., Becke, M. E., Nentwig, C. G., *et al.* (2001). No stress—no whiplash? Prevalence of "whiplash" symptoms following exposure to a placebo rear-end collision. *International Journal of Legal Medicine*, *114*(6), 316–322.

   Simotas, A. C. & Shen, T. (2005). Neck pain in demolition derby drivers. *Archives of Physical Medicine and Rehabilitation*, *86*(4), 693–696.

   Schrader, H., Obelieniene, D., Bovim, G., Surkiene, D., *et al.* (1996). Natural evolution of late whiplash syndrome outside the medicolegal context. *Lancet*, *347*(9010), 1207–1211.

   Schrader, H., Stovner, L. J., Obelieniene, D., Surkiene, D., *et al.* (2006). Examination of the diagnostic validity of "headache attributed to whiplash injury": A controlled, prospective study. *European Journal of Neurology*, *13*(11), 1226–1232.

17 Lumley, M. A., Cohen, J. L., Borszcz, G. S., Cano, A., *et al.* (2011). Pain and emotion: A biopsychosocial review of recent research. *Journal of Clinical Psychology*, *67*(9), 942–968.

   Poiraudeau, S., Rannou, F., Baron, G., Le Henanff, A., *et al.* (2006). Fear-avoidance beliefs about back pain in patients with subacute low back pain. *Pain*, *124*(3), 305–311.

   Hashmi, J. A., Baliki, M. N., Huang, L., Baria, A. T., *et al.* (2013). Shape shifting pain: Chronification of back pain shifts brain representation from nociceptive to emotional circuits. *Brain: A Journal of Neurology*, *136*(Pt 9), 2751–2768.

18 Fredrickson, B. L., Grewen, K. M., Coffey, K. A., Algoe, S. B., *et al.* (2013). A functional genomic perspective on human well-being. *Proceedings of the National Academy of Sciences*, *110*(33), 13684–13689.

   Wang, Y., Ge, J., Zhang, H., Wang, H., & Xie, X. (2019). Altruistic behaviors relieve physical pain. *Proceedings of the National Academy of Sciences*, 201911861.

   Baxter, H. J., Johnson, M. H., & Bean, D. (2012). Efficacy of a character strengths and gratitude intervention for people with chronic back pain. *The Australian Journal of Rehabilitation Counselling*, *18*(2), 135–147.

   Chen, L. H., Chen, M.-Y., & Tsai, Y.-M. (2012). Does gratitude always work? Ambivalence over emotional expression inhibits the beneficial effect of gratitude on well-being. *International Journal of Psychology*, *47*(5), 381–392.

   Singer, T. & Bolz, M. (2013). *Compassion. Bridging Practice and Science*. Retrieved August 12, 2020 from www.compassion-training.org.

19 Wood, J. V., Elaine Perunovic, W. Q., & Lee, J. W. (2009). Positive self-statements: Power for some, peril for others. *Psychological Science*, *20*(7), 860–866.

20 Shannon, J. (2019). *Understanding and Treating Personality Disorders: The DSM-V and Beyond*. Continuing Education Program.

21 *Ibid.*

   Thomas, A., Chess, S., & Birch, H. G. (1970). The origin of personality. *Scientific American*, *223*(2), 102–109.

22 Yeager, D. S., Johnson, R., Spitzer, B. J., Trzesniewski, K. H., Powers, J., & Dweck, C. S. (2014). The far-reaching effects of believing people can change: Implicit theories of personality shape stress, health, and achievement during adolescence. *Journal of Personality and Social Psychology*, *106*(6), 867–884.

23 Laghai, A. & Joseph, S. (2000). Attitudes towards emotional expression: Factor structure, convergent validity and associations with personality. *British Journal of Medical Psychology*, *73*(3), 381–384.

   Wu, Y., Lu, J., Chen, N., & Xiang, B. (2018). The influence of extraversion on emotional expression: A moderated mediation model. *Social Behavior and Personality: An International Journal*, *46*(4), 641–652.

24 Muscatello, M. R. A., Bruno, A., Mento, C., Pandolfo, G., & Zoccali, R. A. (2016). Personality traits and emotional patterns in irritable bowel syndrome. *World Journal of Gastroenterology*, *22*(28), 6402–6415.

25 Marras, W. S., Davis, K. G., Heaney, C. A., Maronitis, A. B., & Allread, W. G. (2000). The influence of psychosocial stress, gender, and personality on mechanical loading of the lumbar spine. *Spine*, *25*(23), 3045–3054.

26 Gustin, S. M., Burke, L. A., Peck, C. C., Murray, G. M., & Henderson, L. A. (2016). Pain and personality: Do individuals with different forms of chronic pain exhibit a mutual personality? *Pain Practice*, *16*(4), 486–494.

   Goswami, R., Anastakis, D. J., Katz, J., & Davis, K. D. (2016). A longitudinal study of pain, personality, and brain plasticity following peripheral nerve injury. *Pain*, *157*(3).

   Ablin, J. N., Zohar, A. H., Zaraya-Blum, R., & Buskila, D. (2016). Distinctive personality profiles of fibromyalgia and chronic fatigue syndrome patients. *PeerJ*, *4*, e2421–e2421.

   Echevarria Baez, M., Miller, S., & Banou, E. (2016). Psychological and personality differences between male and female veterans in an inpatient interdisciplinary chronic pain program. *The Journal of Pain*, *17*(4), S105.

   Conrad, R., Schilling, G., Bausch, C., Nadstawek, J., *et al.* (2007). Temperament and character personality profiles and personality disorders in chronic pain patients. *Pain*, *133*(1).

   Cosio, D. (2018, March 4). *Is There a Chronic Pain Personality Profile?* Retrieved August 12, 2020 from www.practicalpainmanagement.com/treatments/psychological/there-chronic-pain-personality-profile.

27 Oshio, A., Taku, K., Hirano, M., & Saeed, G. (2018). Resilience and big five personality traits: A meta-analysis. *Personality and Individual Differences*, *127*, 54–60.

   Habashi, M. M., Graziano, W. G., & Hoover, A. E. (2016). Searching for the prosocial personality: A big five approach to linking personality and prosocial behavior. *Personality and Social Psychology Bulletin*, *42*(9), 1177–1192.

   Komarraju, M., Karau, S. J., Schmeck, R. R., & Avdic, A. (2011). The big five personality traits, learning styles, and academic achievement. *Digit Ratio (2D:4D) and Individual Differences Research*, *51*(4), 472–477.

Goodwin, R. D. & Friedman, H. S. (2006). Health status and the five-factor personality traits in a nationally representative sample. *Journal of Health Psychology, 11*(5), 643–654.

Rhodes, R. E. & Smith, N. E. I. (2006). Personality correlates of physical activity: A review and meta-analysis. *British Journal of Sports Medicine, 40*(12), 958.

Dixon-Gordon, K. L., Whalen, D. J., Layden, B. K., & Chapman, A. L. (2015). A systematic review of personality disorders and health outcomes. *Canadian Psychology/Psychologie Canadienne, 56*(2), 168–190.

Smith, T. W. & Spiro, I., A. (2002). Personality, health, and aging: Prolegomenon for the next generation. *Journal of Research in Personality, 36*(4), 363–394.

Quirk, S. E., Berk, M., Chanen, A. M., Koivumaa-Honkanen, H., *et al.* (2016). Population prevalence of personality disorder and associations with physical health comorbidities and health care service utilization: A review. *Personality Disorders, 7*(2), 136–146.

Huang, I.-C., Lee, J. L., Ketheeswaran, P., Jones, C. M., Revicki, D. A., & Wu, A. W. (2017). Does personality affect health-related quality of life? A systematic review. *PLOS ONE, 12*(3), e0173806.

Soldz, S. & Vaillant, G. E. (1999). The big five personality traits and the life course: A 45-year longitudinal study. *Journal of Research in Personality, 33*(2), 208–232.

Mols, F. & Denollet, J. (2010). Type D personality in the general population: A systematic review of health status, mechanisms of disease, and work-related problems. *Health and Quality of Life Outcomes, 8*(1), 9.

Bucher, M. A., Suzuki, T., & Samuel, D. B. (2019). A meta-analytic review of personality traits and their associations with mental health treatment outcomes. *Clinical Psychology Review, 70*, 51–63.

28 Kaufman, S. B., Yaden, D. B., Hyde, E., & Tsukayama, E. (2019). The light vs. dark triad of personality: Contrasting two very different profiles of human nature. *Frontiers in Psychology, 10*, 467.

29 Shannon (2019).

30 Corrigan, P. (2004). How stigma interferes with mental health care. *The American Psychologist, 59*(7), 614–625.

31 Fobian, A. D. & Elliott, L. (2019). A review of functional neurological symptom disorder etiology and the integrated etiological summary model. *Journal of Psychiatry & Neuroscience: JPN, 44*(1), 8–18.

32 Nathanson, D. L. (1994). *Shame and Pride: Affect, Sex, and the Birth of the Self.* New York: Norton.

33 Conrad, *et al.* (2007).

O'Leary, D. (2018). Why bioethics should be concerned with medically unexplained symptoms. *The American Journal of Bioethics, 18*(5), 6–15.

Rosendal, M., Olde Hartman, T. C., Aamland, A., van der Horst, H., *et al.* (2017). "Medically unexplained" symptoms and symptom disorders in primary care: Prognosis-based recognition and classification. *BMC Family Practice, 18*(1), 18.

Johansen, M.-L. & Risor, M. B. (2017). What is the problem with medically unexplained symptoms for GPs? A meta-synthesis of qualitative studies. *Patient Education and Counseling, 100*(4), 647–654.

34 Kobasa, S. C. (1979). Stressful life events, personality, and health: An inquiry into hardiness. *Journal of Personality and Social Psychology, 37*(1), 1–11.

Langer, E. J. & Rodin, J. (1976). The effects of choice and enhanced personal responsibility for the aged: A field experiment in an institutional setting. *Journal of Personality and Social Psychology, 34*(2), 191–198.

35 Grau, J. W. (2014). Learning from the spinal cord: How the study of spinal cord plasticity informs our view of learning. *Associative Perspectives on the Neurobiology of Learning, 108*, 155–171.

36 Sarter, M., Givens, B., & Bruno, J. P. (2001). The cognitive neuroscience of sustained attention: Where top-down meets bottom-up. *Brain Research. Brain Research Reviews, 35*(2), 146–160.

Thiele, A. & Bellgrove, M. A. (2018). Neuromodulation of attention. *Neuron, 97*(4), 769–785.

Taylor, A. G., Goehler, L. E., Galper, D. I., Innes, K. E., & Bourguignon, C. (2010). Top-down and bottom-up mechanisms in mind-body medicine: Development of an integrative framework for psychophysiological research. *Explore, 6*(1), 29.

Park, G. & Thayer, J. F. (2014). From the heart to the mind: Cardiac vagal tone modulates top-down and bottom-up visual perception and attention to emotional stimuli. *Frontiers in Psychology, 5*, 278.

Langner, R. & Eickhoff, S. B. (2013). Sustaining attention to simple tasks: A meta-analytic review of the neural mechanisms of vigilant attention. *Psychological Bulletin, 139*(4), 870–900.

Hauck, M., Domnick, C., Lorenz, J., Gerloff, C., & Engel, A. K. (2015). Top-down and bottom-up modulation of pain-induced oscillations. *Frontiers in Human Neuroscience, 9*, 375–375.

37 Brosschot, J. F. (2002). Cognitive-emotional sensitization and somatic health complaints. *Scandinavian Journal of Psychology, 43*(2), 113–121.

38 Zusman, M. (2002). Forebrain-mediated sensitization of central pain pathways: "Non-specific" pain and a new image for MT. *Manual Therapy, 7*, 80–88.

39 Visintainer, M. A., Volpicelli, J. R., & Seligman, M. E. (1982). Tumor rejection in rats after inescapable or escapable shock. *Science, 216*(4544), 437.

40 Kuper, H., Marmot, M., & Hemingway, H. (2002). Systematic review of prospective cohort studies of psychosocial factors in the etiology and prognosis of coronary heart disease. *Seminars in Vascular Medicine, 2*(3), 267–314.

Väänänen, A., Kumpulainen, R., Kevin, M. V., Ala-Mursula, L., *et al.* (2008). Work-family characteristics as determinants of sickness absence: A large-scale cohort study of three occupational grades. *Journal of Occupational Health Psychology, 13*(2), 181–196.

41 Glanz, K. & Schwartz, M. D. (2008). Stress, Coping, and Health Behavior. In *Health Behavior and Health Education: Theory, Research, and Practice* (Fourth edition, pp.211–236). San Francisco, CA: Jossey-Bass.

42 Kirmayer, L. & Gomez-Carrillo, A. (2019). Agency, embodiment and enactment in psychosomatic theory and practice. *Medical Humanities, 45*, 1–14. p.3.

43 Smith, C. A., Haynes, K. N., Lazarus, R. S., & Pope, L. K. (1993). In search of the "hot" cognitions: Attributions, appraisals, and their relation to emotion. *Journal of Personality and Social Psychology, 65*(5), 916–929.
   Lazarus, R. S. & Folkman, S. (1999). *Stress, Appraisal, and Coping*. New York: Springer.
   Lazarus, R. S. (2013). *Fifty Years of the Research and Theory of R.S. Lazarus: An Analysis of Historical and Perennial Issues*. Mahwah, NJ: Erlbaum.
   Pearlin, L. I. & Schooler, C. (1978). The structure of coping. *Journal of Health and Social Behavior, 19*(1), 2–21.

44 Bandura, A. (1977). Self-efficacy: Toward a unifying theory of behavioral change. *Psychological Review, 84*(2), 191–215.
   Bandura, A. (2002). Social cognitive theory in cultural context. *Applied Psychology, 51*(2), 269–290.
   Bandura, A. (2004). Health promotion by social cognitive means. *Health Education and Behavior, 31*(2), 143–164.
   Bandura, A. (2018). Toward a psychology of human agency: Pathways and reflections. *Perspectives on Psychological Science, 13*(2), 130–136.

45 Dobson, F., Bennell, K. L., French, S. D., Nicolson, P. J. A., *et al.* (2016). Barriers and facilitators to exercise participation in people with hip and/or knee osteoarthritis: Synthesis of the literature using behavior change theory. *American Journal of Physical Medicine & Rehabilitation, 95*(5).

46 Alcoholics Anonymous. (2001). *Alcoholics Anonymous* (Fourth edition). New York City: Alcoholics Anonymous World Services. p.420.

47 Van Arsdale, R. & Van Arsdale, D. (2004). *The Way of the Beloved: A Spiritual Path for Couples*. Questa, NM: Open Door Publishing.

48 Halifax, J. (2018). *Standing at the Edge: Finding Freedom where Fear and Courage Meet* (First edition). New York: Flatiron Books. p.2.

CHAPTER 7

1 Moraes, L. J., Miranda, M. B., Loures, L. F., Mainieri, A. G., & Mármora, C. H. C. (2018). A systematic review of psychoneuroimmunology-based interventions. *Psychology, Health & Medicine, 23*(6), 635–652.

2 Muehsam, D., Lutgendorf, S., Mills, P. J., Rickhi, B., *et al.* (2017). The embodied mind: A review on functional genomic and neurological correlates of mind-body therapies. *Neuroscience and Biobehavioral Reviews, 73*, 165–181.
   Taylor, A. G., Goehler, L. E., Galper, D. I., Innes, K. E., & Bourguignon, C. (2010). Top-down and bottom-up mechanisms in mind-body medicine: Development of an integrative framework for psychophysiological research. *Explore, 6*(1), 29.

3 Benson, H., Beary, J. F., & Carol, M. P. (1974). The relaxation response. *Psychiatry, 37*.
   Benson, H., Greenwood, M. M., & Klemchuk, H. (1975). The relaxation response: Psychophysiologic aspects and clinical applications. *The International Journal of Psychiatry in Medicine, 6*(1–2), 87–98.

4 McCorry, L. K. (2007). Physiology of the autonomic nervous system. *American Journal of Pharmaceutical Education, 71*(4), 78–78.

5 Selye, H. (1978). *The Stress of Life* (Revised edition). New York: McGraw-Hill.
   Tachè, Y. (2014). Hans Selye and the stress response: From "the first mediator" to the identification of the hypothalamic corticotropin-releasing factor. *Ideggyogyaszati Szemle, 67*(3–4), 95–98.

6 Bracha, H. S. (2004). Freeze, flight, fight, fright, faint: Adaptationist perspectives on the acute stress response spectrum. *CNS Spectrums, 9*(9), 679–685.
   Roelofs, K., Hagenaars, M. A., & Stins, J. (2010). Facing freeze: Social threat induces bodily freeze in humans. *Psychological Science, 21*(11), 1575–1581.

7 Porges, S. W. (2009). The polyvagal theory: New insights into adaptive reactions of the autonomic nervous system. *Cleveland Clinic Journal of Medicine, 76*(Suppl 2), S86–S90.

8 Christensen, J. S., Wild, H., Kenzie, E. S., Wakeland, W., Budding, D., & Lillas, C. (2020). Diverse autonomic nervous system stress response patterns in childhood sensory modulation. *Frontiers in Integrative Neuroscience, 14*, 6.
   Berntson, G. G., Cacioppo, J. T., & Quigley, K. S. (1991). Autonomic determinism: The modes of autonomic control, the doctrine of autonomic space, and the laws of autonomic constraint. *Psychological Review, 98*(4), 459–487.

9 Christensen, *et al.* (2020).
   Berntson, G. G. & Cacioppo, J. T. (2004). Heart Rate Variability: Stress and Psychiatric Conditions. In M. Malik & A. J. Camm (Eds) *Dynamic Electrocardiography* (pp.57–64). Oxford: Blackwell Publishing.

10 Beissner, F., Meissner, K., Bär, K.-J., & Napadow, V. (2013). The autonomic brain: An activation likelihood estimation meta-analysis for central processing of autonomic function. *The Journal of Neuroscience, 33*(25), 10503.

11 Christensen, *et al.* (2020).

12   Corrigan, F., Fisher, J., & Nutt, D. (2010). Autonomic dysregulation and the Window of Tolerance model of the effects of complex emotional trauma. *Journal of Psychopharmacology, 25*(1), 17–25.

Silverman, M. N., Heim, C. M., Nater, U. M., Marques, A. H., & Sternberg, E. M. (2010). Neuroendocrine and immune contributors to fatigue. *PM&R, 2*(5), 338–346.

Fagundes, C. P., Glaser, R., & Kiecolt-Glaser, J. K. (2013). Stressful early life experiences and immune dysregulation across the lifespan. *Brain, Behavior, and Immunity, 27*, 8–12.

Abboud, François M., Harwani, Sailesh C., & Chapleau, Mark W. (2012). Autonomic neural regulation of the immune system. *Hypertension, 59*(4), 755–762.

13   Porges (2009).

Christensen, *et al.* (2020).

14   Kolacz, J., Kovacic, K. K., & Porges, S. W. (2019). Traumatic stress and the autonomic brain-gut connection in development: Polyvagal theory as an integrative framework for psychosocial and gastrointestinal pathology. *Developmental Psychobiology, 61*(5), 796–809.

Porges, S. W. & Kolacz, J. (n.d.). Neurocardiology through the Lens of the Polyvagal Theory. In R. J. Gelpi & B. Buchholz *Neurocardiology: Pathophysiological Aspects and Clinical Implications.* Amsterdam: Elsevier.

Cheshire, W. P. (2012). Highlights in clinical autonomic neuroscience: New insights into autonomic dysfunction in autism. *Autonomic Neuroscience, 171*(1), 4–7.

15   Ziemssen, T. & Siepmann, T. (2019). The investigation of the cardiovascular and sudomotor autonomic nervous system: A review. *Frontiers in Neurology, 10*, 53–53.

16   McEwen, B. S. & Wingfield, J. C. (2003). The concept of allostasis in biology and biomedicine. *Hormones and Behavior, 43*(1), 2–15.

Karatsoreos, I. N. & McEwen, B. S. (2011). Psychobiological allostasis: Resistance, resilience and vulnerability. *Trends in Cognitive Sciences, 15*(12), 576–584.

McEwen, B. S. & Gianaros, P. J. (2011). Stress- and allostasis-induced brain plasticity. *Annual Review of Medicine, 62*(1), 431–445.

Mariotti, A. (2015). The effects of chronic stress on health: New insights into the molecular mechanisms of brain-body communication. *Future Science OA, 1*(3), FSO23–FSO23.

Miller, G. E., Chen, E., & Zhou, E. S. (2007). If it goes up, must it come down? Chronic stress and the hypothalamic-pituitary-adrenocortical axis in humans. *Psychological Bulletin, 133*(1), 25–45.

Miller, G. E., Cohen, S., & Ritchey, A. K. (2002). Chronic psychological stress and the regulation of pro-inflammatory cytokines: A glucocorticoid-resistance model. *Health Psychology, 21*(6), 531–541.

Cohen, S., Janicki-Deverts, D., & Miller, G. E. (2007). Psychological stress and disease. *JAMA, 298*(14), 1685–1687.

Aschbacher, K., Kornfeld, S., Picard, M., Puterman, E., *et al.* (2014). Chronic stress increases vulnerability to diet-related abdominal fat, oxidative stress, and metabolic risk. *Psychoneuroendocrinology, 46*, 14–22.

Tian, R., Hou, G., Li, D., & Yuan, T.-F. (2014). A possible change process of inflammatory cytokines in the prolonged chronic stress and its ultimate implications for health. *The Scientific World Journal, 2014*, 780616.

Radley, J., Morilak, D., Viau, V., & Campeau, S. (2015). Chronic stress and brain plasticity: Mechanisms underlying adaptive and maladaptive changes and implications for stress-related CNS disorders. *Neuroscience and Biobehavioral Reviews, 58*, 79–91.

17   Taylor, *et al.* (2010).

Streeter, C. C., Gerbarg, P. L., Saper, R. B., Ciraulo, D. A., & Brown, R. P. (2012). Effects of yoga on the autonomic nervous system, gamma-aminobutyric-acid, and allostasis in epilepsy, depression, and post-traumatic stress disorder. *Medical Hypotheses, 78*(5), 571–579.

18   Pfau, M. L. & Russo, S. J. (2015). Peripheral and central mechanisms of stress resilience. *Neurobiology of Stress, 1*, 66–79.

19   Ranjbar, N. & Erb, M. (2019). Adverse childhood experiences and trauma-informed care in rehabilitation clinical practice. *Archives of Rehabilitation Research and Clinical Translation*, 100003.

20   Ellis, B. J. & Del Giudice, M. (2019). Developmental adaptation to stress: An evolutionary perspective. *Annual Review of Psychology, 70*(1), 111–139.

21   Wadsworth, M. E. (2015). Development of maladaptive coping: A functional adaptation to chronic, uncontrollable stress. *Child Development Perspectives, 9*(2), 96–100.

22   Makriyianis, H. M., Adams, E. A., Lozano, L. L., Mooney, T. A., Morton, C., & Liss, M. (2019). Psychological inflexibility mediates the relationship between adverse childhood experiences and mental health outcomes. *Journal of Contextual Behavioral Science, 14*, 82–89.

23   Felitti, V. J., Anda, R. F., Nordenberg, D., Williamson, D. F., *et al.* (1998). Relationship of childhood abuse and household dysfunction to many of the leading causes of death in adults. The Adverse Childhood Experiences (ACE) Study. *American Journal of Preventive Medicine, 14*(4), 245–258.

24   Del Giudice, M. (2018). *Evolutionary Psychopathology: A Unified Approach.* New York: Oxford University Press.

25   Payne, P. & Crane-Godreau, M. A. (2015). The preparatory set: A novel approach to understanding stress, trauma, and the bodymind therapies. *Frontiers in Human Neuroscience, 9*, 178.

26   Sullivan, M. B., Erb, M., Schmalzl, L., Moonaz, S., Noggle Taylor, J., & Porges, S. W. (2018). Yoga therapy and polyvagal

theory: The convergence of traditional wisdom and contemporary neuroscience for self-regulation and resilience. *Frontiers in Human Neuroscience, 12,* 67.

Cottingham, J. T., Porges, S. W., & Richmond, K. (1988). Shifts in pelvic inclination angle and parasympathetic tone produced by Rolfing soft tissue manipulation. *Physical Therapy, 68*(9), 1364–1370.

Cottingham, J. T., Porges, S. W., & Lyon, T. (1988). Effects of soft tissue mobilization (Rolfing pelvic lift) on parasympathetic tone in two age groups. *Physical Therapy, 68*(3), 352–356.

Watanabe, N., Reece, J., & Polus, B. I. (2007). Effects of body position on autonomic regulation of cardiovascular function in young, healthy adults. *Chiropractic & Osteopathy, 15,* 19–19.

Seifert, G., Kanitz, J.-L., Rihs, C., Krause, I., Witt, K., & Voss, A. (2018). Rhythmical massage improves autonomic nervous system function: A single-blind randomised controlled trial. *Journal of Integrative Medicine, 16*(3), 172–177.

Collet, C., Di Rienzo, F., El Hoyek, N., & Guillot, A. (2013). Autonomic nervous system correlates in movement observation and motor imagery. *Frontiers in Human Neuroscience, 7,* 415–415.

27 Collet, *et al.* (2013).

Shafir, T., Tsachor, R. P., & Welch, K. B. (2015). Emotion regulation through movement: Unique sets of movement characteristics are associated with and enhance basic emotions. *Frontiers in Psychology, 6,* 2030.

Tsachor, R. P. & Shafir, T. (2017). A somatic movement approach to fostering emotional resiliency through Laban Movement Analysis. *Frontiers in Human Neuroscience, 11,* 410.

Melzer, A., Shafir, T., & Tsachor, R. P. (2019). How do we recognize emotion from movement? Specific motor components contribute to the recognition of each emotion. *Frontiers in Psychology, 10,* 1389.

28 Rainville, P., Bechara, A., Naqvi, N., & Damasio, A. R. (2006). Basic emotions are associated with distinct patterns of cardiorespiratory activity. *International Journal of Psychophysiology, 61*(1), 5–18.

Kop, W. J., Synowski, S. J., Newell, M. E., Schmidt, L. A., Waldstein, S. R., & Fox, N. A. (2011). Autonomic nervous system reactivity to positive and negative mood induction: The role of acute psychological responses and frontal electrocortical activity. *Biological Psychology, 86*(3), 230–238.

Paulus, M. P. (2013). The breathing conundrum—interoceptive sensitivity and anxiety. *Depression and Anxiety, 30*(4), 315–320.

Homma, I. & Masaoka, Y. (2008). Breathing rhythms and emotions. *Experimental Physiology, 93*(9), 1011–1021.

29 Payne & Crane-Godreau (2015).

30 Sullivan, *et al.* (2018).

Sullivan, M. B., Moonaz, S., Weber, K., Taylor, J. N., & Schmalzl, L. (2018). Toward an explanatory framework for yoga therapy informed by philosophical and ethical perspectives. *Alternative Therapies in Health and Medicine, 24*(1), 38–47.

31 Kogler, L., Müller, V. I., Chang, A., Eickhoff, S. B., *et al.* (2015). Psychosocial versus physiological stress—Meta-analyses on deactivations and activations of the neural correlates of stress reactions. *NeuroImage, 119,* 235–251.

32 Goyal, M., Singh, S., Sibinga, E. M. S., Gould, N. F., *et al.* (2014). Meditation programs for psychological stress and well-being: A systematic review and meta-analysis. *JAMA Internal Medicine, 174*(3), 357–368.

Zou, Y., Zhao, X., Hou, Y.-Y., Liu, T., *et al.* (2017). Meta-analysis of effects of voluntary slow breathing exercises for control of heart rate and blood pressure in patients with cardiovascular diseases. *The American Journal of Cardiology, 120*(1), 148–153.

Mather, M. & Thayer, J. F. (2018). How heart rate variability affects emotion regulation brain networks. *Emotion-Cognition Interactions, 19,* 98–104.

Course-Choi, J., Saville, H., & Derakshan, N. (2017). The effects of adaptive working memory training and mindfulness meditation training on processing efficiency and worry in high worriers. *Behaviour Research and Therapy, 89,* 1–13.

Sharma, H. (2015). Meditation: Process and effects. *Ayu, 36*(3), 233–237.

33 McEwen, B. S. (2008). Central effects of stress hormones in health and disease: Understanding the protective and damaging effects of stress and stress mediators. *European Journal of Pharmacology, 583*(2–3), 174–185.

34 Jankord, R. & Herman, J. P. (2008). Limbic regulation of hypothalamo-pituitary-adrenocortical function during acute and chronic stress. *Annals of the New York Academy of Sciences, 1148,* 64–73.

35 Miller, *et al.* (2007).

36 Porges, S. W. (2004). Neuroception: A subconscious system for detecting threats and safety. *Zero Three, 24,* 19–24.

37 Damasio, A. & Carvalho, G. B. (2013). The nature of feelings: Evolutionary and neurobiological origins. *Nature Reviews Neuroscience, 14*(2), 143–152.

38 Feingold, K. R., Anawalt, B., Boyce, A., Chrousos, G., *et al.* (Eds) (2000). *Endotext.* Retrieved August 13, 2020 from www.ncbi.nlm.nih.gov/books/NBK278943.

39 Berger, J. M., Singh, P., Khrimian, L., Morgan, D. A., *et al.* (2019). Mediation of the acute stress response by the skeleton. *Cell Metabolism, 30*(5), 890–902.e8.

Zoch, M. L., Clemens, T. L., & Riddle, R. C. (2016). New insights into the biology of osteocalcin. *Bone, 82,* 42–49.

40 Selye (1978).

41 Lazarus, R. S. & Folkman, S. (1999). *Stress, Appraisal, and Coping.* New York: Springer.

42 Schneiderman, N., Ironson, G., & Siegel, S. D. (2005). Stress and health: Psychological, behavioral, and biological determinants. *Annual Review of Clinical Psychology, 1,* 607–628.

43 Schwabe, L. (2013). Stress and the engagement of multiple memory systems: Integration of animal and human studies. *Hippocampus, 23*(11), 1035–1043.

44 Peters, M. L., Godaert, G. L. R., Ballieux, R. E., & Heijnen, C. J. (2003). Moderation of physiological stress responses by personality traits and daily hassles: Less flexibility of immune system responses. *Biological Psychology, 65*(1), 21–48.
Crum, A. J., Salovey, P., & Achor, S. (2013). Rethinking stress: The role of mindsets in determining the stress response. *Journal of Personality and Social Psychology, 104*(4), 716–733.

45 Keller, A., Litzelman, K., Wisk, L. E., Maddox, T., *et al.* (2012). Does the perception that stress affects health matter? The association with health and mortality. *Health Psychology, 31*(5), 677–684.
Richardson, S., Shaffer, J. A., Falzon, L., Krupka, D., Davidson, K. W., & Edmondson, D. (2012). Meta-analysis of perceived stress and its association with incident coronary heart disease. *The American Journal of Cardiology, 110*(12), 1711–1716.
Jamieson, J. P., Nock, M. K., & Mendes, W. B. (2012). Mind over matter: Reappraising arousal improves cardiovascular and cognitive responses to stress. *Journal of Experimental Psychology. General, 141*(3), 417–422.

46 Poulin, M. J., Brown, S. L., Dillard, A. J., & Smith, D. M. (2013). Giving to others and the association between stress and mortality. *American Journal of Public Health, 103*(9), 1649–1655.

47 Hannibal, K. E. & Bishop, M. D. (2014). Chronic stress, cortisol dysfunction, and pain: A psychoneuroendocrine rationale for stress management in pain rehabilitation. *Physical Therapy, 94*(12), 1816–1825.

48 Furman, D., Campisi, J., Verdin, E., Carrera-Bastos, P., *et al.* (2019). Chronic inflammation in the etiology of disease across the life span. *Nature Medicine, 25*(12), 1822–1832.

49 Miller, *et al.* (2002).
Cohen, S., Doyle, W. J., & Skoner, D. P. (1999). Psychological stress, cytokine production, and severity of upper respiratory illness. *Psychosomatic Medicine, 61*(2), 175–180.

50 Liu, Y.-Z., Wang, Y.-X., & Jiang, C.-L. (2017). Inflammation: The common pathway of stress-related diseases. *Frontiers in Human Neuroscience, 11*, 316–316.

51 Segerstrom, S. C. & Miller, G. E. (2004). Psychological stress and the human immune system: A meta-analytic study of 30 years of inquiry. *Psychological Bulletin, 130*(4), 601–630.

52 Cohen, S., Janicki-Deverts, D., Doyle, W. J., Miller, G. E., *et al.* (2012). Chronic stress, glucocorticoid receptor resistance, inflammation, and disease risk. *Proceedings of the National Academy of Sciences of the United States of America, 109*(16), 5995–5999.

53 Deretic, V., Saitoh, T., & Akira, S. (2013). Autophagy in infection, inflammation and immunity. *Nature Reviews Immunology, 13*(10), 722–737.
Buckley, C. D. (2011). Why does chronic inflammation persist: An unexpected role for fibroblasts. *The Role of Non-Immune Tissues in Guiding the Action of the Immune System, 138*(1), 12–14.

54 Eisenberger, N. I., Moieni, M., Inagaki, T. K., Muscatell, K. A., & Irwin, M. R. (2017). In sickness and in health: The co-regulation of inflammation and social behavior. *Neuropsychopharmacology, 42*(1), 242–253.

55 Kolacz, *et al.* (2019).

56 Lozupone, C. A., Stombaugh, J. I., Gordon, J. I., Jansson, J. K., & Knight, R. (2012). Diversity, stability and resilience of the human gut microbiota. *Nature, 489*(7415), 220–230.

57 Dominguez-Bello, M. G., Costello, E. K., Contreras, M., Magris, M., *et al.* (2010). Delivery mode shapes the acquisition and structure of the initial microbiota across multiple body habitats in newborns. *Proceedings of the National Academy of Sciences of the United States of America, 107*(26), 11971–11975.

58 Moloney, R. D., Desbonnet, L., Clarke, G., Dinan, T. G., & Cryan, J. F. (2014). The microbiome: Stress, health and disease. *Mammalian Genome: Official Journal of the International Mammalian Genome Society, 25*(1–2), 49–74.

59 Foster, J. A., Rinaman, L., & Cryan, J. F. (2017). Stress and the gut-brain axis: Regulation by the microbiome. *Neurobiology of Stress, 7*, 124–136.

60 Porges, S. W. (2011). *The Polyvagal Theory: Neurophysiological Foundations of Emotions, Attachment, Communication, and Self-Regulation (The Norton Series on Interpersonal Neurobiology)* (First edition). New York: W. W. Norton.

61 Johnson, R. L. & Wilson, C. G. (2018). A review of vagus nerve stimulation as a therapeutic intervention. *Journal of Inflammation Research, 11*, 203–213.

62 Nijjar, P. S., Puppala, V. K., Dickinson, O., Duval, S., *et al.* (2014). Modulation of the autonomic nervous system assessed through heart rate variability by a mindfulness based stress reduction program. *International Journal of Cardiology, 177*(2), 557–559.
Tang, Y.-Y., Ma, Y., Fan, Y., Feng, H., *et al.* (2009). Central and autonomic nervous system interaction is altered by short-term meditation. *Proceedings of the National Academy of Sciences, 106*(22), 8865.

63 Chin, M. S. & Kales, S. N. (2019). Understanding mind–body disciplines: A pilot study of paced breathing and dynamic muscle contraction on autonomic nervous system reactivity. *Stress and Health, 35*(4), 542–548.
Russo, M. A., Santarelli, D. M., & O'Rourke, D. (2017). The physiological effects of slow breathing in the healthy human. *Breathe, 13*(4), 298–309.
Zaccaro, A., Piarulli, A., Laurino, M., Garbella, E., *et al.* (2018). How breath-control can change your life: A systematic review on psycho-physiological correlates of slow breathing. *Frontiers in Human Neuroscience, 12*, 353.

Farb, N., Daubenmier, J., Price, C. J., Gard, T., *et al.* (2015). Interoception, contemplative practice, and health. *Frontiers in Psychology*, 6, 763.

64 Sandercock, G. R. H., Bromley, P. D., & Brodie, D. A. (2005). Effects of exercise on heart rate variability: Inferences from meta-analysis. *Medicine and Science in Sports and Exercise*, 37(3), 433–439.

Nolan, R. P., Jong, P., Barry-Bianchi, S. M., Tanaka, T. H., & Floras, J. S. (2008). Effects of drug, biobehavioral and exercise therapies on heart rate variability in coronary artery disease: A systematic review. *European Journal of Cardiovascular Prevention & Rehabilitation*, 15(4), 386–396.

Zou, L., Sasaki, J. E., Wei, G.-X., Huang, T., *et al.* (2018). Effects of mind-body exercises (tai chi/yoga) on heart rate variability parameters and perceived stress: A systematic review with meta-analysis of randomized controlled trials. *Journal of Clinical Medicine*, 7(11), 404.

65 Tsakiris, M. & Preester, H. de (Eds) (2019). *The Interoceptive Mind: From Homeostasis to Awareness* (First edition). Oxford: Oxford University Press.

Price, C. J. & Hooven, C. (2018). Interoceptive awareness skills for emotion regulation: Theory and approach of mindful awareness in body-oriented therapy (MABT). *Frontiers in Psychology*, 9, 798–798.

Haase, L., Stewart, J. L., Youssef, B., May, A. C., *et al.* (2016). When the brain does not adequately feel the body: Links between low resilience and interoception. *Biological Psychology*, 113, 37–45.

66 Park, S. K., Tucker, K. L., O'Neill, M. S., Sparrow, D., *et al.* (2009). Fruit, vegetable, and fish consumption and heart rate variability: The Veterans Administration Normative Aging Study. *The American Journal of Clinical Nutrition*, 89(3), 778–786.

Hansen, A. L., Dahl, L., Olson, G., Thornton, D., *et al.* (2014). Fish consumption, sleep, daily functioning, and heart rate variability. *Journal of Clinical Sleep Medicine*, 10(5), 567–575.

Luyer, M. D., Greve, J. W. M., Hadfoune, M., Jacobs, J. A., Dejong, C. H., & Buurman, W. A. (2005). Nutritional stimulation of cholecystokinin receptors inhibits inflammation via the vagus nerve. *The Journal of Experimental Medicine*, 202(8), 1023–1029.

67 Bonaz, B., Bazin, T., & Pellissier, S. (2018). The vagus nerve at the interface of the microbiota-gut-brain axis. *Frontiers in Neuroscience*, 12, 49–49.

68 Gimeno-Blanes, F. J., Blanco-Velasco, M., Barquero-Pérez, Ó., García-Alberola, A., & Rojo-Álvarez, J. L. (2016). Sudden cardiac risk stratification with electrocardiographic indices—A review on computational processing, technology transfer, and scientific evidence. *Frontiers in Physiology*, 7, 82–82.

69 Kim, H.-G., Cheon, E.-J., Bai, D.-S., Lee, Y. H., & Koo, B.-H. (2018). Stress and heart rate variability: A meta-analysis and review of the literature. *Psychiatry Investigation*, 15(3), 235–245.

70 Voss, P., Thomas, M. E., Cisneros-Franco, J. M., & de Villers-Sidani, É. (2017). Dynamic brains and the changing rules of neuroplasticity: Implications for learning and recovery. *Frontiers in Psychology*, 8, 1657–1657.

71 Hölzel, B. K., Carmody, J., Vangel, M., Congleton, C., *et al.* (2011). Mindfulness practice leads to increases in regional brain gray matter density. *Psychiatry Research: Neuroimaging*, 191(1), 36–43.

Lazar, S. W., Bush, G., Gollub, R. L., Fricchione, G. L., Khalsa, G., & Benson, H. (2000). Functional brain mapping of the relaxation response and meditation. *NeuroReport*, 11(7).

Lazar, S. W., Kerr, C. E., Wasserman, R. H., Gray, J. R., *et al.* (2005). Meditation experience is associated with increased cortical thickness. *Neuroreport*, 16.

Davidson, R. J., Kabat-Zinn, J., Schumacher, J., Rosenkranz, M., *et al.* (2003). Alterations in brain and immune function produced by mindfulness meditation. *Psychosomatic Medicine*, 65(4), 564–570.

72 Cramer, S. C., Sur, M., Dobkin, B. H., O'Brien, C., *et al.* (2011). Harnessing neuroplasticity for clinical applications. *Brain: A Journal of Neurology*, 134(Pt 6), 1591–1609.

73 Tang, Y.-Y., Lu, Q., Fan, M., Yang, Y., & Posner, M. I. (2012). Mechanisms of white matter changes induced by meditation. *Proceedings of the National Academy of Sciences*, 109(26), 10570.

74 Kempermann, G., Gage, F. H., Aigner, L., Song, H., *et al.* (2018). Human adult neurogenesis: Evidence and remaining questions. *Cell Stem Cell*, 23(1), 25–30.

75 Altman, J. & Das, G. D. (1965). Autoradiographic and histological evidence of postnatal hippocampal neurogenesis in rats. *The Journal of Comparative Neurology*, 124(3), 319–335.

76 Eriksson, P. S., Perfilieva, E., Björk-Eriksson, T., Alborn, A. M., *et al.* (1998). Neurogenesis in the adult human hippocampus. *Nature Medicine*, 4(11), 1313–1317.

Boldrini, M., Fulmore, C. A., Tartt, A. N., Simeon, L. R., *et al.* (2018). Human hippocampal neurogenesis persists throughout aging. *Cell Stem Cell*, 22(4), 589–599.e5.

77 Kempermann, *et al.* (2018).

78 Moreno-Jiménez, E. P., Flor-García, M., Terreros-Roncal, J., Rábano, A., *et al.* (2019). Adult hippocampal neurogenesis is abundant in neurologically healthy subjects and drops sharply in patients with Alzheimer's disease. *Nature Medicine*, 25(4), 554–560.

79 Weinhold, B. (2006). Epigenetics: The science of change. *Environmental Health Perspectives*, 114(3), A160–A167.

80 Lee, R. S., Tamashiro, K. L. K., Yang, X., Purcell, R. H., *et al.* (2010). Chronic corticosterone exposure increases expression and decreases deoxyribonucleic acid methylation of Fkbp5 in mice. *Endocrinology*, 151(9), 4332–4343.

Romens, S. E., McDonald, J., Svaren, J., & Pollak, S. D. (2015). Associations between early life stress and gene methylation in children. *Child Development*, *86*(1), 303–309.

McGowan, P. O., Sasaki, A., D'Alessio, A. C., Dymov, S., *et al.* (2009). Epigenetic regulation of the glucocorticoid receptor in human brain associates with childhood abuse. *Nature Neuroscience*, *12*(3), 342–348.

Youssef, N. A., Lockwood, L., Su, S., Hao, G., & Rutten, B. P. F. (2018). The effects of trauma, with or without PTSD, on the transgenerational DNA methylation alterations in human offsprings. *Brain Sciences*, *8*(5), 83.

Morita, K., Saito, T., Ohta, M., Ohmori, T., *et al.* (2005). Expression analysis of psychological stress-associated genes in peripheral blood leukocytes. *Neuroscience Letters*, *381*(1–2), 57–62.

81   Black, D. S., Cole, S. W., Irwin, M. R., Breen, E., *et al.* (2013). Yogic meditation reverses NF-κB and IRF-related transcriptome dynamics in leukocytes of family dementia caregivers in a randomized controlled trial. *Psychoneuroendocrinology*, *38*(3), 348–355.

Ren, H., Collins, V., Clarke, S. J., Han, J.-S., *et al.* (2012). Epigenetic changes in response to tai chi practice: A pilot investigation of DNA methylation marks. *Evidence-Based Complementary and Alternative Medicine: ECAM*, *2012*, 841810–841810.

Rathore, M. & Abraham, J. (2018). Implication of asana, pranayama and meditation on telomere stability. *International Journal of Yoga*, *11*(3), 186–193.

82   Benedetti, F. (2014). *Placebo Effects* (Second edition). Oxford: Oxford University Press.

83   Jonas, W. B. (2019). The myth of the placebo response. *Frontiers in Psychiatry*, *10*, 577.

84   *Ibid.* p.1.

85   *Ibid.*

86   Kaplan, R. M. & Irvin, V. L. (2015). Likelihood of null effects of large NHLBI clinical trials has increased over time. *PloS One*, *10*(8), e0132382–e0132382.

87   Zou, K., Wong, J., Abdullah, N., Chen, X., *et al.* (2016). Examination of overall treatment effect and the proportion attributable to contextual effect in osteoarthritis: Meta-analysis of randomised controlled trials. *Annals of the Rheumatic Diseases*, *75*(11), 1964–1970.

88   Previtali, D., Merli, G., Di Laura Frattura, G., Candrian, C., Zaffagnini, S., & Filardo, G. (2020). The long-lasting effects of "placebo injections" in knee osteoarthritis: A meta-analysis. *Cartilage*, 1947603520906597.

89   Benedetti, F. (2019). The dangerous side of placebo research: Is hard science boosting pseudoscience? *Clinical Pharmacology and Therapeutics*, *106*(6), 1166–1168.

90   Sohn, H., Narain, D., Meirhaeghe, N., & Jazayeri, M. (2019). Bayesian computation through cortical latent dynamics. *Neuron*, *103*(5), 934–947.e5.

91   Purcell, N., Zamora, K., Gibson, C., Tighe, J., *et al.* (2019). Patient experiences with integrated pain care: A qualitative evaluation of one VA's biopsychosocial approach to chronic pain treatment and opioid safety. *Global Advances in Health and Medicine*, *8*, 2164956119838845.

92   Roberts, C. S., Baker, F., Hann, D., Runfola, J., *et al.* (2005). Patient-physician communication regarding use of complementary therapies during cancer treatment. *Journal of Psychosocial Oncology*, *23*(4), 35–60.

Rausch, S. M., Winegardner, F., Kruk, K. M., Phatak, V., *et al.* (2011). Complementary and alternative medicine: Use and disclosure in radiation oncology community practice. *Supportive Care in Cancer*, *19*(4), 521–529.

93   Petrovic, P., Kalso, E., Petersson, K. M., & Ingvar, M. (2002). Placebo and opioid analgesia—Imaging a shared neuronal network. *Science*, *295*, 1737–1740.

94   Amanzio, M. & Benedetti, F. (1999). Neuropharmacological dissection of placebo analgesia: Expectation-activated opioid systems versus conditioning-activated specific subsystems. *The Journal of Neuroscience*, *19*(1), 484–494.

95   Benedetti, F., Pollo, A., Lopiano, L., Lanotte, M., Vighetti, S., & Rainero, I. (2003). Conscious expectation and unconscious conditioning in analgesic, motor, and hormonal placebo/nocebo responses. *The Journal of Neuroscience*, *23*(10), 4315–4323.

Colloca, L. & Benedetti, F. (2005). Placebos and painkillers: Is mind as real as matter? *Nature Reviews Neuroscience*, *6*, 545–552.

Colloca, L. & Barsky, A. J. (2020). Placebo and nocebo effects. *New England Journal of Medicine*, *382*(6), 554–561.

96   Ader, R. (2003). Conditioned immunomodulation: Research needs and directions. *Brain, Behavior, and Immunity*, *17*(Suppl 1), S51–57.

97   Benedetti, F. (2005). Neurobiological mechanisms of the placebo effect. *Journal of Neuroscience*, *25*(45), 10390–10402.

98   de la Fuente-Fernández, R., Ruth, T. J., Sossi, V., Schulzer, M., Calne, D. B., & Stoessl, A. J. (2001). Expectation and dopamine release: Mechanism of the placebo effect in Parkinson's disease. *Science*, *293*(5532), 1164–1166.

Pollo, A., Torre, E., Lopiano, L., Rizzone, M., *et al.* (2002). Expectation modulates the response to subthalamic nucleus stimulation in Parkinsonian patients. *Neuroreport*, *13*(11), 1383–1386.

99   Pollo, A., Vighetti, S., Rainero, I., & Benedetti, F. (2003). Placebo analgesia and the heart. *Pain*, *102*(1–2), 125–133.

100 Häuser, W., Hansen, E., & Enck, P. (2012). Nocebo phenomena in medicine: Their relevance in everyday clinical practice. *Deutsches Ärzteblatt International*, *109*(26), 459–465.

101 Kennedy, W. P. (1961). The nocebo reaction. *Medical World*, *95*, 203–205.

102 Drici, M. D., Raybaud, F., De Lunardo, C., Iacono, P., & Gustovic, P. (1995). Influence of the behaviour pattern on the nocebo response of healthy volunteers. *British Journal of Clinical Pharmacology*, *39*(2), 204–206.

103 de Craen, A. J., Roos, P. J., de Vries, A. L., & Kleijnen, J. (1996). Effect of colour of drugs: Systematic review of perceived effect of drugs and of their effectiveness. *BMJ (Clinical Research Ed.)*, 313(7072), 1624–1626.
Buckalew, L. W. & Coffield, K. E. (1982). An investigation of drug expectancy as a function of capsule color and size and preparation form. *Journal of Clinical Psychopharmacology*, 2(4), 245–248.
Espay, A. J., Norris, M. M., Eliassen, J. C., Dwivedi, A., et al. (2015). Placebo effect of medication cost in Parkinson disease: A randomized double-blind study. *Neurology*, 84(8), 794–802.

104 Planès, S., Villier, C., & Mallaret, M. (2016). The nocebo effect of drugs. *Pharmacology Research & Perspectives*, 4(2), e00208–e00208.

105 Evers, A. W. M., Colloca, L., Blease, C., Annoni, M., et al. (2018). Implications of placebo and nocebo effects for clinical practice: Expert consensus. *Psychotherapy and Psychosomatics*, 87(4), 204–210.
Testa, M. & Rossettini, G. (2016). Enhance placebo, avoid nocebo: How contextual factors affect physiotherapy outcomes. *Manual Therapy*, 24, 65–74.
Bishop, F. L., Coghlan, B., Geraghty, A. W., Everitt, H., et al. (2017). What techniques might be used to harness placebo effects in non-malignant pain? A literature review and survey to develop a taxonomy. *BMJ Open*, 7(6).
Kaptchuk, T. J., Friedlander, E., Kelley, J. M., Sanchez, M. N., et al. (2010). Placebos without deception: A randomized controlled trial in irritable bowel syndrome. *PloS One*, 5(12), e15591.
Carvalho, C., Caetano, J. M., Cunha, L., Rebouta, P., Kaptchuk, T. J., & Kirsch, I. (2016). Open-label placebo treatment in chronic low back pain: A randomized controlled trial. *Pain*, 157(12), 2766–2772.
Colloca & Barsky (2020).

106 Benz, L. N. & Flynn, T. W. (2013). Placebo, nocebo, and expectations: Leveraging positive outcomes. *Journal of Orthopaedic and Sports Physical Therapy*, 43(7), 439–441.

107 Erb, M. & Sullivan, M. B. (2017). I shall please—Placebo and yoga therapy. *Yoga Therapy Today* (Spring). Retrieved August 13, 2020 from https://cdn.ymaws.com/www.iayt.org/resource/resmgr/docs_pubs_ytt/2017_YTT_Pubs/10.YTT_Spring2017_Features_P.pdf. p.32.

108 Colloca & Barsky (2020).

109 Rossettini, G., Carlino, E., & Testa, M. (2018). Clinical relevance of contextual factors as triggers of placebo and nocebo effects in musculoskeletal pain. *BMC Musculoskeletal Disorders*, 19(1), 27. p.2.

110 Rossettini, G., Camerone, E. M., Carlino, E., Benedetti, F., & Testa, M. (2020). Context matters: The psychoneurobiological determinants of placebo, nocebo and context-related effects in physiotherapy. *Archives of Physiotherapy*, 10(1), 11.

111 Stilwell, P. & Harman, K. (2019). An enactive approach to pain: Beyond the biopsychosocial model. *Phenomenology and the Cognitive Sciences*.

112 Benedetti (2019).

113 Zou, et al. (2016).
Purcell, et al. (2019).
Diener, I., Kargela, M., & Louw, A. (2016). Listening is therapy: Patient interviewing from a pain science perspective. *Physiotherapy Theory and Practice*, 32(5), 356–367.
Bishop, M. D., Mintken, P., Bialosky, J. E., & Cleland, J. A. (2019). Factors shaping expectations for complete relief from symptoms during rehabilitation for patients with spine pain. *Physiotherapy Theory and Practice*, 35(1), 70–79.
McDevitt, A. W., Mintken, P. E., Cleland, J. A., & Bishop, M. D. (2018). Impact of expectations on functional recovery in individuals with chronic shoulder pain. *The Journal of Manual & Manipulative Therapy*, 26(3), 136–146.
Bishop, M. D., Mintken, P. E., Bialosky, J. E., & Cleland, J. A. (2013). Patient expectations of benefit from interventions for neck pain and resulting influence on outcomes. *The Journal of Orthopaedic and Sports Physical Therapy*, 43(7), 457–465.

114 Ongaro, G. & Ward, D. (2017). An enactive account of placebo effects. *Biology & Philosophy*, 32(4), 507–553. p.507.

115 *Ibid.* p.508.

116 Rowlands, M. (2010). *The New Science of the Mind: From Extended Mind to Embodied Phenomenology.* Cambridge, MA: MIT Press.

117 Thompson, E. (2010). *Mind in Life: Biology, Phenomenology, and the Sciences of Mind.* Cambridge, MA: Belknap Press of Harvard University Press.

118 Beauvais, F. (2017). Possible contribution of quantum-like correlations to the placebo effect: Consequences on blind trials. *Theoretical Biology & Medical Modelling*, 14(1), 12–12.
Heelan, P. A. (2013). Phenomenology, ontology, and quantum physics. *Foundations of Science*, 18(2), 379–385.

119 Rovelli, C. & Smolin, L. (n.d.). Science is not about certainty: A philosophy of physics. *Edge.Org*. Retrieved August 13, 2020 from www.edge.org/conversation/carlo_rovelli-science-is-not-about-certainty-a-philosophy-of-physics.

120 Simpkin, A. L. & Schwartzstein, R. M. (2016). Tolerating uncertainty—The next medical revolution? *New England Journal of Medicine*, 375(18), 1713–1715.

121 Remen, R. N. (1999). Helping, fixing or serving? *Shambhala Sun*. Retrieved August 13, 2020 from www.uc.edu/content/dam/uc/honors/docs/communityengagement/HelpingFixingServing.pdf.

SECTION TWO INTRODUCTION

1   Wayne, P. M., Yeh, G. Y., & Mehta, D. H. (2020). A spoonful of mind-body medicine: If a little is good, is more better? *The Journal of Alternative and Complementary Medicine, 26*(1), 4–7.

CHAPTER 8

1   Singh Ospina, N., Phillips, K. A., Rodriguez-Gutierrez, R., Castaneda-Guarderas, A., *et al.* (2018). Eliciting the patient's agenda: Secondary analysis of recorded clinical encounters. *Journal of General Internal Medicine, 34*(1), 36–40.
2   *Ibid.*
3   Jacobs, D. F. & Silvernail, J. L. (2011). Therapist as operator or interactor? Moving beyond the technique. *The Journal of Manual & Manipulative Therapy, 19*(2), 120–121.
4   Porges, S. (2017). Vagal Pathways: Portals to Compassion. In E. M. Seppala, E. Simon-Thomas, S. L. Brown, M. C. Worline, C. D. Cameron, & J. R. Doty (Eds) *The Oxford Handbook of Compassion Science* (pp.189–202). New York: Oxford University Press.
5   Brody, H. (1994). "My story is broken; can you help me fix it?": Medical ethics and the joint construction of narrative. *Literature and Medicine, 13*(1), 79–92.
    Engel, G. (1988). How Much Longer Must Medicine's Science Be Bound by a Seventeenth Century World View? In K. L. White (Ed.) *The Task of Medicine: Dialogue at Wickenburg* (pp.113–136). Menlo Park, CA: Henry J. Kaiser Family Foundation.
6   Stilwell, P. & Harman, K. (2019). An enactive approach to pain: Beyond the biopsychosocial model. *Phenomenology and the Cognitive Sciences.*
7   Porges (2017).
8   Kleining, G. & Witt, H. (2000). The qualitative heuristic approach: A methodology for discovery in psychology and the social sciences. Rediscovering the method of introspection as an example. *Forum Qualitative Sozialforschung/ Forum: Qualitative Social Research, Qualitative Research: National, Disciplinary, Methodical and Empirical Examples 1*(1).
9   Anderson, K. O., Green, C. R., & Payne, R. (2009). Racial and ethnic disparities in pain: Causes and consequences of unequal care. *The Journal of Pain, 10*(12), 1187–1204.
10 Singer, T., Critchley, H., & Preuschoff, K. (2009). A common role of insula in feelings, empathy and uncertainty. *Trends in Cognitive Sciences, 13*, 334–340.
    Fukushima, H., Terasawa, Y., & Umeda, S. (2011). Association between interoception and empathy: Evidence from heartbeat-evoked brain potential. *International Journal of Psychophysiology, 79*(2), 259–265.
    Panksepp, J. (2006). The Core Emotional Systems of the Mammalian Brain: The Fundamental Substrates of Human Emotions. In *About a Body: Working with the Embodied Mind in Psychotherapy.* Hove; New York: Routledge.
    Singer, T. (2012). The past, present and future of social neuroscience: A European perspective. *Neuroimaging: Then, Now and the Future, 61*(2), 437–449.
    Bornemann, B. & Singer, T. (2013). A Cognitive Neuroscience Perspective: The ReSource Model of Compassion. In *Compassion—Bridging Practice and Science* (pp.178–191). Munich: Max Planck Society.
    Craig, A. D. (2003). Interoception: The sense of the physiological condition of the body. *Current Opinion in Neurobiology, 13*(4), 500–505.
11 Pärnamets, P., Espinosa, L., & Olsson, A. (2018). Physiological synchrony predicts observational threat learning in humans. *Proceedings of the Royal Society B 287*, 20192779.
    Vanutelli, M., Gatti, L., Angioletti, L., & Balconi, M. (2017). Affective synchrony and autonomic coupling during cooperation: A hyperscanning study. *BioMed Research International, 2017.*
    Seppala, E. M., Hutcherson, C. A., Nguyen, D. T., Doty, J. R., & Gross, J. J. (2014). Loving-kindness meditation: A tool to improve healthcare provider compassion, resilience, and patient care. *Journal of Compassionate Health Care, 1*(1), 5.
    Luken, M. & Sammons, A. (2016). Systematic review of mindfulness practice for reducing job burnout. *The American Journal of Occupational Therapy, 70*(2), 7002250020p1–7002250020p10.
    Jha, A. P., Stanley, E. A., Kiyonaga, A., Wong, L., & Gelfand, L. (2010). Examining the protective effects of mindfulness training on working memory capacity and affective experience. *Emotion, 10*(1), 54–64.
12 Diener, I., Kargela, M., & Louw, A. (2016). Listening is therapy: Patient interviewing from a pain science perspective. *Physiotherapy Theory and Practice, 32*(5), 356–367.
    Ferreira, P. H., Ferreira, M. L., Maher, C. G., Refshauge, K. M., Latimer, J., & Adams, R. D. (2013). The therapeutic alliance between clinicians and patients predicts outcome in chronic low back pain. *Physical Therapy, 93*(4), 470–478.
    Hall, A. M., Ferreira, P. H., Maher, C. G., Latimer, J., & Ferreira, M. L. (2010). The influence of the therapist-patient relationship on treatment outcome in physical rehabilitation: A systematic review. *Physical Therapy, 90*(8), 1099–1110.
13 Baldwin, S. A., Wampold, B. E., & Imel, Z. E. (2007). Untangling the alliance-outcome correlation: Exploring the relative importance of therapist and patient variability in the alliance. *Journal of Consulting and Clinical Psychology, 75*(6), 842–852.

14   Ferreira, *et al.* (2013).
     Hall, *et al.* (2010).
     Hush, J. M., Cameron, K., & Mackey, M. (2011). Patient satisfaction with musculoskeletal physical therapy care: A systematic review. *Physical Therapy*, *91*(1), 25–36.
     Schönberger, M., Humle, F., Zeeman, P., & Teasdale, T. W. (2006). Working alliance and patient compliance in brain injury rehabilitation and their relation to psychosocial outcome. *Neuropsychological Rehabilitation*, *16*(3), 298–314.
     Fuentes, J., Armijo-Olivo, S., Funabashi, M., Miciak, M., *et al.* (2014). Enhanced therapeutic alliance modulates pain intensity and muscle pain sensitivity in patients with chronic low back pain: An experimental controlled study. *Physical Therapy*, *94*(4), 477–489.

15   Fuentes, *et al.* (2014).

16   Ferreira, *et al.* (2013).
     Schönberger, *et al.* (2006).

17   Roter, D. (2000). The medical visit context of treatment decision-making and the therapeutic relationship. *Health Expectations: An International Journal of Public Participation in Health Care and Health Policy*, *3*(1), 17–25. p.23.

18   Miciak, M., Mayan, M., Brown, C., Joyce, A. S., & Gross, D. P. (2018). The necessary conditions of engagement for the therapeutic relationship in physiotherapy: An interpretive description study. *Archives of Physiotherapy*, *8*, 3–3.

19   Porges, S. W. (2011). *The Polyvagal Theory: Neurophysiological Foundations of Emotions, Attachment, Communication, and Self-Regulation (The Norton Series on Interpersonal Neurobiology)* (First edition). New York: W. W. Norton.

20   Klimecki, O. M., Leiberg, S., Lamm, C., & Singer, T. (2013). Functional neural plasticity and associated changes in positive affect after compassion training. *Cerebral Cortex*, *23*(7), 1552–1561.
     Weng, H. Y., Fox, A. S., Shackman, A. J., Stodola, D. E., *et al.* (2013). Compassion training alters altruism and neural responses to suffering. *Psychological Science*, *24*(7), 1171–1180.
     Jazaieri, H., McGonigal, K., Jinpa, T., Doty, J. R., Gross, J. J., & Goldin, P. R. (2014). A randomized controlled trial of compassion cultivation training: Effects on mindfulness, affect, and emotion regulation. *Motivation and Emotion*, *38*(1), 23–35.
     Singer, T. & Bolz, M. (2013). *Compassion. Bridging Practice and Science*. Retrieved August 17, 2020 from www.compassion-training.org.
     Seppala, E. (Ed.) (2017). *The Oxford Handbook of Compassion Science*. New York: Oxford University Press.
     Batt-Rawden, S. A., Chisolm, M. S., Anton, B., & Flickinger, T. E. (2013). Teaching empathy to medical students: An updated, systematic review. *Academic Medicine: Journal of the Association of American Medical Colleges*, *88*(8), 1171–1177.
     Stepien, K. A. & Baernstein, A. (2006). Educating for empathy. A review. *Journal of General Internal Medicine*, *21*(5), 524–530.
     Jeffrey, D. & Downie, R. (2016). Empathy—Can it be taught? *The Journal of the Royal College of Physicians of Edinburgh*, *46*(2), 107–112.

21   Halifax, J. (2012). A heuristic model of enactive compassion. *Current Opinion in Supportive and Palliative Care*, *6*(2), 228–235.

22   Jeffrey & Downie (2016).
     Shea, S. & Lionis, C. (2017). The call for compassion in health care. In *The Oxford Handbook of Compassion Science* (pp.457–473). New York: Oxford University Press.
     Crawford, P., Brown, B., Kvangarsnes, M., & Gilbert, P. (2014). The design of compassionate care. *Journal of Clinical Nursing*, *23*(23–24), 3589–3599.
     Brown, B., Crawford, P., Gilbert, P., Gilbert, J., & Gale, C. (2014). Practical compassions: Repertoires of practice and compassion talk in acute mental healthcare. *Sociology of Health and Illness*, *36*(3), 383–399.
     Prosko, S. (2019). Compassion in Pain Care. In *Yoga and Science in Pain Care: Treating the Person in Pain* (pp.235–256). London: Singing Dragon.

23   Gilbert, P. & Mascaro, J. (2017). Compassion Fears, Blocks and Resistances: An Evolutionary Investigation. In E. M. Seppala, E. Simon-Thomas, S. L. Brown, M. C. Worline, C. D. Cameron, & J. R. Doty (Eds) *The Oxford Handbook of Compassion Science* (pp.399–418). New York: Oxford University Press.

24   Prosko (2019).

25   Low, M. (2017). A novel clinical framework: The use of dispositions in clinical practice. A person centred approach. *Journal of Evaluation in Clinical Practice*, *23*(5), 1062–1070.

26   Brody (1994).

27   The Center for Mind-Body Medicine. (2019). *Guiding Principles*. Live Presentation presented at the Advanced Professional Training Program in Mind-Body Medicine, Rohnert Park, CA.

28   *Ibid.*

29   Felitti, V. J., Anda, R. F., Nordenberg, D., Williamson, D. F., *et al.* (1998). Relationship of childhood abuse and household dysfunction to many of the leading causes of death in adults. The Adverse Childhood Experiences (ACE) Study. *American Journal of Preventive Medicine*, *14*(4), 245–258.

30   Dube, S. R. (2018). Continuing conversations about adverse childhood experiences (ACEs) screening: A public health perspective. *Child Abuse & Neglect*, *85*, 180–184.

Finkelhor, D. (2018). Screening for adverse childhood experiences (ACEs): Cautions and suggestions. *Child Abuse and Neglect, 85,* 174–179.

Felitti, V. J. (2017). Future applications of the adverse childhood experiences research. *Journal of Child and Adolescent Trauma, 10,* 205–206.

31   Ranjbar, N. & Erb, M. (2019). Adverse childhood experiences and trauma-informed care in rehabilitation clinical practice. *Archives of Rehabilitation Research and Clinical Translation,* 100003.

32   Hoffmann, T. C., Lewis, J., & Maher, C. G. (2020). Shared decision making should be an integral part of physiotherapy practice. *Physiotherapy, 107,* 43–49.

33   Sobell, L. C. & Sobell, M. B. (2013). *Motivational Techniques and Skills for Health and Mental Health Coaching/Counseling.* Retrieved June 3, 2020 from www.nova.edu/gsc/forms/mi-techniques-skills.pdf.

CHAPTER 9

1   Charon, R. (2001). Narrative medicine: A model for empathy, reflection, profession, and trust. *JAMA, 286*(15), 1897–1902.

Charon, R. (2008). *Narrative Medicine: Honoring the Stories of Illness.* Oxford: Oxford University Press.

Charon, R. & Wyer, P. (2008). Narrative evidence based medicine. *The Lancet, 371*(9609), 296–297.

2   Richards, D. P. (2020). Don't call my experience a patient "story." *TheBMJopinion.* Retrieved August 17, 2020 from https://blogs.bmj.com/bmj/2020/01/09/dawn-p-richards-dont-call-my-experience-a-patient-story.

3   Charon (2001).

4   Lewis, B. E. (2011). Narrative medicine and healthcare reform. *Journal of Medical Humanities, 32*(1), 9–20. p.9.

5   Baines, R., Denniston, C., & Munro, J. (2019, July 8). The transformative power of patient narratives in healthcare education. *TheBMJopinion.* Retrieved August 17, 2020 from https://blogs.bmj.com/bmj/2019/07/08/the-transformative-power-of-patient-narratives-in-healthcare-education.

6   Hsu, J. (2008). The Secrets of STORYTELLING: Our love for telling tales reveals the workings of the mind. *Scientific American Mind, 19*(4). Retrieved August 17, 2020 from https://pdfs.semanticscholar.org/83ef/ba087fc7016fedd9b9a9ec501a62f97a7aa7.pdf.

7   Chongde, L. & Tsingan, L. (2003). Multiple intelligence and the structure of thinking. *Theory and Psychology, 13,* 829–845.

8   Hahn, J. (2016). Structure of a Dissertation for a Participatory Phenomenology Design. In K. D. Strang (Ed.) *The Palgrave Handbook of Research Design in Business and Management.* New York: Palgrave Macmillan.

9   Lima, D. D., Alves, V. L. P., & Turato, E. R. (2014). The phenomenological-existential comprehension of chronic pain: Going beyond the standing healthcare models. *Philosophy, Ethics, and Humanities in Medicine, 9,* 2. p.1.

10   Laing, R. D. (1967). The Politics of Experience. In *Psychology.* New York: Pantheon Books.

11   Hinyard, L. J. & Kreuter, M. W. (2007). Using narrative communication as a tool for health behavior change: A conceptual, theoretical, and empirical overview. *Health Education and Behavior, 34*(5), 777–792.

Diener, I., Kargela, M., & Louw, A. (2016). Listening is therapy: Patient interviewing from a pain science perspective. *Physiotherapy Theory and Practice, 32*(5), 356–367.

12   Muehsam, D., Lutgendorf, S., Mills, P. J., Rickhi, B., *et al.* (2017). The embodied mind: A review on functional genomic and neurological correlates of mind-body therapies. *Neuroscience and Biobehavioral Reviews, 73,* 165–181.

Taylor, A. G., Goehler, L. E., Galper, D. I., Innes, K. E., & Bourguignon, C. (2010). Top-down and bottom-up mechanisms in mind-body medicine: Development of an integrative framework for psychophysiological research. *Explore, 6*(1), 29.

13   van der Kolk, B. A. (1994). The body keeps the score: Memory and the evolving psychobiology of posttraumatic stress. *Harvard Review of Psychiatry, 1*(5), 253–265.

van der Kolk, B. A. (2014). *The Body Keeps the Score: Brain, Mind, and Body in the Healing of Trauma.* New York: Viking.

14   Holopainen, R., Piirainen, A., Heinonen, A., Karppinen, J., & O'Sullivan, P. (2018). From "Non-encounters" to autonomic agency. Conceptions of patients with low back pain about their encounters in the health care system. *Musculoskeletal Care, 16*(2), 269–277.

15   Sullivan, M. B., Moonaz, S., Weber, K., Taylor, J. N., & Schmalzl, L. (2018). Toward an explanatory framework for yoga therapy informed by philosophical and ethical perspectives. *Alternative Therapies in Health and Medicine, 24*(1), 38–47.

16   *Ibid.* pp.2–3.

Dowling, M. (2007). From Husserl to van Manen. A review of different phenomenological approaches. *International Journal of Nursing Studies, 44*(1), 131–142. p.132.

17   Gawande, A. (2018, June 2). Curiosity and what equality really means. *The New Yorker.* Retrieved August 17, 2020 from www.newyorker.com/news/news-desk/curiosity-and-the-prisoner.

18   Laozi & Mitchell, S. (2006). *Tao Te Ching: A New English Version.* New York: HarperCollins. p.15.

19   Baldwin, S. A., Wampold, B. E., & Imel, Z. E. (2007). Untangling the alliance-outcome correlation: Exploring the relative importance of therapist and patient variability in the alliance. *Journal of Consulting and Clinical Psychology, 75*(6), 842–852.

20   Miller, S. D., Hubble, M. A., Chow, D., & Seidel, J. (2015). Beyond measures and monitoring: Realizing the potential of feedback-informed treatment. *Psychotherapy, 52*(4), 449–457.

21   Charon & Wyer (2008). p.296.

22   Uribe, F. M. (2018, November 5). Believing without evidence is always morally wrong. *Aeon, Online*. Retrieved August 17, 2020 from https://aeon.co/ideas/believing-without-evidence-is-always-morally-wrong.

23   Sententiae Antiquae. (n.d.). Head and heart: A quotation falsely attributed to Aristotle. Retrieved August 17, 2020 from https://sententiaeantiquae.com/2017/05/27/head-and-heart-a-quotation-falsely-attributed-to-aristotle.

24   Lewis (2011). p.9.

CHAPTER 10

1   Schwartz, M. S. (2010). A new improved universally accepted official definition of biofeedback: Where did it come from? Why? Who did It? Who is it for? What's next? *Biofeedback, 38*(3), 88–90. p.90.

2   Benson, H., Greenwood, M. M., & Klemchuk, H. (1975). The relaxation response: Psychophysiologic aspects and clinical applications. *The International Journal of Psychiatry in Medicine, 6*(1–2), 87–98.
     Lazar, S. W., Bush, G., Gollub, R. L., Fricchione, G. L., Khalsa, G., & Benson, H. (2000). Functional brain mapping of the relaxation response and meditation. *NeuroReport, 11*(7).

3   Stetter, F. & Kupper, S. (2002). Autogenic training: A meta-analysis of clinical outcome studies. *Applied Psychophysiology and Biofeedback, 27*(1), 45–98.
     Seo, E., Hong, E., Choi, J., Kim, Y., Brandt, C., & Im, S. (2018). Effectiveness of autogenic training on headache: A systematic review. *Complementary Therapies in Medicine, 39*, 62–67.

4   Frank, D. L., Khorshid, L., Kiffer, J. F., Moravec, C. S., & McKee, M. G. (2010). Biofeedback in medicine: Who, when, why and how? *Mental Health in Family Medicine, 7*(2), 85–91.

5   Cohen, S., Janicki-Deverts, D., & Miller, G. E. (2007). Psychological stress and disease. *JAMA, 298*(14), 1685–1687.

6   Frank, *et al.* (2010).
     Tan, G., Shaffer, F., Lyle, R., Teo, I., & Association for Applied Psychophysiology and Biofeedback. (2017). *Evidence-Based Practice in Biofeedback and Neurofeedback*. Wheat Ridge, CO: Association for Applied Psychophysiology and Biofeedback.

7   Tan, G., Shaffer, F., Lyle, R., & Teo, I. (2017). *Evidence-Based Practice in Biofeedback and Neurofeedback* (Third edition). Overland Park, KS: The Association for Applied Psychophysiology and Biofeedback, Inc.

8   Benedetti, F. (2013). Placebo and the new physiology of the doctor-patient relationship. *Physiological Reviews, 93*(3), 1207–1246.
     Daniali, H. & Flaten, M. A. (2019). A qualitative systematic review of effects of provider characteristics and nonverbal behavior on pain, and placebo and nocebo effects. *Frontiers in Psychiatry, 10*, 242–242.

9   Vahey, R. & Becerra, R. (2015). Galvanic skin response in mood disorders: A critical review. *International Journal of Psychology and Psychological Therapy, 15*(2), 275–304.

10   Schwartz, M. S. & Andrasik, F. (2017). *Biofeedback: A Practitioner's Guide*. New York: Guilford Press.

11   Peper, E., Tylova, H., Gibney, K., Harvey, R., & Combatalade, D. (2008). *Biofeedback Mastery—An Experiential Teaching and Self-Training Manual*. Wheat Ridge, CO: Association for Applied Psychophysiology and Biofeedback.

12   Skinner, B. F. (1938). *The Behavior of Organisms: An Experimental Analysis*. New York: Appleton-Century.

13   Schwartz & Andrasik (2017). p.5.

14   Lehrer, P. & Eddie, D. (2013). Dynamic processes in regulation and some implications for biofeedback and biobehavioral interventions. *Applied Psychophysiology and Biofeedback, 38*(2), 143–155.
     Thayer, J. F. & Sternberg, E. (2006). Beyond heart rate variability. *Annals of the New York Academy of Sciences, 1088*(1), 361–372.

15   Thayer, J. F., Åhs, F., Fredrikson, M., Sollers, J. J., & Wager, T. D. (2012). A meta-analysis of heart rate variability and neuroimaging studies: Implications for heart rate variability as a marker of stress and health. *Neuroscience and Biobehavioral Reviews, 36*(2), 747–756.
     Liddell, B. J., Kemp, A. H., Steel, Z., Nickerson, A., *et al.* (2016). Heart rate variability and the relationship between trauma exposure age, and psychopathology in a post-conflict setting. *BMC Psychiatry, 16*, 133–133.
     Chalmers, J. A., Quintana, D. S., Abbott, M. J.-A., & Kemp, A. H. (2014). Anxiety disorders are associated with reduced heart rate variability: A meta-analysis. *Frontiers in Psychiatry, 5*, 80.
     Hillebrand, S., Gast, K. B., de Mutsert, R., Swenne, C. A., *et al.* (2013). Heart rate variability and first cardiovascular event in populations without known cardiovascular disease: Meta-analysis and dose-response meta-regression. *EP Europace, 15*(5), 742–749.
     Koenig, J., Kemp, A. H., Beauchaine, T. P., Thayer, J. F., & Kaess, M. (2016). Depression and resting state heart rate variability in children and adolescents—A systematic review and meta-analysis. *Clinical Psychology Review, 46*, 136–150.

16   Shaffer, F. & Ginsberg, J. P. (2017). An overview of heart rate variability metrics and norms. *Frontiers in Public Health, 5*, 258.

Gevirtz, R., Lehrer, P., & Schwartz, M. (n.d.). Cardiorespiratory Biofeedback. In *Biofeedback: A Practitioner's Guide* (Fourth edition, pp.196–213). New York: The Guilford Press.

17   Holzman, J. B. & Bridgett, D. J. (2017). Heart rate variability indices as bio-markers of top-down self-regulatory mechanisms: A meta-analytic review. *Neuroscience and Biobehavioral Reviews, 74*(Pt A), 233–255.

Di Bello, M., Carnevali, L., Petrocchi, N., Thayer, J. F., Gilbert, P., & Ottaviani, C. (2020). The compassionate vagus: A meta-analysis on the connection between compassion and heart rate variability. *Neuroscience and Biobehavioral Reviews, 116*, 21–30.

18   Kim, H.-G., Cheon, E.-J., Bai, D.-S., Lee, Y. H., & Koo, B.-H. (2018). Stress and heart rate variability: A meta-analysis and review of the literature. *Psychiatry Investigation, 15*(3), 235–245.

19   Thayer, *et al.* (2012).

Chalmers, *et al.* (2014).

Hillebrand, *et al.* (2013).

Kim, *et al.* (2018).

Williams, D. P., Koenig, J., Carnevali, L., Sgoifo, A., *et al.* (2019). Heart rate variability and inflammation: A meta-analysis of human studies. *Brain, Behavior, and Immunity, 80*, 219–226.

Mccraty, R. & Shaffer, F. (2015). Heart rate variability: New perspectives on physiological mechanisms, assessment of self-regulatory capacity, and health risk. *Global Advances in Health and Medicine, 4*(1), 46–61.

Beauchaine, T. P. & Thayer, J. F. (2015). Heart rate variability as a transdiagnostic biomarker of psychopathology. *Psychophysiological Science and the Research Domain Criteria, 98*(2, Part 2), 338–350.

Goessl, V. C., Curtiss, J. E., & Hofmann, S. G. (2017). The effect of heart rate variability biofeedback training on stress and anxiety: A meta-analysis. *Psychological Medicine, 47*(15), 2578–2586.

Tracy, L. M., Ioannou, L., Baker, K. S., Gibson, S. J., Georgiou-Karistianis, N., & Giummarra, M. J. (2016). Meta-analytic evidence for decreased heart rate variability in chronic pain implicating parasympathetic nervous system dysregulation. *Pain, 157*(1), 7–29.

Karavidas, M. K., Lehrer, P. M., Vaschillo, E., Vaschillo, B., *et al.* (2007). Preliminary results of an open label study of heart rate variability biofeedback for the treatment of major depression. *Applied Psychophysiology and Biofeedback, 32*(1), 19–30.

20   Sætren, S. S., Sütterlin, S., Lugo, R. G., Prince-Embury, S., & Makransky, G. (2019). A multilevel investigation of resiliency scales for children and adolescents: The relationships between self-perceived emotion regulation, vagally mediated heart rate variability, and personal factors associated with resilience. *Frontiers in Psychology, 10*, 438–438.

21   Peper, *et al.* (2008).

22   Steffen, P. R., Austin, T., DeBarros, A., & Brown, T. (2017). The impact of resonance frequency breathing on measures of heart rate variability, blood pressure, and mood. *Frontiers in Public Health, 5*, 222.

23   Lehrer, P. M., Vaschillo, E., & Vaschillo, B. (2000). Resonant frequency biofeedback training to increase cardiac variability: Rationale and manual for training. *Applied Psychophysiology and Biofeedback, 25*(3), 177–191.

Vaschillo, E. G., Vaschillo, B., & Lehrer, P. M. (2006). Characteristics of resonance in heart rate variability stimulated by biofeedback. *Applied Psychophysiology and Biofeedback, 31*(2), 129–142.

24   Thayer & Sternberg (2006).

Hildebrandt, L. K., McCall, C., Engen, H. G., & Singer, T. (2016). Cognitive flexibility, heart rate variability, and resilience predict fine-grained regulation of arousal during prolonged threat. *Psychophysiology, 53*(6), 880–890.

Shaffer, F., McCraty, R., & Zerr, C. L. (2014). A healthy heart is not a metronome: An integrative review of the heart's anatomy and heart rate variability. *Frontiers in Psychology, 5*, 1040.

25   Steinbrook, R. (2006). Imposing personal responsibility for health. *New England Journal of Medicine, 355*(8), 753–756.

Resnik, D. B. (2007). Responsibility for health: Personal, social, and environmental. *Journal of Medical Ethics, 33*(8), 444.

26   Artiga, S. & Hinton, E. (2018, May 10). Beyond health care: The role of social determinants in promoting health and health equity. *KFF*. Retrieved August 17, 2020 from www.kff.org/disparities-policy/issue-brief/beyond-health-care-the-role-of-social-determinants-in-promoting-health-and-health-equity.

CHAPTER 11

1   Wasserman, K. (1984). Coupling of external to internal respiration. *American Review of Respiratory Disease, 129*(2P2), S21–S24.

Gnaiger, E., Steinlechner-Maran, R., Méndez, G., Eberl, T., & Margreiter, R. (1995). Control of mitochondrial and cellular respiration by oxygen. *Journal of Bioenergetics and Biomembranes, 27*(6), 583–596.

2   Bonham, A. C. (1995). Neurotransmitters in the CNS control of breathing. *Respiration Physiology, 101*(3), 219–230.

Törk, I., McRitchie, D., Rikard-Bell, G., & Paxinos, G. (2002). Autonomic Regulatory Centers in the Medulla Oblongata. In G. Paxino (Ed.) *The Human Nervous System*. San Diego: Academic Press.

3   Porges, S. W. (2011). *The Polyvagal Theory: Neurophysiological Foundations of Emotions, Attachment, Communication, and Self-Regulation (The Norton Series on Interpersonal Neurobiology)* (First edition). New York: W. W. Norton.

4   Shaffer, F. & Ginsberg, J. P. (2017). An overview of heart rate variability metrics and norms. *Frontiers in Public Health*, *5*, 258.
     Shaffer, F., McCraty, R., & Zerr, C. L. (2014). A healthy heart is not a metronome: An integrative review of the heart's anatomy and heart rate variability. *Frontiers in Psychology*, *5*, 1040.

5   Kalsbeek, A., Bruinstroop, E., Yi, C. X., Klieverik, L. P., La Fleur, S. E., & Fliers, E. (2010). Hypothalamic control of energy metabolism via the autonomic nervous system. *Annals of the New York Academy of Sciences*, *1212*, 114–129.
     Kalsbeek, A., Bruinstroop, E., Yi, C.-X., Klieverik, L., Liu, J., & Fliers, E. (2014). Hormonal control of metabolism by the hypothalamus-autonomic nervous system-liver axis. *Frontiers of Hormone Research*, *42*, 1–28.

6   Lundberg, J. O., Farkas-Szallasi, T., Weitzberg, E., Rinder, J., *et al.* (1995). High nitric oxide production in human paranasal sinuses. *Nature Medicine*, *1*(4), 370–373.

7   Ricciardolo, F. (2003). Multiple roles of nitric oxide in the airways. *Thorax*, *58*, 175–182.
     Proud, D. (2005). Nitric oxide and the common cold. *Current Opinion in Allergy and Clinical Immunology*, *5*, 37–42.
     Akaike, T. & Maeda, H. (2000). Nitric oxide and virus infection. *Immunology*, *101*(3), 300–308.
     Belvisi, M. G., David Stretton, C., Yacoub, M., & Barnes, P. J. (1992). Nitric oxide is the endogenous neurotransmitter of bronchodilator nerves in humans. *European Journal of Pharmacology*, *210*(2), 221–222.

8   Russo, M. A., Santarelli, D. M., & O'Rourke, D. (2017). The physiological effects of slow breathing in the healthy human. *Breathe*, *13*(4), 298–309.

9   Farhi, D. (1996). *The Breathing Book: Good Health and Vitality Through Essential Breath Work* (First edition). New York: Henry Holt.

10   Bordoni, B., Purgol, S., Bizzarri, A., Modica, M., & Morabito, B. (2018). The influence of breathing on the central nervous system. *Cureus*, *10*(6), e2724.

11   Porges (2011).

12   Ma, X., Yue, Z.-Q., Gong, Z.-Q., Zhang, H., *et al.* (2017). The effect of diaphragmatic breathing on attention, negative affect and stress in healthy adults. *Frontiers in Psychology*, *8*.

13   Brown, R., Gerbarg, P., & Muench, F. (2013). Breathing practices for treatment of psychiatric and stress-related medical conditions. *The Psychiatric Clinics of North America*, *36*, 121–140.

14   Lehrer, P. M., Vaschillo, E., & Vaschillo, B. (2000). Resonant frequency biofeedback training to increase cardiac variability: Rationale and manual for training. *Applied Psychophysiology and Biofeedback*, *25*(3), 177–191.

15   Farhi (1996). p.72.

16   Paccione, C. & Jacobsen, H. (2019). Motivational non-directive resonance breathing as a treatment for chronic widespread pain. *Frontiers in Psychology*, *10*, 1207.

17   *Ibid.*

18   Gerritsen, R. J. S. & Band, G. P. H. (2018). Breath of life: The respiratory vagal stimulation model of contemplative activity. *Frontiers in Human Neuroscience*, *12*, 397–397.

19   Brown, *et al.* (2013).

20   Jerath, R., Edry, J. W., Barnes, V. A., & Jerath, V. (2006). Physiology of long pranayamic breathing: Neural respiratory elements may provide a mechanism that explains how slow deep breathing shifts the autonomic nervous system. *Medical Hypotheses*, *67*(3), 566–571.
     Schmalzl, L., Powers, C., & Henje Blom, E. (2015). Neurophysiological and neurocognitive mechanisms underlying the effects of yoga-based practices: Towards a comprehensive theoretical framework. *Frontiers in Human Neuroscience*, *9*, 235.

21   Shaffer & Ginsberg (2017).
     Brown, *et al.* (2013).
     Jerath, *et al.* (2006).

22   McCraty, R. (2017). New frontiers in heart rate variability and social coherence research: Techniques, technologies, and implications for improving group dynamics and outcomes. *Frontiers in Public Health*, *5*, 267.

23   Farhi (1996).
     Semin, G. R., & Cacioppo, J. T. (2008). Grounding Social Cognition: Synchronization, Coordination, and Co-Regulation. In *Embodied Grounding: Social, Cognitive, Affective, and Neuroscientific Approaches* (pp.119–147). New York: Cambridge University Press.

24   Boulding, R., Stacey, R., Niven, R., & Fowler, S. J. (2016). Dysfunctional breathing: A review of the literature and proposal for classification. *European Respiratory Review*, *25*(141), 287.

25   Vassilakopoulos, T., Roussos, C., & Zakynthinos, S. (2004). The immune response to resistive breathing. *European Respiratory Journal*, *24*(6), 1033.
     Nardi, A. E., Freire, R. C., & Zin, W. A. (2009). Panic disorder and control of breathing. *Dyspnea: Mechanisms of Respiratory Sensation*, *167*(1), 133–143.
     Conrad, A., Müller, A., Doberenz, S., Kim, S., *et al.* (2007). Psychophysiological effects of breathing instructions for stress management. *Applied Psychophysiology and Biofeedback*, *32*(2), 89–98.

26   Roth, W. T. (2005). Physiological markers for anxiety: Panic disorder and phobias. *Presidential and Vice-Presidential Addresses, Invited Keynote Lectures and Special Didactic Lectures: 12th World Congress of Psychophysiology: The Olympics of the Brain*, *58*(2), 190–198.

27   Boulding, *et al.* (2016).

Somers, V. K., Mark, A. L., Zavala, D. C., & Abboud, F. M. (1989). Influence of ventilation and hypocapnia on sympathetic nerve responses to hypoxia in normal humans. *Journal of Applied Physiology, 67*(5), 2095–2100.

Sharma, S., Hashmi, M., & Rawat, D. (2020, February 16). Hypocarbia. *StatPearls.* Retrieved August 17, 2020 from www.ncbi.nlm.nih.gov/books/NBK493167.

28 Sanborn, M. R., Edsell, M. E., Kim, M. N., Mesquita, R., *et al.* (2015). Cerebral hemodynamics at altitude: Effects of hyperventilation and acclimatization on cerebral blood flow and oxygenation. *Wilderness and Environmental Medicine, 26*(2), 133–141.

29 Lewis, D. (2011). *The Tao of Natural Breathing: For Health, Well-Being and Inner Growth.* Berkeley, CA: Rodmell Press.

30 *Ibid.*

31 Steffen, P. R., Austin, T., DeBarros, A., & Brown, T. (2017). The impact of resonance frequency breathing on measures of heart rate variability, blood pressure, and mood. *Frontiers in Public Health, 5,* 222.

32 Brown, R. P. & Gerbarg, P. L. (2005). Sudarshan kriya yogic breathing in the treatment of stress, anxiety, and depression: Part II—Clinical applications and guidelines. *The Journal of Alternative and Complementary Medicine, 11*(4), 711–717.

33 Farhi (1996).
Bordoni, *et al.* (2018).
Brown, *et al.* (2013).
Brown & Gerbarg (2005).

34 Brown & Gerbarg (2005).

35 Brown, *et al.* (2013).
Brown & Gerbarg (2005).

36 Brown & Gerbarg (2005).

37 Bordoni, *et al.* (2018).

38 Jafari, H., Courtois, I., Van den Bergh, O., Vlaeyen, J. W. S., & Van Diest, I. (2017). Pain and respiration: A systematic review. *Pain, 158*(6), 995–1006.

39 Paccione & Jacobsen (2019).
Maletic, V. & Raison, C. L. (2009). Neurobiology of depression, fibromyalgia and neuropathic pain. *Frontiers in Bioscience (Landmark Edition), 14,* 5291–5338.

40 Bastian, B., Jetten, J., Hornsey, M. J., & Leknes, S. (2014). The positive consequences of pain: A biopsychosocial approach. *Personality and Social Psychology Review, 18*(3), 256–279.

41 Naparstek, B. (n.d.). *Ease Pain* [CD]. Cleveland, OH: Health Journeys.

42 Bordoni, *et al.* (2018).

43 Nummenmaa, L., Glerean, E., Hari, R., & Hietanen, J. K. (2014). Bodily maps of emotions. *Proceedings of the National Academy of Sciences, 111*(2), 646.

44 Nummenmaa, L., Hari, R., Hietanen, J. K., & Glerean, E. (2018). Maps of subjective feelings. *Proceedings of the National Academy of Sciences, 115*(37), 9198.

45 Brown, *et al.* (2013).

CHAPTER 12

1   Conrad, A., Müller, A., Doberenz, S., Kim, S., *et al.* (2007). Psychophysiological effects of breathing instructions for stress management. *Applied Psychophysiology and Biofeedback, 32*(2), 89–98.

2   Taylor, A. G., Goehler, L. E., Galper, D. I., Innes, K. E., & Bourguignon, C. (2010). Top-down and bottom-up mechanisms in mind-body medicine: Development of an integrative framework for psychophysiological research. *Explore (New York, N.Y.), 6*(1), 29.
Schmalzl, L., Powers, C., & Henje Blom, E. (2015). Neurophysiological and neurocognitive mechanisms underlying the effects of yoga-based practices: Towards a comprehensive theoretical framework. *Frontiers in Human Neuroscience, 9*(235).

3   Lutz, A., Jha, A. P., Dunne, J. D., & Saron, C. D. (2015). Investigating the phenomenological matrix of mindfulness-related practices from a neurocognitive perspective. *The American Psychologist, 70*(7), 632–658.

4   Kabat-Zinn, J. (2003). Mindfulness-based interventions in context: Past, present, and future. *Clinical Psychology: Science and Practice, 10*(2), 144–156. p.145.

5   National Center for Complementary and Integrative Health. (n.d.). *National Health Interview Survey 2017.* Retrieved August 24, 2020 from https://nccih.nih.gov/research/statistics/NHIS/2017.

6   National Center for Complementary and Integrative Health. (n.d.). *Meditation: In Depth.* Retrieved August 24, 2020 from https://nccih.nih.gov/health/meditation/overview.htm.

7   Hussain, D. & Bhushan, B. (2010). Psychology of meditation and health: Present status and future directions. *International Journal of Psychology and Psychological Therapy, 10*(3), 439–451.

8   Loizzo, J. (2014). Meditation research, past, present, and future: Perspectives from the Nalanda contemplative science tradition. *Annals of the New York Academy of Sciences, 1307*(1), 43–54.
Kabat-Zinn, J. (2005). *Wherever You Go, There You Are: Mindfulness Meditation in Everyday Life.* New York: Hyperion.

9   Chiesa, A. & Serretti, A. (2009). Mindfulness-based stress reduction for stress management in healthy people: A review and meta-analysis. *The Journal of Alternative and Complementary Medicine, 15*(5), 593–600.

Khoury, B., Sharma, M., Rush, S. E., & Fournier, C. (2015). Mindfulness-based stress reduction for healthy individuals: A meta-analysis. *Journal of Psychosomatic Research, 78*(6), 519–528.

Bohlmeijer, E., Prenger, R., Taal, E., & Cuijpers, P. (2010). The effects of mindfulness-based stress reduction therapy on mental health of adults with a chronic medical disease: A meta-analysis. *Journal of Psychosomatic Research, 68*(6), 539–544.

Anheyer, D., Haller, H., Barth, J., Lauche, R., Dobos, G., & Cramer, H. (2017). Mindfulness-Based Stress Reduction for Treating Low Back Pain: A Systematic Review and Meta-Analysis. *Annals of Internal Medicine, 166*(11), 799–807.

10   Kabat-Zinn, J. (2016). *Coming to Our Senses: Healing Ourselves and the World Through Mindfulness.* New York: Hachette.

11   Fritschi, L., Brown, A. L., Rokho, K., Schewla, D., & Kephalopoulos, S. (2011). *Burden of Disease from Environmental Noise: Quantification of Healthy Life Years Lost in Europe.* Retrieved August 24, 2020 from www.euro.who.int/__data/assets/pdf_file/0008/136466/e94888.pdf.

Gaston, K. J., Bennie, J., Davies, T. W., & Hopkins, J. (2013). The ecological impacts of nighttime light pollution: A mechanistic appraisal. *Biological Reviews, 88*(4), 912–927.

12   Bernstein, A., Vago, D. R., & Barnhofer, T. (2019). Understanding mindfulness, one moment at a time: An introduction to the special issue. *Current Opinion in Psychology, 28*, vi–x.

13   Gordon, J. (2017). *Mind-Body Medicine Professional Training Program.* Washington, DC: The Center for Mind-Body Medicine.

14   Bormann, J. E., Thorp, S. R., Smith, E., Glickman, M., *et al.* (2018). Individual treatment of posttraumatic stress disorder using mantram repetition: A randomized clinical trial. *American Journal of Psychiatry, 175*(10), 979–988.

15   Dunne, J. D., Thompson, E., & Schooler, J. (2019). Mindful meta-awareness: Sustained and non-propositional. *Mindfulness, 28*, 307–311.

16   Naparstek, B. (n.d.). *Guided Imagery for Posttraumatic Stress: Healing Trauma.* Cleveland, OH: Health Journeys.

17   Kabat-Zinn (2005).

18   Siegel, D. J. (2008). *Reflections on The Mindful Brain.* Retrieved August 24, 2020 from https://communityofmindfulparenting.com/documents/research/Siegel-Mindfulness.pdf.

19   Schooler, J. W., Smallwood, J., Christoff, K., Handy, T. C., Reichle, E. D., & Sayette, M. A. (2011). Meta-awareness, perceptual decoupling and the wandering mind. *Trends in Cognitive Sciences, 15*(7), 319–326.

20   Kucyi, A., Salomons, T. V., & Davis, K. D. (2013). Mind wandering away from pain dynamically engages antinociceptive and default mode brain networks. *Proceedings of the National Academy of Sciences of the United States of America, 110*(46), 18692–18697.

21   Raichle, M. E. (2015). The brain's default mode network. *Annual Review of Neuroscience, 38*(1), 433–447.

22   Baliki, M. N., Geha, P. Y., Apkarian, A. V., & Chialvo, D. R. (2008). Beyond feeling: Chronic pain hurts the brain, disrupting the default-mode network dynamics. *The Journal of Neuroscience, 28*(6), 1398–1403.

Weissman-Fogel, I., Moayedi, M., Tenenbaum, H. C., Goldberg, M. B., Freeman, B. V., & Davis, K. D. (2011). Abnormal cortical activity in patients with temporomandibular disorder evoked by cognitive and emotional tasks. *Pain, 152*(2), 384–396.

Napadow, V., Kim, J., Clauw, D. J., & Harris, R. E. (2012). Decreased intrinsic brain connectivity is associated with reduced clinical pain in fibromyalgia. *Arthritis and Rheumatism, 64*(7), 2398–2403.

Baliki, M. N., Petre, B., Torbey, S., Herrmann, K. M., *et al.* (2012). Corticostriatal functional connectivity predicts transition to chronic back pain. *Nature Neuroscience, 15*(8), 1117–1119.

Hamilton, J. P., Farmer, M., Fogelman, P., & Gotlib, I. H. (2015). Depressive rumination, the default-mode network, and the dark matter of clinical neuroscience. *Depression, 78*(4), 224–230.

23   Marchetti, I., Koster, E. H. W., Sonuga-Barke, E. J., & De Raedt, R. (2012). The default mode network and recurrent depression: A neurobiological model of cognitive risk factors. *Neuropsychology Review, 22*(3), 229–251.

Li, B., Liu, L., Friston, K. J., Shen, H., *et al.* (2013). A treatment-resistant default mode subnetwork in major depression. *Sources of Treatment Resistance in Depression: Inflammation and Functional Connectivity, 74*(1), 48–54.

Bartova, L., Meyer, B. M., Diers, K., Rabl, U., *et al.* (2015). Reduced default mode network suppression during a working memory task in remitted major depression. *Journal of Psychiatric Research, 64*, 9–18.

Michalak, J., Hölz, A., & Teismann, T. (2011). Rumination as a predictor of relapse in mindfulness-based cognitive therapy for depression. *Psychology and Psychotherapy: Theory, Research and Practice, 84*(2), 230–236.

24   Wiech, K. (2016). Deconstructing the sensation of pain: The influence of cognitive processes on pain perception. *Science, 354*(6312), 584.

Zhang, S., Wu, W., Huang, G., Liu, Z., *et al.* (2014). Resting-state connectivity in the default mode network and insula during experimental low back pain. *Neural Regeneration Research, 9*(2), 135–142.

25   Schooler, *et al.* (2011).

26   Raichle (2015).

27   Hasenkamp, W. & Barsalou, L. W. (2012). Effects of meditation experience on functional connectivity of distributed brain networks. *Frontiers in Human Neuroscience, 6*.

Hasenkamp, W., Wilson-Mendenhall, C. D., Duncan, E., & Barsalou, L. W. (2012). Mind wandering and attention during focused meditation: A fine-grained temporal analysis of fluctuating cognitive states. *Neuroergonomics: The Human Brain in Action and at Work, 59*(1), 750–760.

28 Fox, K. C. R., Dixon, M. L., Nijeboer, S., Girn, M., *et al.* (2016). Functional neuroanatomy of meditation: A review and meta-analysis of 78 functional neuroimaging investigations. *Neuroscience and Biobehavioral Reviews, 65*, 208–228.

Goyal, M., Singh, S., Sibinga, E. M. S., Gould, N. F., *et al.* (2014). Meditation programs for psychological stress and well-being: A systematic review and meta-analysis. *JAMA Internal Medicine, 174*(3), 357–368.

Hilton, L., Hempel, S., Ewing, B. A., Apaydin, E., *et al.* (2016). Mindfulness meditation for chronic pain: Systematic review and meta-analysis. *Annals of Behavioral Medicine, 51*(2), 199–213.

29 Hasenkamp, Wilson-Mendenhall, Duncan, & Barsalou (2012).

30 Yates, J., Immergut, M., & Graves, J. (2017). *The Mind Illuminated: A Complete Meditation Guide Integrating Buddhist Wisdom and Brain Science for Greater Mindfulness.* New York; London; Toronto; Sydney; New Delhi: Touchstone.

31 Killingsworth, M. A. & Gilbert, D. T. (2010). A wandering mind is an unhappy mind. *Science, 330*(6006), 932.

32 Sweeney, A. M. & Moyer, A. (2015). Self-affirmation and responses to health messages: A meta-analysis on intentions and behavior. *Health Psychology, 34*(2), 149–159.

33 Galante, J., Galante, I., Bekkers, M.-J., & Gallacher, J. (2014). Effect of kindness-based meditation on health and well-being: A systematic review and meta-analysis. *Journal of Consulting and Clinical Psychology, 82*(6), 1101–1114.

34 Begley, S. (2007). *How a New Science Reveals Our Extraordinary Potential to Transform Ourselves.* New York: Ballantine Books.

35 Fox, *et al.* (2016).

Tang, Y. Y., Hölzel, B. K., & Posner, M. I. (2015). The neuroscience of mindfulness meditation. *Nature Reviews Neuroscience, 16*(4), 213–225.

36 Lazar, S. W., Kerr, C. E., Wasserman, R. H., Gray, J. R., *et al.* (2005). Meditation experience is associated with increased cortical thickness. *Neuroreport, 16.*

37 Hölzel, B. K., Carmody, J., Evans, K. C., Hoge, E. A., *et al.* (2010). Stress reduction correlates with structural changes in the amygdala. *Social Cognitive and Affective Neuroscience, 5*(1), 11–17.

38 Hölzel, B. K., Carmody, J., Vangel, M., Congleton, C., *et al.* (2011). Mindfulness practice leads to increases in regional brain gray matter density. *Psychiatry Research: Neuroimaging, 191*(1), 36–43.

39 Younge, J. O., Gotink, R. A., Baena, C. P., Roos-Hesselink, J. W., & Hunink, M. M. (2014). Mind-body practices for patients with cardiac disease: A systematic review and meta-analysis. *European Journal of Preventive Cardiology, 22*(11), 1385–1398.

Kwekkeboom, K. L. & Bratzke, L. C. (2016). A systematic review of relaxation, meditation, and guided imagery strategies for symptom management in heart failure. *The Journal of Cardiovascular Nursing, 31*(5), 457–468.

Curiati, J. A., Bocchi, E., Freire, J. O., Arantes, A. C., *et al.* (2005). Meditation reduces sympathetic activation and improves the quality of life in elderly patients with optimally treated heart failure: A prospective randomized study. *Journal of Alternative and Complementary Medicine, 11*(3), 465–472.

Galvin, J. A., Benson, H., Deckro, G. R., Fricchione, G. L., & Dusek, J. A. (2006). The relaxation response: Reducing stress and improving cognition in healthy aging adults. *Complementary Therapies in Clinical Practice, 12*(3), 186–191.

Levine, G. N., Lange, R. A., Bairey-Merz, C. N., Davidson, R. J., *et al.* (2017). Meditation and cardiovascular risk reduction. *Journal of the American Heart Association, 6*(10), e002218.

40 Lee, D. J., Kulubya, E., Goldin, P., Goodarzi, A., & Girgis, F. (2018). Review of the neural oscillations underlying meditation. *Frontiers in Neuroscience, 12*, 178.

Steinhubl, S. R., Wineinger, N. E., Patel, S., Boeldt, D. L., *et al.* (2015). Cardiovascular and nervous system changes during meditation. *Frontiers in Human Neuroscience, 9*, 145.

41 Kaliman, P. (2019). Epigenetics and meditation. *Mindfulness, 28*, 76–80.

Ornish, D., Magbanua, M. J. M., Weidner, G., Weinberg, V., *et al.* (2008). Changes in prostate gene expression in men undergoing an intensive nutrition and lifestyle intervention. *Proceedings of the National Academy of Sciences of the United States of America, 105*(24), 8369–8374.

Carlson, L. E., Beattie, T. L., Giese-Davis, J., Faris, P., *et al.* (2015). Mindfulness-based cancer recovery and supportive-expressive therapy maintain telomere length relative to controls in distressed breast cancer survivors. *Cancer, 121*(3), 476–484.

42 Davidson, R. J., Kabat-Zinn, J., Schumacher, J., Rosenkranz, M., *et al.* (2003). Alterations in brain and immune function produced by mindfulness meditation. *Psychosomatic Medicine, 65*(4), 564–570.

Black, D. S. & Slavich, G. M. (2016). Mindfulness meditation and the immune system: A systematic review of randomized controlled trials. *Annals of the New York Academy of Sciences, 1373*(1), 13–24.

Falkenberg, R. I., Eising, C., & Peters, M. L. (2018). Yoga and immune system functioning: A systematic review of randomized controlled trials. *Journal of Behavioral Medicine, 41*(4), 467–482.

Bower, J. E. & Irwin, M. R. (2016). Mind-body therapies and control of inflammatory biology: A descriptive review. *Brain, Behavior, and Immunity, 51*, 1–11.

Creswell, J. D., Taren, A. A., Lindsay, E. K., Greco, C. M., *et al.* (2016). Alterations in resting-state functional connectivity link mindfulness meditation with reduced interleukin-6: A randomized controlled trial. *Biological Psychiatry, 80*(1), 53–61.

43 Blanck, P., Perleth, S., Heidenreich, T., Kröger, P., *et al.* (2018). Effects of mindfulness exercises as stand-alone intervention on symptoms of anxiety and depression: Systematic review and meta-analysis. *Behaviour Research and Therapy, 102*, 25–35.

Boccia, M., Piccardi, L., & Guariglia, P. (2015). The meditative mind: A comprehensive meta-analysis of MRI studies. *BioMed Research International, 2015*, 419808.

Montero-Marin, J., Garcia-Campayo, J., Pérez-Yus, M. C., Zabaleta-del-Olmo, E., & Cuijpers, P. (2019). Meditation techniques v. relaxation therapies when treating anxiety: A meta-analytic review. *Psychological Medicine, 49*(13), 2118–2133.

Hoge, E. A., Bui, E., Marques, L., Metcalf, C. A., *et al.* (2013). Randomized controlled trial of mindfulness meditation for generalized anxiety disorder: Effects on anxiety and stress reactivity. *The Journal of Clinical Psychiatry, 74*(8), 786–792.

Sevinc, G., Hölzel, B. K., Greenberg, J., Gard, T., *et al.* (2019). Strengthened hippocampal circuits underlie enhanced retrieval of extinguished fear memories following mindfulness training. *Biological Psychiatry, 86*(9), 693–702.

44 Hussain & Bhushan (2010).

Anheyer, *et al.* (2017).

Hilton, *et al.* (2016).

Zeidan, F., Emerson, N. M., Farris, S. R., Ray, J. N., *et al.* (2015). Mindfulness meditation-based pain relief employs different neural mechanisms than placebo and sham mindfulness meditation-induced analgesia. *The Journal of Neuroscience, 35*(46), 15307.

Zeidan, F., Adler-Neal, A. L., Wells, R. E., Stagnaro, E., *et al.* (2016). Mindfulness-meditation-based pain relief is not mediated by endogenous opioids. *The Journal of Neuroscience, 36*(11), 3391–3397.

Zeidan, F., Salomons, T., Farris, S. R., Emerson, N. M., *et al.* (2018). Neural mechanisms supporting the relationship between dispositional mindfulness and pain. *Pain, 159*(12), 2477–2485.

Harrison, R., Zeidan, F., Kitsaras, G., Ozcelik, D., & Salomons, T. V. (2019). Trait mindfulness is associated with lower pain reactivity and connectivity of the default mode network. *The Journal of Pain, 20*(6), 645–654.

Grant, J. A., Courtemanche, J., Duerden, E. G., Duncan, G. H., & Rainville, P. (2010). Cortical thickness and pain sensitivity in zen meditators. *Emotion, 10*(1), 43–53.

Ball, E. F., Nur Shafina Muhammad Sharizan, E., Franklin, G., & Rogozińska, E. (2017). Does mindfulness meditation improve chronic pain? A systematic review. *Current Opinion in Obstetrics & Gynecology, 29*(6), 359–366.

Bawa, F. L. M., Mercer, S. W., Atherton, R. J., Clague, F., *et al.* (2015). Does mindfulness improve outcomes in patients with chronic pain? Systematic review and meta-analysis. *British Journal of General Practice, 65*(635), e387.

Rajguru, P., Kolber, M. J., Garcia, A. N., Smith, M. T., Patel, C. K., & Hanney, W. J. (2014). Use of mindfulness meditation in the management of chronic pain: A systematic review of randomized controlled trials. *American Journal of Lifestyle Medicine, 9*(3), 176–184.

Zeidan, F. & Vago, D. R. (2016). Mindfulness meditation-based pain relief: A mechanistic account. *Annals of the New York Academy of Sciences, 1373*(1), 114–127.

45 Luberto, C. M., Shinday, N., Song, R., Philpotts, L. L., *et al.* (2018). A systematic review and meta-analysis of the effects of meditation on empathy, compassion, and prosocial behaviors. *Mindfulness, 9*(3), 708–724.

Lutz, A., Brefczynski-Lewis, J., Johnstone, T., & Davidson, R. J. (2008). Regulation of the neural circuitry of emotion by compassion meditation: Effects of meditative expertise. *PloS One, 3*(3), e1897–e1897.

46 Greenberg, J., Romero, V. L., Elkin-Frankston, S., Bezdek, M. A., Schumacher, E. H., & Lazar, S. W. (2019). Reduced interference in working memory following mindfulness training is associated with increases in hippocampal volume. *Brain Imaging and Behavior, 13*(2), 366–376.

Tang, Y.-Y., Ma, Y., Wang, J., Fan, Y., *et al.* (2007). Short-term meditation training improves attention and self-regulation. *Proceedings of the National Academy of Sciences of the United States of America, 104*(43), 17152–17156.

Gard, T., Hölzel, B. K., & Lazar, S. W. (2014). The potential effects of meditation on age-related cognitive decline: A systematic review. *Annals of the New York Academy of Sciences, 1307*, 89–103.

47 Pascoe, M. C., Thompson, D. R., & Ski, C. F. (n.d.). Meditation and endocrine health and wellbeing. *Trends in Endocrinology & Metabolism, 31*(7), 469–477.

48 Zeng, X., Chiu, C. P. K., Wang, R., Oei, T. P. S., & Leung, F. Y. K. (2015). The effect of loving-kindness meditation on positive emotions: A meta-analytic review. *Frontiers in Psychology, 6*, 1693–1693.

Shonin, E., Van Gordon, W., Garcia-Campayo, J., & Griffiths, M. D. (2017). Can compassion help cure health-related disorders? *The British Journal of General Practice, 67*(657), 177–178.

Shonin, D. E., Van Gordon, W., Compare, A., Zanganeh, M., & Griffiths, M. (2014). Buddhist-derived loving-kindness and compassion meditation for the treatment of psychopathology: A systematic review. *Mindfulness, 6*, 1161–1180.

Wilson, A. C., Mackintosh, K., Power, K., & Chan, S. W. Y. (2019). Effectiveness of self-compassion related therapies: A systematic review and meta-analysis. *Mindfulness, 10*(6), 979–995.

Kreplin, U., Farias, M., & Brazil, I. A. (2018). The limited prosocial effects of meditation: A systematic review and meta-analysis. *Scientific Reports, 8*(1), 2403.

Bluth, K. & Neff, K. D. (2018). New frontiers in understanding the benefits of self-compassion. *Self and Identity, 17*(6), 605–608.

49 Corrigan, F., Fisher, J., & Nutt, D. (2010). Autonomic dysregulation and the Window of Tolerance model of the effects of complex emotional trauma. *Journal of Psychopharmacology*, *25*(1), 17–25.

50 Cebolla, A., Demarzo, M., Martins, P., Soler, J., & Garcia-Campayo, J. (2017). Unwanted effects: Is there a negative side of meditation? A multicentre survey. *PloS One*, *12*(9), e0183137–e0183137.

Van Dam, N. T., van Vugt, M. K., Vago, D. R., Schmalzl, L., *et al.* (2018). Mind the hype: A critical evaluation and prescriptive agenda for research on mindfulness and meditation. *Perspectives on Psychological Science*, *13*(1), 36–61.

51 National Center for Complementary and Integrative Health. (n.d.). *NCCIH Timeline*. Retrieved August 24, 2020 from https://nccih.nih.gov/about/nccih-timeline.

52 Barnes, P. M., Powell-Griner, E., McFann, K., & Nahin, R. L. (2004, May 27). *Complementary and Alternative Medicine Use Among Adults: United States. 2002*. Retrieved August 24, 2020 from https://nccih.nih.gov/sites/nccam.nih.gov/files/news/camstats/2002/report.pdf.

53 National Center for Complementary and Integrative Health. (2018). *Complementary, Alternative, or Integrative Health: What's In a Name? NCCIH Publication No. D347*. Retrieved August 24, 2020 from https://nccih.nih.gov/health/integrative-health.

Clarke, T. C., Barnes, P. M., Black, L. I., Stussman, B. J., & Nahin, R. L. (2018). *Use of Yoga, Meditation, and Chiropractors Among U.S. Adults Aged 18 and Over*. Retrieved August 24, 2020 from www.cdc.gov/nchs/data/databriefs/db325-h.pdf.

54 Vieten, C., Wahbeh, H., Cahn, B. R., MacLean, K., *et al.* (2018). Future directions in meditation research: Recommendations for expanding the field of contemplative science. *PloS One*, *13*(11), e0205740–e0205740.

55 Bazarko, D., Cate, R. A., Azocar, F., & Kreitzer, M. J. (2013). The impact of an innovative mindfulness-based stress reduction program on the health and well-being of nurses employed in a corporate setting. *Journal of Workplace Behavioral Health*, *28*(2), 107–133.

Gilmartin, H., Goyal, A., Hamati, M. C., Mann, J., Saint, S., & Chopra, V. (2017). Brief mindfulness practices for healthcare providers—A systematic literature review. *The American Journal of Medicine*, *130*(10), 1219.e1–1219.e17.

CHAPTER 13

1   Haase, L., Stewart, J. L., Youssef, B., May, A. C., *et al.* (2016). When the brain does not adequately feel the body: Links between low resilience and interoception. *Biological Psychology*, *113*, 37–45.

2   Kain, K. L., Levine, P. A., & Terrell, S. J. (2018). *Nurturing Resilience: Helping Clients Move Forward From Developmental Trauma*. Berkeley, CA: North Atlantic Books.

3   Google Books Ngram Viewer. (n.d.) *Sensation*. Retrieved August 24, 2020 from <iframe name="ngram_chart" src="https://books.google.com/ngrams/interactive_chart?content=Sensation&year_start=1800&year_end=2000&corpus=15&smoothing=3&share=&direct_url=t1%3B%2CSensation%3B%2Cc0" width=900 height=500 marginwidth=0 marginheight=0 hspace=0 vspace=0 frameborder=0 scrolling=no></iframe>.

4   Wiktionary. (n.d.). *Sensatio*. Retrieved August 24, 2020 from https://en.wiktionary.org/wiki/sensatio.

5   Dunn, W. (2009). *Living Sensationally: Understanding Your Senses*. London; Philadelphia: Jessica Kingsley Publishers. p.18.

6   Greven, C. U., Lionetti, F., Booth, C., Aron, E. N., et al. (2019). Sensory processing sensitivity in the context of environmental sensitivity: A critical review and development of research agenda. *Neuroscience & Biobehavioral Reviews*, *98*, 287–305.

7   Moore, K. (2005). *The Sensory Connection Program*. Farmington, MA: Therapro Inc. p.7.

8   Khalsa, S. S., Adolphs, R., Cameron, O. G., Critchley, H. D., *et al.* (2018). Interoception and mental health: A roadmap. *Biological Psychiatry. Cognitive Neuroscience and Neuroimaging*, *3*(6), 501–513.

Chick, C. F., Rounds, J. D., Hill, A. B., & Anderson, A. K. (2019). My body, your emotions: Viscerosomatic modulation of facial expression discrimination. *Biological Psychology*, 107779.

Gao, Q., Ping, X., & Chen, W. (2019). Body influences on social cognition through interoception. *Frontiers in Psychology*, *10*, 2066.

9   Calì, G., Ambrosini, E., Picconi, L., Mehling, W. E., & Committeri, G. (2015). Investigating the relationship between interoceptive accuracy, interoceptive awareness, and emotional susceptibility. *Frontiers in Psychology*, *6*, 1202–1202.

de Jong, M., Lazar, S. W., Hug, K., Mehling, W. E., *et al.* (2016). Effects of mindfulness-based cognitive therapy on body awareness in patients with chronic pain and comorbid depression. *Frontiers in Psychology*, *7*, 967–967.

10 Hanley, A. W., Mehling, W. E., & Garland, E. L. (2017). Holding the body in mind: Interoceptive awareness, dispositional mindfulness and psychological well-being. *Journal of Psychosomatic Research*, *99*, 13–20.

11 Talbot, K., Madden, V. J., Jones, S. L., & Moseley, G. L. (2019). The sensory and affective components of pain: Are they differentially modifiable dimensions or inseparable aspects of a unitary experience? A systematic review. *British Journal of Anaesthesia*, *123*(2), e263–e272.

12 Nummenmaa, L., Glerean, E., Hari, R., & Hietanen, J. K. (2014). Bodily maps of emotions. *Proceedings of the National Academy of Sciences*, *111*(2), 646.

Nummenmaa, L., Hari, R., Hietanen, J. K., & Glerean, E. (2018). Maps of subjective feelings. *Proceedings of the National Academy of Sciences of the United States of America*, *115*(37), 9198–9203.

13 Carter, L. & Ogden, J. (2020). Evaluating interoceptive crossover between emotional and physical symptoms. *Psychology, Health & Medicine*, 1–10.

14 Stern, E. R., Grimaldi, S. J., Muratore, A., Murrough, J., *et al.* (2017). Neural correlates of interoception: Effects of interoceptive focus and relationship to dimensional measures of body awareness. *Human Brain Mapping*, *38*(12), 6068–6082.

Farb, N., Daubenmier, J., Price, C. J., Gard, T., *et al.* (2015). Interoception, contemplative practice, and health. *Frontiers in Psychology*, *6*, 763.

Muehsam, D., Lutgendorf, S., Mills, P. J., Rickhi, B., *et al.* (2017). The embodied mind: A review on functional genomic and neurological correlates of mind-body therapies. *Neuroscience and Biobehavioral Reviews*, *73*, 165–181.

15 Carter & Ogden (2020).

Adolfi, F., Couto, B., Richter, F., Decety, J., *et al.* (2017). Convergence of interoception, emotion, and social cognition: A twofold fMRI meta-analysis and lesion approach. *Cortex*, *88*, 124–142.

Garfinkel, S. N. & Critchley, H. D. (2013). Interoception, emotion and brain: New insights link internal physiology to social behaviour. Commentary on: "Anterior insular cortex mediates bodily sensibility and social anxiety" by Terasawa *et al.* (2012). *Social Cognitive and Affective Neuroscience*, *8*(3), 231–234.

16 Craig, A. D. (2015). *How Do You Feel? An Interoceptive Moment with Your Neurobiological Self*. Princeton, NJ: Princeton University Press.

17 Porges, S. W. (2004). Neuroception: A subconscious system for detecting threats and safety. *Zero Three*, *24*, 19–24.

18 Fittipaldi, S., Abrevaya, S., Fuente, A. de la, Pascariello, G. O., *et al.* (2020). A multidimensional and multi-feature framework for cardiac interoception. *NeuroImage*, 116677.

19 Dunn, B. D., Galton, H. C., Morgan, R., Evans, D., *et al.* (2010). Listening to your heart: How interoception shapes emotion experience and intuitive decision making. *Psychological Science*, *21*(12), 1835–1844.

20 Celikel, F. C. & Saatcioglu, O. (2006). Alexithymia and anxiety in female chronic pain patients. *Annals of General Psychiatry*, *5*(1), 13.

Lumley, M. A., Smith, J. A., & Longo, D. J. (2002). The relationship of alexithymia to pain severity and impairment among patients with chronic myofascial pain: Comparisons with self-efficacy, catastrophizing, and depression. *Journal of Psychosomatic Research*, *53*(3), 823–830.

Saariaho, A. S., Saariaho, T. H., Mattila, A. K., Karukivi, M. R., & Joukamaa, M. I. (2013). Alexithymia and depression in a chronic pain patient sample. *General Hospital Psychiatry*, *35*(3), 239–245.

Herbert, B. M., Herbert, C., & Pollatos, O. (2011). On the relationship between interoceptive awareness and alexithymia: Is interoceptive awareness related to emotional awareness? *Journal of Personality*, *79*(5), 1149–1175.

Van der Maas, L. C. C., Köke, A., Pont, M., Bosscher, R. J., *et al.* (2015). Improving the multidisciplinary treatment of chronic pain by stimulating body awareness: A cluster-randomized trial. *The Clinical Journal of Pain*, *31*(7), 660–669.

Schabrun, S. M., Elgueta-Cancino, E. L., & Hodges, P. W. (2017). Smudging of the motor cortex is related to the severity of low back pain. *Spine*, *42*(15), 1172–1178.

Senkowski, D. & Heinz, A. (2016). Chronic pain and distorted body image: Implications for multisensory feedback interventions. *Neuroscience and Biobehavioral Reviews*, *69*, 252–259.

Moseley, G. L. (2008). I can't find it! Distorted body image and tactile dysfunction in patients with chronic back pain. *Pain*, *140*(1), 239–243.

Lotze, M. & Moseley, G. L. (2007). Role of distorted body image in pain. *Current Rheumatology Reports*, *9*(6), 488–496.

Kuehn, E. & Pleger, B. (2018). How visual body perception influences somatosensory plasticity. *Neural Plasticity*, *2018*, 7909684–7909684.

Pleger, B., Draganski, B., Schwenkreis, P., Lenz, M., *et al.* (2014). Complex regional pain syndrome type I affects brain structure in prefrontal and motor cortex. *PloS One*, *9*(1), e85372–e85372.

21 Lesser, I. M. (1981). A review of the alexithymia concept. *Psychosomatic Medicine*, *43*(6), 531–543.

Luminet, O., Bagby, R. M., & Taylor, G. J. (Eds) (2018). *Alexithymia: Advances in Research, Theory, and Clinical Practice*. Cambridge; New York: Cambridge University Press.

22 Landsman-Dijkstra, J. J. A., van Wijck, R., Groothoff, J. W., & Rispens, P. (2004). The short-term effects of a body awareness program: Better self-management of health problems for individuals with chronic a-specific psychosomatic symptoms. *Patient Education and Counseling*, *55*(2), 155–167.

Gyllensten, A. L., Hansson, L., & Ekdahl, C. (2003). Outcome of basic body awareness therapy. A randomized controlled study of patients in psychiatric outpatient care. *Advances in Physiotherapy*, *5*(4), 179–190.

Gyllensten, A. L. & Gard, G. (2018). Best Practice: Basic Body Awareness Therapy—Evidence and Experiences. In M. Probst & H. Skjaerven (Eds) *Physiotherapy in Mental Health and Psychiatry—A Scientific and Clinical-Based Approach*. London: Elsevier.

23 Mehling, W. E., Wrubel, J., Daubenmier, J. J., Price, C. J., *et al.* (2011). Body awareness: A phenomenological inquiry into the common ground of mind-body therapies. *Philosophy, Ethics, and Humanities in Medicine: PEHM*, *6*, 6.

24 Felitti, V. J. & Anda, R. F. (2014). The Lifelong Effects of Adverse Childhood Experiences. In R. Alexander & D. Esernio-Jenssen (Eds) *Chadwick's Child Maltreatment: Sexual Abuse & Psychological Maltreatment, Encyclopedic* (Fourth edition, Volume 2). Florissant, MO: STM Learning, Inc.

25 Woods-Jaeger, B. A., Cho, B., Sexton, C. C., Slagel, L., & Goggin, K. (2018). Promoting resilience: Breaking the intergenerational cycle of adverse childhood experiences. *Health Education and Behavior*, *45*(5), 772–780.

26 Kain, *et al.* (2018).

27 Bowlby, J. (2008). *A Secure Base: Clinical Applications of Attachment Theory (Routledge Classics)*. London: Routledge.

28 Schore, A. N. (2019). *The Development of the Unconscious Mind (A Norton Professional Book and the Norton Series on Interpersonal Neurobiology)* (First edition). New York: W. W. Norton.

29 Porges, S. W. (2009). The polyvagal theory: New insights into adaptive reactions of the autonomic nervous system. *Cleveland Clinic Journal of Medicine*, *76*(Suppl 2), S86–S90.

30 Porges, S. W. (2011). *The Polyvagal Theory: Neurophysiological Foundations of Emotions, Attachment, Communication, and Self-Regulation (The Norton Series on Interpersonal Neurobiology)* (First edition). New York: W. W. Norton.

31 Thayer, J. F. & Lane, R. D. (2000). A model of neurovisceral integration in emotion regulation and dysregulation. *Journal of Affective Disorders*, *61*(3), 201–216.
    Smith, R., Thayer, J. F., Khalsa, S. S., & Lane, R. D. (2017). The hierarchical basis of neurovisceral integration. *Neuroscience and Biobehavioral Reviews*, *75*, 274–296.

32 Payne, P., Levine, P. A., & Crane-Godreau, M. A. (2015). Somatic experiencing: Using interoception and proprioception as core elements of trauma therapy. *Frontiers in Psychology*, *6*, 93.

33 Ogden, P. & Fisher, J. (2015). *Sensorimotor Psychotherapy: Interventions for Trauma and Attachment*. New York: W. W. Norton. p.824.

34 Corrigan, F., Fisher, J., & Nutt, D. (2010). Autonomic dysregulation and the window of tolerance model of the effects of complex emotional trauma. *Journal of Psychopharmacology*, *25*(1), 17–25.

35 Kolacz, J. & Porges, S. W. (2018). Chronic diffuse pain and functional gastrointestinal disorders after traumatic stress: Pathophysiology through a polyvagal perspective. *Frontiers in Medicine*, *5*, 145.
    Scaer, R. C. (2001). The neurophysiology of dissociation and chronic disease. *Applied Psychophysiology and Biofeedback*, *26*(1), 73–91.
    Tracy, L. M., Ioannou, L., Baker, K. S., Gibson, S. J., Georgiou-Karistianis, N., & Giummarra, M. J. (2016). Meta-analytic evidence for decreased heart rate variability in chronic pain implicating parasympathetic nervous system dysregulation. *Pain*, *157*(1), 7–29.
    Streeter, C. C., Gerbarg, P. L., Saper, R. B., Ciraulo, D. A., & Brown, R. P. (2012). Effects of yoga on the autonomic nervous system, gamma-aminobutyric-acid, and allostasis in epilepsy, depression, and post-traumatic stress disorder. *Medical Hypotheses*, *78*(5), 571–579.
    Barakat, A., Vogelzangs, N., Licht, C. M. M., Geenen, R., *et al.* (2012). Dysregulation of the autonomic nervous system and its association with the presence and intensity of chronic widespread pain. *Arthritis Care & Research*, *64*(8), 1209–1216.
    Koenig, J. & Thayer, J. F. (2016). Sex differences in healthy human heart rate variability: A meta-analysis. *Neuroscience and Biobehavioral Reviews*, *64*, 288–310.
    Koenig, J., Jarczok, M. N., Ellis, R. J., Hillecke, T. K., & Thayer, J. F. (2014). Heart rate variability and experimentally induced pain in healthy adults: A systematic review. *European Journal of Pain*, *18*(3), 301–314.
    Koenig, J., Kemp, A. H., Beauchaine, T. P., Thayer, J. F., & Kaess, M. (2016). Depression and resting state heart rate variability in children and adolescents—A systematic review and meta-analysis. *Clinical Psychology Review*, *46*, 136–150.
    Azam, M. A., Katz, J., Mohabir, V., & Ritvo, P. (2016). Individuals with tension and migraine headaches exhibit increased heart rate variability during post-stress mindfulness meditation practice but a decrease during a post-stress control condition—A randomized, controlled experiment. *International Journal of Psychophysiology*, *110*, 66–74.
    Meeus, M., Goubert, D., De Backer, F., Struyf, F., *et al.* (2013). Heart rate variability in patients with fibromyalgia and patients with chronic fatigue syndrome: A systematic review. *Seminars in Arthritis and Rheumatism*, *43*(2), 279–287.
    Staud, R. (2008). Heart rate variability as a biomarker of fibromyalgia syndrome. *Future Rheumatology*, *3*(5), 475–483.
    Nelson, S., Simons, L. E., & Logan, D. (2018). The incidence of adverse childhood experiences (ACEs) and their association with pain-related and psychosocial impairment in youth with chronic pain. *The Clinical Journal of Pain*, *34*(5), 402–408.
    Lê-Scherban, F., Wang, X., Boyle-Steed, K. H., & Pachter, L. M. (2018). Intergenerational associations of parent adverse childhood experiences and child health outcomes. *Pediatrics*, *141*(6).
    Jones, G. T., Power, C., & Macfarlane, G. J. (2009). Adverse events in childhood and chronic widespread pain in adult life: Results from the 1958 British Birth Cohort Study. *Pain*, *143*(1–2), 92–96.
    Anda, R., Tietjen, G., Schulman, E., Felitti, V., & Croft, J. (2010). Adverse childhood experiences and frequent headaches in adults. *Headache*, *50*(9), 1473–1481.
    Felitti, V. J. (2009). Adverse childhood experiences and adult health. *Academic Pediatrics*, *9*(3), 131–132.
    Kopec, J. A. & Sayre, E. C. (2005). Stressful experiences in childhood and chronic back pain in the general population. *The Clinical Journal of Pain*, *21*(6), 478–483.
    Davis, D. A., Luecken, L. J., & Zautra, A. J. (2005). Are reports of childhood abuse related to the experience of chronic pain in adulthood? A meta-analytic review of the literature. *The Clinical Journal of Pain*, *21*(5), 398–405.
    Imbierowicz, K. & Egle, U. T. (2003). Childhood adversities in patients with fibromyalgia and somatoform pain disorder. *European Journal of Pain*, *7*(2), 113–119.

Lampe, A., Doering, S., Rumpold, G., Sölder, E., *et al.* (2003). Chronic pain syndromes and their relation to childhood abuse and stressful life events. *Journal of Psychosomatic Research, 54*(4), 361–367.

McBeth, J., Macfarlane, G. J., Benjamin, S., & Silman, A. J. (2001). Features of somatization predict the onset of chronic widespread pain: Results of a large population-based study. *Arthritis and Rheumatism, 44*(4), 940–946.

Martinez, J. C., Bajorek, E. M., & Burge, S. (n.d.). *Associations Between Adverse Childhood Experiences and Pain, Health, and Functioning in Patients with Chronic Low Back Pain.* Presented at The University of Texas Health Science Center at San Antonio. Retrieved August 24, 2020 from https://iims.uthscsa.edu/sites/iims/files/RRNet/Martinez_%20JC.pdf.

36   National Institute for the Clinical Application of Behavioral Medicine (2019). *How to Help Your Clients Understand Their Window of Tolerance [Infographic].* Retrieved January 8, 2021 from https://www.nicabm.com/trauma-how-to-help-your-clients-understand-their-window-of-tolerance.

37   Arnsten, A. F. T., Raskind, M. A., Taylor, F. B., & Connor, D. F. (2015). The effects of stress exposure on prefrontal cortex: Translating basic research into successful treatments for post-traumatic stress disorder. *Stress Resilience, 1*, 89–99.

38   Benson, H., Greenwood, M. M., & Klemchuk, H. (1975). The relaxation response: Psychophysiologic aspects and clinical applications. *The International Journal of Psychiatry in Medicine, 6*(1–2), 87–98.

39   Esterov, D. & Greenwald, B. D. (2017). Autonomic dysfunction after mild traumatic brain injury. *Brain Sciences, 7*(8).

40   Dalgleish, T., Moradi, A. R., Taghavi, M. R., Neshat-Doost, H. T., & Yule, W. (2001). An experimental investigation of hypervigilance for threat in children and adolescents with post-traumatic stress disorder. *Psychological Medicine, 31*(3), 541–547.

Kimble, M. O., Fleming, K., Bandy, C., Kim, J., & Zambetti, A. (2010). Eye tracking and visual attention to threating stimuli in veterans of the Iraq war. *Journal of Anxiety Disorders, 24*(3), 293–299.

Vythilingam, M., Blair, K. S., Mccaffrey, D., Scaramozza, M., *et al.* (2007). Biased emotional attention in post-traumatic stress disorder: A help as well as a hindrance? *Psychological Medicine, 37*(10), 1445–1455.

41   Porges, S. W. (2017). *The Pocket Guide to the Polyvagal Theory: The Transformative Power of Feeling Safe (The Norton Series on Interpersonal Neurobiology)* (First edition). New York: W. W Norton & Company.

42   Kolacz & Porges (2018).

Sullivan, M. B., Erb, M., Schmalzl, L., Moonaz, S., Noggle Taylor, J., & Porges, S. W. (2018). Yoga therapy and polyvagal theory: The convergence of traditional wisdom and contemporary neuroscience for self-regulation and resilience. *Frontiers in Human Neuroscience, 12*, 67.

43   Kolacz & Porges (2018).

Porges, S. W. & Kolacz, J. (n.d.). Neurocardiology through the Lens of the Polyvagal Theory. In R. J. Gelpi & B. Buchholz (Eds) *Neurocardiology: Pathophysiological Aspects and Clinical Implications.* Amsterdam: Elsevier.

44   Van der Maas, *et al.* (2015).

Marchi, L., Marzetti, F., Orrù, G., Lemmetti, S., *et al.* (2019). Alexithymia and psychological distress in patients with fibromyalgia and rheumatic disease. *Frontiers in Psychology, 10*, 1735.

45   de Jong, *et al.* (2016).

46   Herbert, *et al.* (2011).

Domschke, K., Stevens, S., Pfleiderer, B., & Gerlach, A. L. (2010). Interoceptive sensitivity in anxiety and anxiety disorders: An overview and integration of neurobiological findings. *Clinical Psychology Review, 30*(1), 1–11.

Aaron, R. V., Fisher, E. A., de la Vega, R., Lumley, M. A., & Palermo, T. M. (2019). Alexithymia in individuals with chronic pain and its relation to pain intensity, physical interference, depression, and anxiety: A systematic review and meta-analysis. *Pain, 160*(5).

Paulus, M. P. & Stein, M. B. (2010). Interoception in anxiety and depression. *Brain Structure and Function, 214*(5), 451–463.

Pollatos, O., Gramann, K., & Schandry, R. (2007). Neural systems connecting interoceptive awareness and feelings. *Human Brain Mapping, 28*(1), 9–18.

Avery, J. A., Drevets, W. C., Moseman, S. E., Bodurka, J., Barcalow, J. C., & Simmons, W. K. (2014). Major depressive disorder is associated with abnormal interoceptive activity and functional connectivity in the insula. *Neurostimulation Treatments for Depression, 76*(3), 258–266.

Di Lernia, D., Serino, S., & Riva, G. (2016). Pain in the body. Altered interoception in chronic pain conditions: A systematic review. *Neuroscience and Biobehavioral Reviews, 71*, 328–341.

47   Diego, M. A. & Field, T. (2009). Moderate pressure massage elicits a parasympathetic nervous system response. *International Journal of Neuroscience, 119*(5), 630–638.

CHAPTER 14

1   Achterberg, J., Dossey, B. M., & Kolkmeier, L. (1994). *Rituals of Healing: Using Imagery for Health and Wellness.* New York: Bantam Books. p.244.

2   Tusek, D. L., Church, J. M., Strong, S. A., Grass, J. A., & Fazio, V. W. (1997). Guided imagery: A significant advance in the care of patients undergoing elective colorectal surgery. *Diseases of the Colon and Rectum, 40*(2), 172–178.

3   Tusek, D. L., Cwynar, R., & Cosgrove, D. M. (1999). Effect of guided imagery on length of stay, pain and anxiety in cardiac surgery patients. *The Journal of Cardiovascular Management, 10*(2), 22–28.

4   Scherwitz, L. W., McHenry, P., & Herrero, R. (2005). Interactive guided imagery SM therapy with medical patients: Predictors of health outcomes. *The Journal of Alternative and Complementary Medicine, 11*(1), 69–83.

5   Peper, E., Gibney, K. H., & Holt, C. F. (2002). *Make Health Happen: Training Yourself to Create Wellness*. Dubuque, IA: Kendall/Hunt.

6   Daselaar, S. M., Porat, Y., Huijbers, W., & Pennartz, C. M. A. (2010). Modality-specific and modality-independent components of the human imagery system. *NeuroImage, 52*(2), 677–685.

7   Hadjibalassi, M., Lambrinou, E., Papastavrou, E., & Papathanassoglou, E. (2018). The effect of guided imagery on physiological and psychological outcomes of adult ICU patients: A systematic literature review and methodological implications. *Australian Critical Care, 31*(2), 73–86.

8   Holmes, E. A. & Mathews, A. (2010). Mental imagery in emotion and emotional disorders. *Clinical Psychology Review, 30*(3), 349–362.

9   Daselaar, *et al.* (2010).

10   *Ibid.*

11   Hadjibalassi, *et al.* (2018).

12   Charette, S., Fiola, J. L., Charest, M.-C., Villeneuve, E., *et al.* (2015). Guided imagery for adolescent post-spinal fusion pain management: A pilot study. *Pain Management Nursing, 16*(3), 211–220.
      Zech, N., Hansen, E., Bernardy, K., & Häuser, W. (2017). Efficacy, acceptability and safety of guided imagery/hypnosis in fibromyalgia—A systematic review and meta-analysis of randomized controlled trials. *European Journal of Pain, 21*(2), 217–227.
      Bernardy, K., Füber, N., Klose, P., & Häuser, W. (2011). Efficacy of hypnosis/guided imagery in fibromyalgia syndrome—A systematic review and meta-analysis of controlled trials. *BMC Musculoskeletal Disorders, 12*(1), 133.
      Kwekkeboom, K. L., Kneip, J., & Pearson, L. (2003). A pilot study to predict success with guided imagery for cancer pain. *Pain Management Nursing, 4*(3), 112–123.
      Baird, C. L., Murawski, M. M., & Wu, J. (2010). Efficacy of guided imagery with relaxation for osteoarthritis symptoms and medication intake. *Pain Management Nursing, 11*(1), 56–65.
      Chen, Y. L. & Francis, A. J. P. (2010). Relaxation and imagery for chronic, nonmalignant pain: Effects on pain symptoms, quality of life, and mental health. *Pain Management Nursing, 11*(3), 159–168.
      Posadzki, P. & Ernst, E. (2011). Guided imagery for musculoskeletal pain: A systematic review. *The Clinical Journal of Pain, 27*(7).
      Lee, C., Crawford, C., Teo, L., Spevak, C., & Active Self-Care Therapies for Pain (PACT) Working Group. (2014). An analysis of the various chronic pain conditions captured in a systematic review of active self-care complementary and integrative medicine therapies for the management of chronic pain symptoms. *Pain Medicine, 15*(Suppl 1), S96–S103.

13   Eremin, O., Walker, M. B., Simpson, E., Heys, S. D., *et al.* (2009). Immuno-modulatory effects of relaxation training and guided imagery in women with locally advanced breast cancer undergoing multimodality therapy: A randomised controlled trial. *The Breast, 18*(1), 17–25.
      Trakhtenberg, E. C. (2008). The effects of guided imagery on the immune system: A critical review. *International Journal of Neuroscience, 118*(6), 839–855.

14   O'Toole, M. S., Bovbjerg, D. H., Renna, M. E., Lekander, M., Mennin, D. S., & Zachariae, R. (2018). Effects of psychological interventions on systemic levels of inflammatory biomarkers in humans: A systematic review and meta-analysis. *Brain, Behavior, and Immunity, 74*, 68–78.

15   Loft, M. H. & Cameron, L. D. (2013). Using mental imagery to deliver self-regulation techniques to improve sleep behaviors. *Annals of Behavioral Medicine, 46*(3), 260–272.

16   Nir, Y. & Tononi, G. (2010). Dreaming and the brain: From phenomenology to neurophysiology. *Trends in Cognitive Sciences, 14*(2), 88–100.

17   Somerville, K. & Cooper, M. (2007). Using imagery to identify and characterise core beliefs in women with bulimia nervosa, dieting and non-dieting women. *Eating Behaviors, 8*(4), 450–456.

18   Roffe, L., Schmidt, K., & Ernst, E. (2005). A systematic review of guided imagery as an adjuvant cancer therapy. *Psycho-Oncology, 14*(8), 607–617.
      Freeman, L., Cohen, L., Stewart, M., White, R., *et al.* (2008). The experience of imagery as a post-treatment intervention in patients with breast cancer: Program, process, and patient recommendations. *Oncology Nursing Forum, 35*(6), E116–121.
      Watanabe, E., Fukuda, S., Hara, H., Maeda, Y., Ohira, H., & Shirakawa, T. (2006). Differences in relaxation by means of guided imagery in a healthy community sample. *Alternative Therapies in Health and Medicine, 12*(2), 60–66.
      Yoo, H. J., Ahn, S. H., Kim, S. B., Kim, W. K., & Han, O. S. (2005). Efficacy of progressive muscle relaxation training and guided imagery in reducing chemotherapy side effects in patients with breast cancer and in improving their quality of life. *Supportive Care in Cancer, 13*(10), 826–833.

19   Kwekkeboom, K. L. & Bratzke, L. C. (2016). A systematic review of relaxation, meditation, and guided imagery strategies for symptom management in heart failure. *The Journal of Cardiovascular Nursing, 31*(5), 457–468.

20   Zach, S., Dobersek, U., Filho, E., Inglis, V., & Tenenbaum, G. (2018). A meta-analysis of mental imagery effects on post-injury functional mobility, perceived pain, and self-efficacy. *Psychology of Sport and Exercise, 34*, 79–87.

21 Jacobson, A. F., Umberger, W. A., Palmieri, P. A., Alexander, T. S., *et al.* (2016). Guided imagery for total knee replacement: A randomized, placebo-controlled pilot study. *The Journal of Alternative and Complementary Medicine, 22*(7), 563–575.

22 Casement, M. D. & Swanson, L. M. (2012). A meta-analysis of imagery rehearsal for post-trauma nightmares: Effects on nightmare frequency, sleep quality, and posttraumatic stress. *Clinical Psychology Review, 32*(6), 566–574.

23 Apóstolo, J. L. A. & Kolcaba, K. (2009). The effects of guided imagery on comfort, depression, anxiety, and stress of psychiatric inpatients with depressive disorders. *Archives of Psychiatric Nursing, 23*(6), 403–411.

24 Muse, K., McManus, F., Hackmann, A., Williams, M., & Williams, M. (2010). Intrusive imagery in severe health anxiety: Prevalence, nature and links with memories and maintenance cycles. *Behaviour Research and Therapy, 48*(8), 792–798.

25 Conroy, D. & Hagger, M. S. (2018). Imagery interventions in health behavior: A meta-analysis. *Health Psychology, 37*(7), 668–679.

26 Freeman, M., Ayers, C., Kondo, K., Noonan, K., *et al.* (2019). *Guided Imagery, Biofeedback, and Hypnosis: A Map of the Evidence.* Retrieved August 24, 2020 from www.hsrd.research.va.gov/publications/esp/guided-imagery.pdf.

27 Hétu, S., Grégoire, M., Saimpont, A., Coll, M.-P., *et al.* (2013). The neural network of motor imagery: An ALE meta-analysis. *Neuroscience and Biobehavioral Reviews, 37*(5), 930–949.
Bowering, K. J., O'Connell, N. E., Tabor, A., Catley, M. J., *et al.* (2013). The effects of graded motor imagery and its components on chronic pain: A systematic review and meta-analysis. *The Journal of Pain, 14*(1), 3–13.

28 Zimmermann-Schlatter, A., Schuster, C., Puhan, M. A., Siekierka, E., & Steurer, J. (2008). Efficacy of motor imagery in post-stroke rehabilitation: A systematic review. *Journal of NeuroEngineering and Rehabilitation, 5*(1), 8.
Pichiorri, F., Morone, G., Petti, M., Toppi, J., *et al.* (2015). Brain-computer interface boosts motor imagery practice during stroke recovery. *Annals of Neurology, 77*(5), 851–865.
Ietswaart, M., Johnston, M., Dijkerman, H. C., Joice, S., *et al.* (2011). Mental practice with motor imagery in stroke recovery: Randomized controlled trial of efficacy. *Brain, 134*(5), 1373–1386.
Im, H., Ku, J., Kim, H. J., & Kang, Y. J. (2016). Virtual reality-guided motor imagery increases corticomotor excitability in healthy volunteers and stroke patients. *Annals of Rehabilitation Medicine, 40*(3), 420–431.
Alves, S. S., Ocamoto, G. N., de Camargo, P. S., Santos, A. T. S., & Terra, A. M. S. V. (2018). Effects of virtual reality and motor imagery techniques using Fugl Meyer Assessment scale in post-stroke patients. *International Journal of Therapy and Rehabilitation, 25*(11), 587–596.
Johnson, N. N., Carey, J., Edelman, B. J., Doud, A., *et al.* (2018). Combined rTMS and virtual reality brain–computer interface training for motor recovery after stroke. *Journal of Neural Engineering, 15*(1), 016009.

29 Moseley, G. L. (Ed.) (2012). *The Graded Motor Imagery Handbook.* Adelaide: Noigroup Publ.

30 Eaves, D. L., Riach, M., Holmes, P. S., & Wright, D. J. (2016). Motor imagery during action observation: A brief review of evidence, theory and future research opportunities. *Frontiers in Neuroscience, 10*, 514.

CHAPTER 15

1 Finocchiaro, M. S. & Schmitz, C. L. (1984). Exercise: A holistic approach for the treatment of the adolescent psychiatric patient. *Issues in Mental Health Nursing, 6*(3–4), 237–243.

2 Debarnot, U., Sperduti, M., Di Rienzo, F., & Guillot, A. (2014). Experts bodies, experts minds: How physical and mental training shape the brain. *Frontiers in Human Neuroscience, 8.*

3 Lewthwaite, R. (2010). Grand challenge for movement science and sport psychology: Embracing the social-cognitive–affective–motor nature of motor behavior. *Frontiers in Psychology, 1.*

4 Davis, J. I. & Markman, A. B. (2012). Embodied cognition as a practical paradigm: Introduction to the topic, the future of embodied cognition. *Topics in Cognitive Science, 4*(4), 685–691.
Koziol, L. F., Budding, D. E., & Chidekel, D. (2012). From movement to thought: Executive function, embodied cognition, and the cerebellum. *The Cerebellum, 11*(2), 505–525.

5 Wolpert, D. (n.d.). *The Real Reason for Brains.* In D. Wolpert (2011). *The Real Reason for Brains* [Video file]. Retrieved August 24, 2020 from www.ted.com/talks/daniel_wolpert_the_real_reason_for_brains?language=en.

6 Fuchs, T. & Koch, S. C. (2014). Embodied affectivity: On moving and being moved. *Frontiers in Psychology, 5.*

7 Zacharatos, H., Gatzoulis, C., & Chrysanthou, Y. L. (2014). Automatic emotion recognition based on body movement analysis: A survey. *IEEE Computer Graphics and Applications, 34*, 35–45.

8 Darwin, C. (1872). *The Expression of the Emotions in Man and Animals* (Neudr. Bruxelles, 1969). London: Murray.

9 Shafir, T., Tsachor, R. P., & Welch, K. B. (2016). Emotion regulation through movement: Unique sets of movement characteristics are associated with and enhance basic emotions. *Frontiers in Psychology, 6.*
Liao, Y., Shonkoff, E. T., & Dunton, G. F. (2015). The acute relationships between affect, physical feeling states, and physical activity in daily life: A review of current evidence. *Frontiers in Psychology, 6*, 1975.

10 Kolář, P. & Andelova, V. (2013). *Clinical Rehabilitation.* Prague: Rehabilitation Prague School.

11   Bartenieff, I. & Lewis, D. (1980). *Body Movement: Coping with the Environment*. New York: Gordon and Breach Science Publishers.
     Tsachor, R. P. & Shafir, T. (2017). A somatic movement approach to fostering emotional resiliency through Laban Movement Analysis. *Frontiers in Human Neuroscience, 11*, 410.

12   Penedo, F. J. & Dahn, J. R. (2005). Exercise and well-being: A review of mental and physical health benefits associated with physical activity. *Current Opinion in Psychiatry, 18*(2), 189–193.

13   Dum, R. P., Levinthal, D. J., & Strick, P. L. (2016). Motor, cognitive, and affective areas of the cerebral cortex influence the adrenal medulla. *Proceedings of the National Academy of Sciences, 113*(35), 9922–9927.

14   Kasai, T. (2016). Fluid retention and rostral fluid shift in sleep-disordered breathing. *Current Hypertension Reviews, 12*(1), 32–42.

15   Penedo & Dahn (2005).

16   Debarnot, *et al.* (2014).
     Dayan, E. & Cohen, L. G. (2011). Neuroplasticity subserving motor skill learning. *Neuron, 72*(3), 443–454.
     Desai, R., Tailor, A., & Bhatt, T. (2015). Effects of yoga on brain waves and structural activation: A review. *Complementary Therapies in Clinical Practice, 21*(2), 112–118.

17   Debarnot, *et al.* (2014).
     Davis & Markman (2012).
     Engel, A. K., Maye, A., Kurthen, M., & König, P. (2013). Where's the action? The pragmatic turn in cognitive science. *Trends in Cognitive Sciences, 17*(5), 202–209.
     Koziol, *et al.* (2012).
     Gottwald, J. M., Achermann, S., Marciszko, C., Lindskog, M., & Gredebäck, G. (2016). An embodied account of early executive-function development: Prospective motor control in infancy is related to inhibition and working memory. *Psychological Science, 27*(12), 1600–1610.
     Leisman, G., Moustafa, A., & Shafir, T. (2016). Thinking, walking, talking: Integratory motor and cognitive brain function. *Frontiers in Public Health, 4*.
     Dijkstra, K. & Post, L. (2015). Mechanisms of embodiment. *Frontiers in Psychology, 6*.
     Brown, S., Martinez, M. J., & Parsons, L. M. (2005). The neural basis of human dance. *Cerebral Cortex, 16*(8), 1157–1167.
     Connors, B. L., Rende, R., & Colton, T. J. (2013). Predicting individual differences in decision-making process from signature movement styles: An illustrative study of leaders. *Frontiers in Psychology, 4*, 658.
     Wheeler, M. J., Green, D. J., Ellis, K. A., Cerin, E., *et al.* (2019). Distinct effects of acute exercise and breaks in sitting on working memory and executive function in older adults: A three-arm, randomised cross-over trial to evaluate the effects of exercise with and without breaks in sitting on cognition. *British Journal of Sports Medicine, 54*(13), 776.
     Moser, M.-B., Rowland, D. C., & Moser, E. I. (2015). Place cells, grid cells, and memory. *Cold Spring Harbor Perspectives in Biology, 7*(2), a021808.
     Adami, R., Pagano, J., Colombo, M., Platonova, N., *et al.* (2018). Reduction of movement in neurological diseases: Effects on neural stem cells characteristics. *Frontiers in Neuroscience, 12*, 336.

18   Tunçgenç, B. & Cohen, E. (2016). Movement synchrony forges social bonds across group divides. *Frontiers in Psychology, 7*.
     Tomei, A. & Grivel, J. (2014). Body posture and the feeling of social closeness: An exploratory study in a naturalistic setting. *Current Psychology, 33*(1), 35–46.

19   Young, I. M. (1980). Throwing like a girl: A phenomenology of feminine body comportment motility and spatiality. *Human Studies, 3*(1), 137–156.

20   Melzer, A., Shafir, T., & Tsachor, R. P. (2019). How do we recognize emotion from movement? Specific motor components contribute to the recognition of each emotion. *Frontiers in Psychology, 10*.

21   Chinellato, E., Castiello, U., & Sartori, L. (2015). Motor interference in interactive contexts. *Frontiers in Psychology, 6*.
     Giudice, M. D., Manera, V., & Keysers, C. (2009). Programmed to learn? The ontogeny of mirror neurons. *Developmental Science, 12*(2), 350–363.

22   Shafir, *et al.* (2016).
     Tsachor & Shafir (2017).
     Damasio, A. R. (1999). *The Feeling of What Happens: Body and Emotion in the Making of Consciousness* (Vol. 1). New York: Harcourt Brace.
     Damasio, A. & Carvalho, G. B. (2013). The nature of feelings: Evolutionary and neurobiological origins. *Nature Reviews Neuroscience, 14*(2), 143–152.
     Damasio, A. R., Grabowski, T. J., Bechara, A., Damasio, H., *et al.* (2000). Subcortical and cortical brain activity during the feeling of self-generated emotions. *Nature Neuroscience, 3*(10), 1049–1056.
     James, W. (1884). What is an emotion? *Mind, 9*(34), 188–205.
     Michalak, J., Troje, N. F., Fischer, J., Vollmar, P., Heidenreich, T., & Schulte, D. (2009). Embodiment of sadness and depression-gait patterns associated with dysphoric mood. *Psychosomatic Medicine, 71*(5), 580–587.
     Venture, G., Kadone, H., Zhang, T., Grèzes, J., Berthoz, A., & Hicheur, H. (2014). Recognizing emotions conveyed by human gait. *International Journal of Social Robotics, 6*(4), 621–632.

23 Pekrun, R., Elliot, A. J., & Maier, M. A. (2009). Achievement goals and achievement emotions. *Journal of Educational Psychology, 101*(1), 115–135.

24 Wikström-Grotell, C. & Eriksson, K. (2012). Movement as a basic concept in physiotherapy—A human science approach. *Physiotherapy Theory and Practice, 28*(6), 428–438.

25 Lewthwaite (2010).

26 Guéguen, N., Meineri, S., & Charles-Sire, V. (2010). Improving medication adherence by using practitioner nonverbal techniques: A field experiment on the effect of touch. *Journal of Behavioral Medicine, 33*(6), 466–473.

27 Aveyard, B., Sykes, M., & Doherty, D. (2002). Therapeutic touch in dementia care. *Nursing Older People, 14*.
    McCann, K. & McKenna, H. P. (1993). An examination of touch between nurses and elderly patients in a continuing care setting in Northern Ireland. *Journal of Advanced Nursing, 18*(5), 838–846.

28 Eddy, M. (2016). *Mindful Movement: The Evolution of the Somatic Arts and Conscious Action.* Bristol: Intellect Press.

29 Grossberg, S. (2013). Adaptive resonance theory: How a brain learns to consciously attend, learn, and recognize a changing world. *Neural Networks, 37*, 1–47.

30 Ogden, P. (2015). *Sensorimotor Psychotherapy: Interventions for Trauma and Attachment (Norton Series on Interpersonal Neurobiology).* New York: W. W. Norton.

31 Kroll, H. (2017). *Keynote: Forging Pathways, Alexander Technique and Pain.* Presented at the Alexander Technique International Annual Meeting, Islandwood Campus, Bainbridge Island, WA.

32 Eaves, D. L., Riach, M., Holmes, P. S., & Wright, D. J. (2016). Motor imagery during action observation: A brief review of evidence, theory and future research opportunities. *Frontiers in Neuroscience, 10*.

33 Lafleur, M. F., Jackson, P. L., Malouin, F., Richards, C. L., Evans, A. C., & Doyon, J. (2002). Motor learning produces parallel dynamic functional changes during the execution and imagination of sequential foot movements. *NeuroImage, 16*(1), 142–157.
    Jackson, P. L., Lafleur, M. F., Malouin, F., Richards, C. L., & Doyon, J. (2003). Functional cerebral reorganization following motor sequence learning through mental practice with motor imagery. *NeuroImage, 20*(2), 1171–1180.

34 Debarnot, *et al.* (2014).

35 Barreto-Silva, V., Bigliassi, M., Chierotti, P., & Altimari, L. R. (2018). Psychophysiological effects of audiovisual stimuli during cycle exercise. *European Journal of Sport Science, 18*(4), 560.

36 Monticone, M., Ferrante, S., Rocca, B., Baiardi, P., Farra, F. D., & Foti, C. (2013). Effect of a long-lasting multidisciplinary program on disability and fear-avoidance behaviors in patients with chronic low back pain: Results of a randomized controlled trial. *The Clinical Journal of Pain, 29*(11), 929–938.

37 *Ibid.*
    Luque-Suarez, A., Martinez-Calderon, J., & Falla, D. (2019). Role of kinesiophobia on pain, disability and quality of life in people suffering from chronic musculoskeletal pain: A systematic review. *British Journal of Sports Medicine, 53*(9), 554–559.
    Karos, K., Meulders, A., Gatzounis, R., Seelen, H. A. M., Geers, R. P. G., & Vlaeyen, J. W. S. (2017). Fear of pain changes movement: Motor behaviour following the acquisition of pain-related fear. *European Journal of Pain, 21*(8), 1432–1442.
    Guck, T. P., Burke, R. V., Rainville, C., Hill-Taylor, D., & Wallace, D. P. (2015). A brief primary care intervention to reduce fear of movement in chronic low back pain patients. *Translational Behavioral Medicine, 5*(1), 113–121.

38 Luque-Suarez, *et al.* (2019).
    Luque-Suarez, A., Falla, D., Morales-Asencio, J. M., & Martinez-Calderon, J. (2018). Is kinesiophobia and pain catastrophising at baseline associated with chronic pain and disability in whiplash-associated disorders? A systematic review. *British Journal of Sports Medicine, 7*.
    Yahia, A., Yangui, N., Mallek, A., Ghroubi, S., & Elleuch, M. H. (2017). Kinesiophobia, functional disability and physical deconditioning evaluation in chronic low back pain. *Annals of Physical and Rehabilitation Medicine, 60*, e19–e20.
    Ishak, N. A., Zahari, Z., & Justine, M. (2017). Kinesiophobia, pain, muscle functions, and functional performances among older persons with low back pain. *Pain Research and Treatment, 20*, 3489617.

39 Butler, D. S. & Moseley, G. L. (2013). *Explain Pain.* Adelaide: NOI Group Publications.
    Leeuw, M., Goossens, M. E. J. B., Linton, S. J., Crombez, G., Boersma, K., & Vlaeyen, J. W. S. (2007). The fear-avoidance model of musculoskeletal pain: Current state of scientific evidence. *Journal of Behavioral Medicine, 30*(1), 77–94.

40 Monticone, M., Cedraschi, C., Ambrosini, E., Rocca, B., *et al.* (2015). Cognitive-behavioural treatment for subacute and chronic neck pain. *Cochrane Database of Systematic Reviews, (5)*, Art. No.: CD010664.
    Monticone, M., Ambrosini, E., Rocca, B., Cazzaniga, D., Liquori, V., & Foti, C. (2016). Group-based task-oriented exercises aimed at managing kinesiophobia improved disability in chronic low back pain. *European Journal of Pain, 20*(4), 541–551.
    Bailey, K. M., Carleton, R. N., Vlaeyen, J. W. S., & Asmundson, G. J. G. (2010). Treatments addressing pain-related fear and anxiety in patients with chronic musculoskeletal pain: A preliminary review. *Cognitive Behaviour Therapy, 39*(1), 46–63.

41 Skjaerven, L. H. (2018). Perspectives on Human Movement, the Phenomenon of Movement Quality and How to Promote Movement Quality Through Movement Awareness as Physiotherapy in Mental Health. In *Physiotherapy in Mental Health and Psychiatry: A Scientific and Clinical Based Approach* (pp.23–31). Edinburgh: Elsevier.

42 Park, J., Krause-Parello, C. A., & Barnes, C. M. (2020). A narrative review of movement-based mind-body interventions: Effects of yoga, tai chi, and qigong for back pain patients. *Holistic Nursing Practice, 34*(1).

Murillo-García, Á., Villafaina, S., Adsuar, J. C., Gusi, N., & Collado-Mateo, D. (2018). Effects of dance on pain in patients with fibromyalgia: A systematic review and meta-analysis. *Evidence-Based Complementary and Alternative Medicine,* 8709748.

Büssing, A., Ostermann, T., Lüdtke, R., & Michalsen, A. (2012). Effects of yoga interventions on pain and pain-associated disability: A meta-analysis. *The Journal of Pain, 13*(1), 1–9.

Schmalzl, L., Crane-Godreau, M. A., & Payne, P. (2014). Movement-based embodied contemplative practices: Definitions and paradigms. *Frontiers in Human Neuroscience, 8,* 205.

Woodman, J., Ballard, K., Hewitt, C., & MacPherson, H. (2018). Self-efficacy and self-care-related outcomes following Alexander Technique lessons for people with chronic neck pain in the ATLAS randomised, controlled trial. *European Journal of Integrative Medicine, 17,* 64–71.

Little, P., Lewith, G., Webley, F., Evans, M., *et al.* (2008). Randomised controlled trial of Alexander Technique lessons, exercise, and massage (ATEAM) for chronic and recurrent back pain. *BMJ, 337,* a884.

43 D'Mello, S., Dale, R., & Graesser, A. (2012). Disequilibrium in the mind, disharmony in the body. *Cognition and Emotion, 26*(2), 362–374. p.372.

44 Penedo & Dahn (2005).

Stewart, K. J., Turner, K. L., Bacher, A. C., DeRegis, J. R., *et al.* (2003). Are fitness, activity, and fatness associated with health-related quality of life and mood in older persons? *Journal of Cardiopulmonary Rehabilitation, 23*(2), 115–121.

Bartholomew, J. B., Morrison, D., & Ciccolo, J. T. (2005). Effects of acute exercise on mood and well-being in patients with major depressive disorder. *Medicine and Science in Sports and Exercise, 37*(12), 2032–2037.

Cooney, G. M., Dwan, K., Grieg, C., Lawlor, D. A., *et al.* (2013). Exercise for depression. *Cochrane Database of Systematic Reviews, 9,* CD004366.

Schuch, F. B., Vancampfort, D., Firth, J., Rosenbaum, S., *et al.* (2018). Physical activity and incident depression: A meta-analysis of prospective cohort studies. *American Journal of Psychiatry, 175*(7), 631–648.

Mather, A. S., Rodriguez, C., Guthrie, M. F., McHarg, A. M., Reid, I. C., & McMurdo, M. E. T. (2002). Effects of exercise on depressive symptoms in older adults with poorly responsive depressive disorder: Randomised controlled trial. *British Journal of Psychiatry, 180*(5), 411–415.

Teychenne, M., Abbott, G., Lamb, K. E., Rosenbaum, S., & Ball, K. (2017). Is the link between movement and mental health a two-way street? Prospective associations between physical activity, sedentary behaviour and depressive symptoms among women living in socioeconomically disadvantaged neighbourhoods. *Preventive Medicine, 102,* 72–78.

White, R. L., Babic, M. J., Parker, P. D., Lubans, D. R., Astell-Burt, T., & Lonsdale, C. (2017). Domain-specific physical activity and mental health: A meta-analysis. *American Journal of Preventive Medicine, 52*(5), 653–666.

Ackerley, R., Aimonetti, J.-M., & Ribot-Ciscar, E. (2017). Emotions alter muscle proprioceptive coding of movements in humans. *Scientific Reports, 7*(1).

Schmidt, K.-H., Beck, R., Rivkin, W., & Diestel, S. (2016). Self-control demands at work and psychological strain: The moderating role of physical fitness. *International Journal of Stress Management, 23*(3), 255–275.

Yorks, D. M., Frothingham, C. A., & Schuenke, M. D. (2017). Effects of group fitness classes on stress and quality of life of medical students. *The Journal of the American Osteopathic Association, 117*(11), e17.

Collins, A., Hill, L. E., Chandramohan, Y., Whitcomb, D., Droste, S. K., & Reul, J. M. H. (2009). Exercise improves cognitive responses to psychological stress through enhancement of epigenetic mechanisms and gene expression in the dentate gyrus. *PLoS ONE, 4*(1), e4330.

45 Skowronek, I. B. & Handler, L. (2014). Can yoga reduce symptoms of anxiety and depression? *Journal of Family Practice, 63*(7), 398–407.

Sullivan, M. B., Erb, M., Porges, S. W., Moonaz, S., Schmalzl, L., & Taylor, J. N. (2018). Yoga therapy and polyvagal theory: The convergence of traditional wisdom and contemporary neuroscience for self-regulation and resilience. *Frontiers in Human Neuroscience, 12.*

van der Kolk, B. A., Stone, L., West, J., Rhodes, A., Emerson, D., Suvak, M., & Spinazzola, J. (2014). Yoga as an adjunctive treatment for posttraumatic stress disorder: A randomized controlled trial. *The Journal of Clinical Psychiatry, 75*(6), e559–e565.

46 Levine, P. A. (2010). *In an Unspoken Voice: How the Body Releases Trauma and Restores Goodness.* Berkeley, CA: North Atlantic Books.

47 Kain, K. L., Levine, P. A., & Terrell, S. J. (2018). *Nurturing Resilience.* Berkeley, CA: North Atlantic Books.

48 Herman, J. L. (1997). *Trauma and Recovery* (Revised edition). New York: Basic Books.

49 Cohen, R. L. (1981). On the generality of some memory laws. *Scandinavian Journal of Psychology, 22*(1), 267–281.

Madan, C. R. & Singhal, A. (2012). Using actions to enhance memory: Effects of enactment, gestures, and exercise on human memory. *Frontiers in Psychology, 3.*

50 Morsella, E. & Krauss, R. M. (2004). The role of gestures in spatial working memory and speech. *The American Journal of Psychology, 117*(3), 411–424.

51 Kelly, S. D., Barr, D. J., Church, R. B., & Lynch, K. (1999). Offering a hand to pragmatic understanding: The role of speech and gesture in comprehension and memory. *Journal of Memory and Language, 40*(4), 577–592.

Thompson, L. A. (1995). Encoding and memory for visible speech and gestures. *Psychology and Aging, 10*(2), 215–228.

Cook, S. W., Yip, T. K., & Goldin-Meadow, S. (2010). Gesturing makes memories that last. *Journal of Memory and Language, 63*(4), 465–475.

Cook, S. W., Yip, T. K., & Goldin-Meadow, S. (2012). Gestures, but not meaningless movements, lighten working memory load when explaining math. *Language and Cognitive Processes, 27*(4), 594.

52 Moser, *et al.* (2015).

53 Sleiman, S. F., Henry, J., Al-Haddad, R., Hayek, L. E., *et al.* (n.d.). Exercise promotes the expression of brain derived neurotrophic factor (BDNF) through the action of the ketone body b-hydroxybutyrate. *Cell Biology, 21.*

54 Maejima, H., Ninuma, S., Okuda, A., Inoue, T., & Hayashi, M. (2018). Exercise and low-level GABAA receptor inhibition modulate locomotor activity and the expression of BDNF accompanied by changes in epigenetic regulation in the hippocampus. *Neuroscience Letters, 685,* 18–23.

van Praag, H., Kempermann, G., & Gage, F. H. (1999). Running increases cell proliferation and neurogenesis in the adult mouse dentate gyrus. *Nature Neuroscience, 2*(3), 266–270.

van Praag, H., Christie, B. R., Sejnowski, T. J., & Gage, F. H. (1999). Running enhances neurogenesis, learning, and long-term potentiation in mice. *Proceedings of the National Academy of Sciences, 96*(23), 13427–13431.

Moon, H. Y., Becke, A., Berron, D., Becker, B., *et al.* (2016). Running-induced systemic cathepsin B secretion is associated with memory function. *Cell Metabolism, 24*(2), 332–340.

55 Carey, J. R., Bhatt, E., & Nagpal, A. (2005). Neuroplasticity promoted by task complexity. *Exercise and Sport Sciences Reviews, 33*(1), 8.

Muir, A. L. & Jones, L. M. (2009). Is neuroplasticity promoted by task complexity? *New Zealand Journal of Physiotherapy, 37,* 3.

56 Debarnot, *et al.* (2014).

Dayan & Cohen (2011).

57 Fisher, B. E., Petzinger, G. M., Nixon, K., Hogg, E., *et al.* (2004). Exercise-induced behavioral recovery and neuroplasticity in the 1-methyl-4-phenyl-1,2,3,6-tetrahydropyridine-lesioned mouse basal ganglia. *Journal of Neuroscience Research, 77*(3), 378–390.

Fisher, B. E., Li, Q., Nacca, A., Salem, G. J., *et al.* (2013). Treadmill exercise elevates striatal dopamine D2 receptor binding potential in patients with early Parkinson's disease. *NeuroReport, 24*(10), 509–514.

Choi, S. H., Bylykbashi, E., Chatila, Z. K., Lee, S. W., *et al.* (2018). Combined adult neurogenesis and BDNF mimic exercise effects on cognition in an Alzheimer's mouse model. *Science, 361*(6406), eaan8821.

58 Williams, D. M., Dunsiger, S., Jennings, E. G., & Marcus, B. H. (2012). Does affective valence during and immediately following a 10-min walk predict concurrent and future physical activity? *Annals of Behavioral Medicine, 44*(1), 43–51.

Teixeira, P. J., Carraça, E. V., Markland, D., Silva, M. N., & Ryan, R. M. (2012). Exercise, physical activity, and self-determination theory: A systematic review. *International Journal of Behavioral Nutrition and Physical Activity, 9,* 78.

59 Rhodes, R. E. & Dickau, L. (2012). Experimental evidence for the intention-behavior relationship in the physical activity domain: A meta-analysis. *Health Psychology, 31*(6), 724–727.

60 Forrest, L. N., Smith, A. R., Fussner, L. M., Dodd, D. R., & Clerkin, E. M. (2016). Using implicit attitudes of exercise importance to predict explicit exercise dependence symptoms and exercise behaviors. *Psychology of Sport and Exercise, 22,* 91–97.

61 Conroy, D. E., Hyde, A. L., Doerksen, S. E., & Ribeiro, N. F. (2010). Implicit attitudes and explicit motivation prospectively predict physical activity. *Annals of Behavioral Medicine, 39*(2), 112–118.

62 Ekelund, U., Steene-Johannessen, J., Brown, W. J., Fagerland, M. W., *et al.* (2016). Does physical activity attenuate, or even eliminate, the detrimental association of sitting time with mortality? A harmonised meta-analysis of data from more than 1 million men and women. *The Lancet, 388*(10051), 1302–1310.

Rosenbaum, S., Tiedemann, A., Sherrington, C., Curtis, J., & Ward, P. B. (2014). Physical activity interventions for people with mental illness: A systematic review and meta-analysis. *The Journal of Clinical Psychiatry, 75*(9), 964–974.

63 Jenkins, E. M., Nairn, L. N., Skelly, L. E., Little, J. P., & Gibala, M. J. (2019). Do stair climbing exercise "snacks" improve cardiorespiratory fitness? *Applied Physiology, Nutrition, and Metabolism, 44*(6), 681–684.

64 Adami, *et al.* (2018).

65 Batson, G. (2007). Revisiting overuse injuries in dance in view of motor learning and somatic models of distributed practice. *Journal of Dance Medicine and Science, 11*(3), 70–75.

66 Melzer, *et al.* (2019).

Lago-Rodríguez, A., Cheeran, B., Koch, G., Hortobágyi, T., & Fernandez-del-Olmo, M. (2014). The role of mirror neurons in observational motor learning: An integrative review. *European Journal of Human Movement, 32.* 82–103.

67 Davis, M. & Hadiks, D. (1994). Nonverbal aspects of therapist attunement. *Journal of Clinical Psychology, 50*(3), 393–405.

Macaulay, H. L., Toukmanian, S. G., & Gordon, K. M. (2007). Attunement as the core of therapist-expressed empathy. *Canadian Journal of Counselling and Psychotherapy, 41*(4).

Kojima, H., Froese, T., Oka, M., Iizuka, H., & Ikegami, T. (2017). A sensorimotor signature of the transition to conscious social perception: Co-regulation of active and passive touch. *Frontiers in Psychology, 8,* 1778.

Amighi, J. K., Loman, S., Lewis, P., & Sossin, K. M. (1999). *The Meaning of Movement: Developmental and Clinical Perspectives of the Kestenberg Movement Profile.* London: Gordon & Breach.

Allsop, J. S., Vaitkus, T., Marie, D., & Miles, L. K. (2016). Coordination and collective performance: Cooperative goals boost interpersonal synchrony and task outcomes. *Frontiers in Psychology, 7.*

Lameira, A. R., Eerola, T., & Ravignani, A. (2019). Coupled whole-body rhythmic entrainment between two chimpanzees. *Scientific Reports, 9*(1), 18914.

68   Stolper, E., van Royen, P., & Dinant, G. J. (2010). The "sense of alarm" ("gut feeling") in clinical practice. A survey among European general practitioners on recognition and expression. *European Journal of General Practice, 16*(2), 72–74.

Langridge, N., Roberts, L., & Pope, C. (2015). The clinical reasoning processes of extended scope physiotherapists assessing patients with low back pain. *Manual Therapy, 20*(6), 745–750.

69   O'Keeffe, M., Cullinane, P., Hurley, J., Leahy, I., *et al.* (2016). What influences patient-therapist interactions in musculoskeletal physical therapy? Qualitative systematic review and meta-synthesis. *Physical Therapy, 96*(5), 609–922.

70   Langridge, *et al.* (2015).

Huhn, K., Gilliland, S. J., Black, L. L., Wainwright, S. F., & Christensen, N. (2019). Clinical reasoning in physical therapy: A concept analysis. *Physical Therapy, 99*(4), 440–456.

71   Bartenieff & Lewis (1980).

Bartenieff, I. (1962). Effort observation and effort assessment in rehabilitation. *National Notation Conference.* Presented at the Dance Notation Bureau, New York.

72   Schmidt, N. B., Richey, J. A., Zvolensky, M. J., & Maner, J. K. (2008). Exploring human freeze responses to a threat stressor. *Journal of Behavior Therapy and Experimental Psychiatry, 39*(3), 292–304.

73   Knuth, A., Stewart, L. R., Brent, C., & Salerno, R. (2018). Psychological aspects of rehabilitation as perceived by physical therapists. *Journal of Physical Fitness, Medicine and Treatment in Sports, 2*(1).

74   Hara, M., Pozeg, P., Rognini, G., Higuchi, T., *et al.* (2015). Voluntary self-touch increases body ownership. *Frontiers in Psychology, 6.*

75   Spencer, L., Adams, T. B., Malone, S., Roy, L., & Yost, E. (2006). Applying the transtheoretical model to exercise: A systematic and comprehensive review of the literature. *Health Promotion Practice, 7*(4), 428–443.

CHAPTER 16

1   Chiesa, A., Serretti, A., & Jakobsen, J. C. (2013). Mindfulness: Top-down or bottom-up emotion regulation strategy? *Clinical Psychology Review, 33*(1), 82–96.

Taylor, A. G., Goehler, L. E., Galper, D. I., Innes, K. E., & Bourguignon, C. (2010). Top-down and bottom-up mechanisms in mind-body medicine: Development of an integrative framework for psychophysiological research. *Explore, 6*(1), 29.

2   Glanz, K., Rimer, B., & Viswanath, K. (2008). *Health Behavior and Health Education: Theory, Research and Practice* (Fourth edition). San Francisco, CA: Jossey-Bass.

Aron, A. R. (2007). The neural basis of inhibition in cognitive control. *The Neuroscientist, 13*(3), 214–228.

3   Watson, J. A., Ryan, C. G., Cooper, L., Ellington, D., *et al.* (2019). Pain neuroscience education for adults with chronic musculoskeletal pain: A mixed-methods systematic review and meta-analysis. *The Journal of Pain, 20*(10), 1140.e1–1140.e22. p.3.

4   *Ibid.*

Dahlhamer, J., Lucas, J., Zelaya, C., Nahin, R., *et al.* (2018). Prevalence of chronic pain and high-impact chronic pain among adults—United States, 2016. *MMWR. Morbidity and Mortality Weekly Report, 67*, 1001–1006.

5   Dahlhamer, *et al.* (2018).

6   Pitcher, M. H., Von Korff, M., Bushnell, M. C., & Porter, L. (2019). Prevalence and profile of high-impact chronic pain in the United States. *The Journal of Pain, 20*(2), 146–160.

7   Buchbinder, R., van Tulder, M., Öberg, B., Costa, L. M., *et al.* (2018). Low back pain: A call for action. *Lancet, 391*(10137), 2384–2388.

8   Pitcher, *et al.* (2019).

9   Foster, N. E., Anema, J. R., Cherkin, D., Chou, R., *et al.* (2018). Prevention and treatment of low back pain: Evidence, challenges, and promising directions. *Lancet, 391*(10137), 2368–2383.

10   Centers for Disease Control and Prevention. (2018). *Opioid Overdose.* Retrieved August 25, 2020 from www.cdc.gov/drugoverdose/data/prescribing.html.

11   Scherrer, J. F., Svrakic, D. M., Freedland, K. E., Chrusciel, T., *et al.* (2014). Prescription opioid analgesics increase the risk of depression. *Journal of General Internal Medicine, 29*(3), 491–499.

12   Gudin, J. A., Laitman, A., & Nalamachu, S. (2015). Opioid related endocrinopathy. *Pain Medicine, 16*(Suppl 1), S9–15.

13   Chu, L. F., Angst, M. S., & Clark, D. (2008). Opioid-induced hyperalgesia in humans: Molecular mechanisms and clinical considerations. *The Clinical Journal of Pain, 24*(6), 479–496.

14   Garland, E. L., Bryan, C. J., Nakamura, Y., Froeliger, B., & Howard, M. O. (2017). Deficits in autonomic indices of emotion regulation and reward processing associated with prescription opioid use and misuse. *Psychopharmacology, 234*(4), 621–629.

Stein, D. J., van Honk, J., Ipser, J., Solms, M., & Panksepp, J. (2007). Opioids: From physical pain to the pain of social isolation. *CNS Spectrums, 12*(9), 669–674.

15 Chu, *et al.* (2008).

16 Ashworth, J., Green, D. J., Dunn, K. M., & Jordan, K. P. (2013). Opioid use among low back pain patients in primary care: Is opioid prescription associated with disability at 6-month follow-up? *Pain, 154*(7), 1038–1044.
Carnide, N., Hogg-Johnson, S., Côté, P., Irvin, E., *et al.* (2017). Early prescription opioid use for musculoskeletal disorders and work outcomes. *The Clinical Journal of Pain, 33*(7), 647–658.

17 Institute of Medicine (US) Committee on Advancing Pain Research, Care, and Education. (2011). *Relieving Pain in America: A Blueprint for Transforming Prevention, Care, Education, and Research.* Retrieved August 25, 2020 from www.ncbi.nlm.nih.gov/books/NBK91497.

18 International Society for the Study of Pain. (2018). *Fact Sheet: Promoting Chronic Pain Self-Management Education.* Washington, DC: International Society for the Study of Pain.

19 Buchbinder, *et al.* (2018).

20 International Society for the Study of Pain. (2018).

21 Heathcote, L. C., Pate, J. W., Park, A. L., Leake, H. B., *et al.* (2019). Pain neuroscience education on YouTube. *PeerJ, 7*, e6603–e6603.

22 International Society for the Study of Pain. (2018). *2018 Global Year for Excellence in Pain Education: Patient Education.* Retrieved August 25, 2020 from www.iasp-pain.org/Advocacy/GYAP.aspx?ItemNumber=7066.

23 International Society for the Study of Pain. (2018). *IASP Terminology.* Retrieved August 25, 2020 from www.iasp-pain.org/Education/Content.aspx?ItemNumber=1698#Pain.

24 Galambos, A., Szabó, E., Nagy, Z., Édes, A. E., *et al.* (2019). A systematic review of structural and functional MRI studies on pain catastrophizing. *Journal of Pain Research, 12*, 1155–1178.
Marcuzzi, A., Wrigley, P. J., Dean, C. M., Graham, P. L., & Hush, J. M. (2018). From acute to persistent low back pain: A longitudinal investigation of somatosensory changes using quantitative sensory testing—An exploratory study. *Pain Reports, 3*(2).

25 Stewart, M. & Loftus, S. (2018). Sticks and stones: The impact of language in musculoskeletal rehabilitation. *Journal of Orthopaedic and Sports Physical Therapy, 48*(7), 519–522. p.519.

26 Cohen, M., Quintner, J., & van Rysewyk, S. (2018). Reconsidering the International Association for the Study of Pain definition of pain. *Pain Reports, 3*(2), e634–e634.
Treede, R.-D. (2018). The International Association for the Study of Pain definition of pain: As valid in 2018 as in 1979, but in need of regularly updated footnotes. *Pain Reports, 3*(2), e643–e643.

27 Loeser, J. (1980). Perspectives on Pain. In P. Turner, C. Padgham., & A. Hedges (Eds) *Clinical Pharmacology and Therapeutics.* London: Palgrave Macmillan.
Waddell, G. (1987). 1987 Volvo award in clinical sciences. A new clinical model for the treatment of low-back pain. *Spine, 12*(7), 632–644.
Waddell, G. (1992). Biopsychosocial analysis of low back pain. *Common Low Back Pain: Prevention of Chronicity, 6*(3), 523–557.

28 Cohen, *et al.* (2018).

29 Moayedi, M. & Davis, K. D. (2013). Theories of pain: From specificity to gate control. *Journal of Neurophysiology, 109*(1), 5–12.

30 *Ibid.*

31 Buchbinder, *et al.* (2018).

32 *Ibid.*

33 Tonosu, J., Oka, H., Higashikawa, A., Okazaki, H., Tanaka, S., & Matsudaira, K. (2017). The associations between magnetic resonance imaging findings and low back pain: A 10-year longitudinal analysis. *PloS One, 12*(11), e0188057–e0188057.

34 Buchbinder, *et al.* (2018).
Deyo, R. A., Mirza, S. K., Turner, J. A., & Martin, B. I. (2009). Overtreating chronic back pain: Time to back off? *Journal of the American Board of Family Medicine, 22*(1), 62–68.
Maher, C., Underwood, M., & Buchbinder, R. (2017). Non-specific low back pain. *Lancet, 389*(10070), 736–747.

35 Louw, A., Zimney, K., Puentedura, E. J., & Diener, I. (2016). The efficacy of pain neuroscience education on musculoskeletal pain: A systematic review of the literature. *Physiotherapy Theory and Practice, 32*(5), 332–355.

36 Louw, A. & Puentedura, E. (2013). *Therapeutic Neuroscience Education: Teaching Patients About Pain: A Guide for Clinicians.* Louisville, KY: International Spine and Pain Institute.

37 Darlow, B., Brown, M., Thompson, B., Hudson, B., *et al.* (2018). Living with osteoarthritis is a balancing act: An exploration of patients' beliefs about knee pain. *BMC Rheumatology, 2.*

38 *Ibid.*

39 Louw, A., Zimney, K., O'Hotto, C., & Hilton, S. (2016). The clinical application of teaching people about pain. *Physiotherapy Theory and Practice, 32*(5), 385–395.

40 Moayedi & Davis (2013).

41 Louw, A., Puentedura, E. J., Zimney, K., & Schmidt, S. (2016). Know pain, know gain? A perspective on pain neuroscience education in physical therapy. *The Journal of Orthopaedic and Sports Physical Therapy, 46*(3), 131–134.

42   Hashmi, J. A., Baliki, M. N., Huang, L., Baria, A. T., *et al.* (2013). Shape shifting pain: Chronification of back pain shifts brain representation from nociceptive to emotional circuits. *Brain: A Journal of Neurology, 136*(Pt 9), 2751–2768.

43   Leknes, S. & Bastian, B. (2014). The benefits of pain. *Review of Philosophy and Psychology, 5.*
     Bastian, B., Jetten, J., Hornsey, M. J., & Leknes, S. (2014). The positive consequences of pain: A biopsychosocial approach. *Personality and Social Psychology Review, 18*(3), 256–279.

44   Sternbach, R. (Ed.) (1978). *The Psychology of Pain.* New York: Raven Press.
     Mullen, P. D., Laville, E. A., Biddle, A. K., & Lorig, K. (1987). Efficacy of psychoeducational interventions on pain, depression, and disability in people with arthritis: A meta-analysis. *The Journal of Rheumatology, 14*(Suppl 15), 33–39.
     Schwartz, D. P., DeGood, D. E., & Shutty, M. S. (1985). Direct assessment of beliefs and attitudes of chronic pain patients. *Archives of Physical Medicine and Rehabilitation, 66*(12), 806–809.
     Engel, J. M. (1994). Cognitive-behavioral treatment of chronic recurrent pain. *Occupational Therapy International, 1*(2), 82–89.
     Devine, E. C. & Westlake, S. K. (1995). The effects of psychoeducational care provided to adults with cancer: Meta-analysis of 116 studies. *Oncology Nursing Forum, 22*(9), 1369–1381.
     Mulligan, K. & Newman, S. (2003). Psychoeducational interventions in rheumatic diseases: A review of papers published from September 2001 to August 2002. *Current Opinion in Rheumatology, 15*(2), 156–159.
     Hawley, D. J. (1995). Psycho-educational interventions in the treatment of arthritis. *Bailliere's Clinical Rheumatology, 9*(4), 803–823.
     Goldberg, W. (1985). A behavioral approach to managing chronic low back pain. *Canadian Family Physician Medecin de Famille Canadien, 31,* 542–545.

45   Heathcote, *et al.* (2019).

46   Louw, *et al.* (2016).

47   Heathcote, *et al.* (2019).

48   Louw & Puentedura (2013).

49   *Ibid.*

50   Stilwell, P. & Harman, K. (2019). An enactive approach to pain: Beyond the biopsychosocial model. *Phenomenology and the Cognitive Sciences, 18,* 637–665.
     Thacker, M. (2015). Is pain in the brain? *Pain and Rehabilitation, 3.*
     Dunagan, J. (2010). Politics for the neurocentric age. *Journal of Futures Studies, 15.*

51   Smart, K. M., Blake, C., Staines, A., Thacker, M., & Doody, C. (2012). Mechanisms-based classifications of musculoskeletal pain: Part 1 of 3: Symptoms and signs of central sensitisation in patients with low back (±leg) pain. *Manual Therapy, 17*(4), 336–344.

52   Moayedi & Davis (2013).

53   Smart, *et al.* (2012).

54   Albrecht, D. S., Granziera, C., Hooker, J. M., & Loggia, M. L. (2016). In vivo imaging of human neuroinflammation. *ACS Chemical Neuroscience, 7*(4), 470–483.

55   Smart, *et al.* (2012).

56   Louw, *et al.* (2016).

57   Smart, *et al.* (2012).

58   Moseley, L. (2007). Reconceptualising pain according to modern pain science. *Physical Therapy Reviews, 12,* 169–178.

59   Pinho-Ribeiro, F. A., Verri, W. A., & Chiu, I. M. (2017). Nociceptor sensory neuron-immune interactions in pain and inflammation. *Trends in Immunology, 38*(1), 5–19.
     Chapman, C. R., Tuckett, R. P., & Song, C. W. (2008). Pain and stress in a systems perspective: Reciprocal neural, endocrine, and immune interactions. *The Journal of Pain, 9*(2), 122–145.
     Drummond, P. D. (2013). Sensory-Autonomic Interactions in Health and Disease. In R. M. Buijs & D. F. Swaab (Eds) *Handbook of Clinical Neurology (Volume 117).* Amsterdam: Elsevier B.V. pp.309–319.
     Zhuo, M. (2016). Neural mechanisms underlying anxiety-chronic pain interactions. *Trends in Neurosciences, 39*(3), 136–145.
     Benarroch, E. E. (2006). Pain-autonomic interactions. *Neurological Sciences, 27*(2), s130–s133.

60   Tegner, H., Frederiksen, P., Esbensen, B. A., & Juhl, C. (2018). Neurophysiological pain education for patients with chronic low back pain: A systematic review and meta-analysis. *The Clinical Journal of Pain, 34*(8), 778–786.

61   Stewart & Loftus (2018).

62   Louw & Puentedura (2013).

63   Brinjikji, W., Luetmer, P., Comstock, B., Bresnahan, B., *et al.* (2015). Systematic literature review of imaging features of spinal degeneration in asymptomatic populations. *American Journal of Neuroradiology, 36*(4), 811–816.

64   Moayedi & Davis (2013).

65   Smart, *et al.*(2012).

66   Watson, *et al.* (2019).

67   Heathcote, *et al.* (2019).

68   Louw, *et al.* (2016).

69   Diener, I., Kargela, M., & Louw, A. (2016). Listening is therapy: Patient interviewing from a pain science perspective. *Physiotherapy Theory and Practice, 32*(5), 356–367.

70 Noijam. (2018). *Integrating Explain Pain and Cognitive Functional Therapy in Persistent Low Back Pain.* Retrieved August 25, 2020 from https://noijam.com/2018/11/29/integrating-explain-pain-and-cognitive-functional-therapy-in-persistent-low-back-pain.

71 Louw, *et al.* (2016).

72 Louw, A. (2019). *Pain Education Doesn't Work: Not By Itself.* Presented at the International Spine and Pain Institute/Evidence in Motion, July 2019.

73 Linton, S. J., Flink, I. K., & Vlaeyen, J. W. S. (2018). Understanding the etiology of chronic pain from a psychological perspective. *Physical Therapy, 98*(5), 315–324.
Main, C. J. & George, S. Z. (2011). Psychosocial influences on low back pain: Why should you care? *Physical Therapy, 91*(5), 609–613.
Nicholas, M. K., Linton, S. J., Watson, P. J., Main, C. J., & "Decade of the Flags" Working Group. (2011). Early identification and management of psychological risk factors ("yellow flags") in patients with low back pain: A reappraisal. *Physical Therapy, 91*(5), 737–753.

74 Ranjbar, N. & Erb, M. (2019). Adverse childhood experiences and trauma-informed care in rehabilitation clinical practice. *Archives of Rehabilitation Research and Clinical Translation,* 100003.

75 Keefe, F. J., Main, C. J., & George, S. Z. (2018). Advancing psychologically informed practice for patients with persistent musculoskeletal pain: Promise, pitfalls, and solutions. *Physical Therapy, 98*(5), 398–407.

76 Martinez-Calderon, J., Flores-Cortes, M., Morales-Asencio, J. M., & Luque-Suarez, A. (2020). Conservative interventions reduce fear in individuals with chronic low back pain: A systematic review. *Archives of Physical Medicine and Rehabilitation, 101*(2), 329–358.

77 Lumley, M. A. & Schubiner, H. (2019). Psychological therapy for centralized pain: An integrative assessment and treatment model. *Psychosomatic Medicine, 81*(2), 114–124.

78 Louw (2019).

79 Heathcote, *et al.* (2019).

80 Louw (2019).

81 Riley, S. P., Bialosky, J., & Coronado, R. A. (2020). Are changes in fear-avoidance beliefs and self-efficacy mediators of discharge function and pain in patients with acute and chronic low back pain? *Journal of Orthopaedic and Sports Physical Therapy,* 1–29.

82 Costal, L. da C. M., Maherl, C. G., McAuleyl, J. H., Hancockl, M. J., & Smeetsl, R. J. E. M. (2011). Self-efficacy is more important than fear of movement in mediating the relationship between pain and disability in chronic low back pain. *European Journal of Pain, 15*(2), 213–219.

83 Louw (2019).

84 Kolb, D. A. (2015). *Experiential Learning: Experience as the Source of Learning and Development* (Second edition). Upper Saddle River, NJ: Pearson Education, Inc.

85 George, S. Z., Wittmer, V. T., Fillingim, R. B., & Robinson, M. E. (2010). Comparison of graded exercise and graded exposure clinical outcomes for patients with chronic low back pain. *The Journal of Orthopaedic and Sports Physical Therapy, 40*(11), 694–704.

86 Bisra, K., Liu, Q., Nesbit, J., Salimi, F., & Winne, P. (2018). Inducing self-explanation: A meta-analysis. *Educational Psychology Review, 30,* 1–23.

87 Williams, J. J. & Lombrozo, T. (2010). The role of explanation in discovery and generalization: Evidence from category learning. *Cognitive Science, 34*(5), 776–806.

88 Louw, *et al.* (2016).

89 *Ibid.*

90 *Ibid.*

91 Davies, S., Quintner, J., Parsons, R., Parkitny, L., *et al.* (2011). Preclinic group education sessions reduce waiting times and costs at public pain medicine units. *Pain Medicine, 12*(1), 59–71.
Moreno Rodriguez, R., López, J., Garrote, I., & Goicoechea, C. (2018). Effects on self-efficacy for managing chronic pain and fatigue of rheumatoid arthritis following a group educational programme (based) on occupational therapy. *International Physical Medicine & Rehabilitation Journal, 3.*

92 Wood, L., Hendrick, P., & Quraishi, N. (2016). A systematic review of pain and disability outcomes of pain neuroscience education (PNE) in the management of chronic low back pain. *The Spine Journal, 16*(4), S51.
Malfliet, A., Kregel, J., Coppieters, I., De Pauw, R., *et al.* (2018). Effect of pain neuroscience education combined with cognition-targeted motor control training on chronic spinal pain: A randomized clinical trial. *JAMA Neurology, 75*(7), 808–817.
Nijs, J., Meeus, M., Cagnie, B., Roussel, N. A., *et al.* (2014). A modern neuroscience approach to chronic spinal pain: Combining pain neuroscience education with cognition-targeted motor control training. *Physical Therapy, 94*(5), 730–738.

93 Schemer, L., Vlaeyen, J. W. S., Doerr, J. M., Skoluda, N., *et al.* (2018). Treatment processes during exposure and cognitive-behavioral therapy for chronic back pain: A single-case experimental design with multiple baselines. *Behaviour Research and Therapy, 108,* 58–67.

94 Louw (2019).

95 *Ibid.*

96   Wood, L. & Hendrick, P. A. (2019). A systematic review and meta-analysis of pain neuroscience education for chronic low back pain: Short- and long-term outcomes of pain and disability. *European Journal of Pain*, *23*(2), 234–249.

97   Traeger, A. C., Lee, H., Hübscher, M., Skinner, I. W., *et al.* (2019). Effect of intensive patient education vs placebo patient education on outcomes in patients with acute low back pain: A randomized clinical trial. *JAMA Neurology*, *76*(2), 161–169.

98   Ecclestone, K. & Hayes, D. (2019). *The Dangerous Rise of Therapeutic Education*. London and New York: Routledge Education Classic Editions.

99   Stilwell & Harman (2019).
     Gatchel, R. J., Peng, Y. B., Peters, M. L., Fuchs, P. N., & Turk, D. C. (2007). The biopsychosocial approach to chronic pain: Scientific advances and future directions. *Psychological Bulletin*, *133*(4), 581–624.

100 Stewart & Loftus (2018). p.519.

101 *Ibid.*

102 Barsky, A. J. (2017). The iatrogenic potential of the physician's words. *JAMA*, *318*(24), 2425–2426.
     Karran, E. L., Medalian, Y., Hillier, S. L., & Moseley, G. L. (2017). The impact of choosing words carefully: An online investigation into imaging reporting strategies and best practice care for low back pain. *PeerJ*, *5*, e4151.
     Bossen, J. K. J., Hageman, M. G. J. S., King, J. D., & Ring, D. C. (2013). Does rewording MRI reports improve patient understanding and emotional response to a clinical report? *Clinical Orthopaedics and Related Research*, *471*(11), 3637–3644.

103 Louw (2019).

104 Moseley, L. & Moen, D. (n.d.). *Understanding Your Pain*. Retrieved August 25, 2020 from www.tamethebeast.org.

105 Tegner, *et al.* (2018).

CHAPTER 17

1   Butler, A. C., Chapman, J. E., Forman, E. M., & Beck, A. T. (2006). The empirical status of cognitive-behavioral therapy: A review of meta-analyses. *Clinical Psychology Review*, *26*(1), 17–31.
     David, D., Cristea, I., & Hofmann, S. G. (2018). Why cognitive behavioral therapy is the current gold standard of psychotherapy. *Frontiers in Psychiatry*, *9*, 4–4.

2   Cohen, S. R. & Mount, B. M. (2000). Pain with life-threatening illness: Its perception and control are inextricably linked with quality of life. *Pain Research and Management*, *5*, 971487.

3   O'Sullivan, P. B., Caneiro, J. P., O'Keeffe, M., Smith, A., *et al.* (2018). Cognitive functional therapy: An integrated behavioral approach for the targeted management of disabling low back pain. *Physical Therapy*, *98*(5), 408–423.
     Hodges, P. W. & Tucker, K. (2011). Moving differently in pain: A new theory to explain the adaptation to pain. *Pain*, *152*(Suppl 3), S90–98.

4   Bair, M. J., Robinson, R. L., Katon, W., & Kroenke, K. (2003). Depression and pain comorbidity: A literature review. *Archives of Internal Medicine*, *163*(20), 2433–2445.

5   Druss, B. G., Rosenheck, R. A., & Sledge, W. H. (2000). Health and disability costs of depressive illness in a major U.S. corporation. *The American Journal of Psychiatry*, *157*(8), 1274–1278.
     Currie, S. R. & Wang, J. (2004). Chronic back pain and major depression in the general Canadian population. *Pain*, *107*(1–2), 54–60.

6   Cowell, I., O'Sullivan, P., O'Sullivan, K., Poyton, R., McGregor, A., & Murtagh, G. (2018). Perceptions of physiotherapists towards the management of non-specific chronic low back pain from a biopsychosocial perspective: A qualitative study. *Musculoskeletal Science & Practice*, *38*, 113–119.
     Brunner, E., Dankaerts, W., Meichtry, A., O'Sullivan, K., & Probst, M. (2018). Physical therapists' ability to identify psychological factors and their self-reported competence to manage chronic low back pain. *Physical Therapy*, *98*(6), 471–479.
     Young, D., Callaghan, M., Hunt, C., Briggs, M., & Griffiths, J. (2019). Psychologically informed approaches to chronic low back pain: Exploring musculoskeletal physiotherapists' attitudes and beliefs. *Musculoskeletal Care*, *17*(2), 272–276.
     Synnott, A., O'Keeffe, M., Bunzli, S., Dankaerts, W., O'Sullivan, P., & O'Sullivan, K. (2015). Physiotherapists may stigmatise or feel unprepared to treat people with low back pain and psychosocial factors that influence recovery: A systematic review. *Journal of Physiotherapy*, *61*(2), 68–76.

7   Linton, S. J. & Shaw, W. S. (2011). Impact of psychological factors in the experience of pain. *Physical Therapy*, *91*(5), 700–711.

8   Denneny, D., Frijdal (nee Klapper), A., Bianchi-Berthouze, N., Greenwood, J., *et al.* (2020). The application of psychologically informed practice: Observations of experienced physiotherapists working with people with chronic pain. *Physiotherapy*, *106*, 163–173.
     Hasenbring, M. I., Fehrmann, E., & Ebenbichler, G. (2020). Embodied pain: There is a need to reflect interactions between cognitions, behavior, and neuromuscular activity in chronic pain. *The Clinical Journal of Pain*, *36*(3).

9   Holopainen, R., Simpson, P., Piirainen, A., Karppinen, J., *et al.* (2020). Physiotherapists' perceptions of learning and implementing a biopsychosocial intervention to treat musculoskeletal pain conditions: A systematic review and metasynthesis of qualitative studies. *Pain*, *161*(6), 1150–1168.

10 Öst, L.-G. (2014). The efficacy of acceptance and commitment therapy: An updated systematic review and meta-analysis. *Behaviour Research and Therapy, 61*, 105–121.
    A-Tjak, J. G. L., Davis, M. L., Morina, N., Powers, M. B., Smits, J. A. J., & Emmelkamp, P. M. G. (2015). A meta-analysis of the efficacy of acceptance and commitment therapy for clinically relevant mental and physical health problems. *Psychotherapy and Psychosomatics, 84*(1), 30–36.

11 O'Sullivan, *et al.* (2018).
    Vibe Fersum, K., O'Sullivan, P., Skouen, J. S., Smith, A., & Kvåle, A. (2013). Efficacy of classification-based cognitive functional therapy in patients with non-specific chronic low back pain: A randomized controlled trial. *European Journal of Pain, 17*(6), 916–928.

12 Gu, J., Strauss, C., Bond, R., & Cavanagh, K. (2015). How do mindfulness-based cognitive therapy and mindfulness-based stress reduction improve mental health and wellbeing? A systematic review and meta-analysis of mediation studies. *Clinical Psychology Review, 37*, 1–12.
    Parra-Delgado, M. & Latorre-Postigo, J. (2013). Effectiveness of mindfulness-based cognitive therapy in the treatment of fibromyalgia: A randomised trial. *Cognitive Therapy and Research, 37*, 1015–1026.
    de Jong, M., Lazar, S. W., Hug, K., Mehling, W. E., *et al.* (2016). Effects of mindfulness-based cognitive therapy on body awareness in patients with chronic pain and comorbid depression. *Frontiers in Psychology, 7*, 967–967.

13 Lumley, M. A., Schubiner, H., Lockhart, N. A., Kidwell, K. M., *et al.* (2017). Emotional awareness and expression therapy, cognitive behavioral therapy, and education for fibromyalgia: A cluster-randomized controlled trial. *Pain, 158*(12), 2354–2363.
    Lumley, M. A. & Schubiner, H. (2019). Psychological therapy for centralized pain: An integrative assessment and treatment model. *Psychosomatic Medicine, 81*(2), 114–124.

14 Hayes, S. C. (2019). *A Liberated Mind: How to Pivot Toward What Matters.* New York: Avery.

15 Hayes, S. C. (2016). Acceptance and commitment therapy, relational frame theory, and the third wave of behavioral and cognitive therapies—Republished article. *Special 50th Anniversary Issue: Honoring the Past and Looking to the Future: Updates on Seminal Behavior Therapy Publications on Current Therapies and Future Directions, Part II, 47*(6), 869–885.

16 Boone, M. S., Mundy, B., Morrissey Stahl, K., & Genrich, B. E. (2015). Acceptance and commitment therapy, functional contextualism, and clinical social work. *Journal of Human Behavior in the Social Environment, 25*(6), 643–656.

17 McCracken, L. M. & Vowles, K. E. (2014). Acceptance and commitment therapy and mindfulness for chronic pain: Model, process, and progress. *American Psychologist, 69*(2), 178–187.
    Buhrman, M., Skoglund, A., Husell, J., Bergström, K., *et al.* (2013). Guided internet-delivered acceptance and commitment therapy for chronic pain patients: A randomized controlled trial. *Behaviour Research and Therapy, 51*(6), 307–315.
    Wetherell, J. L., Afari, N., Rutledge, T., Sorrell, J. T., *et al.* (2011). A randomized, controlled trial of acceptance and commitment therapy and cognitive-behavioral therapy for chronic pain. *Pain, 152*(9), 2098–2107.

18 Yıldız, E. (2020). The effects of acceptance and commitment therapy on lifestyle and behavioral changes: A systematic review of randomized controlled trials. *Perspectives in Psychiatric Care, 56*(3), 657–690.

19 Finkenauer, C., Engels, R., & Baumeister, R. (2005). Parenting behaviour and adolescent behavioural and emotional problems: The role of self-control. *International Journal of Behavioral Development, 29*(1), 58–69. pp.58–59.

20 Converse, B. A., Juarez, L., & Hennecke, M. (2019). Self-control and the reasons behind our goals. *Journal of Personality and Social Psychology, 116*(5), 860–883.

21 *Ibid.*

22 Hennecke, M., Czikmantori, T., & Brandstätter, V. (2018). Doing despite disliking: Self-regulatory strategies in everyday aversive activities. *European Journal of Personality, 33*(1), 104–128.

23 *Ibid.*

24 Lutz, A., Jha, A. P., Dunne, J. D., & Saron, C. D. (2015). Investigating the phenomenological matrix of mindfulness-related practices from a neurocognitive perspective. *The American Psychologist, 70*(7), 632–658.

25 Russek, L. & McManus, C. (2015). A practical guide to integrating behavioral and psychologically informed approaches into physical therapist management of patients with chronic pain. *Orthopaedic Practice, 27*(1), 8–16.

26 Khoo, E.-L., Small, R., Cheng, W., Hatchard, T., *et al.* (2019). Comparative evaluation of group-based mindfulness-based stress reduction and cognitive behavioural therapy for the treatment and management of chronic pain: A systematic review and network meta-analysis. *Evidence Based Mental Health, 22*(1), 26.

27 Torre, J. B. & Lieberman, M. D. (2018). Putting feelings into words: Affect labeling as implicit emotion regulation. *Emotion Review, 10*(2), 116–124.

28 *Ibid.*
    Bushnell, M. C., Čeko, M., & Low, L. A. (2013). Cognitive and emotional control of pain and its disruption in chronic pain. *Nature Reviews Neuroscience, 14*, 502.
    Taylor, A. G., Goehler, L. E., Galper, D. I., Innes, K. E., & Bourguignon, C. (2010). Top-down and bottom-up mechanisms in mind-body medicine: Development of an integrative framework for psychophysiological research. *Explore, 6*(1), 29.

29   Wood, J. V., Elaine Perunovic, W. Q., & Lee, J. W. (2009). Positive self-statements: Power for some, peril for others. *Psychological Science*, *20*(7), 860–866.

Wood, A. M., Froh, J. J., & Geraghty, A. W. A. (2010). Gratitude and well-being: A review and theoretical integration. *Positive Clinical Psychology*, *30*(7), 890–905.

30   Benedetti, F. (2005). Neurobiological mechanisms of the placebo effect. *Journal of Neuroscience*, *25*(45), 10390–10402.

Benedetti, F. (2014). *Placebo Effects*. Oxford: Oxford University Press.

31   de Craen, A. J., Roos, P. J., de Vries, A. L., & Kleijnen, J. (1996). Effect of colour of drugs: Systematic review of perceived effect of drugs and of their effectiveness. *BMJ (Clinical Research Ed.)*, *313*(7072), 1624–1626.

32   Buckalew, L. W. & Coffield, K. E. (1982). An investigation of drug expectancy as a function of capsule color and size and preparation form. *Journal of Clinical Psychopharmacology*, *2*(4), 245–248.

33   Espay, A. J., Norris, M. M., Eliassen, J. C., Dwivedi, A., *et al.* (2015). Placebo effect of medication cost in Parkinson disease: A randomized double-blind study. *Neurology*, *84*(8), 794–802.

34   Berthelot, J.-M., Nizard, J., & Maugars, Y. (2018). The negative Hawthorne effect: Explaining pain overexpression. *Joint Bone Spine*, *86*(4), 445–449.

35   *Ibid.*

36   Burke, M. J. (2019). "It's all in your head"—Medicine's silent epidemic. *JAMA Neurology*, *76*(12), 1417–1418.

CHAPTER 18

1   Engel, G. L. (1977). The need for a new medical model: A challenge for biomedicine. *Science*, *196*(4286), 129–136.

Hiatt, J. F. (1986). Spirituality, medicine, and healing. *Southern Medical Journal*, *79*(6), 736–743.

McKee, D. D. & Chappel, J. N. (1992). Spirituality and medical practice. *The Journal of Family Practice*, *35*(2), 201, 205–208.

Sulmasy, D. P. (2002). A biopsychosocial-spiritual model for the care of patients at the end of life. *The Gerontologist*, *42*(Spec No 3), 24–33.

Taylor, L. E. V., Stotts, N. A., Humphreys, J., Treadwell, M. J., & Miaskowski, C. (2013). A biopsychosocial-spiritual model of chronic pain in adults with sickle cell disease. *Pain Management Nursing*, *14*(4), 287–301.

Puchalski, C. M., Vitillo, R., Hull, S. K., & Reller, N. (2014). Improving the spiritual dimension of whole person care: Reaching national and international consensus. *Journal of Palliative Medicine*, *17*(6), 642–656.

2   *Ibid.* p.644.

3   *Ibid.*

Koenig, H. G., McCullough, M. E., & Larson, D. B. (2001). *Handbook of Religion and Health*. Oxford; New York: Oxford University Press.

Koenig, H. G. (2012). Religion, spirituality, and health: The research and clinical implications. *ISRN Psychiatry*, *2012*, 1–33.

King, M. B. & Koenig, H. G. (2009). Conceptualising spirituality for medical research and health service provision. *BMC Health Services Research*, *9*(1).

Steinhauser, K. E., Fitchett, G., Handzo, G. F., Johnson, K. S., *et al.* (2017). State of the science of spirituality and palliative care research part I: Definitions, measurement, and outcomes. *Journal of Pain and Symptom Management*, *54*(3), 428–440.

Vaillant, G. (2008). Positive emotions, spirituality and the practice of psychiatry. *Mens Sana Monographs*, *6*(1), 48.

4   Cole, S. W., Levine, M. E., Arevalo, J. M. G., Ma, J., Weir, D. R., & Crimmins, E. M. (2015). Loneliness, eudaimonia, and the human conserved transcriptional response to adversity. *Psychoneuroendocrinology*, *62*, 11–17.

Keyes, C. L. & Simoes, E. J. (2012). To flourish or not: Positive mental health and all-cause mortality. *American Journal of Public Health*, *102*(11), 2164–2172.

Boyle, P. A., Barnes, L. L., Buchman, A. S., & Bennett, D. A. (2009). Purpose in life is associated with mortality among community-dwelling older persons. *Psychosomatic Medicine*, *71*(5), 574–579.

Krause, N. (2009). Meaning in life and mortality. *The Journals of Gerontology Series B: Psychological Sciences and Social Sciences*, *64B*(4), 517–527.

Schleicher, H., Alonso, C., Shirtcliff, E. A., Muller, D., Loevinger, B. L., & Coe, C. L. (2005). In the face of pain: The relationship between psychological well-being and disability in women with fibromyalgia. *Psychotherapy and Psychosomatics*, *74*(4), 231–239.

Dezutter, J., Casalin, S., Wachholtz, A., Luyckx, K., Hekking, J., & Vandewiele, W. (2013). Meaning in life: An important factor for the psychological well-being of chronically ill patients? *Rehabilitation Psychology*, *58*(4), 334–341.

Koizumi, M., Ito, H., Kaneko, Y., & Motohashi, Y. (2008). Effect of having a sense of purpose in life on the risk of death from cardiovascular diseases. *Journal of Epidemiology*, *18*(5), 191–196.

Alimujiang, A., Wiensch, A., Boss, J., Fleischer, N. L., *et al.* (2019). Association between life purpose and mortality among US adults older than 50 years. *JAMA Network Open*, *2*(5), e194270–e194270.

5   Koenig, *et al.* (2001).

Koenig (2012).

King & Koenig (2009).

6 Zimmer, Z., Jagger, C., Chiu, C.-T., Ofstedal, M. B., Rojo, F., & Saito, Y. (2016). Spirituality, religiosity, aging and health in global perspective: A review. *SSM: Population Health, 2*, 373–381.

Hackney, C. & Sanders, G. S. (2003). Religiosity and mental health: A meta-analysis of recent studies. *Journal for the Scientific Study of Religion, 42*(1), 43–55.

7 Ryan, R. M. & Deci, E. L. (2001). On happiness and human potentials: A review of research on hedonic and eudaimonic well-being. *Annual Review of Psychology, 52*(1), 141–166.

Huta, V. & Waterman, A. S. (2014). Eudaimonia and its distinction from hedonia: Developing a classification and terminology for understanding conceptual and operational definitions. *Journal of Happiness Studies, 15*(6), 1425–1456.

Ryff, C. D. & Keyes, C. L. (1995). The structure of psychological well-being revisited. *Journal of Personality and Social Psychology, 69*(4), 719–727.

8 Koenig, *et al.* (2001).

Koenig (2012).

Lysne, C. J. & Wachholtz, A. B. (2010). Pain, spirituality, and meaning making: What can we learn from the literature? *Religions, 2*(1), 1–16.

Nsamenang, S. A., Hirsch, J. K., Topciu, R., Goodman, A. D., & Duberstein, P. R. (2016). The interrelations between spiritual well-being, pain interference and depressive symptoms in patients with multiple sclerosis. *Journal of Behavioral Medicine, 39*(2), 355–363.

Seybold, K. S. (2007). Physiological mechanisms involved in religiosity/spirituality and health. *Journal of Behavioral Medicine, 30*(4), 303–309.

Wachholtz, A. B. & Pearce, M. J. (2009). Does spirituality as a coping mechanism help or hinder coping with chronic pain? *Current Pain and Headache Reports, 13*(2), 127–132.

Wachholtz, A. B., Pearce, M. J., & Koenig, H. (2007). Exploring the relationship between spirituality, coping, and pain. *Journal of Behavioral Medicine, 30*(4), 311–318.

Witvliet, C., Ludwig, T., & Vander Laan, K. (2001). Granting forgiveness or harboring grudges: Implications for emotion, physiology, and health. *Psychological Science, 12*(2), 117–123.

Worthington, E. L., Witvliet, C. V. O., Pietrini, P., & Miller, A. J. (2007). Forgiveness, health, and well-being: A review of evidence for emotional versus decisional forgiveness, dispositional forgivingness, and reduced unforgiveness. *Journal of Behavioral Medicine, 30*(4), 291–302.

Klimecki, O. M., Leiberg, S., Lamm, C., & Singer, T. (2013). Functional neural plasticity and associated changes in positive affect after compassion training. *Cerebral Cortex, 23*(7), 1552–1561.

Pace, T. W. W., Negi, L. T., Adame, D. D., Cole, S. P., *et al.* (2009). Effect of compassion meditation on neuroendocrine, innate immune and behavioral responses to psychosocial stress. *Psychoneuroendocrinology, 34*(1), 87–98.

Wood, A. M., Froh, J. J., & Geraghty, A. W. A. (2010). Gratitude and well-being: A review and theoretical integration. *Clinical Psychology Review, 30*(7), 890–905.

Hill, P. L., Allemand, M., & Roberts, B. W. (2013). Examining the pathways between gratitude and self-rated physical health across adulthood. *Personality and Individual Differences, 54*(1), 92–96.

Newberg, A. B. (2014). The neuroscientific study of spiritual practices. *Frontiers in Psychology, 5*, 215–215.

9 Grant & Glueck. (n.d.). *The Harvard Grant and Glueck Study.* Retrieved August 27, 2020 from www.adultdevelopmentstudy.org/grantandglueckstudy.

10 Cole, *et al.* (2015).

Keyes & Simoes (2012).

Boyle, *et al.* (2009).

Krause (2009).

Schleicher, *et al.* (2005).

Dezutter, *et al.* (2013).

Ryff, C. D. (2014). Psychological well-being revisited: Advances in the science and practice of eudaimonia. *Psychotherapy and Psychosomatics, 83*(1), 10–28.

Ryff, C. D., Singer, B. H., & Dienberg Love, G. (2004). Positive health: Connecting well-being with biology. *Philosophical Transactions of the Royal Society B: Biological Sciences, 359*(1449), 1383–1394.

Dezutter, J., Luyckx, K., & Wachholtz, A. (2015). Meaning in life in chronic pain patients over time: Associations with pain experience and psychological well-being. *Journal of Behavioral Medicine, 38*(2), 384–396.

Fredrickson, B. L., Grewen, K. M., Algoe, S. B., Firestine, A. M., *et al.* (2015). Psychological well-being and the human conserved transcriptional response to adversity. *PloS One, 10*(3), e0121839.

Fredrickson, B. L., Grewen, K. M., Coffey, K. A., Algoe, S. B., *et al.* (2013). A functional genomic perspective on human well-being. *Proceedings of the National Academy of Sciences, 110*(33), 13684–13689.

11 Wachholtz, A. B. & Pargament, K. I. (2005). Is spirituality a critical ingredient of meditation? Comparing the effects of spiritual meditation, secular meditation, and relaxation on spiritual, psychological, cardiac, and pain outcomes. *Journal of Behavioral Medicine, 28*(4), 369–384.

Wachholtz, A. B. & Pargament, K. I. (2008). Migraines and meditation: Does spirituality matter? *Journal of Behavioral Medicine, 31*(4), 351–366.

12 Mallinson, J. & Singleton, M. (2017). *Roots of Yoga.* London: Penguin Books.

13   Sullivan, M. B., Moonaz, S., Weber, K., Taylor, J. N., & Schmalzl, L. (2018). Toward an explanatory framework for yoga therapy informed by philosophical and ethical perspectives. *Alternative Therapies in Health and Medicine*, *24*(1), 38–47.

14   Yoga Alliance. (n.d.). *Yoga in America Study*. Retrieved August 27, 2020 from www.yogaalliance. org/2016YogaInAmericaStudy.
     NHIS. (n.d.). *NHIS 2018 Statistics on Use of Complementary Health*. Retrieved August 27, 2020 from https://nccih. nih.gov/research/statistics/NHIS/2017.
     Clarke, T. C., Black, L. I., Stussman, B. J., Barnes, P. M., & Nahin, R. L. (2015). Trends in the use of complementary health approaches among adults: United States, 2002–2012. *National Health Statistics Reports*, *79*, 1.
     Sharp, D., Lorenc, A., Morris, R., Feder, G., *et al.* (2018). Complementary medicine use, views, and experiences: A national survey in England. *BJGP Open*, bjgpopen18X101614.

15   Yoga Alliance. (n.d.).
     NHIS. (n.d.).
     Clarke, *et al.* (2015).
     Sharp, *et al.* (2018).

16   Ivtzan, I. & Jegatheeswaran, S. (2015). The yoga boom in Western society: Practitioners' spiritual vs. physical intentions and their impact on psychological wellbeing. *Journal of Yoga and Physical Therapy*, *5*(3).
     Smith, J. A., Greer, T., Sheets, T., & Watson, S. (2011). Is there more to yoga than exercise? *Alternative Therapies in Health and Medicine*, *17*(3), 22.
     Gaiswinkler, L. & Unterrainer, H. F. (2016). The relationship between yoga involvement, mindfulness and psychological well-being. *Complementary Therapies in Medicine*, *26*, 123–127.

17   Ivtzan & Jegatheeswaran (2015).
     Park, C. L., Riley, K. E., Bedesin, E., & Stewart, V. M. (2016). Why practice yoga? Practitioners' motivations for adopting and maintaining yoga practice. *Journal of Health Psychology*, *21*(6), 887–896.

18   Koenig (2012).
     Vaillant (2008).
     Pressman, S. D., Jenkins, B. N., & Moskowitz, J. T. (2019). Positive affect and health: What do we know and where next should we go? *Annual Review of Psychology*, *70*, 627–650.

19   Varela, F. J., Thompson, E., & Rosch, E. (2017). *The Embodied Mind: Cognitive Science and Human Experience*. Cambridge, MA: MIT Press.

20   Frankl, V. E. (2006). *Man's Search for Meaning*. Boston, MA: Beacon Press.

21   Levin, J. (2016). Prevalence and religious predictors of healing prayer use in the USA: Findings from the Baylor Religion Survey. *Journal of Religion and Health*, *55*(4), 1136–1158.
     Kaufman, J. A. (2018). Nature, mind, and medicine: A model for mind-body healing. *Explore*, *14*(4), 268–276.
     Mygind, L., Kjeldsted, E., Hartmeyer, R. D., Mygind, E., Bølling, M., & Bentsen, P. (2019). Immersive nature-experiences as health promotion interventions for healthy, vulnerable, and sick populations? A systematic review and appraisal of controlled studies. *Frontiers in Psychology*, *10*, 943.

22   Grant & Glueck (n.d.).

23   Cole, S. W., Hawkley, L. C., Arevalo, J. M., Sung, C. Y., Rose, R. M., & Cacioppo, J. T. (2007). Social regulation of gene expression in human leukocytes. *Genome Biology*, *8*(9), R189.
     Cole, S. W. (2014). Human social genomics. *PLoS Genetics*, *10*(8).

CHAPTER 19

1   Knill, P. J., Barba, H. N., & Fuchs, M. N. (1995). *Minstrels of Soul: Intermodal Expressive Therapy*. Toronto: Palmerston Press.
    McNiff, S. (1994). *Art as Medicine: Creating a Therapy of the Imagination*. London: Piatkus.

2   Malchiodi, C. A. (Ed.) (2003). *Handbook of Art Therapy*. New York: Guilford Press.

3   Hovey, R. B., Khayat, V. C., & Feig, E. (2017). Listening to and letting pain speak: Poetic reflections. *British Journal of Pain*, *12*(2), 95–103.

4   Taylor, A. G., Goehler, L. E., Galper, D. I., Innes, K. E., & Bourguignon, C. (2010). Top-down and bottom-up mechanisms in mind-body medicine: Development of an integrative framework for psychophysiological research. *Explore*, *6*(1), 29.

5   Chervonsky, E. & Hunt, C. (2017). Suppression and expression of emotion in social and interpersonal outcomes: A meta-analysis. *Emotion*, *17*(4), 669–683.
    Clift, S., Camic, P. M., & Royal Society for Public Health (Eds) (2016). *Oxford Textbook of Creative Arts, Health, and Wellbeing: International Perspectives on Practice, Policy, and Research* (First edition). Oxford: Oxford University Press.

6   Pordeus, V. (2018). *Restoring the Art of Healing*. Retrieved September 4, 2020 from www.researchgate.net/ publication/324122048_restoring_the_art_of_healing_vitor_pordeus_md. p.29.

7   *Ibid.*

8   *Ibid.* p.40.

9   Antelo, F. (2013). Pain and the paintbrush: The life and art of Frida Kahlo. *The Virtual Mentor: VM*, *15*(5), 460–465.

10 Courtney, C. A., O'Hearn, M. A., & Franck, C. C. (2016). Frida Kahlo: Portrait of chronic pain. *Physical Therapy*, *97*(1), 90–96.

11 Lambert, P., Betts, D., Rollins, J., Sonke, J., & Swanson, K. (2017). *Art, Health, and Well-Being in America*. Retrieved September 4, 2020 from www.americansforthearts.org/node/101238.

12 Stuckey, H. L. & Nobel, J. (2010). The connection between art, healing, and public health: A review of current literature. *American Journal of Public Health*, *100*(2), 254–263.

13 Moon, B. L. (2009). *Existential Art Therapy: The Canvas Mirror* (Third edition). Springfield, IL: Charles C. Thomas. p.11.

14 McNiff, S. (2004). *Art Heals: How Creativity Cures the Soul*. Boston: Shambhala.

15 Porges, S. W. (2011). *The Polyvagal Theory: Neurophysiological Foundations of Emotions, Attachment, Communication, and Self-Regulation (The Norton Series on Interpersonal Neurobiology)* (First edition). New York: W. W. Norton.

16 Betensky, M. G. (1995). *What Do You See? Phenomenology of Therapeutic Art Expression* (pp.xii, 196). London: Jessica Kingsley Publishers.

17 Hovey, *et al.* (2017). p.96.

18 Stuckey & Nobel (2010).
Broadbent, E., Schoones, J. W., Tiemensma, J., & Kaptein, A. A. (2018). A systematic review of patients' drawing of illness: Implications for research using the Common Sense Model. *Health Psychology Review*, 1–21.

19 Hovey, *et al.* (2017).
Stuckey & Nobel (2010).

20 Kaimal, G., Ray, K., & Muniz, J. (2016). Reduction of cortisol levels and participants' responses following art making. *Art Therapy*, *33*(2), 74–80.

21 Hass-Cohen, N., Clyde Findlay, J., Carr, R., & Vanderlan, J. (2014). "Check, change what you need to change and/or keep what you want": An art therapy neurobiological-based trauma protocol. *Art Therapy*, *31*(2), 69–78.

22 Klagsbrun, J., Rappaport, L., Marcow-Speiser, V., Post, P., Stepakoff, S., & Karman, S. (2005). Focusing and expressive arts therapy as a complementary treatment for women with breast cancer. *Journal of Creativity in Mental Health*, *1*, 107–137.

23 *Ibid.*

24 Tarr, J., Cornish, F., & Gonzalez-Polledo, E. (2018). Beyond the binaries: Reshaping pain communication through arts workshops. *Sociology of Health and Illness*, *40*(3), 577–592.

25 Stuckey & Nobel (2010).

26 Geller, J. S. (2019). Group medical visits: Introducing the "group inclusion effect" and key principles for maximization. *The Journal of Alternative and Complementary Medicine*, *25*(7), 673–674.

27 Kwong, M.-K., Ho, R. T.-H., & Huang, Y.-T. (2019). A creative pathway to a meaningful life: An existential expressive arts group therapy for people living with HIV in Hong Kong. *The Arts in Psychotherapy*, *63*, 9–17.

28 *Ibid.*

29 Lynch, M., Sloane, G., Sinclair, C., & Bassett, R. (2013). Resilience and art in chronic pain. *Arts and Health*, *5*(1), 51–67. p.59.

30 Vick, R. & Sexton-Radek, K. (2005). Art and migraine: Researching the relationship between artmaking and pain experience. *Art Therapy: Journal of the American Art Therapy Association*, *22*.

31 Smyth, J. M. & Pennebaker, J. W. (2008). Exploring the boundary conditions of expressive writing: In search of the right recipe. *British Journal of Health Psychology*, *13*(1), 1–7.

32 Pennebaker, J. W. & Evans, J. F. (2014). *Expressive Writing: Words that Heal*. Enumclaw, WA: Idyll Arbor, Inc.

33 Mosher, C. E., DuHamel, K. N., Lam, J., Dickler, M., *et al.* (2012). Randomised trial of expressive writing for distressed metastatic breast cancer patients. *Psychology and Health*, *27*(1), 88–100.

34 Frattaroli, J. (2006). Experimental disclosure and its moderators: A meta-analysis. *Psychological Bulletin*, *132*(6), 823–865.

35 *Ibid.*

36 Harris, A. H. S. (2006). Does expressive writing reduce health care utilization? A meta-analysis of randomized trials. *Journal of Consulting and Clinical Psychology*, *74*(2), 243–252.

37 Niles, A. N., Haltom, K. E. B., Mulvenna, C. M., Lieberman, M. D., & Stanton, A. L. (2014). Randomized controlled trial of expressive writing for psychological and physical health: The moderating role of emotional expressivity. *Anxiety, Stress, and Coping*, *27*(1), 1–17.

38 Knowles, E. D., Wearing, J. R., & Campos, B. (2011). Culture and the health benefits of expressive writing. *Social Psychological and Personality Science*, *2*(4), 408–415.

39 Smyth & Pennebaker (2008). pp.3–4.

40 Sloan, D. M., Feinstein, B. A., & Marx, B. P. (2009). The durability of beneficial health effects associated with expressive writing. *Anxiety, Stress, and Coping*, *22*(5), 509–523.

41 Niles, *et al.* (2014).

42 Smyth & Pennebaker (2008).

43 *Ibid.* p.2.

44 Cusack, K., Jonas, D. E., Forneris, C. A., Wines, C., *et al.* (2016). Psychological treatments for adults with posttraumatic stress disorder: A systematic review and meta-analysis. *Clinical Psychology Review*, *43*, 128–141.

Lenz, A. S. & Hollenbaugh, K. M. (2015). Meta-analysis of trauma-focused cognitive behavioral therapy for treating PTSD and co-occurring depression among children and adolescents. *Counseling Outcome Research and Evaluation*, 6(1), 18–32.

45 Smyth & Pennebaker (2008). p.2.

46 *Ibid.* p.3.

47 *Ibid.* p.3.

CHAPTER 20

1   Porges, S. W. (2011). *The Polyvagal Theory: Neurophysiological Foundations of Emotions, Attachment, Communication, and Self-Regulation (The Norton Series on Interpersonal Neurobiology)* (First edition). New York: W. W. Norton.

2   Van Puyvelde, M., Neyt, X., McGlone, F., & Pattyn, N. (2018). Voice stress analysis: A new framework for voice and effort in human performance. *Frontiers in Psychology*, 9, 1994.
    Eckland, N. S., Leyro, T. M., Mendes, W. B., & Thompson, R. J. (2019). The role of physiology and voice in emotion perception during social stress. *Journal of Nonverbal Behavior*, 43(4), 493–511.

3   Gobl, C. & Ní Chasaide, A. (2003). The role of voice quality in communicating emotion, mood and attitude. *Speech Communication*, 40(1), 189–212.
    Scherer, K. R. (1995). Expression of emotion in voice and music. *Journal of Voice*, 9(3), 235–248.
    Bänziger, T., Grandjean, D., & Scherer, K. (2009). Emotion recognition from expressions in face, voice, and body: The multimodal emotion recognition test (MERT). *Emotion*, 9, 691–704.

4   Roy, N., Bless, D. M., & Heisey, D. (2000). Personality and voice disorders: A multitrait-multidisorder analysis. *Journal of Voice*, 14(4), 521–548.
    Roy, N. & Bless, D. M. (2000). Personality traits and psychological factors in voice pathology. *Journal of Speech, Language, and Hearing Research*, 43(3), 737–748.
    Van Houtte, E., Van Lierde, K., & Claeys, S. (2011). Pathophysiology and treatment of muscle tension dysphonia: A review of the current knowledge. *Journal of Voice*, 25(2), 202–207.

5   Walumbwa, F. O. & Schaubroeck, J. (2009). Leader personality traits and employee voice behavior: Mediating roles of ethical leadership and work group psychological safety. *Journal of Applied Psychology*, 94(5), 1275–1286.

6   Weis, L. & Fine, M. (Eds) (2005). *Beyond Silenced Voices: Class, Race, and Gender in United States Schools* (Revised edition). Albany, NY: State University of New York Press.
    Kim, H. & Markus, H. (2005). Speech and Silence: An Analysis of the Cultural Practice of Talking. In *Beyond Silenced Voices: Class, Race, and Gender in United States Schools* (Revised edition, pp.181–198). Albany, NY: State University of New York Press.

7   Westermeyer, P. (2013). Music and spirituality: Reflections from a Western Christian perspective. *Religions*, 4, 567–583.
    Kidwell, M. D. (2014). Music therapy and spirituality: How can I keep from singing? *Music Therapy Perspectives*, 32(2), 129–135.

8   Cohen, S. M., Kim, J., Roy, N., Asche, C., & Courey, M. (2012). Prevalence and causes of dysphonia in a large treatment-seeking population. *The Laryngoscope*, 122(2), 343–348.

9   Roy, N., Merrill, R. M., Thibeault, S., Parsa, R. A., Gray, S. D., & Smith, E. M. (2004). Prevalence of voice disorders in teachers and the general population. *Journal of Speech, Language, and Hearing Research*, 47(2), 281–293.

10 Dietrich, M., Verdolini Abbott, K., Gartner-Schmidt, J., & Rosen, C. A. (2008). The frequency of perceived stress, anxiety, and depression in patients with common pathologies affecting voice. *Journal of Voice*, 22(4), 472–488.

11 Cacioppo, J. T., Tassinary, L. G., & Berntson, G. G. (2017). *Handbook of Psychophysiology*. New York, NY: Cambridge University Press.

12 Dietrich, *et al.* (2008). p.474.

13 *Ibid.*

14 D'Antoni, M. L., Harvey, P. L., & Fried, M. P. (1995). Alternative medicine: Does it play a role in the management of voice disorders? *Journal of Voice: Official Journal of the Voice Foundation*, 9(3), 308–311.
    Czajkowski, A.-M. & Greasley, A. (2015). Mindfulness for singers: The effects of a targeted mindfulness course on learning vocal technique. *British Journal of Music Education*, 32, 1–23.

15 Dietrich, M. & Verdolini Abbott, K. (2012). Vocal function in introverts and extraverts during a psychological stress reactivity protocol. *Journal of Speech, Language, and Hearing Research*, 55(3), 973–987.

16 Collier, G. & Collier, G. (1985). *Emotional Expression*. New York: Psychology Press.
    King, L. A. & Emmons, R. A. (1990). Conflict over emotional expression: Psychological and physical correlates. *Journal of Personality and Social Psychology*, 58(5), 864–877.
    Bonanno, G. A., Papa, A., Lalande, K., Westphal, M., & Coifman, K. (2004). The importance of being flexible: The ability to both enhance and suppress emotional expression predicts long-term adjustment. *Psychological Science*, 15(7), 482–487.
    Katana, M., Röcke, C., Spain, S. M., & Allemand, M. (2019). Emotion regulation, subjective well-being, and perceived stress in daily life of geriatric nurses. *Frontiers in Psychology*, 10, 1097.

17   Porges, S. W. (2009). The polyvagal theory: New insights into adaptive reactions of the autonomic nervous system. *Cleveland Clinic Journal of Medicine, 76*(Suppl 2), S86–S90.

18   *Ibid.*

19   Porges (2011).

20   *Ibid.*
       Mogenson, G. J., Jones, D. L., & Yim, C. Y. (1980). From motivation to action: Functional interface between the limbic system and the motor system. *Progress in Neurobiology, 14*(2–3), 69–97.

21   Porges (2011).

22   *Ibid.*

23   *Ibid.*

24   Goy, H., Fernandes, D. N., Pichora-Fuller, M. K., & van Lieshout, P. (2013). Normative voice data for younger and older adults. *Journal of Voice: Official Journal of the Voice Foundation, 27*(5), 545–555.
       Hirano, M. & McCormick, K. R. (1986). Clinical examination of voice by Minoru Hirano. *The Journal of the Acoustical Society of America, 80*(4), 1273–1273.
       Hixon, T. J., Shriberg, L. D., & Saxman, J. H. (Eds) (1980). *Introduction to Communication Disorders.* Englewood Cliffs, NJ: Prentice-Hall.

25   Porges (2011).

26   *Ibid.*

27   *Ibid.*

28   Price, C. J. & Hooven, C. (2018). Interoceptive awareness skills for emotion regulation: Theory and approach of mindful awareness in body-oriented therapy (MABT). *Frontiers in Psychology, 9*, 798–798.
       Lumley, M. A., Cohen, J. L., Borszcz, G. S., Cano, A., *et al.* (2011). Pain and emotion: A biopsychosocial review of recent research. *Journal of Clinical Psychology, 67*(9), 942–968.

29   Heinrich-Clauer, V. (2016). Body resonance and the voice. *The Clinical Journal of the International Institute for Bioenergetic Analysis, 26*, 137–161.

30   Gard, T., Noggle, J. J., Park, C. L., Vago, D. R., & Wilson, A. (2014). Potential self-regulatory mechanisms of yoga for psychological health. *Frontiers in Human Neuroscience, 8*, 770.
       Saoji, A. A., Raghavendra, B. R., & Manjunath, N. K. (2018). Effects of yogic breath regulation: A narrative review of scientific evidence. *Journal of Ayurveda and Integrative Medicine, 10*(1), 50–58.

31   Baker, F. & Uhlig, S. (Eds) (2011). *Voicework in Music Therapy: Research and Practice.* London; Philadelphia: Jessica Kingsley Publishers.

32   Bullack, A., Gass, C., Nater, U. M., & Kreutz, G. (2018). Psychobiological effects of choral singing on affective state, social connectedness, and stress: Influences of singing activity and time course. *Frontiers in Behavioral Neuroscience, 12*, 223.
       Gao, J., Leung, H. K., Wu, B. W. Y., Skouras, S., & Sik, H. H. (2019). The neurophysiological correlates of religious chanting. *Scientific Reports, 9*(1), 4262.
       Bernardi, L., Sleight, P., Bandinelli, G., Cencetti, S., *et al.* (2001). Effect of rosary prayer and yoga mantras on autonomic cardiovascular rhythms: Comparative study. *BMJ, 323*(7327), 1446–1449.
       Bernardi, L., Porta, C., & Sleight, P. (2006). Cardiovascular, cerebrovascular, and respiratory changes induced by different types of music in musicians and non-musicians: The importance of silence. *Heart, 92*(4), 445.
       Fox, K. C. R., Dixon, M. L., Nijeboer, S., Girn, M., *et al.* (2016). Functional neuroanatomy of meditation: A review and meta-analysis of 78 functional neuroimaging investigations. *Neuroscience and Biobehavioral Reviews, 65*, 208–228.
       Bernardi, N. F., Snow, S., Peretz, I., Orozco Perez, H. D., Sabet-Kassouf, N., & Lehmann, A. (2017). Cardiorespiratory optimization during improvised singing and toning. *Scientific Reports, 7*(1), 8113.
       Kang, J., Scholp, A., & Jiang, J. (2017). A review of the physiological effects and mechanisms of singing. *Journal of Voice, 32*.
       Zarate, J. M. (2013). The neural control of singing. *Frontiers in Human Neuroscience, 7*, 237.
       Peper, E., Pollock, W., Harvey, R., Yoshino, A., Daubenmier, J., & Anziani, M. (2019). Which quiets the mind more quickly and increases HRV: Toning or mindfulness? *NeuroRegulation, 6*, 128–133.

33   Bliss-Moreau, E., Barrett, L. F., & Owren, M. J. (2010). I like the sound of your voice: Affective learning about vocal signals. *Journal of Experimental Social Psychology, 46*(3), 557–563.

CHAPTER 21

1   American Music Therapy Association. (n.d.). *What is Music Therapy?* Retrieved September 7, 2020 from www.musictherapy.org.

2   Gold, C., Solli, H. P., Krüger, V., & Lie, S. A. (2009). Dose-response relationship in music therapy for people with serious mental disorders: Systematic review and meta-analysis. *Clinical Psychology Review, 29*(3), 193–207.
       Ueda, T., Suzukamo, Y., Sato, M., & Izumi, S.-I. (2013). Effects of music therapy on behavioral and psychological symptoms of dementia: A systematic review and meta-analysis. *Ageing Research Reviews, 12*(2), 628–641.

Zhao, K., Bai, Z. G., Bo, A., & Chi, I. (2016). A systematic review and meta-analysis of music therapy for the older adults with depression. *International Journal of Geriatric Psychiatry*, *31*(11), 1188–1198.

Bieleninik, Ł., Ghetti, C., & Gold, C. (2016). Music therapy for preterm infants and their parents: A meta-analysis. *Pediatrics*, *138*(3), e20160971.

Pelletier, C. L. (2004). The effect of music on decreasing arousal due to stress: A meta-analysis. *Journal of Music Therapy*, *41*(3), 192–214.

Wang, C.-F., Sun, Y.-L., & Zang, H.-X. (2014). Music therapy improves sleep quality in acute and chronic sleep disorders: A meta-analysis of 10 randomized studies. *International Journal of Nursing Studies*, *51*(1), 51–62.

3   Thaut, M., Gardiner, J., Holmberg, D., Horwitz, J., *et al.* (2009). Neurologic Music Therapy Improves Executive Function and Emotional Adjustment in Traumatic Brain Injury Rehabilitation. In S. Dalla Bella, V. B. Penhune, N. Kraus, K. Overy, C. Pantev, & J. S. Snyder (Eds) *The Neurosciences and Music III: Disorders and Plasticity, Volume 1169* (pp.406–571). London: John Wiley & Sons.

Thaut, M. H. & McIntosh, G. C. (2014). Neurologic music therapy in stroke rehabilitation. *Current Physical Medicine and Rehabilitation Reports*, *2*(2), 106–113.

Hegde, S. (2014). Music-based cognitive remediation therapy for patients with traumatic brain injury. *Frontiers in Neurology*, *5*, 34.

Bukowska, A. A., Krężałek, P., Mirek, E., Bujas, P., & Marchewka, A. (2016). Neurologic music therapy training for mobility and stability rehabilitation with Parkinson's disease: A pilot study. *Frontiers in Human Neuroscience*, *9*, 710.

4   Thaut, M. (2005). Rhythm, Music, and the Brain: Scientific Foundations and Clinical Applications. In *Studies on New Music Research: Vol. 7*. New York: Routledge.

Grahn, J. A. (2012). Neural mechanisms of rhythm perception: Current findings and future perspectives. *Topics in Cognitive Science*, *4*(4), 585–606.

5   Aigen, K. (2014). Music-centered dimensions of Nordoff-Robbins Music Therapy. *Music Therapy Perspectives*, *32*(1), 18–29.

Carpente, J. A. (2014). Individual Music-Centered Assessment Profile for Neurodevelopmental Disorders (IMCAP-ND): New developments in music-centered evaluation. *Music Therapy Perspectives*, *32*(1), 56–60.

Mahoney, J. (2016). Current practice in Nordoff-Robbins Music Therapy (NRMT). *Qualitative Inquiries in Music Therapy: A Monograph Series*, *11*(3).

Cohen, N. S. (2018). *Advanced Methods of Music Therapy Practice: The Bonny Method of Guided Imagery and Music, Nordoff-Robbins Music Therapy, Analytical Music Therapy, and Vocal Psychotherapy*. London; Philadelphia: Jessica Kingsley Publishers.

6   Cohen (2018).

McKinney, C. H. & Honig, T. J. (2016). Health outcomes of a series of Bonny Method of guided imagery and music sessions: A systematic review. *Journal of Music Therapy*, *54*(1), 1–34.

7   Aigen, K. (2005). *Music-Centered Music Therapy*. Gilsum, NH: Barcelona Publ.

8   *Ibid.* pp.254–255.

9   O'Kelly, J. (2016). Music therapy and neuroscience: Opportunities and challenges. *Voices: A World Forum for Music Therapy*, *16*(2).

10 Chanda, M. L. & Levitin, D. J. (2013). The neurochemistry of music. *Trends in Cognitive Sciences*, *17*(4), 179–193.

11 *Ibid.*

12 Wheeler, B. (2014). Music in Psychosocial Training and Counseling (MPC). In M. Thaut and B. Hoemberg (Eds) *Handbook of Neurologic Music Therapy*. Oxford: Oxford University Press.

Hanser, S. B. (2016). *Integrative Health Through Music Therapy: Accompanying the Journey from Illness to Wellness*. London: Palgrave Macmillan.

13 Gold, *et al.* (2009).

Aalbers, S., Fusar-Poli, L., Freeman, R., Spreen, M., *et al.* (2017). Music therapy for depression. *Cochrane Database of Systematic Reviews*, (11).

14 Ueda, *et al.* (2013).

McDermott, O., Crellin, N., Ridder, H. M., & Orrell, M. (2013). Music therapy in dementia: A narrative synthesis systematic review. *International Journal of Geriatric Psychiatry*, *28*(8), 781–794.

15 Moore, K. S. (2013). A systematic review on the neural effects of music on emotion regulation: Implications for music therapy practice. *Journal of Music Therapy*, *50*(3), 198–242.

16 Weller, C. M. & Baker, F. A. (2011). The role of music therapy in physical rehabilitation: A systematic literature review. *Nordic Journal of Music Therapy*, *20*(1), 43–61.

17 Klassen, J. A., Liang, Y., Tjosvold, L., Klassen, T. P., & Hartling, L. (2008). Music for pain and anxiety in children undergoing medical procedures: A systematic review of randomized controlled trials. *Ambulatory Pediatrics*, *8*(2), 117–128.

Nilsson, U. (2008). The anxiety- and pain-reducing effects of music interventions: A systematic review. *AORN Journal*, *87*(4), 780–807.

Fitzpatrick, K., Moss, H., & Colman Harmon, D. (2019). The use of music in the chronic pain experience: An investigation into the use of music and music therapy by patients and staff at a hospital outpatient pain clinic. *Music and Medicine*, *11*(1), 6–22.

18 Geretsegger, M., Elefant, C., Mössler, K., & Gold, C. (2014). Music therapy for people with autism spectrum disorder. *Cochrane Database of Systematic Reviews*, (6).

19 Bradt, J., Magee, W., Dileo, C., Wheeler, B., & McGilloway, E. (2010). Music therapy for acquired brain injury. *Cochrane Database of Systematic Reviews*, (7).

20 Mofredj, A., Alaya, S., Tassaioust, K., Bahloul, H., & Mrabet, A. (2016). Music therapy, a review of the potential therapeutic benefits for the critically ill. *Journal of Critical Care*, *35*, 195–199.

21 Porges, S. W. (2008). Music Therapy & Trauma: Insights from the Polyvagal Theory. In *Symposium on Music Therapy & Trauma: Bridging Theory and Clinical Practice*. Retrieved September 7, 2020 from www.semanticscholar.org/paper/Music-Therapy-%26-Trauma%3A-Insights-from-the-Polyvagal-Porges/ae81423342b0b7e2eb2f0d97eb09b5b19c60de54.

22 *Ibid.*

23 *Ibid.*

24 Bullack, A., Gass, C., Nater, U. M., & Kreutz, G. (2018). Psychobiological effects of choral singing on affective state, social connectedness, and stress: Influences of singing activity and time course. *Frontiers in Behavioral Neuroscience*, *12*, 223.

Gao, J., Leung, H. K., Wu, B. W. Y., Skouras, S., & Sik, H. H. (2019). The neurophysiological correlates of religious chanting. *Scientific Reports*, *9*(1), 4262.

Bernardi, L., Sleight, P., Bandinelli, G., Cencetti, S., *et al.* (2001). Effect of rosary prayer and yoga mantras on autonomic cardiovascular rhythms: Comparative study. *BMJ*, *323*(7327), 1446–1449.

Fox, K. C. R., Dixon, M. L., Nijeboer, S., Girn, M., *et al.* (2016). Functional neuroanatomy of meditation: A review and meta-analysis of 78 functional neuroimaging investigations. *Neuroscience and Biobehavioral Reviews*, *65*, 208–228.

25 Cooper, L. (2019). *Using Music as Medicine—Finding the Optimum Music Listening "Dosage."* Retrieved September 7, 2020 from www.britishacademyofsoundtherapy.com/wp-content/uploads/2019/12/Deezer-Health-and-Wellbeing-research-short-.pdf.

26 Hanser (2016).

27 Winner, E. (2007). Development in the Arts: Drawing and Music. In W. Damon & R. M. Lerner (Eds) *Handbook of Child Psychology* (6th ed.). Hoboken, NJ: John Wiley & Sons. pp.322–358.

28 dos Santos Delabary, M., Komeroski, I. G., Monteiro, E. P., Costa, R. R., & Haas, A. N. (2018). Effects of dance practice on functional mobility, motor symptoms and quality of life in people with Parkinson's disease: A systematic review with meta-analysis. *Aging Clinical and Experimental Research*, *30*(7), 727–735.

Koch, S., Kunz, T., Lykou, S., & Cruz, R. (2014). Effects of dance movement therapy and dance on health-related psychological outcomes: A meta-analysis. *The Arts in Psychotherapy*, *41*(1), 46–64.

CHAPTER 22

1 Minich, D. M. & Bland, J. S. (2013). Personalized lifestyle medicine: Relevance for nutrition and lifestyle recommendations. *The Scientific World Journal*, *2013*, 129841–129841.

2 Rapozo, D. C. M., Bernardazzi, C., & de Souza, H. S. P. (2017). Diet and microbiota in inflammatory bowel disease: The gut in disharmony. *World Journal of Gastroenterology*, *23*(12), 2124–2140.

3 Centers for Disease Control and Prevention. (2019). *Chronic Diseases in America*. Retrieved September 7, 2020 from www.cdc.gov/chronicdisease/resources/infographic/chronic-diseases.htm.

4 Marczak, L., O'Rourke, K., Shepard, D., & Institute for Health Metrics and Evaluation. (2016). When and why people die in the United States, 1990–2013. *JAMA*, *315*(3), 241–241.

5 Ford, E. S., Bergmann, M. M., Kröger, J., Schienkiewitz, A., Weikert, C., & Boeing, H. (2009). Healthy living is the best revenge: Findings from the European Prospective Investigation into Cancer and Nutrition-Potsdam study. *Archives of Internal Medicine*, *169*(15), 1355–1362.

Gopinath, B., Rochtchina, E., Flood, V. M., & Mitchell, P. (2010). Healthy living and risk of major chronic diseases in an older population. *Archives of Internal Medicine*, *170*(2), 208–209.

6 Cohen, S., Janicki-Deverts, D., & Miller, G. E. (2007). Psychological stress and disease. *JAMA*, *298*(14), 1685–1687.

7 Treede, R.-D., Rief, W., Barke, A., Aziz, Q., *et al.* (2019). Chronic pain as a symptom or a disease: The IASP Classification of Chronic Pain for the International Classification of Diseases (ICD-11). *Pain*, *160*(1).

8 Nelson, S. M., Cunningham, N. R., & Kashikar-Zuck, S. (2017). A conceptual framework for understanding the role of adverse childhood experiences in pediatric chronic pain. *The Clinical Journal of Pain*, *33*(3), 264–270.

Campbell, J. A., Walker, R. J., & Egede, L. E. (2016). Associations between adverse childhood experiences, high-risk behaviors, and morbidity in adulthood. *American Journal of Preventive Medicine*, *50*(3), 344–352.

Rehkopf, D. H., Headen, I., Hubbard, A., Deardorff, J., *et al.* (2016). Adverse childhood experiences and later life adult obesity and smoking in the United States. *Annals of Epidemiology*, *26*(7), 488–492.e5.

9 De Gregori, M., Muscoli, C., Schatman, M. E., Stallone, T., *et al.* (2016). Combining pain therapy with lifestyle: The role of personalized nutrition and nutritional supplements according to the SIMPAR Feed Your Destiny approach. *Journal of Pain Research*, *9*, 1179–1189.

10 Halfon, N., Larson, K., & Slusser, W. (2013). Associations between obesity and comorbid mental health, developmental, and physical health conditions in a nationally representative sample of US children aged 10 to 17. *Academic Pediatrics*, *13*(1), 6–13.

Dominick, C. H., Blyth, F. M., & Nicholas, M. K. (2012). Unpacking the burden: Understanding the relationships between chronic pain and comorbidity in the general population. *Pain*, *153*(2), 293–304.

Nilsen, T. I. L., Holtermann, A., & Mork, P. J. (2011). Physical exercise, body mass index, and risk of chronic pain in the low back and neck/shoulders: Longitudinal data from the Nord-Trøndelag Health Study. *American Journal of Epidemiology*, *174*(3), 267–273.

Peltonen, M., Lindroos, A. K., & Torgerson, J. S. (2003). Musculoskeletal pain in the obese: A comparison with a general population and long-term changes after conventional and surgical obesity treatment. *Pain*, *104*(3), 549–557.

11 Treede, *et al.* (2019).

12 Baker, T. A., Clay, O. J., Johnson-Lawrence, V., Minahan, J. A., *et al.* (2017). Association of multiple chronic conditions and pain among older black and white adults with diabetes mellitus. *BMC Geriatrics*, *17*(1), 255.

13 Furman, D., Campisi, J., Verdin, E., Carrera-Bastos, P., *et al.* (2019). Chronic inflammation in the etiology of disease across the life span. *Nature Medicine*, *25*(12), 1822–1832.

14 De Gregori, *et al.* (2016).

15 Cohen, S., Janicki-Deverts, D., Doyle, W. J., Miller, G. E., *et al.* (2012). Chronic stress, glucocorticoid receptor resistance, inflammation, and disease risk. *Proceedings of the National Academy of Sciences of the United States of America*, *109*(16), 5995–5999.

16 Zhang, J.-M. & An, J. (2007). Cytokines, inflammation, and pain. *International Anesthesiology Clinics*, *45*(2), 27–37.

17 Blaser, M. J. (2017). The theory of disappearing microbiota and the epidemics of chronic diseases. *Nature Reviews Immunology*, *17*(8), 461–463.

Nelson, H. H. & Kelsey, K. T. (2016). Epigenetic epidemiology as a tool to understand the role of immunity in chronic disease. *Epigenomics*, *8*(8), 1007–1009.

Marchand, F., Perretti, M., & McMahon, S. B. (2005). Role of the immune system in chronic pain. *Nature Reviews Neuroscience*, *6*(7), 521–532.

18 Galland, L. (2010). Diet and inflammation. *Nutrition in Clinical Practice: Official Publication of the American Society for Parenteral and Enteral Nutrition*, *25*(6), 634–640.

Zhou, X., Du, L., Shi, R., Chen, Z., Zhou, Y., & Li, Z. (2019). Early-life food nutrition, microbiota maturation and immune development shape life-long health. *Critical Reviews in Food Science and Nutrition*, *59*(Suppl 1), S30–S38.

Arabi, S., Molazadeh, M., & Rezaei, N. (2019). *Nutrition, Immunity, and Autoimmune Diseases*. Cham: Springer.

19 Shanahan, F., van Sinderen, D., O'Toole, P. W., & Stanton, C. (2017). Feeding the microbiota: Transducer of nutrient signals for the host. *Gut*, *66*(9), 1709–1717.

Cryan, J. F. & Dinan, T. G. (2012). Mind-altering microorganisms: The impact of the gut microbiota on brain and behaviour. *Nature Reviews Neuroscience*, *13*(10), 701–712.

20 Vighi, G., Marcucci, F., Sensi, L., Di Cara, G., & Frati, F. (2008). Allergy and the gastrointestinal system. *Clinical and Experimental Immunology*, *153*(Suppl 1), 3–6.

21 Mittal, R., Debs, L. H., Patel, A. P., Nguyen, D., *et al.* (2017). Neurotransmitters: The critical modulators regulating gut-brain axis. *Journal of Cellular Physiology*, *232*(9), 2359–2372.

22 Azzouz, L. L. & Sharma, S. (2020). Physiology, large intestine. *StatPearls*. Retrieved September 7, 2020 from www.ncbi.nlm.nih.gov/books/NBK507857.

Kiela, P. R. & Ghishan, F. K. (2016). Physiology of intestinal absorption and secretion. *Best Practice & Research. Clinical Gastroenterology*, *30*(2), 145–159.

23 Liang, S., Wu, X., & Jin, F. (2018). Gut-brain psychology: Rethinking psychology from the microbiota-gut-brain axis. *Frontiers in Integrative Neuroscience*, *12*, 33.

24 Vuong, H. E., Yano, J. M., Fung, T. C., & Hsiao, E. Y. (2017). The microbiome and host behavior. *Annual Review of Neuroscience*, *40*, 21–49.

Rousseaux, C., Thuru, X., Gelot, A., Barnich, N., *et al.* (2007). Lactobacillus acidophilus modulates intestinal pain and induces opioid and cannabinoid receptors. *Nature Medicine*, *13*(1), 35–37.

25 Cryan & Dinan (2012).

Alcock, J., Maley, C. C., & Aktipis, C. A. (2014). Is eating behavior manipulated by the gastrointestinal microbiota? Evolutionary pressures and potential mechanisms. *BioEssays: News and Reviews in Molecular, Cellular and Developmental Biology*, *36*(10), 940–949.

26 Oriach, C. S., Robertson, R. C., Stanton, C., Cryan, J. F., & Dinan, T. G. (2016). Food for thought: The role of nutrition in the microbiota-gut-brain axis. *Gut Microbiota and Nutrition: Where Are We Now?*, *6*, 25–38.

27 Dinan, T. G. & Cryan, J. F. (2012). Regulation of the stress response by the gut microbiota: Implications for psychoneuroendocrinology. *Psychoneuroendocrinology*, *37*(9), 1369–1378.

28 Szychlinska, M. A., Di Rosa, M., Castorina, A., Mobasheri, A., & Musumeci, G. (2019). A correlation between intestinal microbiota dysbiosis and osteoarthritis. *Heliyon*, *5*(1), e01134.

Schott, E. M., Farnsworth, C. W., Grier, A., Lillis, J. A., *et al.* (2018). Targeting the gut microbiome to treat the osteoarthritis of obesity. *JCI Insight*, *3*(8), e95997.

Taneja, V. (2014). Arthritis susceptibility and the gut microbiome. *The Gut Microbiome*, *588*(22), 4244–4249.

Kabeerdoss, J., Sandhya, P., & Danda, D. (2016). Gut inflammation and microbiome in spondyloarthritis. *Rheumatology International, 36*(4), 457–468.

29   Minich & Bland (2013).

30   *Ibid.*

31   Goncalves, M. D., Lu, C., Tutnauer, J., Hartman, T. E., *et al.* (2019). High-fructose corn syrup enhances intestinal tumor growth in mice. *Science, 363*(6433), 1345–1349.

Imamura, F., O'Connor, L., Ye, Z., Mursu, J., *et al.* (2015). Consumption of sugar sweetened beverages, artificially sweetened beverages, and fruit juice and incidence of type 2 diabetes: Systematic review, meta-analysis, and estimation of population attributable fraction. *BMJ (Clinical Research Ed.), 351*, h3576–h3576.

Poti, J. M., Braga, B., & Qin, B. (2017). Ultra-processed food intake and obesity: What really matters for health-processing or nutrient content? *Current Obesity Reports, 6*(4), 420–431.

32   Hall, K. D., Ayuketah, A., Brychta, R., Cai, H., *et al.* (2019). Ultra-processed diets cause excess calorie intake and weight gain: An inpatient randomized controlled trial of ad libitum food intake. *Cell Metabolism, 30*(1), 67–77.

33   *Ibid.*

34   De Gregori, *et al.* (2016).

35   Dai, Z., Niu, J., Zhang, Y., Jacques, P., & Felson, D. T. (2017). Dietary intake of fibre and risk of knee osteoarthritis in two US prospective cohorts. *Annals of the Rheumatic Diseases, 76*(8), 1411–1419.

36   Nelson, A. D. & Camilleri, M. (2015). Chronic opioid induced constipation in patients with nonmalignant pain: Challenges and opportunities. *Therapeutic Advances in Gastroenterology, 8*(4), 206–220.

37   Calder, P. C. (2010). Omega-3 fatty acids and inflammatory processes. *Nutrients, 2*(3), 355–374.

Rajaei, E., Mowla, K., Ghorbani, A., Bahadoram, S., Bahadoram, M., & Dargahi-Malamir, M. (2015). The effect of omega-3 fatty acids in patients with active rheumatoid arthritis receiving DMARDs therapy: Double-blind randomized controlled trial. *Global Journal of Health Science, 8*(7), 18–25.

38   National Institutes of Health, Office of Dietary Supplements. (2019). *Omega-3 Fatty Acids*. Retrieved September 7, 2020 from https://ods.od.nih.gov/factsheets/Omega3FattyAcids-Consumer.

39   Nichols, P. D., Petrie, J., & Singh, S. (2010). Long-chain omega-3 oils—an update on sustainable sources. *Nutrients, 2*(6).

40   Simopoulos, A. P. (2016). An increase in the omega-6/omega-3 fatty acid ratio increases the risk for obesity. *Nutrients, 8*(3), 128–128.

41   Simopoulos, A. P. (2011). Importance of the omega-6/omega-3 balance in health and disease: Evolutionary aspects of diet. In *World Review of Nutrition and Dietetics (Vol. 102)* (pp.10–21).

42   Simopoulos (2016).

43   Bower, A., Marquez, S., & de Mejia, E. G. (2016). The health benefits of selected culinary herbs and spices found in the traditional Mediterranean diet. *Critical Reviews in Food Science and Nutrition, 56*(16), 2728–2746.

Serafini, M. & Peluso, I. (2016). Functional foods for health: The interrelated antioxidant and anti-inflammatory role of fruits, vegetables, herbs, spices and cocoa in humans. *Current Pharmaceutical Design, 22*(44), 6701–6715.

Vázquez-Fresno, R., Rosana, A. R. R., Sajed, T., Onookome-Okome, T., Wishart, N. A., & Wishart, D. S. (2019). Herbs and spices: Biomarkers of intake based on human intervention studies—A systematic review. *Genes and Nutrition, 14*, 18.

44   Kuptniratsaikul, V., Dajpratham, P., Taechaarpornkul, W., Buntragulpoontawee, M., *et al.* (2014). Efficacy and safety of Curcuma domestica extracts compared with ibuprofen in patients with knee osteoarthritis: A multicenter study. *Clinical Interventions in Aging, 9*, 451–458.

45   Kizhakkedath, R. (2013). Clinical evaluation of a formulation containing Curcuma longa and Boswellia serrata extracts in the management of knee osteoarthritis. *Molecular Medicine Reports, 8*(5), 1542–1548.

46   Belcaro, G., Dugall, M., Luzzi, R., Ledda, A., *et al.* (2014). Meriva®+Glucosamine versus Condroitin+Glucosamine in patients with knee osteoarthritis: An observational study. *European Review for Medical and Pharmacological Sciences, 18*(24), 3959–3963.

Harris, S. R., Morrow, K., Titgemeier, B., & Goldberg, D. (2017). Dietary supplement use in older adults. *Current Nutrition Reports, 6*(2), 122–133.

47   Shoba, G., Joy, D., Joseph, T., Majeed, M., Rajendran, R., & Srinivas, P. S. (1998). Influence of piperine on the pharmacokinetics of curcumin in animals and human volunteers. *Planta Medica, 64*(4), 353–356.

48   Mashhadi, N. S., Ghiasvand, R., Askari, G., Hariri, M., Darvishi, L., & Mofid, M. R. (2013). Anti-oxidative and anti-inflammatory effects of ginger in health and physical activity: Review of current evidence. *International Journal of Preventive Medicine, 4*(Suppl 1), S36–S42.

49   Ozgoli, G., Goli, M., & Moattar, F. (2009). Comparison of effects of ginger, mefenamic acid, and ibuprofen on pain in women with primary dysmenorrhea. *Journal of Alternative and Complementary Medicine, 15*(2), 129–132.

Rahnama, P., Montazeri, A., Huseini, H. F., Kianbakht, S., & Naseri, M. (2012). Effect of Zingiber officinale R. rhizomes (ginger) on pain relief in primary dysmenorrhea: A placebo randomized trial. *BMC Complementary and Alternative Medicine, 12*, 92–92.

Black, C. D., Herring, M. P., Hurley, D. J., & O'Connor, P. J. (2010). Ginger (Zingiber officinale) reduces muscle pain caused by eccentric exercise. *The Journal of Pain, 11*(9), 894–903.

50   Guldiken, B., Ozkan, G., Catalkaya, G., Ceylan, F. D., Ekin Yalcinkaya, I., & Capanoglu, E. (2018). Phytochemicals of herbs and spices: Health versus toxicological effects. *Third International Symposium on Phytochemicals in Medicine and Food (3-ISPMF)*, *119*, 37–49.

51   Puterbaugh, J. S. (2009). The emperor's tailors: The failure of the medical weight loss paradigm and its causal role in the obesity of America. *Diabetes, Obesity and Metabolism*, *11*(6), 557–570.

52   Hardcastle, S. & Hagger, M. S. (2011). "You can't do it on your own": Experiences of a motivational interviewing intervention on physical activity and dietary behaviour. *Psychology of Sport and Exercise*, *12*(3), 314–323.

53   O'Brien, G. & Davies, M. (2006). Nutrition knowledge and body mass index. *Health Education Research*, *22*(4), 571–575.

54   Allen, A. P., Dinan, T. G., Clarke, G., & Cryan, J. F. (2017). A psychology of the human brain-gut-microbiome axis. *Social and Personality Psychology Compass*, *11*(4), e12309–e12309.

55   Perkins, S. J., Keville, S., Schmidt, U., & Chalder, T. (2005). Eating disorders and irritable bowel syndrome: Is there a link? *Journal of Psychosomatic Research*, *59*(2), 57–64.

56   *Ibid.*

57   *Ibid.*

58   *Ibid.*

59   Kolacz, J. & Porges, S. W. (2018). Chronic diffuse pain and functional gastrointestinal disorders after traumatic stress: Pathophysiology through a polyvagal perspective. *Frontiers in Medicine*, *5*, 145.

60   Hall, *et al.* (2019).

61   Ifland, J., Preuss, H. G., Marcus, M. T., Rourke, K. M., Taylor, W., & Theresa Wright, H. (2015). Clearing the confusion around processed food addiction. *Journal of the American College of Nutrition*, *34*(3), 240–243.

62   Gibson, E. L. (2012). The psychobiology of comfort eating: Implications for neuropharmacological interventions. *Behavioural Pharmacology*, *23*(5, 6).

63   Porges, S. W. (2011). *The Polyvagal Theory: Neurophysiological Foundations of Emotions, Attachment, Communication, and Self-Regulation (The Norton Series on Interpersonal Neurobiology)* (First edition). New York: W. W. Norton.
     Mogenson, G. J., Jones, D. L., & Yim, C. Y. (1980). From motivation to action: Functional interface between the limbic system and the motor system. *Progress in Neurobiology*, *14*(2–3), 69–97.
     Mathes, W. F., Brownley, K. A., Mo, X., & Bulik, C. M. (2009). The biology of binge eating. *Appetite*, *52*(3), 545–553.

64   Miura, A. (2013). *Essential Japanese Vocabulary: Learn to Avoid Common (and Embarrassing!) Mistakes*. Clarendon, VT: Tuttle Publishing.
     Kuchisabishii. (n.d.). *Urban Dictionary*. Retrieved September 7, 2020 from www.urbandictionary.com/define.php?term=kuchisabishii.

65   Erb, M. (2019). Ingredients in Pain Care: Nutrition and Yoga. In N. Pearson, S. Prosko, & M. Sullivan (Eds) *Yoga and Science in Pain Care: Treating the Person in Pain*. London: Jessica Kingsley Publishers.

CHAPTER 23

1   APTA. (n.d.). *Guide to Physical Therapist Practice*. Retrieved September 8, 2020 from http://guidetoptpractice.apta.org.

2   Voogt, L., de Vries, J., Meeus, M., Struyf, F., Meuffels, D., & Nijs, J. (2015). Analgesic effects of manual therapy in patients with musculoskeletal pain: A systematic review. *Manual Therapy*, *20*(2), 250–256.

3   Kim, J.-H., van Rijn, R. M., van Tulder, M. W., Koes, B. W., *et al.* (2018). Diagnostic accuracy of diagnostic imaging for lumbar disc herniation in adults with low back pain or sciatica is unknown: A systematic review. *Chiropractic and Manual Therapies*, *26*(1), 37.

4   Bialosky, J. E., Beneciuk, J. M., Bishop, M. D., Coronado, R. A., *et al.* (2018). Unraveling the mechanisms of manual therapy: Modeling an approach. *The Journal of Orthopaedic and Sports Physical Therapy*, *48*(1), 8–18.

5   Voogt, *et al.* (2015).

6   Bialosky, *et al.* (2018).

7   Voogt, *et al.* (2015).

8   Rossettini, G., Carlino, E., & Testa, M. (2018). Clinical relevance of contextual factors as triggers of placebo and nocebo effects in musculoskeletal pain. *BMC Musculoskeletal Disorders*, *19*(1), 27.

9   Bialosky, J. E., Bishop, M. D., George, S. Z., & Robinson, M. E. (2011). Placebo response to manual therapy: Something out of nothing? *The Journal of Manual & Manipulative Therapy*, *19*(1), 11–19.

10   Frisaldi, E., Shaibani, A., & Benedetti, F. (2018). Placebo responders and nonresponders: What's new? *Pain Management*, *8*(6), 405–408.

11   Jacobs, D. F. & Silvernail, J. L. (2011). Therapist as operator or interactor? Moving beyond the technique. *The Journal of Manual and Manipulative Therapy*, *19*(2), 120–121.

12   Gay, C. W., Robinson, M. E., George, S. Z., Perlstein, W. M., & Bishop, M. D. (2014). Immediate changes after manual therapy in resting-state functional connectivity as measured by functional magnetic resonance imaging in participants with induced low back pain. *Journal of Manipulative and Physiological Therapeutics*, *37*(9), 614–627.

13   Bialosky, *et al.* (2018).

14 Gay, *et al.* (2014).

15 Bialosky, *et al.* (2018). p.12.

16 Hashmi, J. A., Baliki, M. N., Huang, L., Baria, A. T., *et al.* (2013). Shape shifting pain: Chronification of back pain shifts brain representation from nociceptive to emotional circuits. *Brain: A Journal of Neurology, 136*(Pt 9), 2751–2768.

17 Hemington, K. S., Rogachov, A., Cheng, J. C., Bosma, R. L., *et al.* (2018). Patients with chronic pain exhibit a complex relationship triad between pain, resilience, and within- and cross-network functional connectivity of the default mode network. *Pain, 159*(8), 1621–1630.

18 Kovanur-Sampath, K., Mani, R., Cotter, J., Gisselman, A. S., & Tumilty, S. (2017). Changes in biochemical markers following spinal manipulation—a systematic review and meta-analysis. *Musculoskeletal Science and Practice, 29,* 120–131.

19 Colombi, A. & Testa, M. (2019). The effects induced by spinal manipulative therapy on the immune and endocrine systems. *Medicina, 55*(8), 448.

20 Kovanur-Sampath, *et al.* (2017).

21 Geneen, L., Moore, R., Clarke, C., Martin, D., Colvin, L., & Smith, B. (2017). Physical activity and exercise for chronic pain in adults: An overview of Cochrane Reviews. *Cochrane Database of Systematic Reviews,* (4).

22 International Association for the Study of Pain. (2017). IASP council adopts task force recommendation for third mechanistic descriptor of pain. *IASP Publications and News.* Retrieved September 8, 2020 from www.iasp-pain.org/PublicationsNews/NewsDetail.aspx?ItemNumber=6862.

23 Louw, A., Nijs, J., & Puentedura, E. J. (2017). A clinical perspective on a pain neuroscience education approach to manual therapy. *Journal of Manual and Manipulative Therapy, 25*(3), 160–168. p.162.

24 Weisman, A., Quintner, J., Galbraith, M., & Masharawi, Y. (2020). Why are assumptions passed off as established knowledge? *Medical Hypotheses, 140,* 109693.

25 Trouvin, A.-P. & Perrot, S. (2019). New concepts of pain. *Generalised Musculoskeletal Problems, 33*(3), 101415.

26 Toro-Velasco, C., Arroyo-Morales, M., Fernández-de-las-Peñas, C., Cleland, J. A., & Barrero-Hernández, F. J. (2009). Short-term effects of manual therapy on heart rate variability, mood state, and pressure pain sensitivity in patients with chronic tension-type headache: A pilot study. *Journal of Manipulative and Physiological Therapeutics, 32*(7), 527–535.

    Delaney, J. P. A., Leong, K. S., Watkins, A., & Brodie, D. (2002). The short-term effects of myofascial trigger point massage therapy on cardiac autonomic tone in healthy subjects. *Journal of Advanced Nursing, 37*(4), 364–371.

    Smith, M., Leong, K., Watkins, A., & Brodie, D. (2014). Manual Medicine and the Autonomic Nervous System: Assessing Autonomic Function in Humans. In H. H. King, W. Jänig, and M. M. Patterson (Eds) *The Science and Clinical Application of Manual Therapy.* London: Elsevier Health Sciences UK.

27 Amoroso Borges, B. L., Bortolazzo, G. L., & Neto, H. P. (2018). Effects of spinal manipulation and myofascial techniques on heart rate variability: A systematic review. *Journal of Bodywork and Movement Therapies, 22*(1), 203–208.

28 Silva, D., Osório, R., & Fernandes, A. (2018). Influence of neural mobilization in the sympathetic slump position on the behavior of the autonomic nervous system. *Research on Biomedical Engineering, 34,* 329–336.

29 Picchiottino, M., Leboeuf-Yde, C., Gagey, O., & Hallman, D. M. (2019). The acute effects of joint manipulative techniques on markers of autonomic nervous system activity: A systematic review and meta-analysis of randomized sham-controlled trials. *Chiropractic and Manual Therapies, 27*(1), 17.

30 *Ibid.*

31 Gong, W. (2013). Effects of cervical joint manipulation on joint position sense of normal adults. *Journal of Physical Therapy Science, 25*(6), 721–723.

    Gong, W. (2018). The effects of pelvis, lumbar spine and cervical spine manipulation on joint position sense in healthy adults. *Journal of International Academy of Physical Therapy Research, 9*(1), 1381–1386.

32 Babatunde, F., MacDermid, J., & MacIntyre, N. (2017). Characteristics of therapeutic alliance in musculoskeletal physiotherapy and occupational therapy practice: A scoping review of the literature. *BMC Health Services Research, 17*(1), 375–375.

33 Rossettini, *et al.* (2018). p.1.

34 *Ibid.*

35 *Ibid.*

36 Hertenstein, M. J. & Weiss, S. J. (Eds) (2011). *The Handbook of Touch: Neuroscience, Behavioral, and Health Perspectives.* New York: Springer.

37 Montagu, A. (1986). *Touching: The Human Significance of the Skin* (Third edition). New York: Perennial Library. p.396.

38 Ellingsen, D.-M., Leknes, S., Løseth, G., Wessberg, J., & Olausson, H. (2016). The neurobiology shaping affective touch: Expectation, motivation, and meaning in the multisensory context. *Frontiers in Psychology, 6,* 1986–1986.

39 Kelly, M. A., Nixon, L., McClurg, C., Scherpbier, A., King, N., & Dornan, T. (2018). Experience of touch in health care: A meta-ethnography across the health care professions. *Qualitative Health Research, 28*(2), 200–212.

40 *Ibid.*

41 Tommaso, G., Viceconti, A., Minacci, M., Testa, M., & Rossettini, G. (2019). Manual therapy: Exploiting the role of human touch. *Musculoskeletal Science and Practice, 44,* 102044.

42   Ellingsen, *et al.* (2016).

43   *Ibid.*

44   Moseley, G. L. & Flor, H. (2012). Targeting cortical representations in the treatment of chronic pain: A review. *Neurorehabilitation and Neural Repair, 26*(6), 646–652.

45   Tommaso, *et al.* (2019). p.3.

46   Simonsmeier, B. A. & Buecker, S. (2017). Interrelations of imagery use, imagery ability, and performance in young athletes. *Journal of Applied Sport Psychology, 29*(1), 32–43.
     Schuster, C., Hilfiker, R., Amft, O., Scheidhauer, A., *et al.* (2011). Best practice for motor imagery: A systematic literature review on motor imagery training elements in five different disciplines. *BMC Medicine, 9*(1), 75.

47   Lengacher, C. A., Bennett, M. P., Gonzalez, L., Gilvary, D., *et al.* (2008). Immune responses to guided imagery during breast cancer treatment. *Biological Research for Nursing, 9*(3), 205–214.

48   Gonzales, E. A., Ledesma, R. J. A., McAllister, D. J., Perry, S. M., Dyer, C. A., & Maye, J. P. (2010). Effects of guided imagery on postoperative outcomes in patients undergoing same-day surgical procedures: A randomized, single-blind study. *AANA Journal, 78*(3), 181–188.

49   Forward, J. B., Greuter, N. E., Crisall, S. J., & Lester, H. F. (2015). Effect of structured touch and guided imagery for pain and anxiety in elective joint replacement patients—A randomized controlled trial: M-TIJRP. *The Permanente Journal, 19*(4), 18–28.

50   Louw, *et al.* (2017).

51   Mintken, P. E., Rodeghero, J., & Cleland, J. A. (2018). Manual therapists—Have you lost that loving feeling?! *The Journal of Manual & Manipulative Therapy, 26*(2), 53–54.
     Lluch Girbés, E., Meeus, M., Baert, I., & Nijs, J. (2015). Balancing "hands-on" with "hands-off" physical therapy interventions for the treatment of central sensitization pain in osteoarthritis. *Manual Therapy, 20*(2), 349–352.

52   Ameli, R., Sinaii, N., Luna, M. J., Cheringal, J., Gril, B., & Berger, A. (2018). The National Institutes of Health measure of Healing Experience of All Life Stressors (NIH-HEALS): Factor analysis and validation. *PloS One, 13*(12), e0207820. p.10.

53   Sullivan, M. B., Moonaz, S., Weber, K., Taylor, J. N., & Schmalzl, L. (2018). Toward an explanatory framework for yoga therapy informed by philosophical and ethical perspectives. *Alternative Therapies in Health and Medicine, 24*(1), 38–47.

54   Sullivan, M. B., Erb, M., Schmalzl, L., Moonaz, S., Noggle Taylor, J., & Porges, S. W. (2018). Yoga therapy and polyvagal theory: The convergence of traditional wisdom and contemporary neuroscience for self-regulation and resilience. *Frontiers in Human Neuroscience, 12*, 67.

55   Chesler, A. T., Szczot, M., Bharucha-Goebel, D., Čeko, M., *et al.* (2016). The role of PIEZO2 in human mechanosensation. *New England Journal of Medicine, 375*(14), 1355–1364.

CHAPTER 24

1   Taylor, M. J. (2007). What is yoga therapy? An IAYT definition. *Yoga Therapy in Practice, Dec,* 3. p.3.

2   Feuerstein, G. (1998). *The Yoga Tradition.* Prescott, AZ: Hohm Press.

3   Walsh, R. (2015). What is wisdom? Cross-cultural and cross-disciplinary syntheses. *Review of General Psychology, 19*, 278–293.

4   Bhavanani, A. B. (2011). Are we practicing yoga therapy or yogopathy? *Yoga Therapy Today, 7*(2), 26–28.

5   Taylor, J. C. & Taylor, M. J. (2011). Yoga therapeutics: Preparation and support for end of life. *Topics in Geriatric Rehabilitation, 27*(2), 142–150.

6   Wainer, R. S., Whitman, J. M., Cleland, J. A., & Flynn, T. W. (2007). Regional interdependence: A musculoskeletal examination model whose time has come. *Journal of Orthopedic and Sports Physical Therapy, 37*(11), 658–660.

7   *Ibid.*

8   Taylor & Taylor (2011).

9   Alliance to Advance Comprehensive Integrative Pain Management (n.d.) *History.* Retrieved September 8, 2020 from http://painmanagementalliance.org/about-us/history.

10   Wolsko, P. M., Eisenberg, D. M., Davis, R.B., & Phillips, R.S. (2004). Use of mind-body medical therapies: Results of a national survey. *Journal of General Internal Medicine, 19*, 43–50.

11   Taylor & Taylor (2011).

12   Carrera, J. (2006). *Inside the Yoga Sutras.* Buckingham, VA: Integral Yoga Publications.

13   Taylor, M. J. (1998). *Integrating Yoga Therapy into Rehabilitation.* Scottsdale, AZ: Embug Publishing.

14   *Ibid.*

15   Taylor, M. J. (2004). Yoga Therapeutics: An Ancient Practice in a 21st Century Setting. In C. Davis *Complementary Therapies in Rehabilitation: Evidence for Efficacy in Therapy, Prevention, and Wellness* (Second edition). New York: Slack.

16   Taylor, M. J. (2015). Yoga Therapy for Rehabilitation Professionals. In L. Payne, T. Gold, & E. Goldman *Yoga Therapy and Integrative Medicine: Where Ancient Science Meets Modern Medicine* (First edition, pp.263–285). North Bergen, NJ: Basic Health Publications.

17 Kolasinski, S.L., Garfinkel, M., Tsai, A. G., Matz, W., Van Dyke, A., & Schumacher, H. R. Jr. (2005). Iyengar yoga for treating symptoms of OA of the knees: A pilot study. *Journal of Alternative and Complementary Medicine*, *11*(4), 689–693.

18 Stephens, M. (2012). *Yoga Sequencing: Designing Transformative Yoga Classes*. Berkeley, CA: North Atlantic Books.

19 Ekerholt, K. & Bergland, A. (2008). Breathing: A sign of life and a unique area for reflection and action. *Physical Therapy*, *88*, 832–840.

20 Siegel, D. J. (2007). *The Mindful Brain*. New York: W. W. Norton.

21 *Ibid.*

22 *Ibid.*

23 Senge, P. & Society for Organizational Learning (2004). *Presence*. Boston: Society for Organizational Living.

24 Taylor, M. J. (Ed.) (2015). *Fostering Creativity in Rehabilitation* (First edition). New York: Nova Publishing.

25 *Ibid.* p.278.

CHAPTER 25

1   Tomasello, M., Carpenter, M., Call, J., Behne, T., & Moll, H. (2005). Understanding and sharing intentions: The origins of cultural cognition. *Behavioral and Brain Sciences*, *28*(5), 675–691.
    Bugental, D. B. (2000). Acquisition of the algorithms of social life: A domain-based approach. *Psychological Bulletin*, *126*(2), 187–219.

2   House, J., Landis, K., & Umberson, D. (1988). Social relationships and health. *Science*, *241*(4865), 540.
    Sapolsky, R. M. (2004). *Why Zebras Don't Get Ulcers* (Third edition). New York: Times Books.
    Sapolsky, R. M. (2017). *Behave: The Biology of Humans at our Best and Worst*. New York: Penguin Press.
    Weinstein, M., Lane, M. A., & National Research Council (U.S.) (Eds) (2014). *Sociality, Hierarchy, Health Comparative Biodemography: A Collection of Papers*. Washington, DC: The National Academies Press.
    Steptoe, A., Shankar, A., Demakakos, P., & Wardle, J. (2013). Social isolation, loneliness, and all-cause mortality in older men and women. *Proceedings of the National Academy of Sciences of the United States of America*, *110*(15), 5797–5801.
    Kuiper, J. S., Zuidersma, M., Oude Voshaar, R. C., *et al.* (2015). Social relationships and risk of dementia: A systematic review and meta-analysis of longitudinal cohort studies. *Ageing Research Reviews*, *22*, 39–57.
    Valtorta, N. K., Kanaan, M., Gilbody, S., Ronzi, S., & Hanratty, B. (2016). Loneliness and social isolation as risk factors for coronary heart disease and stroke: Systematic review and meta-analysis of longitudinal observational studies. *Heart*, *102*(13), 1009.
    Wang, J., Mann, F., Lloyd-Evans, B., Ma, R., & Johnson, S. (2018). Associations between loneliness and perceived social support and outcomes of mental health problems: A systematic review. *BMC Psychiatry*, *18*(1), 156.

3   Holt-Lunstad, J., Smith, T. B., & Layton, J. B. (2010). Social relationships and mortality risk: A meta-analytic review. *PLoS Medicine*, *7*(7), e1000316.

4   Eisenberg, N. & Beilin, H. (2014). *The Development of Prosocial Behavior*. Saint Louis, MO: Elsevier Science. p.6.

5   Ranjbar, N., Erb, M., Mohammad, O., & Moreno, F. A. (2020). Trauma-informed care and cultural humility in the mental health care of people from minoritized communities. *Focus*, *18*(1), 8–15.

6   Uchino, B. N., Trettevik, R., Kent de Grey, R. G., Cronan, S., Hogan, J., & Baucom, B. R. W. (2018). Social support, social integration, and inflammatory cytokines: A meta-analysis. *Health Psychology*, *37*(5), 462–471.
    Cohen, S. (2004). Social relationships and health. *The American Psychologist*, *59*(8), 676–684.

7   Eisenberger, N. I., Moieni, M., Inagaki, T. K., Muscatell, K. A., & Irwin, M. R. (2017). In sickness and in health: The co-regulation of inflammation and social behavior. *Neuropsychopharmacology*, *42*(1), 242–253.

8   *Ibid.*

9   Porges, S. W. (2011). *The Polyvagal Theory: Neurophysiological Foundations of Emotions, Attachment, Communication, and Self-Regulation (The Norton Series on Interpersonal Neurobiology)* (First edition). New York: W. W. Norton.

10 Porges, S. W. (2003). Social engagement and attachment. *Annals of the New York Academy of Sciences*, *1008*(1), 31–47.
    Seppala, E. (Ed.) (2017). *The Oxford Handbook of Compassion Science*. New York: Oxford University Press.

11 Tervalon, M. & Murray-García, J. (1998). Cultural humility versus cultural competence: A critical distinction in defining physician training outcomes in multicultural education. *Journal of Health Care for the Poor and Underserved*, *9*(2), 117–125.

12 McCraty, R. (2017). New frontiers in heart rate variability and social coherence research: Techniques, technologies, and implications for improving group dynamics and outcomes. *Frontiers in Public Health*, *5*, 267.

13 Abercrombie, P. D. & Hameed, F. A. (2019). Group visits as a path to health equity. *The Journal of Alternative and Complementary Medicine*, *25*(7), 669–670.
    Burnett, M. & Truesdale, A. (2019). Making health care accessible through group visits. *The Journal of Alternative and Complementary Medicine*, *25*(7), 671–672.
    Parikh, M., Rajendran, I., D'Amico, S., Luo, M., & Gardiner, P. (2019). Characteristics and components of medical group visits for chronic health conditions: A systematic scoping review. *The Journal of Alternative and Complementary Medicine*, *25*(7), 683–698.

Chainani-Wu, N., Weidner, G., Purnell, D. M., Frenda, S., *et al.* (2011). Changes in emerging cardiac biomarkers after an intensive lifestyle intervention. *The American Journal of Cardiology, 108*(4), 498–507.

Dusek, J. A., Otu, H. H., Wohlhueter, A. L., Bhasin, M., *et al.* (2008). Genomic counter-stress changes induced by the relaxation response. *PloS One, 3*(7), e2576.

Spiegel, D., Bloom, J. R., Kraemer, H. C., & Gottheil, E. (1989). Effect of psychosocial treatment on survival of patients with metastatic breast cancer. *Lancet, 2*(8668), 888–891.

Weeks, J. (2019). Special focus issue on innovation in group-delivered services [special issue]. *The Journal of Alternative and Complementary Medicine, 25*(7).

Fawzy, F. I., Fawzy, N. W., Hyun, C. S., Elashoff, R., *et al.* (1993). Malignant melanoma. Effects of an early structured psychiatric intervention, coping, and affective state on recurrence and survival 6 years later. *Archives of General Psychiatry, 50*(9), 681–689.

Andersen, B. L., Yang, H.-C., Farrar, W. B., Golden-Kreutz, D. M., *et al.* (2008). Psychologic intervention improves survival for breast cancer patients: A randomized clinical trial. *Cancer, 113*(12), 3450–3458.

Ornish, D., Magbanua, M. J. M., Weidner, G., Weinberg, V., *et al.* (2008). Changes in prostate gene expression in men undergoing an intensive nutrition and lifestyle intervention. *Proceedings of the National Academy of Sciences of the United States of America, 105*(24), 8369–8374.

14 Geller, J. S. (2019). Group medical visits: Introducing the "group inclusion effect" and key principles for maximization. *The Journal of Alternative and Complementary Medicine, 25*(7), 673–674.

15 Umberson, D. & Montez, J. K. (2010). Social relationships and health: A flashpoint for health policy. *Journal of Health and Social Behavior, 51*(Suppl), S54–S66.

16 Geller (2019).

17 Bruns, E. B., Befus, D., Wismer, B., Knight, K., *et al.* (2019). Vulnerable patients' psychosocial experiences in a group-based, integrative pain management program. *The Journal of Alternative and Complementary Medicine, 25*(7), 719–726.

18 O'Brien, W. H., Singh, R. S., Horan, K., Moeller, M. T., Wasson, R., & Jex, S. M. (2019). Group-based acceptance and commitment therapy for nurses and nurse aides working in long-term care residential settings. *The Journal of Alternative and Complementary Medicine, 25*(7), 753–761.

19 Sundquist, J., Palmér, K., Memon, A. A., Wang, X., Johansson, L. M., & Sundquist, K. (2019). Long-term improvements after mindfulness-based group therapy of depression, anxiety and stress and adjustment disorders: A randomized controlled trial. *Early Intervention in Psychiatry, 13*(4), 943–952.

20 Sandlund, C., Hetta, J., Nilsson, G. H., Ekstedt, M., & Westman, J. (2018). Impact of group treatment for insomnia on daytime symptomatology: Analyses from a randomized controlled trial in primary care. *International Journal of Nursing Studies, 85*, 126–135.

21 Mehl-Madrona, L. & Mainguy, B. (2014). Introducing healing circles and talking circles into primary care. *The Permanente Journal, 18*(2), 4–9.

Kirmayer, L., Simpson, C., & Cargo, M. (2003). Healing traditions: Culture, community and mental health promotion with Canadian Aboriginal peoples. *Australasian Psychiatry, 11*(s1), S15–S23.

22 Gordon, J. (2019, June). *The New Medicine.* Live presentation at the Professional Training Program in Mind-Body Medicine, Sonoma County, CA.

23 Weinlander, E. E., Gaza, E. J., & Winget, M. (2020). Impact of mind-body medicine professional skills training on healthcare professional burnout. *Global Advances in Health and Medicine, 9*, 2164956120906396.

Jones, L., Staples, J., Salgado, E., Garabrant, J., *et al.* (2020). 10. Mind-body skills groups: A possible approach for addressing adolescent depression in primary care. *Journal of Adolescent Health, 66*(2), S5–S6.

Gordon, J. S., Staples, J. K., Blyta, A., Bytyqi, M., & Wilson, A. T. (2008). Treatment of posttraumatic stress disorder in postwar Kosovar adolescents using mind-body skills groups: A randomized controlled trial. *Journal of Clinical Psychiatry, 69.*

Maclaughlin, B. W., Wang, D., Noone, A. M., Liu, N., *et al.* (2011). Stress biomarkers in medical students participating in a mind body medicine skills program. *Evidence-Based Complementary and Alternative Medicine, 2011.*

Gordon, J. S. (2014). Mind-body skills groups for medical students: Reducing stress, enhancing commitment, and promoting patient-centered care. *BMC Medical Education, 14*, 198.

Staples, J. K., Abdel Attai, J. A., & Gordon, J. S. (2011). Mind-body skills groups for posttraumatic stress disorder and depression symptoms in Palestinian children and adolescents in Gaza. *International Journal of Stress Management, 18.*

Gordon, J. S., Staples, J. K., Blyta, A., & Bytyqi, M. (2004). Treatment of posttraumatic stress disorder in postwar Kosovo high school students using mind-body skills groups: A pilot study. *Journal of Traumatic Stress, 17.*

Greeson, J. M., Toohey, M. J., & Pearce, M. J. (2015). An adapted, four-week mind-body skills group for medical students: Reducing stress, increasing mindfulness, and enhancing self-care. *Explore, 11*(3), 186–192.

Finkelstein, C., Brownstein, A., Scott, C., & Lan, Y. L. (2007). Anxiety and stress reduction in medical education: An intervention. *Medical Education, 41.*

Saunders, P. A., Tractenberg, R. E., Chaterji, R., Amri, H., *et al.* (2007). Promoting self-awareness and reflection through an experiential mind-body skills course for first year medical students. *Medical Teacher, 29.*

Ranjbar, N., Ricker, M., & Villagomez, A. (2019). The integrative psychiatry curriculum: Development of an innovative model. *Global Advances in Health and Medicine, 8*, 2164956119847118.

Staples, J. K. & Gordon, J. S. (2005). Effectiveness of a mind-body skills training program for healthcare professionals. *Alternative Therapies in Health and Medicine, 11*(4), 36–41.

Richtsmeier Cyr, L. & Farah, K. (2005). Mind-body skills groups for adolescents. *Biofeedback, Summer*, 63–68.

24 Siegel, D. J. (2017). *Mind: A Journey to the Heart of Being Human* (First edition). New York: W. W. Norton.

25 Flores, P. J., & Porges, S. W. (2017). Group psychotherapy as a neural exercise: Bridging polyvagal theory and attachment theory. *International Journal of Group Psychotherapy, 67*(2), 202–222.

26 Weeks, J. (2019). Reversing the fields: Do group-delivered services belong closer to the center of a transformed health care system? *The Journal of Alternative and Complementary Medicine, 25*(7), 666–668.

27 Gordon, J. S. (2019). *The Transformation: Discovering Wholeness and Healing after Trauma*. New York: HarperOne.

CHAPTER 26

1 Burke, M. J. (2019). "It's all in your head"—Medicine's silent epidemic. *JAMA Neurology, 76*(12), 1417–1418.

2 Taylor, A. G., Goehler, L. E., Galper, D. I., Innes, K. E., & Bourguignon, C. (2010). Top-down and bottom-up mechanisms in mind-body medicine: Development of an integrative framework for psychophysiological research. *Explore, 6*(1), 29.

3 Rowlands, M. (2010). *The New Science of the Mind: From Extended Mind to Embodied Phenomenology*. Cambridge, MA: MIT Press.

4 Manea, M. M., Comsa, M., Minca, A., Dragos, D., & Popa, C. (2015). Brain-heart axis—Review article. *Journal of Medicine and Life, 8*(3), 266–271.

Thayer, J. F. & Lane, R. D. (2009). Claude Bernard and the heart-brain connection: Further elaboration of a model of neurovisceral integration. *Neuroscience and Biobehavioral Reviews, 33*(2), 81–88.

Gershon, M, D. (1999). The enteric nervous system: A second brain. *Hospital Practice, 34*(7), 31–52.

Holzer P. (2017) Interoception and Gut Feelings: Unconscious Body Signals' Impact on Brain Function, Behavior and Belief Processes. In H. F. Angel., L. Oviedo, R. Paloutzian, A. Runehov, & R. Seitz (Eds) *Processes of Believing: The Acquisition, Maintenance, and Change in Creditions. New Approaches to the Scientific Study of Religion, Volume 1*. Cham: Springer.

Liu, P., Peng, G., Zhang, N., Wang, B., & Luo, B. (2019). Crosstalk between the gut microbiota and the brain: An update on neuroimaging findings. *Frontiers in Neurology, 10*, 883–883.

Miller, I. (2018). The gut-brain axis: Historical reflections. *Microbial Ecology in Health and Disease, 29*(1), 1542921–1542921.

Kolacz, J. & Porges, S. W. (2018). Chronic diffuse pain and functional gastrointestinal disorders after traumatic stress: Pathophysiology through a polyvagal perspective. *Frontiers in Medicine, 5*, 145.

Kolacz, J., Kovacic, K. K., & Porges, S. W. (2019). Traumatic stress and the autonomic brain-gut connection in development: Polyvagal theory as an integrative framework for psychosocial and gastrointestinal pathology. *Developmental Psychobiology, 61*(5), 796–809.

Porges, S. W. & Kolacz, J. (n.d.). Neurocardiology through the Lens of the Polyvagal Theory. In R. J. Gelpi & B. Buchholz (Eds) *Neurocardiology: Pathophysiological Aspects and Clinical Implications*. Amsterdam: Elsevier.

5 Kaparo, R. (2012). *Awakening Somatic Intelligence: The Art and Practice of Embodied Mindfulness: Transform Pain, Stress, Trauma, and Aging*. Berkeley, CA: North Atlantic Books.

Ussher, J. M. (1997). *Body Talk: The Material and Discursive Regulation of Sexuality, Madness and Reproduction*. London: Routledge.

Barrett, L. (2015). *Beyond the Brain: How Body and Environment Shape Animal and Human Minds*. Princeton, NJ: Princeton University Press.

Semin, G., Garrido, M., & Palma, T. (2013). Interfacing Body, Mind, the Physical, and Social World. In D. Carlston (Ed.) *The Oxford Handbook of Social Cognition* (pp. 637–655). New York: Oxford University Press.

6 Kelso, J. A. S. (1997). *Dynamic Patterns: The Self-Organization of Brain and Behavior*. Cambridge, MA: MIT Press.

7 Siegel, D. J. (2017). *Mind: A Journey to the Heart of Being Human* (First edition). New York: W. W. Norton.

8 Menary, R. (2012). *The Extended Mind*. Cambridge, MA: MIT Press.

9 Borghi, A., Scorolli, C., Caligiore, D., Baldassarre, G., & Tummolini, L. (2013). The embodied mind extended: Using words as social tools. *Frontiers in Psychology, 4*, 214.

10 Leventhal, T. & Brooks-Gunn, J. (2003). Moving to opportunity: An experimental study of neighborhood effects on mental health. *American Journal of Public Health, 93*(9), 1576–1582.

Ludwig, J., Sanbonmatsu, L., Gennetian, L., Adam, E., *et al*. (2011). Neighborhoods, obesity, and diabetes—A randomized social experiment. *New England Journal of Medicine, 365*(16), 1509–1519.

11 Oosterwijk, S., Lindquist, K. A., Anderson, E., Dautoff, R., Moriguchi, Y., & Barrett, L. F. (2012). States of mind: Emotions, body feelings, and thoughts share distributed neural networks. *Neuroimage, 62*(3), 2110–2128.

Corbetta, M., Patel, G., & Shulman, G. L. (2008). The reorienting system of the human brain: From environment to theory of mind. *Neuron, 58*(3), 306–324.

Shafir, T., Tsachor, R. P., & Welch, K. B. (2015). Emotion regulation through movement: Unique sets of movement characteristics are associated with and enhance basic emotions. *Frontiers in Psychology*, 6, 2030.

12 Wold, B. & Mittelmark, M. B. (2018). Health-promotion research over three decades: The social-ecological model and challenges in implementation of interventions. *Scandinavian Journal of Public Health*, 46(Suppl 20), 20–26.

Windley, P. G. & Scheidt, R. J. (1982). An ecological model of mental health among small-town rural elderly. *Journal of Gerontology*, 37(2), 235–242.

13 Campbell, R., Dworkin, E., & Cabral, G. (2009). An ecological model of the impact of sexual assault on women's mental health. *Trauma, Violence, and Abuse*, 10(3), 225–246.

14 Mencken, H. (1921). Prejudices second series: IV the divine afflatus, 155. *New York Evening Mail*. Retrieved September 9, 2020 from www.archive.org/stream/prejudices030184mbp/prejudices030184mbp_djvu.txt.

15 Hill, D. (1968). Depression: Disease, reaction, or posture? *AJP*, 125(4), 445–457.

Riskind, J. H. & Gotay, C. C. (1982). Physical posture: Could it have regulatory or feedback effects on motivation and emotion? *Motivation and Emotion*, 6(3), 273–298.

Kim, Y., Cheon, S.-M., Youm, C., Son, M., & Kim, J. W. (2018). Depression and posture in patients with Parkinson's disease. *Gait and Posture*, 61, 81–85.

Wilkes, C., Kydd, R., Sagar, M., & Broadbent, E. (2017). Upright posture improves affect and fatigue in people with depressive symptoms. *Journal of Behavior Therapy and Experimental Psychiatry*, 54, 143–149.

Tsachor, R. P. & Shafir, T. (2017). A somatic movement approach to fostering emotional resiliency through Laban Movement Analysis. *Frontiers in Human Neuroscience*, 11, 410.

16 Deacon, B. J. (2013). The biomedical model of mental disorder: A critical analysis of its validity, utility, and effects on psychotherapy research. *Clinical Psychology Review*, 33(7), 846–861.

17 Johnstone, L., Boyle, M., Cromby, J., Dillon, J., et al. (2018). *The Power Threat Meaning Framework: Towards the Identification of Patterns in Emotional Distress, Unusual Experiences and Troubled or Troubling Behaviour, as an Alternative to Functional Psychiatric Diagnosis*. Leicester: British Psychological Society. Retrieved September 9, 2020 from www.bps.org.uk/sites/bps.org.uk/files/Policy%20-%20Files/PTM%20Main.pdf.

18 Tarsha, M. S., Park, S., & Tortora, S. (2020). Body-centered interventions for psychopathological conditions: A review. *Frontiers in Psychology*, 10, 2907.

19 Scaer, R. C. (2014). *The Body Bears the Burden: Trauma, Dissociation, and Disease*. New York: Routledge.

Levine, P. A. & Mate, G. (2012). *In an Unspoken Voice*. Berkeley, CA: North Atlantic Books.

van der Kolk, B. A. (2014). *The Body Keeps the Score: Brain, Mind, and Body in the Healing of Trauma*. New York: Viking.

20 Probst, M. (2017). Physiotherapy and Mental Health. In T. Suzuki (Ed.) *Clinical Physical Therapy*. Vienna: InTech.

Probst, M. & Skjaerven, L. H. (Eds) (2018). *Physiotherapy in Mental Health and Psychiatry: A Scientific and Clinical Based Approach*. London: Elsevier.

Pascoe, M. C. & Parker, A. G. (2019). Physical activity and exercise as a universal depression prevention in young people: A narrative review. *Early Intervention in Psychiatry*, 13(4), 733–739.

Pascoe, M., Bailey, A. P., Craike, M., Carter, T., et al. (2020). Physical activity and exercise in youth mental health promotion: A scoping review. *BMJ Open Sport and Exercise Medicine*, 6(1), e000677.

Schuch, F. B., Vancampfort, D., Richards, J., Rosenbaum, S., Ward, P. B., & Stubbs, B. (2016). Exercise as a treatment for depression: A meta-analysis adjusting for publication bias. *Journal of Psychiatric Research*, 77, 42–51.

21 Roeh, A., Kirchner, S. K., Malchow, B., Maurus, I., et al. (2019). Depression in somatic disorders: Is there a beneficial effect of exercise? *Frontiers in Psychiatry*, 10, 141.

22 Shafir, et al. (2015).

Tsachor & Shafir (2017).

23 Marras, W. S., Davis, K. G., Heaney, C. A., Maronitis, A. B., & Allread, W. G. (2000). The influence of psychosocial stress, gender, and personality on mechanical loading of the lumbar spine. *Spine*, 25(23).

Ablin, J. N., Zohar, A. H., Zaraya-Blum, R., & Buskila, D. (2016). Distinctive personality profiles of fibromyalgia and chronic fatigue syndrome patients. *PeerJ*, 4, e2421–e2421.

24 Stevens, A. J., Rucklidge, J. J., & Kennedy, M. A. (2018). Epigenetics, nutrition and mental health. Is there a relationship? *Nutritional Neuroscience*, 21(9), 602–613.

Moore, K., Hughes, C. F., Ward, M., Hoey, L., & McNulty, H. (2018). Diet, nutrition and the ageing brain: Current evidence and new directions. *Proceedings of the Nutrition Society*, 77(2), 152–163.

Jacka, F. N. (2017). Nutritional psychiatry: Where to next? *EBioMedicine*, 17, 24–29.

Pyne, D. B., Verhagen, E. A., & Mountjoy, M. (2014). Nutrition, illness, and injury in aquatic sports. *International Journal of Sport Nutrition and Exercise Metabolism*, 24(4), 460–469.

Nieman, C. D. & Mitmesser, H. S. (2017). Potential impact of nutrition on immune system recovery from heavy exertion: A metabolomics perspective. *Nutrients*, 9(5).

Ignarro, L. J., Balestrieri, M. L., & Napoli, C. (2007). Nutrition, physical activity, and cardiovascular disease: An update. *Cardiovascular Research*, 73(2), 326–340.

25 Schmalzl, L., Crane-Godreau, M. A., & Payne, P. (2014). Movement-based embodied contemplative practices: Definitions and paradigms. *Frontiers in Human Neuroscience*, 8.

Schmalzl, L., Powers, C., & Henje Blom, E. (2015). Neurophysiological and neurocognitive mechanisms underlying the effects of yoga-based practices: Towards a comprehensive theoretical framework. *Frontiers in Human Neuroscience*, *9*, 235.

Kerr, C. E. & Schmalzl, L. (2016). *Neural Mechanisms Underlying Movement-Based Embodied Contemplative Practices*. Lausanne: Frontiers Media SA.

26 Brown, C., Stoffel, V., & Munoz, J. P. (Eds) (2011). *Occupational Therapy in Mental Health: A Vision for Participation*. Philadelphia, PA: F. A. Davis Co.

27 Probst (2017).

Probst & Skjaerven (2018).

28 Wolff, M. S., Michel, T. H., Krebs, D. E., & Watts, N. T. (1991). Chronic pain—Assessment of orthopedic physical therapists' knowledge and attitudes. *Physical Therapy*, *71*(3), 207–214.

Main, C. J. & George, S. Z. (2011). Psychosocial influences on low back pain: Why should you care? *Physical Therapy*, *91*(5), 609–613.

Linton, S. J. & Shaw, W. S. (2011). Impact of psychological factors in the experience of pain. *Physical Therapy*, *91*(5), 700–711.

Craik, R. L. (2011). A convincing case—For the psychologically informed physical therapist. *Physical Therapy*, *91*(5), 606–608.

Flink, I. K., Reme, S., Jacobsen, H. B., Glombiewski, J. *et al.* (2020). Pain psychology in the 21st century: Lessons learned and moving forward. *Scandinavian Journal of Pain*, 20190180.

29 Balas, E. A. (1998). From appropriate care to evidence-based medicine. *Pediatric Annals*, *27*(9), 581–584.

Balas, E. A. & Boren, S. A. (2000). Managing Clinical Knowledge for Health Care Improvement. In J. Bemmel & A. T. McCray (Eds) *Yearbook of Medical Informatics: Patient-Centered Systems* (pp.65–70). Stuttgart: Schattauer Verlagsgesellschaft.

30 Bero, L. A., Grilli, R., Grimshaw, J. M., Harvey, E., Oxman, A. D., & Thomson, M. A. (1998). Closing the gap between research and practice: An overview of systematic reviews of interventions to promote the implementation of research findings. The Cochrane Effective Practice and Organization of Care Review Group. *BMJ*, *317*(7156), 465–468.

31 Dobkin, P. L. & Hassed, C. (2016). Education Teachers. In *Mindful Medical Practitioners: A Guide for Clinicians and Educators*. Cham: Springer.

32 Halifax, J. (2012). A heuristic model of enactive compassion. *Current Opinion in Supportive and Palliative Care*, *6*(2), 228–235.

Schore, A. N. (2007). Psychoanalytic research: Developmental affective neuroscience and clinical practice. *Psychologist Psychoanalyst*, *27*, 6–16.

Fosha, D., Siegel, D. J., & Solomon, M. F. (Eds) (2009). *The Healing Power of Emotion: Affective Neuroscience, Development, and Clinical Practice* (First edition). New York: W. W. Norton.

33 Schuch, *et al.* (2016).

Harvey, S. B., Øverland, S., Hatch, S. L., Wessely, S., Mykletun, A., & Hotopf, M. (2018). Exercise and the prevention of depression: Results of the HUNT cohort study. *American Journal of Psychiatry*, *175*(1), 28–36.

Anderson, E. & Shivakumar, G. (2013). Effects of exercise and physical activity on anxiety. *Frontiers in Psychiatry*, *4*, 27.

De Moor, M. H. M., Beem, A. L., Stubbe, J. H., Boomsma, D. I., & De Geus, E. J. C. (2006). Regular exercise, anxiety, depression and personality: A population-based study. *Preventive Medicine*, *42*(4), 273–279.

Dauwan, M., Begemann, M. J. H., Heringa, S. M., & Sommer, I. E. (2016). Exercise improves clinical symptoms, quality of life, global functioning, and depression in schizophrenia: A systematic review and meta-analysis. *Schizophrenia Bulletin*, *42*(3), 588–599.

Probst, M., Majeweski, M. L., Albertsen, M. N., Catalan-Matamoros, D., *et al.* (2013). Physiotherapy for patients with anorexia nervosa. *Advances in Eating Disorders*, *1*(3), 224–238.

Vancampfort, D., Knapen, J., Probst, M., Scheewe, T., Remans, S., & De Hert, M. (2012). A systematic review of correlates of physical activity in patients with schizophrenia. *Acta Psychiatrica Scandinavica*, *125*(5), 352–362.

Vancampfort, D., Correll, C. U., Probst, M., Sienaert, P., *et al.* (2013). A review of physical activity correlates in patients with bipolar disorder. *The Journal of Affective Disorders*, *145*(3), 285–291.

34 Gordon, J. S. (2009). *Unstuck: Your Guide to the Seven-Stage Journey out of Depression*. New York: Penguin.

Gordon, J. S. (2019). *The Transformation: Discovering Wholeness and Healing after Trauma*. New York: HarperOne.

35 Ernst, G. (2017). Hidden signals: The history and methods of heart rate variability. *Front Public Health*, *5*, 265.

Dale, L. P., Carroll, L. E., Galen, G., Hayes, J. A., Webb, K. W., & Porges, S. W. (2009). Abuse history is related to autonomic regulation to mild exercise and psychological wellbeing. *Applied Psychophysiology and Biofeedback*, *34*(4), 299–308.

36 Tracy, L. M., Ioannou, L., Baker, K. S., Gibson, S. J., Georgiou-Karistianis, N., & Giummarra, M. J. (2016). Meta-analytic evidence for decreased heart rate variability in chronic pain implicating parasympathetic nervous system dysregulation. *Pain*, *157*(1), 7–29.

Karoly, P. & Ruehlman, L. S. (2006). Psychological "resilience" and its correlates in chronic pain: Findings from a national community sample. *Pain*, *123*(1–2), 90–97.

37   Kemp, A. H. & Quintana, D. S. (2013). The relationship between mental and physical health: Insights from the study of heart rate variability. *International Journal of Psychophysiology, 89*(3), 288–296.

Muehsam, D., Lutgendorf, S., Mills, P. J., Rickhi, B., *et al.* (2017). The embodied mind: A review on functional genomic and neurological correlates of mind-body therapies. *Neuroscience and Biobehavioral Reviews, 73*, 165–181.

Azam, M. A., Katz, J., Mohabir, V., & Ritvo, P. (2016). Individuals with tension and migraine headaches exhibit increased heart rate variability during post-stress mindfulness meditation practice but a decrease during a post-stress control condition: A randomized, controlled experiment. *International Journal of Psychophysiology, 110*, 66–74.

Meeus, M., Goubert, D., De Backer, F., Struyf, F., *et al.* (2013). Heart rate variability in patients with fibromyalgia and patients with chronic fatigue syndrome: A systematic review. *Seminars in Arthritis and Rheumatism, 43*(2), 279–287.

Staud, R. (2008). Heart rate variability as a biomarker of fibromyalgia syndrome. *Future Rheumatology, 3*(5), 475–483.

Otis, J. D., Keane, T. M., & Kerns, R. D. (2003). An examination of the relationship between chronic pain and post-traumatic stress disorder. *Journal of Rehabilitation Research and Development, 40*(5), 397–405.

Fishbain, D. A., Pulikal, A., Lewis, J. E., & Gao, J. (2017). Chronic pain types differ in their reported prevalence of post-traumatic stress disorder (PTSD) and there is consistent evidence that chronic pain is associated with PTSD: An evidence-based structured systematic review. *Pain Medicine, 18*(4), 711–735.

Maletic, V. & Raison, C. L. (2009). Neurobiology of depression, fibromyalgia and neuropathic pain. *Frontiers in Bioscience, 14*, 5291–5338.

Coppens, E., Van Wambeke, P., Morlion, B., Weltens, N., *et al.* (2017). Prevalence and impact of childhood adversities and post-traumatic stress disorder in women with fibromyalgia and chronic widespread pain. *European Journal of Pain, 21*(9), 1582–1590.

38   Lieberman, M. D., Eisenberger, N. I., Crockett, M. J., Tom, S. M., Pfeifer, J. H., & Way, B. M. (2007). Putting feelings into words. *Psychological Science, 18*(5), 421–428.

Lieberman, M. D., Inagaki, T. K., Tabibnia, G., & Crockett, M. J. (2011). Subjective responses to emotional stimuli during labeling, reappraisal, and distraction. *Emotion, 11*(3), 468–480.

39   Lumley, M. A., Cohen, J. L., Borszcz, G. S., Cano, A., *et al.* (2011). Pain and emotion: A biopsychosocial review of recent research. *Journal of Clinical Psychology, 67*(9), 942–968.

Van der Maas, L. C. C., Köke, A., Pont, M., Bosscher, R. J., *et al.* (2015). Improving the multidisciplinary treatment of chronic pain by stimulating body awareness: A cluster-randomized trial. *Clinical Journal of Pain, 31*(7), 660–669.

40   de Jong, M., Lazar, S. W., Hug, K., Mehling, W. E., *et al.* (2016). Effects of mindfulness-based cognitive therapy on body awareness in patients with chronic pain and comorbid depression. *Frontiers in Psychology, 7*, 967–967.

Schauder, K. B., Mash, L. E., Bryant, L. K., & Cascio, C. J. (2015). Interoceptive ability and body awareness in autism spectrum disorder. *Journal of Experimental Child Psychology, 131*, 193–200.

Calsius, J., De Bie, J., Hertogen, R., & Meesen, R. (2016). Touching the lived body in patients with medically unexplained symptoms. How an integration of hands-on bodywork and body awareness in psychotherapy may help people with alexithymia. *Frontiers in Psychology, 7*, 253.

41   Creswell, J. D., Way, B. M., Eisenberger, N. I., & Lieberman, M. D. (2007). Neural correlates of dispositional mindfulness during affect labeling. *Psychosomatic Medicine, 69*(6), 560–565.

42   Smyth, J. M. & Pennebaker, J. W. (2010). Exploring the boundary conditions of expressive writing: In search of the right recipe. *British Journal of Health Psychology, 13*(1), 1–7.

43   Ranjbar, N. & Erb, M. (2019). Adverse childhood experiences and trauma-informed care in rehabilitation clinical practice. *Archives of Rehabilitation Research and Clinical Translation*, 100003.

44   Stoller, R. (1984). Psychiatry's mind-brain dialectic, or the Mona Lisa has no eyebrows. *AJP, 141*(4), 554–558. p.554.

45   *Ibid.*

46   *Ibid.*

CHAPTER 27

1   Bateson, N. & Brubeck, S. B. (2016). *Small Arcs of Larger Circles: Framing through Other Patterns* (Second edition). Bridport: Triarchy Press.

2   Epstein, D. J. (2019). *Range: Why Generalists Triumph in a Specialized World.* New York: Riverhead Books.

3   Holopainen, R., Piirainen, A., Karppinen, J., Linton, S. J., & O'Sullivan, P. (2020). An adventurous learning journey. Physiotherapists' conceptions of learning and integrating cognitive functional therapy into clinical practice. *Physiotherapy Theory and Practice*, 1–18.

4   *Ibid.*

5   Fazey, I., Schäpke, N., Caniglia, G., Hodgson, A., et al. (2020). Transforming knowledge systems for life on Earth: Visions of future systems and how to get there. *Energy Research & Social Science, 70*(101724), 1–18.

6   Fazey, *et al.* (2020). p.5.

7   Ho, E. H., Hagmann, D., & Loewenstein, G. (2020). Measuring information preferences. *Management Science.* Retrieved January 8, 2020 from https://doi.org/10.1287/mnsc.2019.3543.

8   Nissen-Lie, H. A., Rønnestad, M. H., Høglend, P. A., Havik, O. E., et al. (2017). Love yourself as a person, doubt yourself as a therapist? *Clinical Psychology and Psychotherapy, 24*(1), 48–60. p.57.

9   *Ibid*. p.58.

10   Miller, S. D., Hubble, M. A., Chow, D., & Seidel, J. (2015). Beyond measures and monitoring: Realizing the potential of feedback-informed treatment. *Psychotherapy, 52*(4), 449–457.

11   Ameli, R., Sinaii, N., Luna, M. J., Cheringal, J., Gril, B., & Berger, A. (2018). The National Institutes of Health measure of Healing Experience of All Life Stressors (NIH-HEALS): Factor analysis and validation. *PloS One, 13*(12), e0207820.

12   Klaber, R. E. & Bailey, S. (2019). Kindness: An underrated currency. *BMJ, 367*, l6099.

13   Eliot, T. (1942). *Little Gidding*. London: Faber and Faber, pt.5.

APPENDIX A

1   Morin, E. (2020). Uncertainty is intrinsic to the human condition. *CNRS News*. Retrieved September 9, 2020 from https://news.cnrs.fr/articles/uncertainty-is-intrinsic-to-the-human-condition.

2   Angner, E. (2020). Epistemic humility—Knowing your limits in a pandemic. *Behavioral Scientist*. Retrieved September 9, 2020 from https://behavioralscientist.org/epistemic-humility-coronavirus-knowing-your-limits-in-a-pandemic.

3   Zimerman, A. L. (2013). Evidence-based medicine: A short history of a modern medical movement. *Virtual Mentor, 15*(1), 71–76.

4   Guyatt, G., Cairns, J., Churchill, D., Cook, D., *et al.* (1992). Evidence-based medicine: A new approach to teaching the practice of medicine. *JAMA, 268*(17), 2420–2425.

5   Luckmann, R. (2001). Evidence-based medicine: How to practice and teach EBM, 2nd Edition: By David L. Sackett, Sharon E. Straus, W. Scott Richardson, William Rosenberg, and R. Brian Haynes, Churchill Livingstone, 2000. *Journal of Intensive Care Medicine, 16*(3), 155–156.

6   Babiker, A. M. I. (2012). A review and practical application of evidence based medicine (EBM): Testicular adrenal rest tumour. *Sudanese Journal of Paediatrics, 12*(2), 27–35.

7   Ioannidis, J. P. A. (2016). Evidence-based medicine has been hijacked: A report to David Sackett. *Journal of Clinical Epidemiology, 73*, 82–86.

     Balas, E. A. (1998). From appropriate care to evidence-based medicine. *Pediatric Annals, 27*(9), 581–584.

     Balas, E. A. (n.d.). Managing Clinical Knowledge for Health Care Improvement. In *Yearbook of Medical Informatics* (pp.65–70). Bethesda, MD: National Library of Medicine.

     Morris, Z. S., Wooding, S., & Grant, J. (2011). The answer is 17 years, what is the question: Understanding time lags in translational research. *Journal of the Royal Society of Medicine, 104*(12), 510–520.

     Ioannidis, J. P. A., Stuart, M. E., Brownlee, S., & Strite, S. A. (2017). How to survive the medical misinformation mess. *European Journal of Clinical Investigation, 47*(11), 795–802.

     Perezgonzalez, J. D. (2018). Book review: Surgery, the ultimate placebo. *Frontiers in Surgery, 5*, 38.

     Abdel Shaheed, C., Maher, C. G., Williams, K. A., Day, R., & McLachlan, A. J. (2016). Efficacy, tolerability, and dose-dependent effects of opioid analgesics for low back pain: A systematic review and meta-analysis. *JAMA Internal Medicine, 176*(7), 958–968.

     Jonas, W. B., Crawford, C., Colloca, L., Kriston, L., *et al.* (2018). Are invasive procedures effective for chronic pain? A systematic review. *Pain Medicine, 20*(7), 1281–1293.

     Kamper, S. J., Logan, G., Copsey, B., Thompson, J., *et al.* (2019). What is usual care for low back pain? A systematic review of healthcare provided to patients with low back pain in family practice and emergency departments. *Pain, 161*(4), 694–702.

     Wyer, P. C. & Silva, S. A. (2009). Where is the wisdom? I—A conceptual history of evidence-based medicine. *Journal of Evaluation in Clinical Practice, 15*(6), 891–898.

     The Scientist. (2019). *The Top Retractions of 2019*. Retrieved September 9, 2020 from www.the-scientist.com/news-opinion/the-top-retractions-of-2019-66852.

     Murad, M. H., Asi, N., Alsawas, M., & Alahdab, F. (2016). New evidence pyramid. *Evidence-Based Medicine, 21*(4), 125–127.

     Phillips, B. (2014). The crumbling of the pyramid of evidence. *Archives of Diseases in Childhood*. Retrieved September 9, 2020 from https://blogs.bmj.com/adc/2014/11/03/the-crumbling-of-the-pyramid-of-evidence.

     Goldman, J. J. & Shih, T. L. (2011). The limitations of evidence-based medicine: Applying population-based recommendations to individual patients. *Virtual Mentor, 13*(1), 26–30.

     Weeks, J. (2019). Perspectives on the American College of Lifestyle Medicine's strategy to "end the tyranny of the RCT." *The Journal of Alternative and Complementary Medicine, 25*(10), 975–978.

     Katz, D. L. & Karlsen, M. C. (2019). The need for a whole systems approach to evidence evaluation: An update from the American College of Lifestyle Medicine. *The Journal of Alternative and Complementary Medicine, 25*(S1), S19–S20.

     Barry, C. A. (2006). The role of evidence in alternative medicine: Contrasting biomedical and anthropological approaches. *Social Science and Medicine, 62*(11), 2646–2657.

     Jonas, W. & Linde, K. (2002). Conducting and Evaluating Clinical Research on Complementary and Alternative Medicine. In *Principles and Practice of Clinical Research* (pp.401–426). San Diego, CA: Academic Press.

     Mandrola, J., Cifu, A., Prasad, V., & Foy, A. (2019). The case for being a medical conservative. *The American Journal of Medicine, 132*(8), 900–901.

Chandran, P. K. G. (2019). The case for being a medical conservative (not always!). *The American Journal of Medicine, 132*(9), e718.

Wasserstein, R. L., Schirm, A. L., & Lazar, N. A. (2019). Moving to a world beyond "p < 0.05." *The American Statistician, 73*(Suppl 1), 1–19.

de Morton, N. A. (2009). The PEDro scale is a valid measure of the methodological quality of clinical trials: A demographic study. *Australian Journal of Physiotherapy, 55*(2), 129–133.

PEDro. (n.d.). *PEDro Statistics*. Retrieved September 9, 2020 from www.pedro.org.au/english/downloads/pedro-statistics.

Amrhein, V., Greenland, S., & McShane, B. (2019). Scientists rise up against statistical significance. *Nature, 567*, 305–307.

Amrhein, V., Trafimow, D., & Greenland, S. (2019). Inferential statistics as descriptive statistics: There is no replication crisis if we don't expect replication. *The American Statistician, 73*(Suppl 1), 262–270.

Braithwaite, R. S. (2020). EBM's six dangerous words. *JAMA, 323*(17), 1676–1677.

Titler, M. (2008). The Evidence for Evidence-Based Practice Implementation. In R. G. Hughes (Ed.) *Patient Safety and Quality: An Evidence-Based Handbook for Nurses*. Rockville, MD: Agency for Healthcare Research and Quality.

Greenhalgh, T., Howick, J., & Maskrey, N. (2014). Evidence based medicine: A movement in crisis? *British Medical Journal, 348*, g3725.

Ferlie, E., Fitzgerald, L., & Wood, M. (2000). Getting evidence into clinical practice: An organisational behaviour perspective. *Journal of Health Services Research and Policy, 5*(2), 96–102.

8   Grey, A., Bolland, M., Avenell, A., Klein, A., & Gunsalus, C. (2020). *Check for Publication Integrity Before Misconduct—A Tool that Focuses on Papers—Not Researcher Behaviour—Can Help Readers, Editors and Institutions Assess Which Publications to Trust.* Retrieved September 9, 2020 from www.nature.com/articles/d41586-019-03959-6.

9   Braithwaite (2020). p.1666.

10   *Ibid.* p.1667.

11   Beidelschies, M., Alejandro-Rodriguez, M., Ji, X., Lapin, B., Hanaway, P., & Rothberg, M. B. (2019). Association of the functional medicine model of care with patient-reported health-related quality-of-life outcomes. *JAMA Network Open, 2*(10), e1914017–e1914017.

APPENDIX B

1   Rosenberg, L. (2011). Addressing trauma in mental health and substance use treatment. *The Journal of Behavioral Health Services & Research, 38*(4), 428–431.

Frans, Ö., Rimmö, P.-A., Åberg, L., & Fredrikson, M. (2005). Trauma exposure and post-traumatic stress disorder in the general population. *Acta Psychiatrica Scandinavica, 111*(4), 291–299.

Mills, K. L., McFarlane, A. C., Slade, T., Creamer, M., *et al.* (2011). Assessing the prevalence of trauma exposure in epidemiological surveys. *Australian and New Zealand Journal of Psychiatry, 45*(5), 407–415.

Felitti, V. J. (2009). Adverse childhood experiences and adult health. *Academic Pediatrics, 9*(3), 131–132.

2   Menschner, C. & Maul, A. (2016, April). *Key Ingredients for Successful Trauma-Informed Care Implementation.* Retrieved September 9, 2020 from www.chcs.org/media/ATC_whitepaper_040616.pdf.

Ranjbar, N. & Erb, M. (2019). Adverse childhood experiences and trauma-informed care in rehabilitation clinical practice. *Archives of Rehabilitation Research and Clinical Translation*, 100003.

3   Ranjbar, N., Erb, M., Mohammad, O., & Moreno, F. A. (2020). Trauma-informed care and cultural humility in the mental health care of people from minoritized communities. *Focus, 18*(1), 8–15.

4   Ranjbar & Erb (2019).

APPENDIX C

1   Villatte, M., Villatte, J. L., & Hayes, S. C. (2016). *Mastering the Clinical Conversation: Language as Intervention*. New York: The Guilford Press.

Index